FIFTH EDITION

CHAITOW'S
MUSCLE ENERGY
TECHNIQUES

CHAITOW'S

THE LEON CHAITOW LIBRARY
OF BODYWORK AND MOVEMENT THERAPIES

FIFTH EDITION

MUSCLE ENERGY TECHNIQUES

Edited by

Sasha Chaitow, PhD

Visiting Lecturer, Department of Physiotherapy
School of Health Rehabilitation Sciences, University of Patras
Greece

Sandy Fritz, MS, NCTMB

Founder, Owner, Director and Head Instructor, Health Enrichment Center
School of Therapeutic Massage
Lapeer, MI, United States

Foreword by

David Lesondak

ELSEVIER

Elsevier
© 2024 Elsevier Limited. All rights reserved.

First edition 1996
Second edition 1999
Third edition 2006
Reprinted 2007, 2008
Fourth edition 2013

Notices

Practitioners and researchers must always rely on their own experience and knowledge in evaluating and using any information, methods, compounds or experiments described herein. Because of rapid advances in the medical sciences in particular, independent verification of diagnoses and drug dosages should be made. To the fullest extent of the law, no responsibility is assumed by Elsevier, authors, editors or contributors for any injury and/or damage to persons or property as a matter of products liability, negligence or otherwise, or from any use or operation of any methods, products, instructions, or ideas contained in the material herein.

ISBN: 978-0-7020-8272-6

Content Strategist: Andrae Akeh
Content Project Manager: Shubham Dixit
Design: Miles Hitchen
Illustration Manager: Akshaya Mohan
Marketing Manager: Belinda Tudin

Printed in India by Replika Press Pvt Ltd

Last digit is the print number: 9 8 7 6 5 4 3 2 1

Working together
to grow libraries in
developing countries

www.elsevier.com • www.bookaid.org

None of the previous editions could have emerged without the patience, and the provision of a warm and loving environment in which to work, by Leon Chaitow's wife Alkmini. All previous editions bear his undying thanks for her unwavering support – his source of strength throughout his many productive years. Her continued encouragement and patience have allowed the present edition to manifest.

This fifth edition is dedicated to Leon Chaitow and his living legacy: every reader, student, colleague, patient and friend who has benefited from, practiced or built upon his work. What is remembered lives.

CONTENTS

CONTRIBUTORS

Ken Crenshaw, BS in Athletic Training, ATC, CSCS
Director of Sports Medicine and Performance
Baseball Operations
Arizona Diamondbacks
Chandler, AZ, United States

Ryan DiPanfilo, BS
Major League Head Athletic Trainer
Arizona Diamondbacks
Phoenix, AZ, United States

Luke Allen Fritz, LMT, Instructor
Health Enrichment Center
School of Therapeutic Massage and Bodywork
Lapeer, MI, United States

Helge Franke, DO, MRO, MSc AT
Director
Practice for Osteopathy and Naturopathy
Siegen, Germany

Gary Fryer, PhD, BSc (Osteo), ND
College of Health and Biomedicine
Victoria University
Melbourne, VIC, Australia

Donald R. Murphy, DC, FRCC
Clinical Assistant Professor
Department of Family Medicine
Alpert Medical School of Brown University
Providence, RI, United States

Craig Liebenson, DC
LA Sports and Spine
Los Angeles, CA, United States

Shraddha Parmar Pradhan, MPTh (Musculoskeletal Sciences), BPTh
Head Physiotherapist
Department of Physiotherapy
Dr. Pradhan Orthopaedic and Physiotherapy Clinic
Pune, Maharashtra, India

Curtis Thor Rigney, DC, MRes
Faculty of Health
Southern Cross University
Lismore, NSW, Australia

Nathan Shaw, ATC, CSCS
Major League Strength Coach
Arizona Diamondbacks
Phoenix, AZ, United States

Ashok Shyam, DNB Orth, ChM Tr and Orth (Edin)
Orthopaedic Surgeon
Sancheti Institute for Orthopaedics and Rehabilitation
Pune, Maharashtra, India

Derek Somerville, MS, RSCC, LMT
Strength and Conditioning Coach
Arizona Diamondbacks
Scottsdale, AZ, United States

Eric Wilson, PT, DSc, DPT, OCS, SCS, CSCS, FAAOMPT
Deputy Program Director
Tactical Sports and OMPT Fellowship
US Air Force
Colorado Springs, CO, United States

FOREWORD

To be asked to write a foreword is always an honour. Being asked to write the foreword to the fifth edition of this book – *Chaitow's Muscle Energy Techniques*, the inaugural volume in the newly christened *Leon Chaitow Library of Bodywork and Movement Therapies* – is an honour that fills me with deep gratitude and profound humility.

Gratitude because this tome possesses a depth and breadth of scholarship that sets a new gold standard for all other manual therapy books that will follow in its wake. All too often manual therapy is disregarded because of a perception of it being little more than folk medicine and/or largely anecdotal. This book puts paid to those notions with rigorous scholarship, comprehensive research (including and especially when the data doesn't say what we'd like it to say) and highly incisive prose. The chapter on the history and development of Muscle Energy Techniques (MET) is doctorate-level stuff, and a fascinating primer on how to fearlessly and scrupulously document an emerging, evolving therapy.

Along with the prose are clear instructions, with illustrations, on techniques for everywhere you want to treat. All written with a deep understanding of the nuances involved when dealing with actual people and not just parts. For the visual learner there is the added benefit of QR code links to quality video versions of these techniques. And here's where the humility comes.

As a manual therapist for three decades, I naturally continue to expand and refine my toolbox. As many approaches as I have studied, MET has always been a part of that toolbox. Yet this volume has put me in touch with how much I had forgotten, not to mention many potential options for treatment I hadn't thought of or been shown. The sheer volume of things that are out there to be known. That alone makes this an enduring gem. Likewise, the aforementioned rigorous scholarship challenges what I think I know and further hones my critical thinking skills. For me, it's a win/win.

This edition also makes room to explore how manual medicine must fit into the new frontier of whole person care. Whether it's the biopsychosocial model or narrative-based medicine, we must always be clear that we are treating a *person* first, not just a sacrotuberous ligament or densified fascia in the region of the quadratus lumborum. As in my foundation in structural integration, the partnership model where the patient actively participates in their treatment is a built-in feature of MET. This approach not only restores agency and empowers those we treat, but also is an accelerant of better outcomes.

If you're serious about the practice of results-oriented bodywork and manual therapy, and you must be if you've read this far, this book should be one of the cornerstones of your reference library. It is in mine.

David Lesondak
University of Pittsburgh Medical Center
Center for Integrative Medicine
Pittsburgh, PA, United States
September 2022

PREFACE

This is the first edition of this book to be published without Leon Chaitow, my father. His passing in September 2018 was not only personally devastating, but also the sheer volume of tributes from around the world revealed his stature and impact across the manual therapy professions to a greater degree than even I was fully aware. Neither we can fulfil the gap left by his loss, nor do we wish to. Yet, in being privileged to know his thought processes and wishes, we can honour his legacy by building on it as he intended.

Precisely a decade ago, while immersed in revising several of his books in parallel, my father quipped to me with his typical humour: 'Next time these need revision, it will be your problem'. Little did either of us know how quickly that day would come. I took my place at his desk, knowing exactly what he would have done, and reached out to one of his closest colleagues and dearest friends, Sandy Fritz, MS, LMT, who graciously agreed to take up his mantle in overseeing the revision of the scientific aspects of this book, while, as Series and Volume Editor, I have overseen the entire process, editing every chapter to ensure that it remains faithful to my father's intentions, vision and voice, part of which includes maintaining the synthesis and plurality of interprofessional voices.

Sandy has spent hundreds of hours working alongside Leon Chaitow since his earliest teaching tours of the United States in the 1980s, and few understand his clinical reasoning and treatment approaches better than she, as well as his concerns regarding education and evidence-informed practice. First as teacher and student, then as colleagues, then trusted friends, she assisted and co-taught at many of his workshops, and is possibly the only practitioner who – in his own words – can demonstrate and teach his approaches as he would himself. He even said she might do it better. Sandy's long career practising, teaching and writing textbooks, as well as mentoring several generations of massage therapists and advising on policy at a national level, is testament to her deep commitment to excellence and progress in the field of massage therapy and related modalities.

I spent decades assisting in many different aspects of my father's work. Sitting in as interpreter on many of his consultations, I also accompanied him and occasionally modelled on many of his workshop tours, assisted with preparation of his teaching material, and since 2008 I took on various duties helping him to manage the *Journal of Bodywork and Movement Therapies*, where I was appointed Managing Editor when his health declined in 2018. In that role I fostered dialogues and published editorials on matters of translational research and research literacy among clinicians from different bodywork professions. Through my appointment at the University of Patras in Greece in 2020, I teach critical appraisal skills and research development to advanced Physiotherapy students – many of them seasoned clinicians – looking to contribute to the evidence base for manual therapy, and I have adapted my father's teaching materials for use in their undergraduate training in manual therapies, MET among them. As an interdisciplinary scholar, my focus is on the communication gaps between professions and in healthcare education, focusing on elements of the history of medicine and the sociology of knowledge. I am especially interested in the role of the Medical Humanities – an important educational discipline – in improving medical and allied health education. This perspective informs my work addressing the bodywork communities, looking to build bridges and provide transferable skills and tools to improve critical thinking skills and interprofessional dialogue.

These were issues that concerned my father deeply. His original texts on clinical reasoning and personalised approaches to treatment reflect his holistic, osteopathic training. His emphasis on interprofessional dialogue and collaboration is reflected in all his edited volumes, including the present title, for which he selected contributing authors who span the breadth of relevant specialties. Whole-person care is an area that both Sandy and I are especially interested in with regard to seeking balance between the bio-, psycho- and social elements of evidence-informed practice, reflected in our addition of a dedicated chapter (Chapter 1) on this aspect alone, in the context of the clinical decision-making process that may include using MET. Most of the contributed chapters also reflect the renewed emphasis on individualised care and the reasoning that must accompany it.

ABOUT THIS BOOK

This book has had a long and exciting journey from its first edition in 1996, that itself developed out of Leon Chaitow's now-legendary Soft Tissue Manipulation (1980) – that blue hardcover book that many manual therapists will remember well. Muscle Energy Techniques (MET) was just one of several chapters in that first iteration that eventually grew into a series, *Advanced Soft Tissue Techniques*, which includes the Elsevier titles *Positional Release* and *Modern Neuromuscular Techniques*, each synthesising approaches from several professions, each resting on the most recent evidence.

The present title was revised in 1999, 2006 and 2013, and Leon Chaitow wrote of the previous edition specifically that it represented both a refinement and an expansion that he was excited to see, because it incorporated a wealth of evidence that had accumulated in the years since its first emergence. That evidence has now grown further, while the formation of new (2022) research networks co-funded by the National Centre for Complementary and Integrative Health (NCCIH) and the National Institute of Neurological Disorders and Stroke (NINDS) promise valuable developments in coming years, as detailed further in Chapters 1 and 3.

In the previous edition, Leon Chaitow also reflected on the significance of the interdisciplinary and interprofessional nature of MET, an evolution tracked closely in the earlier edition of this book, contextualised further in the present edition (Chapters 1 and 3). He saw its adaptability and cross-professional applicability as a great advantage; however, he also emphasised the need to grasp the nuances of the technique, warning that, although the basic application is easy to learn, all too often, the subtleties that make it effective can be overlooked. He stressed the number of variables that the practitioner must consider, ranging from when the choice of technique is appropriate, to the numerous elements in their application, such as choice of resistance barrier, types of contraction, direction, dosage and its place in a multimodal programme. In the preface to the fourth edition he provided a list of questions the therapist should consider in their clinical reasoning process; this has now been moved to Chapter 2, along with further context on their significance.

NEW IN THIS EDITION

Chapter 1 is a wholly new addition by the present editors, reflecting the now-established shift towards whole-person healthcare and consideration of MET application within that framework. It examines common issues in the correct use of the biopsychosocial model, presents the growing discipline of Narrative Medicine in relation to manual therapy practice and provides illustrations and examples for consideration.

Chapter 3, previously titled The History of MET and written by Helge Franke, has been substantially developed and retitled by Sasha Chaitow to reflect contextual considerations of the impact of a discipline's history on its clinical application. A section has also been added on Leon Chaitow's immense contribution to this field and future directions are also considered.

The emphasis on summarising and critically appraising the evidence has been a hallmark of this book from its earliest inception and in Chapter 4 of the present volume Gary Fryer has provided a fully updated literature review that carefully assesses what is new in the evidence base along with its implications for efficacy. He provides valuable definitions and clarifications regarding key terms and issues in relation to research literacy and provides an important discussion of what more must be done in order to produce – and use – better quality research. More specialised, updated citations and cross-references have been added to all the individual chapters. The 'summary of evidence' that Leon Chaitow was well known for has been enriched and updated by Sandy Fritz and is found in Chapter 2, with additional topic-specific summaries throughout the other chapters.

Though the evidence base continues to grow in size, and more slowly, in quality, the techniques themselves that are presented in the chapters originally written by Leon Chaitow (Chapters 2, 5, 6, 7 and 14, previously with different numbering) have not changed, but readers will find that new content includes consideration of patients with hypermobility and more thorough integration of matters of clinical reasoning, the biopsychosocial model and patient preference.

Chapters 8 to 13, each by contributing authors who are chiropractors and spine experts, rehabilitation experts and orthopedists, physiotherapists, massage therapists, and athletic coaches, provide their respective approaches to both clinical reasoning and application of

MET in their scope of practice. In providing snapshots and case notes from their own practice and clinical reasoning processes, the reader is offered a rich selection of perspectives to inform their own approaches. Within these discussions that report from the front lines while demonstrating the fully rounded evidence-informed approach in action, the authors have provided valuable highlights of misconceptions and errors in application. They also tackle some of the most commonly encountered conditions such as low back and neck pain, weighing both the evidence and experience, and in Chapters 8, 11 and 13 readers will find useful perspectives on both, while matters of patient fearfulness and non-compliance are also addressed. The rapidly growing body of fascia research evidence impacts significantly on our understanding of MET and its usage, especially in relation to biotensegrity and its implications for force transmission. Readers will find relevant discussion of this in Chapters 2, 5, 6 and 7.

There are, as with any manual intervention, contraindications and cautions that are spelled out, and it is emphasised that these techniques should only be applied by formally trained practitioners. Nevertheless, MET remains a safe and effective technique that is a valuable addition to the manual therapist's toolbox, and can be applied in a wide range of clinical situations subject to patient preference and cooperation.

As Leon Chaitow concluded in his preface to the previous edition: MET remains a most versatile modality, with overwhelming evidence for its efficacy in a variety of clinical settings. It allows for a collaborative degree of involvement between patient and therapist – making it more than a purely passive treatment method and possessing the added element of patient empowerment. The processes of engagement of the patient in precisely directed efforts – sustained or rhythmically pulsing – have important proprioceptive re-education potentials, as well as providing the clinician with an opportunity to release, mobilise, tone, or stretch soft tissues or joints, as required.

Sasha Chaitow, Corfu, 2022

ACKNOWLEDGEMENTS

This fifth edition would not have been possible without the warm, wise, professional input of Sandy Fritz. Profound thanks must also go to the Elsevier team – especially Poppy Garraway and Chiara Giglio, and Content Project Manager, Shubham Dixit whose calm guidance brought this project to smooth completion.

Each and every contributing author is due special thanks for their confidence in the new editorial team and their contribution of updated material to this edition: Gary Fryer, Donald R. Murphy, Curtis Thor Rigney, Ashok Shyam, Shraddha Parmar, Eric Wilson, Luke Allen Fritz, Ken Crenshaw, Ryan DiPanfilo, Derek Somerville and Nathan Shaw.

Gary Fryer wishes to acknowledge the assistance of Deborah Goggin, MA, ELS, Scientific Writer, A.T. Still University, in the preparation of Chapter 4.

Sasha Chaitow wishes to personally thank David Peters, Mary Law, Andrew Stevenson, Thomas Myers, Ruth Duncan, Leena Gupta, Anna Maria Mazzieri, Mark Gray, Carol Davis, Leslie Young, Dimitris Kostopoulos, Kostas Rizopoulos, Kostas Fousekis and every other colleague and friend of Leon Chaitow who offered genuine support following his passing. Most of all, she thanks Sandy Fritz.

We are deeply grateful to David Lesondak for contributing the foreword to this fifth edition, and for his generous words of wisdom.

Evidence-Informed Muscle Energy Techniques in the Biopsychosocial Framework

Sasha Chaitow, Sandy Fritz

CHAPTER CONTENTS

The purpose of this fifth edition is to offer as clear a picture as possible of the various muscle energy techniques (METs), their clinical applications and clinical potential – supported by currently available evidence, as well as clinically based opinions based on experience. METs are simple to learn; therefore, expertise emerges in the skill and critical thinking of the practitioner.

An ongoing question related to many forms of manual therapy is the validity of the interventions used in the treatment of musculoskeletal pain and dysfunction. It is necessary to pose this same question in relation to MET. Manual therapy methods such as MET have previously been explained in relation to tissue and biomechanical mechanisms. More recent evidence indicates less support for the biomechanical effect. Instead, it is thought that both biological and psychosocial therapeutic mechanisms contribute to therapeutic benefit.

Clear explanations for the mechanisms underpinning the benefits of a variety of manual therapy techniques remain elusive. The most current research supports modest benefits, especially when combined within a multimodal approach to care. There are indications of effects on inflammation mediation, neural adaptation, shifts in tone and density of soft tissue structures and mechanotransduction regularity mechanisms in fascia (Bove et al., 2019). Within the psychosocial realm, improved mobility and change in sensation, even when temporary, can reduce fear of movement, thus leading to improvement in quality of life (Fryer, 2017a, 2017b; Langevin, 2021). While the application of many specific manual therapy treatments can have similar therapeutic benefits, there can be rationales for choosing one method over another. These topics will be explored further throughout the book.

Readers will decide for themselves regarding the relative validity of these perspectives, along with the possible usefulness of MET. Current manual therapy models include engaging the patient in active approaches, such as exercise, with supportive education. These interventions do not replace manual therapy application but expand the therapeutic interaction. Multimodal approaches are indicated for achieving the best results in the treatment of musculoskeletal pain and dysfunction (Cruz-Montecinos et al., 2017; Lederman, 2017; Smith, 2019; Vivanco-Coke et al., 2020).

THE EVIDENCE

Although manual therapy is considered safe, there is limited evidence on its efficacy in treating chronic pain. The lone exception involves chronic low back pain, wherein there is evidence from systematic reviews, a large clinical trial and observational studies. Lesser evidence supports cost effectiveness and patient satisfaction associated with manual therapy for chronic pain. The only clinical practice guideline established by the American Osteopathic Association recommends that Osteopathic Manipulative Treatment (OMT) should be used to treat chronic low back pain in patients with somatic dysfunction (Licciardone et al., 2020). The 2020 British National Institute for Health and Care Excellence (NICE) Guidelines for practice examined the evidence in favour of manual therapies for chronic primary pain. The consultation committee identified evidence for clinically significant short-term benefits of mixed modality manual therapy over usual care for physical function; of soft tissue technique and manipulation/mobilisation (examined separately in comparison to usual care, acupuncture and dry needling) for pain reduction, quality of life, physical function, psychological distress and sleep improvement. Compared to each other, there was moderate evidence for the benefit of mixed modality manual therapy over soft tissue technique for pain reduction, of soft tissue technique over manipulation/mobilisation for mental quality of life in one study and of manipulation/mobilisation over soft tissue technique in two studies. The committee concluded that there was indeed evidence for benefits relating to pain reduction, quality of life, physical function, psychological distress and pain interference, all considered critical outcomes for the policy-making process. However, it also stated that only 15 randomised controlled trials had met the inclusion criteria for the review, and all of them suffered from design flaws (a high risk of bias and imprecision) in addition to significant variations in the mixed manual therapies investigated. These limitations made it impossible to provide a positive recommendation, despite the committee's acknowledgement of the limitations of the review itself.

In each chapter of this book, as with its previous iterations, the editors and contributors have provided the most recent available evidence relating to MET efficacy and its benefits, together with frank acknowledgement of what remains unknown. The development of METs is explored as one of the great success stories of organic interprofessional collaboration, detailed in Chapter 3, while Gary Fryer provides a rich roadmap and review of the most current literature, highlighting key issues regarding the need for improved research design and critical appraisal skills in Chapter 4. The remaining practical chapters provide a balance of evidence and experience, reflecting Leon Chaitow's support of careful adherence to the original characteristics of evidence-*informed* practice, defined and discussed later in this chapter, and extended in Chapter 4.

This can only come about through closer collaboration between researchers and clinicians to ensure the production of research that is both robust and useful, and through improved training in research literacy for its successful application. It is to this end that we welcome the announcement from Dr Helene Langevin (April 2022), of the successful founding of three new interdisciplinary research networks funded by the National Centre for Complementary and Integrative Health (NCCIH) and the National Institute of Neurological Disorders and Stroke (NINDS), to research manual therapies, somatosensation, the biological effects of soft tissue manipulation, the neural mechanisms of force-based manipulation mechanotransduction and their role in the treatment of back pain (Langevin, 2022). Several further research networks have been established to study mind–body interventions and the promotion of emotional and psychosocial well-being. These are exciting developments for the future of manual therapy, and it is hoped that in the next revision of this book, there will be valuable findings for future editors to incorporate.

Nevertheless, as research continues to emerge, in the context of current clinical practice, choosing to use these methods will continue to rest upon the balance between clinical reasoning, current evidence and patient preference.

FINDING BALANCE

Though the development of an evidence base has come a long way since the early days of MET, interpretations of what constitutes evidence-based practice vary across regions and professions, as do the nomenclature, theoretical fundamentals and educational foundations of different bodywork professions. As manual therapy professions seek to consolidate the validity of their practices and modalities, sometimes their 'medical' applications are emphasised more than functionality and the reduction of adaptive load (see Chapter 2 for further discussion of this), which focus on functional well-being and its maintenance.

The focus on evidence-based practice has become especially significant in view of the renewed scrutiny on clinical practice following the COVID-19 pandemic, and in the context of a wider, often silent, chronic pain epidemic. An important motivation driving this is an ongoing effort to disconnect manual therapies from their association with practices seen as having a 'negative association with alternative medicine' (Brower, 2006). Yet, the emphasis on that negative association is almost 20 years old and, in that time, biomedical clinical practice has actively begun to adopt elements of holistic practice with solid evidence underpinning it, while holistic approaches are becoming integrated into mainstream medical education as part of the shift towards person-centred healthcare. Numerous studies have highlighted the acceptance of integrative health practices among biomedical clinicians, educators and students, emphasising the need for closer integration of education in integrative or Complementary and Alternative Medicine (CAM) healthcare 'throughout pre-clinical, clinical, and graduate medical curricula', since the potential for CAM values to improve the effectiveness and patient-satisfaction of conventional medicine is well-established in biomedicine (Winslow & Shapiro, 2002; Consortium of Academic Health Centers for Integrative Medicine (CAHCIM) 2004; Chaterji et al., 2007; Weeks, 2013).

Two paradoxes are occurring as this unfolds: in the biomedical context, this integration of holistic thinking into mainstream medicine is being presented as a new addition with very little consideration of the foundational principles of osteopathic education in particular, and many other integrative healthcare practices to which the holistic approach has been central for the best part of two centuries. At the same time, few allied and integrative health practitioners and schools are aware of the degree of acknowledgement of holistic thinking and the therapeutic practices that go with it within biomedical practice. The reasons include specialised language barriers and partisan practice-based debate as well as the distinct nature of the ideological principles on which these two 'healthcare social worlds' rest (Brosnan & Turner, 2009). As a result, some practitioner communities have come to perceive holism and 'alternative' practices in terms of their 'negative associations' and strive to distance themselves from them, while others uphold them as a proud countercultural heritage, seen as holding out against the forces of allopathic

approaches (Broom & Adamms, 2009). Thus, despite decades of work to professionalise and validate numerous aspects of integrative (complementary, alternative) therapies, the negative association remains, not due to a lack of acknowledgement by the biomedical establishment, nor because integrative therapies are considered inferior, but as a result of fractured communication and historical misperceptions, some of which are explored in Chapter 3. One widespread misperception acting as a hindrance within integrative health professions, in particular, is the question of what evidence-informed practice should entail and what it really looks like in practice.

EVIDENCE-INFORMED PRACTICE

Evidence-*based* medicine was famously defined by David Sackett et al. (1996) as 'the conscientious, explicit, and judicious use of current best evidence in making decisions about the care of individual patients'. Several studies describe the evidence-*informed* approach as being 'fundamental to practice' aiming 'to address the large gap between what is known and what is consistently done' (Glasziou, 2005; McSherry, 2007; Epstein et al., 2009). More specifically, 'evidence-informed decision-making models advocate for research evidence to be considered in conjunction with clinical expertise, patient preferences and values and available resources'. This perspective addresses real-world scenarios and 'interactions between evidence and action… and complex relationships between healthcare interventions and outcomes' (McCormack et al., 2013). These are discussed in direct relation to MET in Chapter 4. Considered in their broader intersection with healthcare, these statements are drawn from an influential study addressing practical questions on how to improve the uptake of evidence in biomedical practice and what this means in real-world healthcare in relation to both policymaking and patient outcomes. The aim is to promote specifically evidence-informed healthcare and, since its publication almost a decade ago, the research database statistics for this study demonstrate its impact on realistic approaches to improving healthcare standards across specialties.

A CDC report commissioned in 2007 details the significance of evidence-*informed* – as opposed to rigidly interpreted evidence-*based* practice – even more clearly. The failings of systematic reviews and meta-analyses – the foundations of policy-making – are well-acknowledged by major stakeholders and calls for significant improvements to their usefulness have been made at the highest levels for well over a decade. Yet, the same report concludes that misinformation regarding the relative value of such reviews continues to circulate in the media and among researchers in diverse fields due to their poor understanding of the speed of advances being made and a general lack of research literacy. Nevertheless, it concludes that 'advocating an unquestioning or inappropriate overreliance on systematic reviews might discourage innovation or promising practices' (Sweet et al., 2007). After establishing that 'evidence-informed' practice and policy would be the desired ideal, it proposes to promote and improve this through 'identifying, mentoring and supporting the champions of evidence-informed policy'. The points listed for improvement (higher-quality basic research and better communication between sectors) are precisely the same as those concerning integrative and allied health professions.

These findings from the main U.S. health authority acknowledge that the quest for knowledge and evidence, as well as the need to reap their benefits, must also reflect the 'real-world interaction between evidence and action'. This is not controversial in biomedicine nor in public health; it is a pragmatic evaluation of the limitations of existing scientific tools, and an equally realistic acknowledgement that clinical experience – based on appropriate training, professional development and intellectual honesty within one's scope of practice – is of equal value to evidence. A 2017 British Medical Journal survey showed that in primary healthcare about 18% of decisions were based on "patient-oriented high-quality evidence" (Ebell et al., 2017), while a very large variance was observed among medical specialities and from one condition to another. The reasons can be summed up as a combination of resistance to change, practical considerations (such as a lack of time), an overreliance on anecdotes and personal clinical experience, and a lack of research literacy.

Thus, as efforts continue to validate and professionalise MT approaches and practices, it is important to realise the degree to which critical biomedical procedures continue to rely on experience and lower-level evidence. Telling examples are found across fields from surgery to paediatrics (Chaitow, 2022), demonstrating that a lack of evidence or the presence of inconsistent, low-quality research are not grounds in and of themselves for abandoning a technique. Balance must

be sought, rather than what has been termed evidence nihilism, defined as 'rigid adherence to a protocol irrespective of patients' concerns' (Mootz, 2005). The utmost priorities should be patient safety and more thorough practitioner training. Once these requirements are satisfied, Sackett's original definition reminds us that clinical experience and patient preference are equally significant and must be afforded equal weight to the evidence base itself. These three elements: the evidence, clinical expertise and patient preference, are the cornerstones of the biopsychosocial (BPS) approach, which is itself the result of attempts to improve and ring-fence the ethics of medical practice.

WHOLE-PERSON HEALTHCARE

The interaction between the practitioner and patient at intake is critical to the future therapeutic relationship…. Almost as important is a need for rapport and trust…. From the patient's perspective it is vital that a sense emerges that the problems brought for consideration have been understood. From the practitioner's perspective it is important that a broad base of understanding be achieved, developed through the asking of appropriate and strategic questions, and through skillful listening. It is therefore essential… that communication is clear and unambiguous… that the patient's expectations and anxieties, especially those regarding treatment, are explored. Unobtrusive observation of the patient's body language… should all be part of the consultation process. These signs can provide subliminal clues that help in understanding the patient's current mind-set, fears, and motivation. Out of the initial consultation a picture should emerge that allows a 'story' to be constructed. Within the story, the individual's unique biochemical, psychosocial, and biomechanical features (both inborn and acquired) will be seen to have adapted to life events in a manner that has resulted in the emergence of the present symptom picture… Put simply, this means: What allowed [the health problem] to happen and become established? What triggered it? And what keeps it going? Are there multiple factors that feed into one another to perpetuate the problem? This aspect of the 'story' needs to be one that the practitioner can use to construct a treatment plan, and which the patient finds intellectually convincing, so that a desire to cooperate with the treatment plan results, including willingness to apply the homework that is likely to be suggested.

Chaitow and Delany (2005)

Writing this in 2004, Leon Chaitow was describing his own style of patient intake, drawing on his long clinical experience as a practising osteopath. He was not, however, aware, that over at the University of Columbia, a new discipline was just beginning to take root at the heart of biomedicine, which would provide robust research validating his approach, formulating it into a fully structured evidence-based protocol for patient intake and medical student education, and bringing about something of a revolution.

Narrative-based medicine (NBM), originating in narrative ethics, a branch of bioethics (Box 1.1), emerged to counter the problem that 'scientifically competent medicine alone cannot help a patient grapple with the loss of health or find meaning in suffering' (Charon, 2001).

In the NBM framework, disease, dysfunction and pain are seen as a narrative inextricable from the person's life, rather than as a list of codes, difficult names and protocols to be followed or corrections to be shared. This is the true definition of whole-person care. By no means does this suggest that therapists and physicians ought not use their expertise or take the necessary steps in the face of red flags, and it cannot be extensively applied in the context of the emergency room. Nevertheless, in all

other healthcare contexts, it provides a firm foundation on which to renew the dynamic between clinician and patient. As noted by Dr Trisha Greenhalgh – an international authority on applying and implementing evidence-based medicine (EBM) – on the value of narrative medicine as early as 1999: '[It] may provide a way of mediating between the very different worlds of patients and health professionals. Whether performed well or badly is likely to have as much influence on the outcome of the illness from the patient's point of view as the more scientific and technical aspects of diagnosis or treatment' (Greenhalgh & Hurwitz, 1999). From this perspective, it is critical to truly ethical practice.

With this as its goal, NBM has been quietly gaining ground since the turn of this century. Founded by internal medicine specialist Dr Rita Charon at Columbia University and taken up by biomedical specialists worldwide, medical curricula are increasingly incorporating it into their training. The discipline aims to refocus the way medicine is being practised through the development of a holistic diagnostic framework based on the patient's own narrative of their condition, with particular attention paid to the body–mind connection. It is obvious that this is examined in parallel with any required biomedical assessments, but rather than 'telling', 'educating' or 'directing' the patient, the process is guided by the patient and his or her articulated needs.

Importantly, NBM does not challenge biomedicine or EBM; it rests on substantive evidence. Moreover, it does not attempt to reinvent the BPS approach; it was developed to improve on it and correct its flaws. Currently, it is succeeding in instilling holistic and humanistic assessment and treatment at the heart of primary healthcare. In such a climate, there is tremendous potential for building proper bridges with integrative and allied health professions with more solid foundations than in the past. Such developments may also make it possible to solve the impasse that some MTs find themselves dealing with in relation to 'hands-on' or 'hands-off' in their efforts to adhere to EBM guidelines (Chaitow, 2021a), because the clinical reasoning process must establish what is appropriate, not based only on the literature, but also on the patient. Further discussion of the impact of patient preference on therapeutic outcomes is found in Chapter 8, with more context-specific remarks in Chapters 7 and 13. Chapter 11 provides highly useful practical tools for the application of

---

BOX 1.1   Summary of Bioethical Principles

- **Respect for patient autonomy**
- **Nonmaleficence:** Do no deliberate harm
- **Beneficence:** Have the patient's best interest as a priority
- **Justice:** Eliminate discrimination in healthcare provision on the basis of sex, race, age, beliefs, sexual orientation or any other factors.

Narrative Ethics involves appraising an individual story and weighing up how the main principles of bioethics apply to the clinical decision-making in response to it. It starts with the individual patient and adapts how the medical knowledge base can be appropriately applied to their particular situation, taking into account the patient profile in comparison to the subjects of research studies alongside their medical profile.

Beauchamp & Childress (1979) and Charon (2016).

classification models and outcome-based targets to assist in streamlining this process in the context of clinical practice.

THE BIOPSYCHOSOCIAL MODEL COMPARED TO NARRATIVE-BASED MEDICINE[1]

Emerging in the 1970s as a counterweight towards reductionist thought in biomedicine, the BPS approach to assessment and treatment also calls for an integrated approach that takes the patient's psychological, social and cultural influences into account when assessing and treating a complaint (Guillemin & Barnards, 2015). Key to its original formulation is a re-examination of the concept of disease: 'disease cannot be defined based on the *function* of physicians, which is a social and institutional phenomenon' (Guillemin & Barnards, 2015). It confronts the assumption that disease always rests on a pathological cause that must be uprooted to achieve a return to health, rather than attempting to understand the spectrum of contributing factors resulting in illness (Wade & Halligan, 2004). It differentiates disease (with a pathological cause) from illness (the absence of wellness, which may not have a biomedical root pathology).

Factors such as social, lifestyle or mental adjustments made to accommodate its effects (such as guarding an injured limb or coming to terms with lost functionality) should not be pathologised or minimised. Instead, the therapist should seek to understand the context of these adaptations and what they mean to the patient and propose therapeutic options that can meet the patient where they are. This is particularly helpful in the assessment and management of chronic pain, as the BPS model allows a tailored approach that 'places the disease back into the patient' (rather than the textbook or medical database), and has been demonstrated to have significantly greater efficacy than surgery (Weiner, 2008). Some evidence suggests a multidisciplinary BPS approach is more effective than physical hands-on treatment (Kamper et al., 2015). It does not clash with the

EBM model but improves on it when the two are integrated and correctly implemented (Smith et al., 2013).

In practice, the BPS approach includes re-educating the patient around the perception of pain. In the context of physical therapy, this has been dubbed the 'first step in pain neuroscience education (PNE)', wherein the personalised treatment plan should include 'a proper explanation of the neurophysiology of pain and the BPS interactions in an interactive and patient-centred manner' (Guzman et al., 2001; Wijma et al., 2016). The key principles of pain science on which this approach rests have strongly influenced priorities in pain research and have greatly affected both physiotherapy and related professions (Guillemin & Barnards, 2015; Parker & Madden, 2020).

Criticisms of the BPS model relate to the difficulty of implementing it in the clinical setting. Researchers and clinicians alike have acknowledged that it has not been effectively integrated into medical education as a technique, nor has it been 'effectively translated into the practical applications demanded by these domains' (Herman, 2005; Seaburn, 2005; Guillemin & Barnards, 2015). These issues are echoed in the most recent feedback from physical therapists expressing a lack of confidence or skills deficit in implementing the BPS model (Alexanders et al., 2015; Singla et al., 2015; Synnott et al., 2015, 2016). One 2013 study demonstrated that while interdisciplinary multimodal approaches to chronic pain with a BPS component can be effective in the context of physical therapy, the evidence in favour of PNE of patients remains conflicted, though poor implementation may be partly responsible (Sanders et al., 2013; Richter et al., 2020).

Extensive literature exploring BPS in physiotherapy suggests that PNE is becoming firmly established, with moderate results that are enhanced when integrated within an interdisciplinary intervention model (Malfliet et al., 2018). In turn, this has raised concerns over the future of manual treatment, since the aim of PNE is to refocus attention from the painful tissue to the neurological interpretation of stimuli resulting in nociception (Moseley, 2003a, 2003b; Jull & Moore, 2012; Blickenstaff & Pearson, 2016; Louw et al., 2016b; Puentedura & Flynn, 2016; Oostendorp 2018). Some strong cases have been made for the integration of both approaches (Louw et al., 2017), others draw attention to the educational component aimed at altering perceptions of pain and behaviours (Hackstaff et al., 2004). The question of how

---

[1]Parts of this and the following section are adapted from Sasha Chaitow's 4 – part series on the biopsychosocial model, Narrative Medicine and related matters published in successive issues of Massage & Bodywork Magazine (Chaitow 2021a, 2021b, 2021c, 2021d).

best to integrate specialised communication and clinical reasoning skills lacking in manual therapy (MT) education is also being targeted. This was argued recently in a significant editorial focusing on the necessity of skills training in basic listening and interpretation in the context of the intake interview and more adept integration of 'the "bio" of MT... within the "psychosocial" of the intervention model'. Kolb et al. (2020) note that 'Now is the time to update outdated teaching models in MT education and provide leadership for integration of other interventions within the BPS model'. Careful interpretation is called for here; this is not a call for the abolition of hands-on practice, but an appeal to better place the modalities in the therapist's toolbox with correctly implemented BPS as a decision-making roadmap.

Despite the benefits of BPS and PNE, the research suggests that they are not as successful as intended when it comes to forming a person-centred therapeutic alliance, and this is the imbalance that NBM has set out to correct (Diener et al., 2016). A significant number of studies on the integration of behaviour modification programmes in healthcare focus on how to facilitate their acceptance and uptake among resistant patients, leading to an asymmetry of power within the therapeutic relationship that is detrimental to the outcome (Hackstaff et al., 2004; Louw et al., 2016a). Nevertheless, despite positive research on BPS when integrated into interdisciplinary interventions, the separation of the 'bio' from the 'psychosocial' remains a widespread problem. One common trap is that of 'essentialising' traits, whereby a member of a particular culture may be subconsciously stereotyped according to gender, race, age, community or any number of other subcategories. The case summary in Box 1.2 provides an example of this. Though we may assume that by acknowledging an individual's cultural context we are demonstrating respect, we may in fact be imposing our own perceptions on them, thus doing the opposite. Equally, expecting that a specific stimulus will derive a specific response (regardless of the evidence) falls into the same trap and cannot have a holistic result (Murphy et al., 2017). This may be the source of frustration expressed by many physical therapists when they find that their best attempts at applying BPS fall short, especially when too much emphasis is placed on what the therapist believes to be important in terms of the psychosocial element, thus neglecting the 'bio' element (Guillemin & Barnards, 2015). Similar issues apply to PNE, compounded by the role inequality,

since 'the power is all on one side' (Irvine & Charon, 2016). Sometimes, this can lead to an uneasy therapeutic relationship; in others, as demonstrated in Box 1.2, it can be catastrophic.

Seen from the perspective of a patient in pain, however meticulously the therapist has curated their manual therapy evidence-base and completed their BPS intake form, if the patient has arrived expecting a form of therapeutic touch, they may not welcome a lesson in neuroplasticity if they do tnot feel their needs have been heard.

According to the principles of narrative medicine, the act of 'diagnostic listening' allows the therapist to support the patient in facing often unanswerable questions regarding their condition and the contributing factors. This step also allows the practitioner to consider the therapeutic options not through prioritising where it sits on the evidence pyramid, but through a process of open, critical assessment that includes consideration of what the patient as an individual is most likely to respond to. If the patient narrative is ignored, then 'the resultant diagnostic workup might be unfocused and therefore more expensive than necessary; the correct diagnosis might be missed; the clinical care might be marked by noncompliance and the search for another opinion; and the therapeutic relationship might be shallow and ineffective' (Charon, 2001). The case studies in Boxes 1.2 and 1.3 illustrate such situations.

Studies of effective implementation of NBM highlight that the keys to building that therapeutic alliance are embedded in the details normally discarded. Learning to use them is not the same as directive coaching or counselling techniques such as motivational interviewing. It is important that NBM neither be construed as a method of psychoanalysis, nor a form of motivational interviewing. Despite superficial similarities, it is not simply a form of sensitive listening, and it does require training to grasp the method, based on carefully honed protocols and principles (Charon et al., 2015, 2016). An overview of the initial steps is provided in Box 1.3. As an extension of clinical intake interviewing, NBM has the potential to support and improve the clinical reasoning process through significantly empowering the patient, while helping the practitioner to develop strategies for balancing EBM requirements with clinical experience and patient preference, so as to develop truly patient-centred practice.

The NBM approach produces a refreshed focus on the elements of the story that reveal the relationship

BOX 1.2	**Case Notes Illustrating the Need for Narrative Ethics (Chaitow, 2021)**

An elderly patient had suffered from mostly controlled ulcerative colitis since early adulthood. The patient also had partially controlled atrial fibrillation, a heart arrhythmia increasing the risk of stroke, and had recently received an unexpected cancer diagnosis that caused the arrhythmia to flare. Days later, the patient experienced two transient ischaemic attacks (TIAs) (often considered a forewarning of a major stroke to come).

The hospital cardiologist and neurologist recommended administration of aspirin or a stronger blood thinner, warning that the risk of stroke was severe. However, the patient was fearful of the bleed risk due to the colitis that had been flaring for some months. After declining the medication, the patient was dismissed by both specialists as 'difficult' and 'stubborn'. Both refused the patient's requests to discuss the relative risks and alternative options. The patient discharged themselves, expressing suicidal ideations.

Within a week, the patient was rushed to the emergency room (ER) with uncontrollable gastric (gut) bleeding and survived emergency surgery with massive blood loss. Post-surgery, the patient was sent home with mild delirium, a hospital-acquired urinary tract infection (UTI) and no medication to control their heart arrhythmia. No information was provided regarding follow-up care apart from the surgical wound care.

A week later, the patient experienced a major stroke, resulting in total hemiparesis of the left side and severe delirium. On arrival back in the ER, the resident physician said to the family: 'What, atrial fibrillation and no blood thinner? Of course they had a stroke, what, were they stupid?' Following a brain scan, and although the patient was conscious, able to converse lucidly and expressing distress, the neurologist recommended permanent, palliative sedation to the family – without a patient interview, mental state assessment, or patient consent – claiming, on the basis of the MRI and visible damage to the white matter, that the patient was not capable of making informed decisions. The family refused, following the patient's explicit wishes to return home and pursue rehabilitation privately. After several weeks of home-based care, the patient regained full lucidity and continued physical rehabilitation from the stroke until the other conditions led to the patient's passing.

Comment

This sad but true story is an example of an impossible ethical dilemma for patient and clinicians alike, in which basic medical ethics were not observed, the physicians allowed the patient's age and fear reactions to cloud their judgement and extreme paternalistic approaches were applied. Considering the biological factors alone, based strictly on the evidence and statistical calculation, the physicians' advice regarding blood thinners was correct, but failed to consider the patient's comorbidities. Their views regarding post-stroke sedation were also correct based only on the brain MRI but not the patient's clinical state. Had these physicians applied narrative ethics, they would firstly have addressed the patient's mental state and psychological condition, paying attention to the reasoning and beliefs beneath the patient's fears in the context of the patient's psychosocial background in a manner that matched the patient's ability to understand it – that fit with their narrative.

There are reflections here of the story recounted in Tyreman (2018), in which the Hungarian physician, Ignaz Semmelweis, faced ridicule and censure for insisting on an intensive hygiene regime to prevent unnecessary deaths before germ theory had been proven. Tyreman uses the story to illustrate resistance to change within medical professions, and its implications. He notes that beyond the importance of 'good science', the emphasis on patient narratives in clinical practice are crucial to understanding irrational responses of the critically ill if one is to practise truly person-centred care.

The founder of Narrative Medicine, Dr Charon, notes that sometimes narrative practices 'are the therapy itself'. This is not the same as talking therapy. Rather, it means that helping the patient to understand, consider their options when facing critical illness, and come to terms with the very fact of what they are facing, will help them make the treatment decision that is right for them. The opportunity to do so is a therapeutic option in itself. While the above comprises an extreme example, it illustrates the precise points where overly rigid emphasis on statistical evidence can have tragic outcomes, as well as the potential for narrative techniques to improve the situation.

Note: These case notes refer to a real patient. Chaitow (2021).

BOX 1.3 The Narrative Medicine Approach

One of the key protocols of Narrative Medicine involves listening – and reading – closely between the lines of a patient's narrative. This narrative goes beyond what is revealed by the case notes, and it bridges several of the gaps also left by the biopsychosocial approach, which can often result in attempts to 'correct' the patient, however gently, but does not always leave room to explore aspects of their story which might reveal the solution.

The following is a sample case study demonstrating how differently it can work to the other approaches.

Close Reading Exercise

The following list is adapted from the College of Physicians and Surgeons of Columbia University Reading Guide for Reflective Practice, developed through several years of training and parallel validation by Dr Charon and her team (Charon et al., 2015).

After familiarising themselves with this list, readers may wish to read the Case Notes, Biopsychosocial Details, and Patient Narrative that follows, first highlighting anything that stands out in general, then reviewing it while attempting to answer the following points. This is not a substitute for full Narrative Medicine training but is intended to provide a sample of what close reading involves. In a clinical setting, patients could be asked to provide a written account of their condition prior to first consultation. The practitioner would then have the requisite time to examine the material and factor it into the clinical reasoning process.

1. **Observation:** What sensory perceptions are expressed in the narrative? What do you or the narrator see, hear, smell, touch or feel?
2. **Perspective:** Whose perspective is the story told from? Is there more than one? Are some implied, rather than stated directly? How are they communicated?
3. **Form:** What is the type (genre) of writing? Is it a story, a poem, a dark comedy, a dialogue? What imagery or symbols are used? Is the story told in chronological order, is it chaotic, does it point to other stories? What is the tone – is it relaxed, friendly, formal?
4. **Voice:** Whose voice is narrating? Is it in the first-person, second-person or third-person? Is the narrator close to you, or are they distant? Are they self-aware (do they seem aware of the implications of their narrative?) Are there other characters or personifications?
5. **Mood:** What is the mood of the narrative (sad, neutral, amused, hurting, calm)? What is your mood after reading it?

6. **Motion:** How does the story move? Does something change between the beginning and end? Does it take you on a journey? Does it move in circles, or does it communicate a feeling of being stuck?

Case Notes

Forty-year-old female, average weight/BMI. Sedentary lifestyle; desk job. Old (10 years) cervical injury (C6 bulge). Hypermobile but functional, not assessed for Ehlers–Danlos, but tested positive (5/5) on the self-reported screening questionnaire (see Chapter 7). Visibly weak periscapular muscles with scapular winging, shoulder instability and frequent mild pain on affected (right) side. Lower back pain for several months following known strain from heavy lifting. No other serious health complaints.

The patient presented with new symptoms including acute pain in the right posterior forearm and hand, refractory to analgesics. She awoke most mornings with acute pain, as well as stiffness and dull pain in most finger joints, occasionally with redness and mild swelling (sausage finger description). Frequent Raynaud syndrome in fingers and toes apparently triggered by minor environmental temperature changes. Rheumatology bloodwork negative; thyroid normal; all other bloodwork normal. No obvious physical or postural trigger and no other recent injuries.

Treatment: Ten minutes infrared radiation; 10 min transcutaneous electrical nerve stimulation (TENS) applied to upper back; 15 min shockwave therapy (patient consulted first); 30 min massage.

Following the session, the patient stated she felt largely relieved of the discomfort, and telephone follow-up during the week confirmed the pain had not returned. Several months later, it had still not returned.

Biopsychosocial Details

This was a highly educated patient who was aware of the basics of physical health and comfortable with scientific terminology. She had struggled with cervical pain for many years, and more recently, lower back pain and generalised joint pain. She had resisted previous advice to adopt a gentle exercise regime. She had no outside assistance for manual household tasks, was strongly independent, and did not like to seek help. This episode had made her fearful, as prior to seeing the physiotherapist she had seen a series of specialists, fearing an autoimmune condition. Though her lab work was clear, she had endured several months of limited functionality and constant low-grade, occasionally acute pain, and was concerned that this

(Continued)

BOX 1.3   The Narrative Medicine Approach—cont'd

might lead to sensitisation. Her sleep pattern was inconsistent and poor, and she worked long hours at her desk. Within the previous year she had experienced a series of family bereavements, ongoing caregiving responsibilities, a partner with chronic pain and mobility issues, and a relocation involving a lot of heavy carrying.

Clinical Encounter

The therapist questioned the patient regarding daily activities, the pain onset and pattern and her openness to following an exercise regimen. He also sought her preferences regarding treatment options. The discussion revealed that she often carried heavy shopping, lifted heavy objects, and her office chair was the likely cause of coccygeal pain and cervical tension. The therapist emphasised the weakness of her back muscles, the compensation occurring due to this and reminded her of previous visits due to cervical pain flares. On inquiry, she was already aware of the anatomical interactions making this muscle weakness an important target for intervention. He restated the reasons and benefits for making certain lifestyle changes, acknowledging her resistance, but did not provide a solution to overcome it.

Follow-Up

Following this session, the patient bought a trolley to carry heavy loads and shopping and abandoned heavier yard work. The following winter, she wore gloves indoors to guard against the Raynaud symptoms that triggered digital joint pain. She bought a new office chair, adjusted her sitting posture and guarded the painful arm, favouring the other whenever possible. Within a few months, she had put on several pounds (going up two dress sizes), continued to avoid exercise and her sleep continued to be patchy. A year after this episode (there had been no recurrences), she still favoured her 'good' arm and to avoid the heavier tasks she had done in the past. Two years later, the symptoms returned, more debilitating than before. A neck MRI revealed reverse cervical lordosis, multiple cervical disc bulges, multiple medium-large osteophytes on all cervical vertebrae from C2 to C7, no central stenosis, but stenosis of several lateral foramina due to osteophytes. Hypermobile EDS was also confirmed, as was diffuse tendonitis in the rotator cuffs and a partial supraspinatus rupture in the dominant shoulder. Long-term physical therapy and targeted therapeutic exercise were advised.

Questions to Consider

• Were the therapist's initial attempts at helping this patient make lifestyle corrections successful?

• Where did the therapist succeed or fall short, and why?
• What would you have done differently?
• What could have been improved in the care provision between the first presentation (with burning pain) and the imaging acquired 2 years later?
• How would you treat this patient based on this information?

Applied Close Reading

Now read the narrative that follows. Before reading onwards, take a few moments to note down your responses to the points above. Having done so, set these notes aside and consider the story from the patient's perspective. Observe the word choices and consider this patient as a whole person.

Patient narrative: That winter I spent several months in excruciating pain. First my back went and I spent 2 months in bed, then I could barely use my hands. It drove me crazy, and the winter was so cold I had to keep carrying in the wood wearing a belt for my back, but my hands would ache day and night. At one point I couldn't type, my fingers kept going blue as soon as the temperature fell. N. said I should wear gloves in my office, but I thought that was ridiculous. Every morning I thought it might be a little better, but my hands have become monsters, they have a mind of their own. I looked at the symptoms and I'm starting to think this has to be R.A. (rheumatoid arthritis). Maybe my body's decided to take revenge on me. I saw a nice rheumatologist. He thought this was probably lupus and sent me for a battery of tests. I felt strangely relieved. After so much death, it was like a new friend had moved in. I knew what would take me. But I was wrong because the tests were clear. Surprised, the rheumatologist said there was nothing wrong with me, and that maybe it was somatised grief and I just needed to give myself time to recover. He'd be right there, but there's no cure for what I'm carrying. The next day I woke up screaming in pain and called him right away. He told me the name of some painkillers which I didn't get. The rest of the week was hell. I woke up screaming in pain almost every morning; it got so bad I was afraid to go to bed. The light-bulb moment came when I shrieked at my partner 'FIRE! My hand is on FIRE!' He immediately insisted that I phone my physiotherapist – the one specialist I had forgotten as I'd gone hunting after rare autoimmune conditions. I argued

BOX 1.3   The Narrative Medicine Approach—cont'd

back, never having experienced the degree of pain that cervical radiculopathy can generate. Indeed, it seemed that my old cervical disc bulge was having a temper tantrum, and my back had turned into a broken jigsaw after everything I'd done to it. One visit to my physio, a new chair and a new pillow delivered me from the agony within a few days. The acute pain has not returned. My neck is beyond redemption.

Two things have stayed with me; how I awoke screaming 'fire', and that unlocked what was wrong. My physiotherapist zeroed into that description, asking me several times to be precise in how I was describing the sensation. The second thing is how he made me laugh. For the tenth time he gently tried to suggest I should moderate my activities and start doing regular exercise. 'But,' I said to him, 'I do so much yard work, the house is huge, the grounds are huge, I chop and carry wood, and I do it all myself. That's plenty of exercise!' Laughing, he replied: 'My dear, that's not exercise. You're an intellectual, but you're also a lumberjack!' I'm grateful he puts up with me even though I'm such a bad patient.

Narrative Approach

Before reading further, highlight any points, words or phrases that stand out, then work through the narrative using the six points for Close Reading listed above. Then read on and compare your observations. There are no right and wrong answers at this stage.

Sample Response to Patient Narrative

General: Notice the use of 'temper tantrum' and 'grumbles' to talk about the chronic neck issue. Hands become 'monsters', her back becomes a 'broken jigsaw'. She seems to want to distance herself from the sites of pain. Elsewhere, she gives her painful body parts a mind of their own (e.g. 'take revenge').

1. **Observation:** The narrative is very tactile. It focuses primarily on physical sensations, with little to nothing visual until 'FIRE' is repeated and becomes central to the narrative. The only sound is of her 'screaming in pain' (repeated) and 'shrieking'. Pain is also given a sound: 'tantrum, grumbling'. She seems to have everything under tight control until it breaks the surface – and then it's explosive. The 'pain' words are much more intense than anywhere else. The rest of the narrative is quite crisp and quiet in comparison. Control issues?

2. **Perspective:** The narrative is mainly told from the patient's perspective, with a little from the therapist's perspective too. The partner seems to have had the most insight, but the patient seems preoccupied and resistant to advice.

3. The **form** is like a journal entry, fairly informal, but self-aware with a sense of expectation that strangers might read it. She explains details about her activities to fill in the gaps. Repeated imagery of body parts as enemies. The story is told in chronological order, but is there a backstory she is not telling? Possibly related to the 'somatised grief' mentioned, but not explored. She says 'there's no cure' for that. Is this the root of the problem? Despite the explosions of graphic, pain-related imagery, the narrative is controlled, there is a sense of having given up on getting help ('no cure', 'beyond redemption') or some deep resistance to it. The sub-story with the rheumatologist and suspected lupus is incredibly cold – as if she is content with such a potentially serious diagnosis. Perhaps this needs exploring. She tells the sub-story of the conversation with the therapist hinting at the one line that got her to change a few things. She liked being compared to a lumberjack.

4. **Voice:** It's all in the first person; some of it is business-like. Some of the more colourful details make it seem quite intimate, but in fact, it's fairly remote. She's creating distance between herself (the controlled voice) and the pain breaking through it and coming closer to us. Almost as if she's offended by it. She says she is a 'bad patient' aware of what the therapist is trying to help her do, aware that she's not going to do it, feeling sorry for his efforts that she's already decided will fail. She doesn't seem to want to help herself – or doesn't want to acknowledge needing help? Does she feel unable to help herself? Is the resistance because she doesn't believe it will work?

5. **Mood:** The mood is neutral in some places, has moments of graphic pain, fleeting moments of darkness and although the mood at the end is almost satisfied and amused, it leaves something unfinished, uncomfortable.

6. **Motion:** The story moves towards a kind of resolution of the immediate problem, and the patient seems happy enough that she's no longer in pain, as if her problem is now resolved. But the backstory seems unresolved, and it may be key to understanding the resistance to help or change.

(Continued)

BOX 1.3   The Narrative Medicine Approach—cont'd

Notes: Little is known about this patient's family and cultural background. Her narrative mentions grief, caregiving, and work. We can guess she is in a rural area (large yard, carrying firewood), but little else. These elements would need to be sensitively explored before taking too much for granted. Deeper knowledge of the patient's narrative and the sources of her non-compliance would allow the therapist to develop a more effective strategy, by guiding the patient herself to explore her reasons for resistance.

Patient Feedback

On being asked to reflect on her narrative based on these comments, the patient provided the following further feedback:

I chose raw and graphic words to describe pain because I want the reader to see me writhing, to have no doubt as to its intensity. It isn't 'mine' – it's 'the' pain – because this experience is unacceptable to me: I just wanted it to stop – but I endured it for months before seeing someone. I didn't take action because I want to distance myself from it, not allow it in.

I liked the therapist's description of me as an 'intellectual lumberjack' because, to me, that meant someone who endures hardship and physical strain as part of life, who is resilient. That sums me up rather well. He's known me for a while and he knows I know what I 'should' be doing. I have an ingrained 'can-do' attitude. I hate exercise. Spending time I can't spare on boring exercises is my idea

of torture. I understand the science, but nobody has yet been able to show me how I can systematically incorporate those lifestyle hacks into my daily routine without getting bored – or admitting I need to do so. It's easier to just ignore the pain; and this was the first time I couldn't.

Questions to Consider

- How would you talk to such a patient?
- Is this someone who gets listed as 'difficult' and gently pushed towards a different therapist, dismissed for what seems like a wilful refusal to take advice?
- Might it be easier to ignore the backstory?
- What are the implications of doing so?
- Is this someone who would respond to attempts at pain education?
- Might they respond better to touch? Which senses seem most responsive, based on her narrative?
- What is it they really need, and is it what *they* think they need?
- How would you work with these issues within your scope of practice?
- Would muscle energy technique be an appropriate intervention for this patient? If not, why not? If so, within what broader treatment plan?

Compare your notes and observations from this section with the notes you made after the 'Biopsychosocial information' section. What has changed? What more have you discovered about this patient? What do you still not know? How would you proceed?

Charon et al. (2015) and Chaitow (2021c).

---

of the individual to their condition, as well as to their BPS context beyond the essentialist paradigm of culture, social class, race, gender, age and so on. This is a vital component with significant ethical implications, given the significance of social justice concerns. Narrative medicine practitioners make the point that, even when applying the BPS approach to the letter, we are still at risk of error if we look at a patient as a member of a group, rather than an individual. Dismissing a 'difficult' patient without looking at their story automatically creates an injustice, even if they are apparently privileged in every other way, as detailed in Box 1.2. Attention to nuance such as choice of words, coherence of the timeline or whether there is a chaotic quality to their storytelling is as relevant as their lab results. The exploration of these

elements should not be conducted with a view to forcing, or even directing change, but in holding space for the patient, and for the therapist to make them part of the dialogue and deliberation when examining the therapeutic options at hand.

The methods for achieving a shift in focus are drawn directly from the skillsets of the humanities disciplines – embedded in biomedical training through the subdiscipline of the Medical Humanities – whose significance for manual therapy professions is explored in Chapter 3. Some similar initiatives are gradually emerging in U.S. osteopathic schools (Hoff et al., 2014; Baltonado & Cymet, 2017; Klugman, 2018; Sexton, 2018) but, more recently, their value has been acknowledged more substantially in osteopathic research (see Chapter 3). The rationale for their inclusion in medical training is compelling: 'Frequently students coming into medical school believe that they can simply learn enough to be certain that banishing ambiguity and doubt, and thereby remaining less touched by the emotion of the work, is a matter of how much you take in and how hard you work...' (Hermann, 2017). In relation to anatomical knowledge: 'in knowing the cadaver in such intimate detail we believe that we are acquiring the knowledge to overcome death' (Chen, 2008). As important as this knowledge is, it should not overshadow the reality of the individual.

Biomedical educators have sought the further integration of humanities-based learning into medical curricula because of the phenomena outlined above, made worse by a form of detachment that appears to be an undesirable corollary of medical training (Fox & Lief, 1963; Newell, 1993; Cassell, 1995; Lipkin et al., 1995; Charon 2001; Hermann, 2017).

The main objectives of the integrated interdisciplinary training are to facilitate the trainee physicians' self-awareness in their role, to develop more humanistic approaches to practice, and to build resilience by working through difficult scenarios of pain, illness, failure and disaster in the safe environment of the literary text long before they are faced with them in their clinic. Aside from developing better listening skills, humility and resilience when facing the pain of others, there is qualitative evidence that training and long-term familiarisation with literary fiction and visual art creates neurobiological change affecting our ability to *mentalise* (perceive and understand one's own behaviour and that of others, maintaining a not-knowing approach) (Schank & Abelson, 1995; Bal & Veltkamp, 2013; Samur et al., 2018; Welstead et al., 2018). These are techniques well-known to humanities scholars, sociologists of education and educators, who are now working in interdisciplinary teams alongside medical faculty to develop such programmes. The results appear promising and provide a valuable model for faculty across the allied and integrative health disciplines.

In terms of the immediate benefits in the clinical encounter, close reading and listening are transferable skills allowing the clinician to see beyond the 'bio' as well as the too normative 'psychosocial' of the BPS model. The patient narratives provide insight into whether or not – and crucially, *why* – they are likely to comply with and maintain new lifestyle habits. They also reveal what deep thinking patterns require a different approach to

well-meaning imposition of impersonal clinical assessment that maintains a subject–object dynamic. Instead, by providing the patient with the space to share their own narrative, and the sense that their experience of illness is seen and respected, the foundations for trust are laid, and ways forward sought with equal input from the patient. This confirms something that many holistic practitioners have discovered through their training or through experience, as with Leon Chaitow who advocated such an approach without giving it a name. Applying evidence-informed practice to whole-person healthcare includes the whole therapeutic encounter, and the NBM approach offers robustly evidence-based tools through which to implement and teach it.

MANUAL THERAPIES: PAST, PRESENT AND FUTURE

Our understanding of manual therapy approaches such as MET will expand along with the evidence base. As this occurs, it is likely that methods developed by the thought leaders of the past, such as Thomas J. Ruddy, Fred Mitchell, Vladimir Janda, Karl Lewit, Philip Greenman and others, upon whose work Leon Chaitow built this text, will remain relevant. This is because, despite changes in the evidence base, the methodology of MET has changed little and reflects the insight of those who pioneered this form of manual therapy. In the context of an improved BPS model of care, reflection on the leaders and teachers from the past indicates that the three elements of the human experience are not new. One only needs to watch a video of Leon Chaitow, or Prof Lewit or Dr Greenman and the others to identify their understanding of patient-centred care. It was conveyed as an implicit skill and rests on the principles of their own training and practice. It says something about current practices that a BPS focus of care needs to be relearned and raises concern about how it was lost in the first place. There is now a solid evidence base supporting both training and practice of this dimension of the clinical encounter, and holistic thinking and practice are being integrated into biomedical practice on a wide scale through significant educational centres. Though osteopathic practitioners in particular benefit from an integrated approach that has been thought to incorporate these skills, it still does not possess a structure, clear conceptual framework or devoted methods (Tyreman, 2018; Maretic & Abbey, 2021).

While ongoing clinical practice and research will expand the understanding of *why* the methods are beneficial, they are unlikely to change *how* the methods are applied. As various practitioners of MET integrate the methods into practice, understanding how these foundations were laid, and revisiting the evolution and development of these methods will offer great insight to enrich truly patient-centred care.

In the following chapter, the core definitions, concepts and variants of MET are presented, with further detail on their role in reducing adaptive load, as well as practical considerations in their application. It is the authors' view that practitioners and patients can only benefit from the continuing integration of such methods into multimodal frameworks closely informed by whole-person medicine that continues to be judiciously evidence-informed, accepting of the diversity and uncertainty that is part of being human.

REFERENCES

Alexanders, J., Anderson, A., Henderson, S., 2015. Musculoskeletal physiotherapists' use of psychological interventions: a systematic review of therapists' perceptions and practice. Physiotherapy 101 (2), 95–102.

Bal, P.M., Veltkamp, M., 2013. How does fiction reading influence empathy? An experimental investigation on the role of emotional transportation. PLoS One 8 (1), e55341.

Baltonado, J., Cymet, T., 2017. Can the humanities humanize health care? J. Amer. Osteopath. Assoc. 117 (4), 273–275.

Beauchamp, T.L., Childress, J.F., 1979. Principles of biomedical ethics. Oxford, New York.

Blickenstaff, C., Pearson, N., 2016. Reconciling movement and exercise with pain neuroscience education: a case for consistent education. Physiother. Theory Pract. 32 (5), 396–407. https://doi.org/10.1080/09593985.2016.1194653.

Bove, G.M., Delany, S.P., Hobson, L., Cruz, G.E., Harris, M.Y., Amin, M., et al., 2019. Manual therapy prevents onset of nociceptor activity, sensorimotor dysfunction, and neural fibrosis induced by a volitional repetitive task. Pain. 160 (3), 632.

British National Institute for Health and Care Excellence. 2022. Chronic pain: assessment and management, evidence review for manual therapy. https://www.nice.org.uk/guidance/ng193/documents/evidence-review-9

Broom, A., Adamms, J., 2009. The status of CAM in biomedical education. In: Brosnan, C., Turner, B.S. (Eds.), Handbook of the Sociology of Medical Education. Routledge, pp. 124.

Brosnan, C., Turner, B.S. eds., 2009. Handbook of the sociology of medical education. Routledge.

Brower, V., 2006. Mind-body research moves towards the mainstream. EMBO Rep 7 (4), 358–361. https://doi.org/10.1038/sj.embor.7400671.

Chaitow, L., Delany, J., 2005. Clinical application of neuromuscular techniques: practical case study exercises. Elsevier.

Chaitow, S., 2021. How do you feel inside? Why Narrative Medicine is critical to Ethical Practice. Part 436. Massage & Bodywork, pp. 46–51.

Chaitow, S., 2021a. Listen, my body electric: narrative medicine and the holistic revolution in biomedicine: part 1. Massage & Bodywork, Golden, Colorado 36 (2), 42–49.

Chaitow, S., 2021b. Solving the biopsychosocial problem: from evidence-based practice to narrative medicine: part 1. Massage & Bodywork, Golden, Colorado 36 (3), 42–49.

Chaitow, S., 2021c. Narrative medicine in practice: part 3. Massage & Bodywork, Golden, Colorado 36 (5), 40–45.

Chaitow, S., 2022. Evidence in the echo chamber. Massage & Bodywork, Golden, Colorado.

Charon, R., 2001. Narrative medicine: a model for empathy, reflection, profession, and trust. JAMA 286 (15), 1897–1902.

Charon, R., 2016. The principles and practice of narrative medicine. Oxford University Press.

Charon, R., Hermann, N., Devlin, M.J., 2015. Close reading and creative writing in clinical education: teaching attention, representation, and affiliation. Acad. Med. 91 (3), 345–350. dx.doi.org/10.1097/ACM.0000000000000827.

Chaterji, R., Tractenberg, R.E., Amri, H., Lumpkin, M., Amorosi, S.B., Haramati, A., 2007. A large-sample survey of first-and second-year medical student attitudes toward complementary and alternative medicine in the curriculum and in practice. Altern. Ther. Health. Med. 13 (1), 30.

Chen, P., 2008. Final exam: a surgeon's reflections on mortality. Vintage.

Consortium of Academic Health Centers for Integrative Medicine (CAHCIM) (2004) *Curriculum in Integrative Medicine: a guide for medical educators*, Minnesota, MN: CAHCIM.

Cruz-Montecinos, C., Godoy-Olave, D., Contreras-Briceño, F.A., Gutiérrez, P., Torres-Castro, R., Miret-Venegas, L., et al., 2017. The immediate effect of soft tissue manual therapy intervention on lung function in severe chronic obstructive pulmonary disease. Int. J. Chron. Obstruct. Pulmon. Dis. 12, 691–696. doi:10.2147/COPD.S127742.

Diener, I., Kargela., M., Louw, A., 2016. Listening is therapy: patient interviewing from a pain science perspective. Physiother. Theory Pract. 32 (5), 356–367. https://doi.org/10.1080/09593985.2016.1194648.

Ebell, M.H., Sokol, R., Lee, A., Simons, C., Early, J., 2017. How good is the evidence to support primary care practice? BMJ Evid. Based Med. 22, 88–92.

Epstein, I., 2009. Promoting harmony where there is commonly conflict: evidence-informed practice as an integrative strategy. Soc. Work Health Care 48, 216–223.

Fox, R., Lief, H., 1963. Training for "detached concern". In: Lief, H. (Ed.), The Psychological Basis of Medical Practice. Harper & Row, New York, pp. 12–35.

Fryer, G., 2017. Integrating osteopathic approaches based on biopsychosocial therapeutic mechanisms. Part 1: The mechanisms. Int. J. Osteopath. Med. 25, 30–41.

Fryer, G., 2017. Integrating osteopathic approaches based on biopsychosocial therapeutic mechanisms. Part 2: clinical approach. Int. J. Osteopath. Med. 26, 36–43.

Glasziou, P., 2005. Evidence-based medicine: does it make a difference? Make it evidence informed with a little wisdom. Brit. Med. J. 330 (7482), 92.

Greenhalgh, T., Hurwitz, B., 1999. Why study narrative? BMJ 318 (7175), 48–50.

Guillemin, M., Barnard, E., 2015. George Libman Engel: the biopsychosocial model and the construction of medical practice. In: Collyer, F. (eds) The Palgrave Handbook of Social Theory in Health, Illness, and Medicine. Palgrave Macmillan, London. https://doi.org/10.1057/9781137355621_15.

Guzman, J., Esmail, R., Karjalainen, K., Malmivaara, A., Irvin, E., Bombardier, C., 2001. Multidisciplinary rehabilitation for chronic low back pain: systematic review. BMJ 322, 1511–1516.

Hackstaff, L., Davis, C., Katz, L., 2004. The case for integrating behavior change, client-centered practice and other evidence-based models into geriatric care management. Soc. Work Health Care 38 (3), 1–19. https://doi.org/10.1300/J010v38n03_01.

Herman, J., 2005. The need for a transitional model: a challenge for biopsychosocial medicine? Fam. Syst. Health 23 (4), 372–376.

Hermann, N., Creativity: what, why, and where? In: Charon, R. et al, 2017. The principles and practice of narrative medicine. New York, Oxford University Press. pp. 211–228.

Hoff, G., Hirsch, N.J., Means, J.J., Streyffeler, L., 2014. A call to include medical humanities in the curriculum of colleges of osteopathic medicine and in applicant selection. J. Amer. Osteopath. Assoc. 114 (10), 798–804.

Irvine, C., Charon, R., 2016. Deliver us from certainty: training for narrative ethics. In: Charon, R. et al, 2016. The principles and practice of narrative medicine. New York, Oxford University Press. pp. 110–129.

Jull, G., Moore, A., 2012. Hands on, hands off? The swings in musculoskeletal physiotherapy practice. Man. Ther. 17, 199–200.

Kamper, S.J., Apeldoorn, A.T., Chiarotto, A., Smeets, R.J., Ostelo, R.W., Guzman, J., van Tulder, M.W., 2015. Multidisciplinary biopsychosocial rehabilitation for chronic low back pain: cochrane systematic review and meta-analysis. BMJ 350, h444. https://doi.org/10.1136/bmj.h444.

Klugman, C.M., 2018. Medical humanities teaching in north american allopathic and osteopathic medical schools. J. Med. Humanit. 39, 473. https://doi.org/10.1007/s10912-017-9491-z.

Kolb, W.H., McDevitt., A.W., Young, J., Shamus, E., 2020. The evolution of manual therapy education: what are we waiting for? J. Man. Manip. Ther. 28 (1), 1–3. doi:10.1080/10669817.2020.1703315.

Langevin, H.M., 2021. Reconnecting the brain with the rest of the body in musculoskeletal pain research. J. Pain. 22 (1), 1–8.

Langevin, H., 2022. Three new research networks will focus on the neural mechanisms of force-based manipulations. National Center for Complementary and Integrative Health. https://www.nccih.nih.gov/about/offices/od/director/past-messages/three-new-research-networks-will-focus-on-the-neural-mechanisms-of-force-based-manipulations?

Lederman, E., 2017. A process approach in osteopathy: beyond the structural model. Int. J. Osteopathic Med. 23, 22–35.

Licciardone, J.C., Schultz, M.J., Amen, B., 2020. Osteopathic manipulation in the management of chronic pain: current perspectives. J. Pain. Res. 13, 1839–1847. doi:10.2147/JPR.S183170.

Louw, A., Nijs, J., Puentedura, E.J., 2017. A clinical perspective on a pain neuroscience education approach to manual therapy. J. Man. Manip. Ther. 25 (3), 160–168. https://doi.org/10.1080/10669817.2017.1323699.

Louw, A., Puentedura, E.L., Zimney, K., 2016a. Teaching patients about pain: It works, but what should we call it? Physiother. Theory Pract. 32 (5), 328–331.

Louw, A., Zimney, K., Puentedura, E.J., Diener, I., 2016b. The efficacy of pain neuroscience education on musculoskeletal pain: a systematic review of the literature. Physiother. Theory Pract. 32, 332–355.

Malfliet, A., Kregel, J., Meeus, M., Roussel, N., Danneels, L., Cagnie, B., et al., 2018. Blended-learning pain neuroscience education for people with chronic spinal pain: randomized controlled multicenter trial. Phys. Ther. 98 (5), 357–368.

Maretic, S., Abbey, H., 2021. "Understanding patients' narratives" A qualitative study of osteopathic educators' opinions about using Medical Humanities poetry in undergraduate education. Int. J. Osteopathic Med. 40, 29–37.

McCormack, B., Rycroft-Malone, J., Decorby, K., Hutchinson, A.M., Bucknall, T., Kent, B., et al., 2013. A realist review of interventions and strategies to promote evidence-informed healthcare: a focus on change agency. Implementation Science 107 (8), 1–12.

McSherry, R., 2007. Developing, exploring and refining a modified whole systems-based model of evidence-informed nursing. School of Health and Social Care. Teesside University, Middlesbrough, England, UK Unpublished Ph.D. Thesis.

Mootz, R.D., 2005. When evidence and practice collide. J. Manipulative Physiol. Ther. 28 (8), 551–553.

Moseley, G.L., 2003a. Joining forces–combining cognition-targeted motor control training with group or individual pain physiology education: a successful treatment for chronic low back pain. J. Man. Manip. Ther. 11, 88–94.

Moseley, G.L., 2003b. Unravelling the barriers to reconceptualization of the problem in chronic pain: The actual and perceived ability of patients and health professionals to understand the neurophysiology. J. Pain 4, 184–189.

Murphy, J.W., Franz, B.A., Choi, J.M., Callaghan, K.A., 2017. Narrative medicine and community-based health care and planning. Springer, New York, pp. 7–8.

National Commission for the Protection of Human Subjects of Biomedical and Behavioral Research, Department of Health, Education, and Welfare. The Belmont Report No. 78-0012.

Newell, R., 1993. Interviewing Skills for Nurses and other healthcare professionals. Routledge.

Oostendorp, R.A.B., 2018. Credibility of manual therapy is at stake 'where do we go from here? J. Man. Manip. Ther. 26 (4), 189–192.

Parker, R., Madden., V.J., 2020. State of the art: what have the pain sciences brought to physiotherapy? S. Afr. J. Physiother. 76 (1), a1390. doi: https://doi.org/10.4102/sajp.v76i1.1390

Puentedura, E.J., Flynn, T., 2016. Combining manual therapy with pain neuroscience education in the treatment of chronic low back pain: a narrative review of the literature. Physiother. Theory Pract. 32 (5), 408–414. https://doi.org/10.1080/09593985.2016.1194663.

Richter, M., Rauscher, C., Kluttig, A., Mallwitz, J., Delank, K.S., 2020. Effect of additional pain neuroscience education in interdisciplinary multimodal pain therapy on current pain. A non-randomized, controlled intervention study. J. Pain Res. 13, 2947–2957. doi:10.2147/JPR.S272943.

Sackett, D.L., Rosenberg, WMC, Gray, J.A.M., Haynes, R.B., Richardson, W.S., 1996. Evidence based medicine: what it is and what it isn't. BMJ 312. https://doi.org/10.1136/bmj.312.7023.71.

Samur, D., Tops, M., Koole, S.L., 2018. Does a single session of reading literary fiction prime enhanced mentalising

performance? Four replication experiments of Kidd and Castano (2013). Cogn. Emot 32 (1), 130–144.

Sanders, T., Foster, N.E., Bishop, A., Ong, B.N., 2013. Biopsychosocial care and the physiotherapy encounter: physiotherapists' accounts of back pain consultations. BMC Musculoskelet. Disord., 65. doi:10.1186/1471-2474-14-65.

Schank, R.C., Abelson, R.P., 1995. Knowledge and memory: the real story. Knowledge and memory: the real story. Adv. Social Cogn. 8, 1–85.

Seaburn, D.B., 2005. Is going "too far" far enough? Fam. Syst. Health. 23 (4), 396–399.

Sexton, P., 2018. Maintaining balance in medical school through medical humanities electives. Missouri Med 115 (1), 35–36.

Singla, M., Jones., M., Edwards, I., Kumar, S., 2015. Physiotherapists' assessment of patients' psychosocial status: are we standing on thin ice? A qualitative descriptive study. Man. Ther. 20 (2), 328–334.

Smith, D., 2019. Reflecting on new models for osteopathy–it's time for change. Int. J. Osteopathic Med. 31, 15–20.

Smith, R.C., Fortin, A.H., Dwamena, F., Frankel, R.M., 2013. An evidence-based patient-centered method makes the biopsychosocial model scientific. Patient Educ. Couns. 91 (3), 265–270. doi:10.1016/j.pec.2012.12.010.

Sweet, M., Moynihan, R., 2007. Improving population health; the uses of systematic reviews. Centers for Disease Control and Prevention (U.S.). https://stacks.cdc.gov/view/cdc/6921.

Synnott, A., O'Keeffe, M., Bunzli, S., Dankaerts, W., O'Sullivan, P., O'Sullivan, K., 2015. Physiotherapists may stigmatise or feel unprepared to treat people with low back pain and psychosocial factors that influence recovery: a systematic review. J. Physiother. 61 (2), 68–76. doi:10.1016/j.phys.2015.02.016.

Synnott, A., O'Keeffe, M., Bunzli, S., Dankaerts, W., O'Sullivan, P., Robinson, K., et al., 2016. Physiotherapists report improved understanding of and attitude toward the cognitive, psychological and social dimensions of chronic low back pain after cognitive functional therapy training: a qualitative study. J. Physiother. 62 (4), 215–221. doi:10.1016/j.jphys.2016.08.002.

Tyreman, S., 2018. Evidence, alternative facts and narrative: a personal reflection on person-centred care and the role of stories in healthcare. Int. J. Osteopathic Med. 28, 1–3.

Vivanco-Coke, S., Silva, A.J., Quiñinao, F.R., Zambra, R.F., Reyes, J.T., 2020. Evaluation of short-term effectiveness of orthopedic manual therapy in signs and symptoms of myofascial pain: a controlled clinical trial. J. Oral Res. 9 (2), 121–128. doi:10.17126/joralres.2020.019.

Wade, D.T., Halligan, P., 2004. Do biomedical models of illness make for good healthcare systems? BMJ 329 (7479), 1398–1401.

Weeks, J., 2013. Consortium of Academic Health Centers for Integrative Medicine Opens Dialogue With Joint Commission on Standards for Nonpharmacological Treatment of Pain... plus more. Integr. Med. 12 (5), 14.

Weiner, B.K., 2008. Spine update: the biopsychosocial model and spine care. Spine 33 (2), 219–223. doi:10.1097/BRS.0b013e3181604572.

Welstead, H.J., Patrick, J., Russ, T.C., Cooney, G., Mulvenna, C.M., Maclean, C., et al., 2018. Mentalising skills in generic mental healthcare settings: can we make our day-to-day interactions more therapeutic? BJPsych Bulletin 42 (3), 102–108.

Wijma, A.J., van Wilgen, C.P., Meeus, M., Nijs, J., 2016. Clinical biopsychosocial physiotherapy assessment of patients with chronic pain: The first step in pain neuroscience education. Physiother Theory Pract 32 (5), 368–384. https://doi.org/10.1080/09593985.2016.1194651.

Winslow, L.C. and Shapiro, H., 2002. Physicians want education about complementary and alternative medicine to enhance communication with their patients. Arch. Intern. Med. 162 (10), 1176–1181.

2

Muscle Energy Techniques

Leon Chaitow, Sandy Fritz, Sasha Chaitow

CHAPTER CONTENTS

WHAT IS MET?

Muscle energy techniques (METs) are a form of soft-tissue or joint manipulations or mobilisations, derived from osteopathic medicine and employed in the treatment of musculoskeletal dysfunction.

In this chapter we look briefly at the protocols of some of the different models of MET (others are described in later chapters), as well as compare these with a similar modality, proprioceptive neuromuscular facilitation (PNF). This introductory overview of MET contains several important elements, all of which will be expanded on in discussions in subsequent chapters.

Leon Chaitow noted that during the teaching of MET to a diverse range of manual therapists, it became increasingly apparent that, while the basic application was easily grasped, the subtleties that make MET's usefulness in clinical settings so powerful are frequently not appreciated or applied. Indeed, what could be simpler than having the patient contract a tight muscle against resistance (or the muscles associated with a restricted joint) and then stretching the muscle (or mobilising the joint)? While the basics are indeed simple, there are multiple variables available in any MET application and, in any given case, the best results will be achieved only if delivery is individualised to the patient and the situation.

For example, it is always essential to determine whether MET is actually the best clinical choice on its own or in combination with other modalities such as high-velocity manipulation, or positional release. If in combination, where should MET be best used in the treatment sequence?

When applying MET methods, the following questions require consideration:

- What resistance barrier should be used – since soft tissues may be moved towards a 'first sign of resistance', or as far as is tolerable, or somewhere in between – before a contraction is initiated?
- Is it best to utilise an isometric or an isotonic contraction?
- Would a resisted isometric contraction be best applied towards, away from the resistance barrier or in some other direction altogether?
- Similarly, if an isotonic stretch is being used, should the process involve a concentric or eccentric action?
- Stated differently, should the restricted structures (the agonists) be involved in any isometric (or isotonic) contraction, or should the focus be on the antagonists?
- Which direction of effort should be requested, and fully or partially resisted?
- What degree of patient effort ('muscle energy') is optimal?
- How long should a contraction (isometric or isotonic) be maintained?
- Is there a place for respiratory assistance in MET use?
- What should be done following the contraction?
- When tissues are subsequently stretched or mobilised, should the patient be requested to assist in the process? Also, how far beyond the new barrier should tissues be taken and how long should they be held there?
- Should the process be repeated?
- What is the place in MET usage for brief, pulsating contractions ('pulsed MET'), and what benefit would such a method offer compared with sustained contractions?
- How can MET variations (such as slow eccentric isotonic stretch [SEIS]) be best applied post surgically, to prevent fibrosis and undue scarring? (see Chapter 10).

It is suggested that the answers to these questions, and to many other aspects of MET application, are likely to determine the success or failure of MET use. A primary question that this book sets out to address is whether there is significant evidence for the answers to any of these questions and, as in all manual therapy, to what extent MET application is evidence-informed. An annotated survey of evidence spanning the last two decades is presented in Box 2.1. A critical review of the current research validation for MET is provided in Chapter 4 with multiple additional examples offered in all chapters. In sum, the evidence is good, and where guidelines or recommendations are based on opinion or experience, this is clearly stated in the text.

BARRIERS AND MET: 'FEATHER-EDGE' OR STRETCHED?

The essence of MET is that it harnesses the energy of the patient (in the form of muscular effort) to achieve a therapeutic effect. MET, at its most basic, involves the careful positioning of an area of the body, followed by the use of an isometric (sometimes isotonic) contraction. The amount of force employed, as well as the direction(s) and duration of the effort, are specific and controlled, as is the subsequent movement of the involved joint, or soft tissues to a new position after (or sometimes during) the cessation of the contraction. This repositioning might involve a degree of stretching or might take advantage of a reduction in resistance to movement, following the contraction, allowing movement to a new barrier without stretching (in acute settings or in joint treatment).

To achieve those requirements of accuracy and appropriate focusing of effort, the ideal barrier from which to commence the sequence needs to be identified. Kappler and Jones (2003) suggest that we consider joint restrictions from a soft tissue perspective. They suggest that as the barrier is engaged, increasing amounts of force are necessary as the degree of free movement decreases. They note that the word *barrier* may be misleading if it is interpreted as a wall or rigid obstacle to be overcome with a push. *More accurately, the limits are identified by pulling against restraints rather than pushing against some anatomic structure:*

'As the joint reaches the barrier, restraints in the form of fascia and increased motor tone of muscles, serve to inhibit further motion.' If this is indeed the case, then methods such as MET – that address the soft tissue restraints – should help to achieve free joint motion. It is at the moment that a 'restraint' to free movement is noted, that the barrier has actually been passed; this is also described as moving from 'ease' towards 'bind'. The 'feather-edge' of resistance is a point that lies a fraction before that sense of 'bind' or restriction is first noted, and it is suggested that any MET contraction effort

BOX 2.1 Reflections and Commentaries on 20 Years of Research

The reports selected for Box 2.1 were chosen for their illustrative value in highlighting a number of key aspects of MET usage in clinical settings. They are presented in chronological order, from older to most recent, to demonstrate the evolution of our understanding of MET.

Note: This is not meant to be a comprehensive listing.

- Wells et al. (1999) investigated the immediate effects of a single session of MET (together with articulation and myofascial release) on the gait of people with Parkinson disease. Twenty subjects with Parkinson disease enrolled in the study, with 10 randomised to an osteopathic manipulative therapy group and 10 to a sham control group. Eight normal subjects free of Parkinson disease also participated. All subjects with Parkinson disease stopped medications for 12 h before starting gait analysis. The treatment group and the eight normal subjects received one standardised session lasting approximately 30 min. The techniques used in the study were direct, articulatory MET and myofascial techniques, targeting the spine, shoulder and joints of the external limbs, including the ankles and wrists. Gait analysis was performed pre- and post-treatment. Those subjects receiving the active treatment protocol had a significant increase in gait parameters relating to stride length and limb velocity for both upper and lower limbs. The study showed that these methods improve gait parameters in people with Parkinson disease. More research is needed to investigate the longer-term effects and which techniques, or combinations of techniques, work best for improving gait in Parkinson disease. A more current study (Yao et al., 2013) confirmed benefits for this condition.

Comment: This small study highlights the potential for MET, together with other modalities, being usefully employed in treatment of patients with serious neurological problems. Since this study was published, ongoing research (Carnevali et al., 2020; Cerritelli et al., 2020; Tramontano et al., 2020) investigated the interface of manual therapy such as MET with neurological stimulation and processing.

- Knebl et al. (2002) conducted a randomised controlled clinical trial testing the effectiveness of a series of shoulder mobilisations known as the Spencer technique, a traditional osteopathic protocol for treating chronic shoulder restriction and pain. In the study, 29 elderly patients with pre-existing shoulder problems were randomly assigned to Spencer treatment, combined with the additional feature of isometric muscle contractions during treatment, or a control group without MET. The placebo group were placed in the same positions as those receiving the active treatment, but without MET ('corrective force') being part of the protocol. Following five treatment sessions, each of 30 min duration, over a period of 14 weeks, both groups showed significant improvement in shoulder range of motion (ROM) and reduced pain by week 14. However, when the subjects returned 5 weeks following the end of the study, the treatment group (those with added MET) were found to have maintained significant improvements in (ROM), while the placebo group did not: 'Those subjects who had received MET demonstrated continued improvement in ROM, while the ROM of the placebo group decreased'.

Comment: (1) The successful use of MET in this population group highlights its ease of application, safety and comfort. (2) The continued improvement of function following the treatment period in the treatment group hints at an ongoing self-regulating process and is deserving of further study. Current research (Iqbal et al., 2020; Schwerla et al., 2020) supports the findings related to management of shoulder pain and limits in motion.

- Lenehan et al. (2003) examined whether a single application of thoracic MET could significantly increase ROM in asymptomatic volunteers with restricted active trunk rotation. Fifty-nine volunteers were randomly assigned to either treatment (MET) or control groups. Blinded pre- and post-active trunk rotation measures were recorded using a reliable measuring device (see Fig. 2.2).

The participant was instructed to place his or her hands on opposite shoulders and to relax. The treating examiner used palpatory assessment to achieve a spinal neutral range, and when this was achieved the restricted rotation barrier was engaged. The treating examiner resisted a five-second isometric contraction of side-bending by the participant. After each isometric effort, a new rotation barrier was engaged, and the participant repeated the isometric contraction. Four repetitions were completed on each volunteer. Immediately following treatment post-test ROM measures were recorded.

Results showed that a significantly increased range of active trunk rotation ($P < .0005$) was achieved in the direction of restricted rotation, but not on the non-restricted side or in the untreated controls. This study supports the use of MET to increase restricted spinal rotation ROM.

Comment: The use of a resisted side-bending contraction, which allowed immediate increased range into previously restricted rotation, is of particular interest and

BOX 2.1   Reflections and Commentaries on 20 Years of Research—cont'd

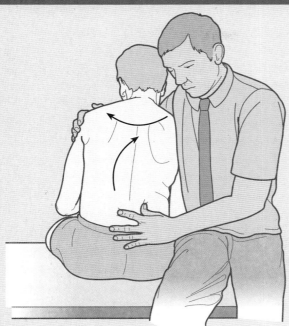

Fig. 2.1 Muscle energy techniques *(MET)* treatment of a restriction involving limitation of L3 flexion, side flexion and rotation to the right. Practitioner palpates for barrier with contacts on the transverse processes of L3.

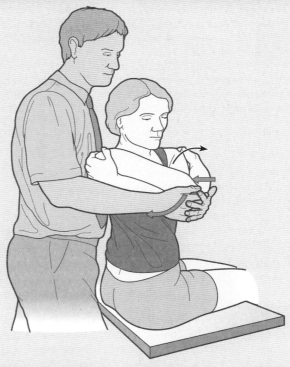

Fig. 2.2 Practitioner eases seated patient into rotation to easy, first-sign-of-resistance barrier. A side-bending isometric contraction is then introduced followed by engagement of new rotation barrier.

significance in this study. This phenomenon is discussed in more detail in Chapter 6, where use of counter-intuitive directions of isometric effort are recommended, in addition to the more obvious possibilities, for example, the use of a resisted rotation contraction, towards or away from the barrier, for a rotation restriction (Figs. 2.1 and 2.2).

• Murphy et al. (2006) described the clinical outcomes of patients with cervical radiculopathy treated non-surgically, including the use of MET or high velocity low amplitude (HVLA) manipulation, together with various exercise strategies, neural mobilisation, self-applied over-the-door traction, ice applications and/or medication (see Chapter 8 for more on Murphy's work).

The overall approach was minimalist in nature; only those treatment approaches that were deemed to be necessary as a result of specific clinical findings were applied. The decision as to which treatments were to be used in any particular patient was made on an individual basis.

The outcomes showed:

Seventeen patients (49%) reported their improvement as 'excellent' and another 14 (40%) did so as 'good'... 24 of 31 (77.4%) patients had a clinically significant improvement from baseline to the end of treatment... [and] at long-term follow-up [improvement] was clinically significant for 25 of the 27 (92.6%) patients.

Comment: This example of patients with serious pain conditions being treated in ways that matched their clinical needs epitomises ideal good practice. The fact that MET played a part in this eclectic therapeutic mix, in those cases where HVLA was deemed unwise, emphasises (1) its relative safety features, (2) its ease of use in highly sensitive settings and (3) the importance of seeing MET as a flexible, safe and effective modality, sometimes used alone, but more often complementing

(Continued)

BOX 2.1 Reflections and Commentaries on 20 Years of Research—cont'd

other manual methods of patient management. Current evidence (Degenhardt et al., 2018; Smith et al., 2019) indicates that the overall incidence of serious adverse events in manual therapies is low.

- Smith & Fryer (2008) tested the usefulness of extending a hamstring muscle stretch, following a MET contraction, from 5 s, as suggested by Greenman, to 30 s, as suggested by Chaitow:

Both techniques appeared to be equally effective in increasing hamstring extensibility, [with] sustained improvement one week following the initial treatment. The findings suggest that altering the duration of the passive stretch component does not have a significant impact on the efficacy of MET for short-term increases in muscle extensibility. Both these post-isometric techniques were superior to passive stretching in this group of subjects.

Comment: Both sustained (30 s) and brief (5 s) post-isometric contraction stretching of the hamstrings produced lasting extensibility in asymptomatic individuals, and more effectively than passive stretching. Whether the brief (5 s) stretching protocol would be equally beneficial in situations involving chronic, indurated muscles remains an open question. The hamstrings have been an ongoing target area for MET research, as seen in Joshi et al. (2017) and Naweed et al. (2020).

- Wright and Drysdale (2008) employed a randomised, controlled protocol in order to evaluate whether either or both of the two MET variations (1) use of the agonist (piriformis itself), supposedly to assess postisometric relaxation effect (PIR), or (2) use of the antagonist, supposedly to assess reciprocal inhibition effects (RI), could significantly enhance hip internal rotation ROM, when applied to the piriformis muscle in asymptomatic young men. The outcomes showed that these methods were equally successful in producing significant increases in ROM ($P < .0001$) (see Fig. 2.3).

Comment: (1) The purported mechanisms (PIR and RI) are disputed as being the means whereby increased ROM is achieved following MET. This is fully discussed in Chapter 4 and elsewhere, including in this chapter. (2) Despite PIR and RI being questioned as the actual mechanisms involved, the results, showing that use of the agonist, or the antagonist, in the isometric contraction, can be equally influential. This has potential clinical relevance; for example, in a setting where one of these contractions proves difficult or painful to perform, the other might offer an alternative choice. Despite the subjects being asymptomatic, these findings point to a

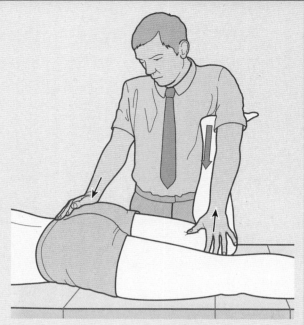

Fig. 2.3 Practitioner eases patient's leg into internal rotation at the hip, until the resistance barrier for piriformis is reached. The patient introduces external hip rotation by lightly bringing the foot/lower leg towards a neutral position against firm resistance from the practitioner.

potential clinical strategy where piriformis ROM is limited, or where pain is present.

- Murphy et al. (2009) describe, in the treatment of 49 patients with lumbar radiculopathy, secondary to herniated disc followed-up for 14.5 months post-cessation of treatment. The use of MET is noted as follows:

Joint manipulation may be used if segmental provocation manoeuvres reproduced all, or part of a patient's pain and centralization of pain was not found on end-range loading examination. This treatment typically involved lying the patient in the side posture position with the side being treated up and applying either a high-velocity, low amplitude 'thrust' or a low-velocity muscle energy manoeuvre.

Outcomes were impressive:

In this study, clinically meaningful improvement in pain was found in 79% of patients, and clinically meaningful improvement in disability was found in 70% of patients.

BOX 2.1   Reflections and Commentaries on 20 Years of Research—cont'd

The authors further comment that:

The fact that outcomes were as good or better at long-term follow-up is significant because it suggests that patients treated according to the [diagnosis-based clinical decision rule] generally do not need ongoing 'maintenance' or 'supportive' care to maintain functional improvement.

Comment: (1) Once again, MET is seen as part of the therapeutic mix, selected according to assessed and perceived clinical needs, and in this clinical setting, not as a stand-alone approach. (2) The practical relevance of integrated protocols such as these is demonstrated by the long-term outcomes. See Chapter 8 for the therapeutic perspective of MET, by the lead author (Dr D. Murphy) of this and the previously reported research study.

- Shadmehr et al. (2009) compared the effects of 10 sessions of static stretching (15 subjects) and 10 sessions of MET (15 subjects) using 50% voluntary isometric contractions of the hamstring to assess the effects on extensibility in asymptomatic young females (aged 20–25 years). Both treatment methods produced significant improvement in the flexibility of the hamstrings ($P < .01$), with no appreciable difference observed between the two methods.

Comment: (1) Once again, we have asymptomatic individuals as the subjects, making interpretation into clinical work difficult. (2) The claim that those treated with MET utilised 50% of available strength requires consideration. A study by Sheard et al. (2009) demonstrated that athletes who were asked to produce varying degrees of voluntary contraction forces were wildly inaccurate in the degree of force that they actually produced. Contraction intensities of between 10% and 100% of maximal voluntary contraction (MVC) have been proposed for use in MET and PNF protocols (Sheard et al., 2009).

The researchers reported that:

Our findings indicate that this group of athletes displayed a poor level of compliance to varying therapist requested contraction intensities with respect to both accuracy and consistency.

This does not negate the outcomes of the Shadmehr study, reported above, but raises a question regarding the use of requests/instructions, such as 'I would like you to push in this direction, with half (or whatever) your available strength'.

- Hunt and Legal (2010) conducted a randomised, single-blinded, controlled study, involving 80 subjects

assessed as presenting with piriformis spasm, together with the presence of myofascial trigger points in that muscle. Twenty-eight subjects were treated using MET, with the objective of relaxing piriformis; 27 subjects were treated with a thrust technique that applied rapid stretch to piriformis; the remainder (controls) were treated by a placebo measure involving a HVLA thrust technique applied to T4. Outcomes involved assessment of pressure pain threshold (using algometry); hip internal rotation range (goniometry); and pain levels using a visual analogue scale (VAS). The MET and HVLA thrust methods both produced an equally significant increase in piriformis extensibility, together with pain relief, compared with the placebo group ($P > .05$).

Comment: MET in treatment of trigger points has been shown in many studies to be an effective means of achieving increased ROM, as well as of trigger point deactivation. Recent research (Alghadir et al., 2020; Wendt & Małgorzata, 2020) also appears to support this.

See Chapters 5 and 6 for additional options involving MET in treatment of piriformis and of myofascial pain.

- Moore et al. (2011) studied the effects of MET in treatment of shoulder ROM of amateur (college) baseball players. A single application of MET was used on the glenohumeral joint (GHJ) horizontal abductors (19 subjects) and the GHJ external rotators, to improve ROM (22 subjects). The results showed single applications of an MET for the GHJ horizontal abductors provides immediate improvements in both GHJ horizontal adduction and internal rotation ROM, in asymptomatic collegiate baseball players.

Comment: (1) ROM increased significantly in both external rotation and horizontal adduction movement, followed a single MET application *involving isometric contraction of only the horizontal abductors*, suggesting a process that offers benefit to other soft tissues than those directly involved in the contraction. This phenomenon will be echoed elsewhere in the book, suggesting that our understanding of the mechanisms involved in MET remain incomplete. (2) How this study of the effects of MET in asymptomatic individuals would translate into settings with symptomatic subjects is open to question; however, the study by Knebl et al. (above) hints at the likelihood of a beneficial influence on dysfunction.

- Rajadurai (2011) conducted a randomised clinical trial to evaluate the effectiveness of MET in reducing pain and improving maximal mouth opening (MMO) in patients with temporomandibular dysfunction (TMD). The sample consisted of 40 participants, aged 20–30 years

(Continued)

BOX 2.1   Reflections and Commentaries on 20 Years of Research—cont'd

(mean age 25.5 ± 2.96) diagnosed with TMD of less than 3 months' duration. Participants were treated with MET, which included postisometric relaxation and reciprocal inhibition (contractions away from, and towards the restriction barrier) on alternate days, for 5 weeks. Before the commencement of the treatment, and at the end of each week, subjects were evaluated for pain intensity using a VAS, and MMO by measuring the inter-incisal distance. There was a significant reduction of pain ($P < .05$) at the end of each week as measured by the VAS. The MMO measurements showed significant and continued improvement in ROM ($P < .05$) at the end of each week when compared to the baseline measurements.

Comment: The successful outcomes achieved via application of MET in treatment of a painful joint restriction, illustrates the potential value of this approach and hints at simple self-application possibilities. Such possibilities are discussed further in Chapter 14. There was no control group in this study, limiting its significance.

- Parmar et al. (2011) evaluated the relative benefits of isolytic MET (isotonic eccentric) stretching compared with standard passive stretching, in order to increase knee ROM and decreased pain in over 50 cases following surgery for hip fracture. It was found that MET was more effective in pain reduction ($P = .003$) and that both methods increased ROM equally ($P \geq .05$).

Comment: As explained in the notes on mechanotransduction elsewhere in this and other chapters, the use of isotonic eccentric contractions is a key part of MET methodology, and this study offers validation in a complex clinical setting.

- Zuil Escobar et al. (2010) evaluated the effects of MET applied to the upper trapezius (see Fig. 2.4) of 35 asymptomatic subjects with latent upper trapezius myofascial trigger points. The subjects were randomised into two groups: one was treated with an MET, while the other was not treated. Pressure pain threshold was evaluated using an analogue algometer before the intervention, 5 min post-intervention and 24 h post-intervention. The treatment group showed a significant increase in pressure pain threshold 5 min after intervention but this disappeared at 24 h post-intervention. Studies investigating MET and efficacy related to treatment of myofascial trigger points are ongoing (Abd El-Azeim et al., 2018; Vivanco-Coke et al., 2020).

Comment: This study highlights several frustrating features of MET research studies, as well as several possibly significant pieces of information. (1) The finding that in a large group of asymptomatic individuals it was possible to

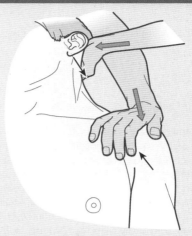

Fig. 2.4 The patient's head and neck are side-flexed and rotated right to the first-sign-of-resistance barrier of upper trapezius. The practitioner offers counter-pressure as the patient attempts to bring the shoulder and neck towards each other in an isometric contraction, after which a new barrier is engaged, or stretching is introduced depending on the status of dysfunction, whether acute or chronic, as explained in the text.

identify latent trigger points in upper trapezius muscles, which clinical experience suggests is one of the most common sites of these features, was of particular interest. (2) The asymptomatic nature of the subjects involved in the study makes it more difficult to relate the outcomes of the study to real-life clinical settings, since few such patients (asymptomatic) present for treatment. (3) The findings suggest that, while briefly beneficial, MET alone may not be the ideal method for treatment of myofascial pain. However, a combined approach may be more beneficial, thus highlighting the importance of integrated approaches that may usefully incorporate MET, such as the integrated neuromuscular inhibition technique (INIT) (Chaitow, 1994) methods detailed in Chapter 14 and now validated following a randomised controlled study in which active trigger points in upper trapezius were successfully treated (Nagrale et al., 2010). INIT continues to be an important point of study. Abd El-Azeim et al. (2018) found that INIT was superior to kinesiotaping. However, a combination of both would seem to be more beneficial. A further study on integrated INIT demonstrated positive results (Chavan et al., 2019), as did a 2020 study on INIT combined with ice massage (Al-Najjar et al., 2020).

It is becoming clearer that combined methods provide more efficacy than any one single approach. The present study, along with the other three mentioned here, appear

BOX 2.1   Reflections and Commentaries on 20 Years of Research—cont'd

to conclude that INIT coupled with conventional treatment plays an important role in reduction of trigger point activity.

- Küçükşen et al. (2013) conducted a comparison study to determine the short- and long-term effectiveness of the MET compared with corticosteroid injections for chronic lateral epicondylitis. The study looked at 82 patients treated with either eight sessions of MET or one corticosteroid injection. A variety of outcome measures were used, and importantly, there was a 1-year follow-up. Measurements were performed before beginning treatment and at 6, 26 and 52 weeks afterwards. Statistically significant improvements were observed in both groups over time. The patients who received a corticosteroid injection showed significantly better effects at 6 weeks, but benefits declined thereafter. Interestingly, at the 26- and 52-week follow-ups, the patients who received MET were statistically significantly better in terms of grip strength and pain scores than those who received the injection.

Comment: This study has multiple points of interest. The 1-year follow-up indicated that MET has the potential for sustained benefits. Many studies indicate that manual therapy tends to offer only short-term results. The comparison to steroid injections is also interesting. Since there are side-effects related to these types of injections, having evidence that MET can provide long-term benefits, as opposed to the more short-lived injection benefits, supports more treatment options. It is also important to note that MET was successful in supporting function and reducing symptoms in an inflammatory-based condition that often becomes more fibrotic in chronic conditions. It may be possible to cautiously extrapolate this information to similar conditions.

- A study by Sewani & Shinde (2017) investigated the effect of hot pack hydrotherapy and MET in subjects with sacroiliac joint dysfunction compared to conventional therapy. Thirty-four subjects aged between 20 and 45 years were allocated into two groups and treated with moist hot packs (MHP), MET, core muscle strengthening and general mobility exercises for 10 days. Assessment was done on the 1st day pre-treatment and 10th day post-treatment. Both groups showed improvement but there was significant improvement in group treated with HMP and MET. A more current study also found that MET along with conventional or other physiotherapy treatment can be helpful in reducing pain and improving function in patients with sacroiliac joint dysfunction (Kansagara & Patel, 2019).

Comment: Effectiveness of MET in treating sacroiliac joint dysfunction needs to be more clearly established with higher quality research. However, the two studies taken together highlight MET as an aspect of multimodal care and the cumulative and synergistic effects of such integration.

- Hidalgo et al. (2017) conducted a systematic review related to non-specific neck pain treatment efficacy using a variety of manual therapy methods, including MET alone or in combination with exercise. The review targeted research from 2000 to 2015. Neck pain types from acute to chronic are included. Methods compared HVLA, mobilisation, mobilisation with movement (MET category) and soft-tissue techniques (ischaemic compression, strain-counterstrain). As described by Zuil Escobar et al. (2010), combined and multimodal interventions yielded better results for pain relief, function, satisfaction with care and general health in comparison to exercise or MT alone for patients with chronic neck pain.

Comment: This systematic review is helpful in that, instead of combining all manual therapy techniques within a single group, the authors sub-categorised them into four distinct groups for comparison with or without exercise. Overall, moderate evidence supports methods such as MET when combined with exercise. The review supports using methods such as MET as part of integrated approaches. Application of clinical reasoning to individual cases determines the most appropriate styles and combinations of manual therapy and exercise. It is becoming more evident that combining different forms of manual therapy with exercise is better than using manual therapy alone, demonstrating that both active and passive forms of therapy are synergetic.

- A systematic review by Thomas et al. (2019) analyses multiple studies to assess the efficacy of MET. The literature search covered the time period between 1981 and 2018. A total of 26 studies were considered eligible and included in the quantitative synthesis: 14 regarding symptomatic patients and 12 regarding asymptomatic subjects. Quality assessment of the studies through the PEDro scale observed a 'moderate to high' quality of included records. The review concludes that METs are effective in improving reported pain, disability and joint ROM in both asymptomatic and symptomatic patients. The studies evaluated in this review have provided evidence that METs are specifically effective for alleviating chronic pain of the lower back and neck and chronic lateral

(Continued)

BOX 2.1   **Reflections and Commentaries on 20 Years of Research—cont'd**

epicondylitis. There is also evidence supporting MET as a beneficial therapy for reducing acute lower back pain and improving the related disability indexes. However, further evidence is needed to confirm MET as an effective treatment for plantar fasciitis and other musculoskeletal disorders.

Comment: As concisely described in the systematic review:

The exact mechanism for MET-induced pain relief is still unknown, although it has been proposed that MET act on joint proprioceptors and mechanorecep-tors that will result in an effect on descending path-ways, changing the motor programming of the target joint. It has also been advocated that the reduction of pain and increased mobility are due to changes in the viscoelastic properties of the soft tissue followed by the application of the technique; the mechanism for increased flexibility has been attributed to an increase in stretch tolerance.

In practice, the clinician may use a variety of MET applications to reduce pain and increase ROM. These are applied to a variety of pathological conditions and on asymptomatic subjects. There is, however, limited knowledge on their effectiveness and which protocol may be the most beneficial. The review did provide guidance to support the clinical reasoning process helpful to determine when

MET approaches are indicated and what combinations of methods to use. Dosing was described by the number of sessions for a typical MET prescription. In this review that number varied from 1 to 18 sessions.

- Park and Lim (2020) looked at proprioceptive neuro-muscular facilitation (PNF) stretching at low intensities, targeting hamstring flexibility to assess the effect of low intensities (40% and 10% of maximum voluntary isometric contraction, MVIC) of PNF stretching on hamstring muscles and to assess the effect of standing toe touch on the duration of hamstring flexibility. Sixty-four healthy adults were divided into four groups: 40% intensity PNF stretching (P40), 10% intensity PNF stretching (P10), 40% intensity PNF stretching with toe touch (P40 with TT) and 10% intensity PNF stretching with toe touch (P10 with TT). Hamstring flexibility was measured using the active knee extension PNF stretching at low intensity, approaching 40% of MVIC, led to more flexibility than 10% MVIC.

Comment: One of the differences between PNF and MET is strength of contraction. PNF is often described at maximal contraction effort and MET more within the parameters of this study of 10%–40% maximum voluntary isometric contraction. PNF was applied more like MET indicating benefit at low intensities. This study points to a potential blending of the two methods rather than using them as distinct and unique disciplines.

---

should commence at this point (Stiles, 2009). Parsons and Marcer (2005) note that active movement stops at the 'physiological barrier' determined by the tension ('bind') in the soft tissues around the joint (e.g. fascia, muscles, ligaments, joint capsule), with normal ranges of movement of a joint ('ease') taking place within these physiological barriers. Factors such as exercise, stretching and age – as well as pathology or dysfunction – can modify the normal physiological range; however, it is usually possible to passively ease a joint's range beyond the physiological barrier by stretching the supporting soft tissues until the anatomical limit of tension is reached (see Fig. 2.5A and B).

Clinically, it is worth considering whether restriction barriers ought to be released, in case they might offer some protective benefit.

The elements that make up standard isometric MET therefore always include:
1. Identification of a resistance barrier

2. The use of an isometric, or sometimes isotonic, contraction
3. A response to that contraction, which appears to facilitate easier movement to a new barrier (or past a new barrier, into stretch by reduced resistance to stretch) or an increased tolerance to the stretch sensation (Magnusson et al., 1996a; Weppler & Magnusson, 2010; Singh & Kaushal, 2020).

A number of facilitating elements have also evolved in the clinical application of MET, including the use of respiratory and visual synkinesis. These are briefly outlined in this chapter and explained further in the clinical chapters (see Chapters 5 to 9 and 11).

Variables

The variables that exist within those three MET elements (barrier identification, isometric or isotonic contraction, subsequent action) include the surprisingly contentious decision regarding how to identify the

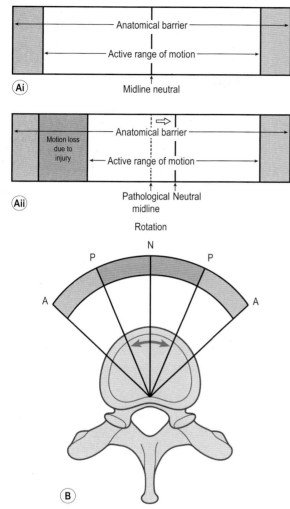

Fig. 2.5 (A) Motion barrier concepts: *Ai,* Normal symmetrical motion. *Aii,* Loss of motion due to injury, with lost motion on one side involving somatic dysfunction. Over time, tissue changes occur (contracture, induration, fibrosis, etc.). Additional adaptations then influence adjacent and distant structures. (Adapted, with permission, from Greenman 1996.) (B) Schematic representation of vertebral rotation barriers. Normal motion occurs between physiological barriers. Any movement beyond anatomical barriers produces physical damage. In muscle energy techniques *(MET),* usage barriers would commonly be short of the physiological barriers, depending on restraints imposed by soft tissue or structural joint changes. *A,* Anatomical barrier; *N,* neutral; *P,* physiological barrier – where passive motion occurs.

resistance or restriction barrier that should be used as the starting point for the isometric or isotonic contraction. There are descriptions of MET where the barrier commences from an easy 'feather-edge' position, as well

as from a position in which the restraining soft tissues are actually stretched (a 'bind' barrier) at the start of the isometric contraction. This latter approach raises several clinical questions:

1. If, as may be the case, the soft tissues held in a stretched position before being required to contract are already hypertonic, and possibly ischaemic, there is a risk that the contraction effort might provoke cramping. This would appear to be a possibility, or even a likelihood, in muscles such as the hamstrings. The author of this chapter suggests that it would be a safer option to employ light contractions, starting with the muscle group at an easy end-of-range barrier, rather than at stretch.

2. The requested contraction effort from the patient would be more easily initiated and achieved, with the muscle (group) in a mid-range or easy end-of-range position, rather than at an end-of-range involving stretch, at the start.

Both comfort and safety issues would appear to support clinical use of the 'ease' barrier rather than a firmer 'bind' barrier, provided the outcomes were not compromised, and clinical experience as well as numerous studies offer support for the 'ease' option.

It is from the identified barrier that the isometric, or possibly isotonic, contraction will be initiated by the patient, on instruction, by the practitioner, with the direction, the degree of force to be employed, and the duration of the contraction, decided and controlled by the practitioner – together with the provision of firm counter-pressure. It is worth emphasising at the outset that the patient's force and '*muscle energy*', – and not that of the practitioner, who offers firm counterforce – should *always* be harnessed; guidelines for ensuring this are provided in later chapters.

Further choices are required following the contraction, including whether a stretch past the barrier should be introduced and, if so, to what extent (amplitude), for how long (duration), and whether the process should be repeated one or more times. Some variables relate to the answers to these questions:

- Is the problem acute or chronic?
- Is the target structure for MET soft tissue or joint?

Some answers to these questions are provided in this chapter, with the issues explored further in Chapters 5 to 7 with evidence offered for the choices that are considered the most appropriate in different settings, *where such evidence exists.* Where it does not, the recommendations are based on clinical experience. In the end, each practitioner's clinical experience will guide therapeutic decision-making, supported by research evidence where this is available, or by the clinical experience of others. This text attempts to offer a broad range of such information from which to choose, and with which to experiment as decisions are made regarding the ideal barrier to employ in different clinical settings.

MET – AN EVOLVING APPROACH

Chapter 3 provides the historical context that helps explain the evolutionary nature of MET, as presented in this text, as well as of the variations that have emerged in a variety of clinical settings in which there is indicative evidence of MET usefulness in treatment of muscle dysfunction (see Chapter 6), joint dysfunction (see Chapter 7), acute spinal trauma (see Chapter 8), chiropractic rehabilitation (see Chapter 9), surgical rehabilitation (see Chapter 10), physical therapy (see Chapter 11), massage (see Chapter 12) and athletic training (see Chapter 13) for example.

ADAPTATION LEADING TO SOMATIC DYSFUNCTION

The tissues of the body respond to applied demands (stressors) originating from previous overuse, misuse, abuse (trauma) and disuse, together with a combination of inherited and acquired features and experiences that will have merged in the individual to create the problem that is being assessed, palpated or observed.

The structures and functions being evaluated represent the unique characteristics of a person's genetic inheritance, involving the biochemical, psychosocial and biomechanical make-up, onto which have been overlaid all the developmental and maturational experiences of life, including acquired habits and patterns of use (e.g. postural or respiratory), ergonomic, work and leisure stresses, as well as the results of injuries, surgeries, emotional burdens and more.

Tissues may gradually change from a state of *normotonicity* to a palpably dysfunctional state, at times involving hypertonicity, and at others hypotonicity, along with altered firing sequences, modified motor control, abnormal postural and/or movement patterns and ultimately dysfunctional chain reactions. What emerges is a picture of impaired or altered function of related components of the somatic framework: skeletal, arthrodial, myofascial,

as well as related vascular, lymphatic and neural features. The outcome can be summarised by the term '*somatic dysfunction*' (Ehrenfeuchter et al., 2011). Such changes almost always demonstrate functional, sometimes visible, often palpable evidence that can frequently be assessed in order to guide the practitioner towards clinical decision-making as to what form of management may be most appropriate.

From an osteopathic perspective Parsons and Marcer (2005) note that '*it is through the summation of both quantitative and qualitative findings that one obtains an indication of the nature and age of the underlying dysfunction. Within the context of acute and chronic somatic dysfunction, MET will be seen to offer tools that can assist in normalization of dysfunction, pain management and rehabilitation*'.

Grieve's Decompensation Model

Gregory Grieve became a chartered physiotherapist in 1952. Grieve (1986) presciently offered a perspective on the evolution of chronic dysfunction in many cases. He described the example of a typical patient, presenting with pain, loss of functional movement or altered patterns of strength, power or endurance. Grieve suggested that, all too commonly, this individual would either have suffered major trauma which had overwhelmed the physiological tolerances of relatively healthy tissues, or might be displaying '*gradual decompensation, demonstrating slow exhaustion of the tissue's adaptive potential, with or without trauma*'. As this process continued, Grieve explained that progressive postural adaptation, influenced by time factors and possibly by trauma, would lead to exhaustion of the body's adaptive potential, thus resulting in dysfunction and, ultimately, symptoms.

Grieve has correctly noted that therapeutic attention to the tissues incriminated in producing symptoms often gives excellent short-term results; however, '*unless treatment is also focused towards restoring function in asymptomatic tissues responsible for the original postural adaptation and subsequent decompensation, the symptoms will recur*'.

MET's influence on such a sequence of adaptive changes might include the ability of carefully applied isometric contractions, elongation influencing resting tone and possibility mild stretch, to positively influence features such as excessive tone, fascial shortening, inflammation and pain (Simons, 2002; Hoeger Bement et al., 2008, 2011; Wang et al., 2020).

Repetitive Lumbar Injury – an Example of Failed Adaptation

In discussing a form of low back pain that is described as repetitive lumbar injury (RLI), Solomonow et al. (2011) outline the aetiology of a complex multi-factorial syndrome that fits the model of adaptive overload. This involves an adaptation sequence in which prolonged cyclic loading of the low back can be shown to induce a process of *creep* – defined as continued deformation of a viscoelastic material under constant load over time – in the spinal tissues (Sánchez-Zuriaga et al., 2010; Larson et al., 2020), reduced muscular activity, triggering spasms and reduced stability, followed by acute inflammation and tissue degradation (Fung et al., 2009), as well as muscular hyperexcitability and hyperstability (Li et al., 2007). These adaptive changes are seen, in animal studies (Solomonow, 2011) and in humans (Solomonow et al., 2003), to be a response to rapid movement, bearing high loads, numerous repetitions and short rest periods, behaviours that are not uncommon in many common work and leisure/athletic activities. The conclusion is that viscoelastic tissues ultimately fail via a process involving the triggering of inflammation, due to overuse, a process that appears to initiate the mechanical and neuromuscular characteristic symptoms of the disorder (Bove et al., 2019).

In contrast, Solomonow et al. (2011) found that low magnitude loads, short loading durations, lengthy rest periods, low movement velocity and few repetitions, did not constitute significant risk factors, yet nevertheless triggered transient stability deficits, and pro-inflammatory tissue degradation. It is suggested that it might be more appropriate to designate these conditions as low risk, instead of no risk (Solomonow et al., 2011).

In perspective, RLI is seen to be a complex multifactorial syndrome, a clear example of adaptation to imposed demands that exceed the ability of the tissues involved to respond. Repeated bending activities in daily living appear to change both structure (ligaments, discs) and function (protective spinal reflexes) (Hodges & Danneels, 2019; Surbeck et al., 2020).

MET can be seen to offer various potential benefits as a therapeutic intervention in such a spectrum of progressive dysfunction. For example, improving restricted mobility (Lenehan et al., 2003; Thomas et al., 2019), possibly reducing excessive inflammatory responses (Fryer & Fossum, 2010; Licciardone et al., 2010), while simultaneously enhancing motor control (Wilson et al., 2003) and balance related to poorly coordinated neuromuscular control, which may alter the normal postural stability of the spine (Hlaing et al., 2020). Altered proprioceptive stimuli elicited increased activation of brain areas involved in threat detection and fear processing in some individuals, which was associated with poor proprioceptive postural control (Goossens et al., 2019). Unless the patterns of use that were fuelling this degenerative process were modified, the MET interventions would offer short-term symptomatic relief at best.

A Therapeutic Formula: Reduce Adaptive Load and Enhance Function

A therapeutic formula is proposed for the clinician who is confronted with chronic adaptive changes of the sort highlighted by Grieve or Solomonow. It is suggested that the focus should be on both reducing adaptive demands – altering the patterns of behaviour that have produced or which are maintaining dysfunction – while at the same time focusing on enhancement of function, working with the self-regulatory systems of the body, so that those adaptive demands can be better managed by the body (Chaitow, 2008). The only other therapeutic possibility would seem to be symptomatic attention. It is in the enhancement of function that MET can be seen to have a potential role. In simple terms, musculoskeletal tissue absorbs or adapts to forces applied to it, and MET can modify these changes (Iqbal et al., 2020). Examples include dysfunctional shoulders of the elderly (Knebl, 2002), following sporting injuries (Curcio et al., 2017) or involving hamstring problems (Smith & Fryer, 2008; Rabia et al., 2019).

Functional Independence

Functional independence is the ideal objective of patient care. This implies the ability to be able to perform the tasks of daily life as well as being socially mobile and active, encompassing household activities, recreational activities and the demands of employment, where appropriate (Waddell & Burton, 2005; Tousignant-Laflamme et al., 2017). Clinical objectives ideally focus on building activity tolerance rather than merely providing symptomatic relief, therefore helping patients to regain independent function. It is within that context that MET operates – as part of a continuum from dysfunction to function – removing or modulating obstacles to recovery (pain, reduced ranges of motion, strength and motor control deficits) and not as an end in itself that is aimed purely at symptomatic relief although, at times, that is a perfectly appropriate clinical objective (LaStayo et al., 2014; Dal Farra et al., 2021).

To be clear, MET is patient-centred and aims to be part of a process that promotes restoration of (ideally pain-free) function. Within that context, attention to local somatic problems that retard functional rehabilitation becomes a priority.

▶ STAR and TART Assessments

Several mnemonics attempt to summarise the findings in somatic dysfunction; none of these is complete, but they are useful as *aides-mémoires*.

In the context of emerging or established somatic dysfunction, two slightly different mnemonics (actually acronyms) are used in osteopathic medicine to remind the clinician of some of the key signs that require evaluation in the process of clinical decision-making, alongside evidence gathered from the patient's history, together with other clinical assessments.

These are STAR and/or TART.

STAR (Dowling, 1998)

Sensibility changes: What subjective changes accompany this dysfunction? Is there pain, stiffness, tenderness, discomfort, weakness, etc.?

Tissue texture abnormality: Are the tissues hot, cold, tense, flabby, oedematous, fibrotic, indurated, in spasm, hypertrophied, etc.?

Asymmetry: Is there an obvious difference compared with contralateral tissues?

Restricted range of motion (ROM): What is the degree (and quality) of pliability, mobility, stability, extensibility, ROM, compared with normal ROM? Does the quality of end-feel offer additionally useful information?

MET methods might be able to modify many of these indicators of dysfunction.

TART (Chase, 2009; Sandhouse, 2011)

Tissue texture abnormality: Are the tissues hot, cold, tense, flabby, oedematous, fibrotic, indurated, in spasm, hypertrophied, etc.?

Asymmetry: Is there an obvious difference compared with contralateral tissues?

ROM abnormality: What is the degree (and quality) of pliability, mobility, stability, extensibility, ROM, compared with normal ROM? Is it hyper- or hypomobile?

Does the quality of end-feel offer additional useful information?

Tenderness: Are these tissues unnaturally sensitive, tender, painful (or numb), etc., on applied pressure, or when actively or passively moved?

MET methods might be able to modify many of these indicators of dysfunction.

Differences? There are subtle differences between the constituent elements of these two acronyms, with STAR offering some subjective feedback relative to *Sensibility*, which is not quite the same as *Tenderness* in the TART sequence. Whatever findings emerge from the assessments these sequences demand need to be overlaid on a background of the medical history of the individual, taken together with the findings from normal clinical tests, examinations and evaluations. In particular, the way MET is applied differs markedly in acute and chronic settings.

Are these features of somatic dysfunction real? While the characteristics of STAR and TART may appear elegantly convincing, the validity of the cluster of signs having relevance has also been tested.

Fryer et al. (2004) were able to confirm that sites in the thoracic paravertebral muscles, identified by deep palpation as displaying 'abnormal tissue texture', also showed greater tenderness than adjacent tissues, thus confirming the *Tenderness* of TART and *Sensibility* of STAR, associated with *Texture* changes in both.

In a follow-up study, Fryer et al. (2005) examined the possibility that tissue texture irregularity of paravertebral sites might be due to greater cross-sectional thickness of the paraspinal muscle bulk. Diagnostic ultrasound showed that this was not the case. A further study (Fryer et al., 2006) examined the electromyography (EMG) activity of deep paraspinal muscles lying below paravertebral thoracic muscles with 'altered texture', which were also more tender than surrounding muscles. This demonstrated increased EMG activity in these dysfunctional muscles (i.e. they were hypertonic). However, in a 2010 study no differences in resting EMG activity were found in the deep paraspinal muscles underlying sites that were identified with palpation as either normal or abnormal. The results of this study do not support previous EMG investigations reported in the osteopathic medical literature, but earlier studies used different methodologies and examined different paraspinal muscles. Based on the current results, factors other than muscle activity may be responsible for the apparent abnormality of these deep tissues. Investigation of these regions for increased tissue fluid and inflammatory mediators is recommended (Fryer et al., 2010).

The asymmetry, tenderness and texture changes, as well as ROM elements of both STAR and TART, remain helpful as assessment somatic dysfunction, manifesting with abnormal barriers to free movement even if conflicting research questions what is felt during palpation.

MUSCLE ENERGY TECHNIQUE AND PROPRIOCEPTIVE NEUROMUSCULAR FACILITATION: SIMILARITIES AND DIFFERENCES

MET and PNF are similar yet different methods. The terms are often used interchangeably. Since the focus of this text is MET, it is valid to compare the treatment approaches. Both involve a patient's muscle contraction against a practitioner's counterforce. MET has osteopathic roots and emerged as a form of osteopathic treatment in which the patient is specifically positioned and then muscles are actively contracted on request in a specific direction against a counterforce. It was first described in 1948 by Fred Mitchell, Sr, DO (Ehrenfeuchter et al., 2011), PNF evolved as part of physical therapy. It uses spiral or diagonal movement patterns to indirectly facilitate movement, with the therapist providing maximal resistance to the stronger motor components, thereby facilitating the weaker components of the patterns (Cifu, 2020). In 1946 Herman Kabat, a neurophysiologist, began to look for natural patterns of movement for rehabilitating the muscles of polio patients. Along with physical therapists Margaret Knott and Dorothy Voss, he developed the PNF method of intervention as a specific sequence of movements performed to stimulate muscle and neurologic functions in rehabilitation (Voss et al., 1985). Further detail on this is found in Chapter 3. PNF stretching has currently narrowed PNF away from the original concept to the point that it is incorrectly perceived simply as a muscle contraction prior to stretching.

MET-PNF Similarities

The definitions given above suggest similarities between MET and PNF:
- Both involve the use of isometric contractions prior to (or during) stretching or movement

- Both have the normalisation of a broad range of orthopaedic conditions (physical therapy) or somatic dysfunction (osteopathy), terms that are clearly interchangeable, as objectives.

It is therefore reasonable to enquire whether there is any actual difference between PNF and MET apart from the names given to what appear to be similar approaches delivered by different professions.

MET-PNF Differences

The most basic distinctions between MET and PNF relate to apparently superficial, yet clinically significant differences:

1. MET, in its original osteopathic setting, aimed to restore joint function to normal. It is only in recent years that soft tissue dysfunction – outside of the context of joint dysfunction – has become a focus. It is in this latter evolution (muscle focus) that the blurring of boundaries between MET and PNF has emerged.

2. PNF identifies the restriction barrier at which the isometric contraction commences quite differently from the way it is identified in MET. In many descriptions of PNF the restriction barrier appears to involve moving the area to an end of range, *where the patient perceives mild discomfort*. For example, Azevedo et al. (2011) identify hamstring end of range as follows: '[The] examiner extended the subject's knee to the point of self-reported mild discomfort'. Note: This barrier definition appears similar to some descriptions of MET, as noted by Shoup (2006), and others, earlier in this chapter.

3. In MET, however, the restriction barrier is most commonly described as the very first perceived sign of tension, resistance, 'bind' (Stiles, 2009) or even short of that (Janda et al., 2006).

4. PNF frequently calls for a far longer and stronger isometric contraction, often employing all available strength, than is used in MET application, where 20% or less of available strength is requested (Greenman, 2003). For example, Glynn and Fiddler (2009) suggest the following in PNF application: 'During the technique the limb is taken to the end of available ROM and the patient is instructed to "hold" the position whilst the physiotherapist applies measured resistance to build up a maximal isometric contraction in the muscle group that requires lengthening'.

5. In this last example, we see the therapist 'applying measured resistance' while the patient 'holds the

position'. This is a reversal of the protocol used in MET where it is *always* the patient, and *not the therapist*, who introduces isometric effort.

It is suggested that the key to safe and clinically effective use of MET lies in understanding and employing 'easy end of range' barriers sometimes described in osteopathy as the 'feather-edge' of the barrier, as well as utilising mild, brief contractions initiated by the patient.

These elements, all of which contribute to MET being a more easily controlled sequence of actions than those described for PNF, as well as potentially being far less stressful for the patient than PNF methods, will be emphasised in those chapters dealing with the clinical use of MET (e.g. Chapters 5 to 7).

Different MET Approaches

How the various METs are applied has varied little since originally described by Dr Mitchell over 50 years ago. The process of application has been refined and nuanced but application foundations remain and have stood the test of time. The descriptions of MET variations listed below are summaries only, which are more detailed, step-by-step, protocols offered in the chapters (e.g. Chapters 5 to 7) where MET in treatment of soft tissue and joint dysfunction are explored.

Note: A series of exercises are described in Chapter 5 to assist with learning the basics of MET application.

A Note on Terminology

1. There is a need for clear and concise language to avoid ambiguity and misinterpretations, for example, when describing apparently simple terms such as 'contract'. Faulkner (2003) points out that the dictionary definition of the verb 'contract' specifically in relation to muscle, is 'to undergo an increase in tension, or force, and become shorter'. Faulkner further notes that an activated muscle always generates force, but that it does not always shorten, for example, when isometrically activated. This leads him to suggest that the term 'isometric contraction' is inaccurate since no external, overall shortening occurs.

2. In an absolute sense he is correct; however, for there to be a simultaneous contraction, and no overall length change, a combination of both shortening and lengthening needs to occur inside the muscle as it contracts. This feature of contraction is explored further below when we evaluate the mechanisms that may be operating in MET and PNF, particularly viscoelasticity.

3. Much of the supporting literature for these techniques derives from the fields of engineering, physiology and neuroscience, as well as physiotherapy and sports science. Searching the research databases such as PubMed reveals the variation in the language used across fields and professions to describe similar phenomena (e.g. interoceptive awareness has a host of synonyms that are not always accurate); methods (e.g. osteopathic manipulative treatment (OMT) as MET combined with other techniques; isometric eccentric contractions, discussed in Chapters 5, 7 and 10; and physiology (e.g. extracellular matrix used interchangeably with fascia). Inaccurate language leads to inaccurate understanding of what neighbouring fields do and hinders progress. Elementary efforts are in progress to streamline this confusing situation (see Chapter 3) but, until they mature, the distance in understanding between the manual therapy professions and other important fields with great potential for interdisciplinary work, remains significant.

The terminology used in the descriptions of MET variations in this book – the words *agonist*, as well as *antagonist*, *acute* and *chronic,* for example – also require definition.

- *Agonist* refers to the muscle or soft tissues that are dysfunctional and are the target for treatment, possibly requiring subsequent stretching.
- *Antagonist* refers to muscles that perform the opposite movement(s) to the agonist.
- *Acute* is defined as anything that is acutely painful, or recently injured (within the previous 3 weeks or so), and therefore still in the remodelling process. Acute tissues are never stretched; however, various forms of isometric or isotonic contraction may be employed in their treatment (see mechanotransduction discussion below). For the purpose of MET, treatment of joints falls into the acute model of care, even if chronically dysfunctional. That is to say, no increased force is used subsequent to isometric contraction in joint treatment, simply movement to a new, easy barrier ('it releases, or it doesn't' is the mantra for joints).
- *Chronic* refers to soft tissues that are not acutely painful, and which have recovered from the acute stages of trauma, possibly manifesting fibrosis.

A number of MET variations exist, including:

- The **basic MET protocol** in which the origin and insertion of the targeted muscle remains constant during the contraction. This approach is regularly used in clinical practice to treat shortened restricted muscles and joints, and in treatment of pain. It involves identification of a restriction barrier. Once the barrier is gently engaged ('first sign of resistance'; feather-edge of resistance' (Stiles, 2009), a light isometric contraction of the agonist, or the antagonist, is introduced by the patient, following instruction as to the direction and degree of force to employ for (usually) 5 to 7 seconds. This is followed by subsequent repositioning of the structures, possibly involving a degree of stretching of the agonist in chronic settings, or simply moving to a new easy end of range, if an acute soft tissue, or any joint restriction is being addressed. The degree of effort called for, as the patient attempts to isometrically move against the practitioner's resisting contact hand(s), should be light, usually less than 20% of available strength, and often far less. The rationale for these variations and choices will be explained fully in later chapters. Choice of the antagonist to contract would be obvious if contraction of the agonist proved painful. The antagonist might also be chosen for active participation for other reasons, for example, as a means of incorporating a variety of soft tissues into an attempt to improve function of a joint (Lewit, 1999; Greenman 2003). In relation to the length of an isometric contraction, Fred Mitchell Jr DO, son of the main developer of MET, and a leading authority on the modality, has observed:

The important thing in MET is getting the correct muscle to contract in the appropriate controlled circumstances – not how long you wait before you say 'stop!' The sensory (spinal) adaptive response in the … proprioceptor mechanism … probably takes no more than one tenth of second. Once that (sensory) adaptive response occurs, passive mobilization, during the post-isometric phase, can usually be accomplished without effort. For joints, more than two seconds of isometric contraction is a waste of energy. For muscle MET, treatment (i.e. the contraction) should take longer.

Mitchell (2009)

- This is, of course, an opinion, albeit an authoritative one, and should be reflected on as such. This is in contrast to a study that evaluated the ideal duration of MET contractions, in which Fryer and Ruszkowski (2004) investigated the influence of contraction duration in MET applied to the atlanto-axial joint in the neck. The results failed to demonstrate a significant benefit in the use of a longer (20 seconds) isometric contraction, compared with a shorter one (5 seconds) when treating the upper neck with MET: 'The use of a 5-second isometric contraction appeared to be more effective than longer contraction durations for increasing cervical range with MET'.

- **Pulsed MET** (Ruddy's rapid resistive duction) calls for the patient to introduce minute repetitive contractions, usually involving the antagonist(s) to restricted soft tissue structures (the 'agonist'), thus facilitating and toning the antagonist, and possibly inhibiting the agonist, with possible additional circulatory and proprioceptive benefits. This method stems from the work of one of the earliest pioneers of MET, Thomas Ruddy, D.O. (Ruddy, 1962) (see Chapters 3 and 5).

- **Rapid eccentric isotonic stretch** is also known as an isolytic stretch because it induces controlled tissue damage, for example, to break down adhesions and fibrosis within the muscle tissue (Kuchera & Kuchera, 1992, Sharvari, 2020). This method contrasts with SEIS that does not damage tissue (Parmar et al., 2011). In application of this method, the practitioner's resistance is greater than the patient's effort, resulting in the *rapid elongation* of the treated muscle while it is contracting.

- **SEIS:** The clinical usefulness of *slowly* stretching a muscle or its antagonist during a contraction has been demonstrated (Jones, 2001; Parmar et al., 2011). The most widely used form of SEIS involves a slow, resisted stretch of the antagonist of shortened soft-tissue structures, a process that tones the antagonist isotonically, after which the agonist is stretched. NOTE: *Confusingly, the slow version of eccentric isotonic stretching is sometimes also termed 'isolytic' (Parmar et al., 2011), and is therefore likely to become common usage, even if inaccurate.*

- **Isokinetic MET** involves multidirectional resisted active movements, designed to tone and balance muscles of an injured joint during rehabilitation. The resistance that the practitioner applies is less than the patient's effort. Therefore, the muscle gradually becomes shorter or is working against resistance. This type of MET is used to build muscle strength, motor control and endurance (Weng et al., 2009).

For more detail of all these methods, including protocols for use of pulsed MET and SEIS see Chapters 5 to 7.

The Addition of Respiratory and Visual Synkinesis

Respiratory synkinesis refers to the suggestion that it is clinically useful to have the patient inhale during most contractions and exhale during release or stretching, albeit with some exceptions. Exceptions are discussed in later chapters (Lewit, 1986, 1999).

Visual synkinesis refers to the clinical value of having the patient look in the direction of contraction, and then the direction of release or stretch. Look up and extensors tone, look down and flexors prepare for activity (Lisberger et al., 1994; Lewit, 1999). Janda (1988) confirms that eye position modifies muscle tone (visual synkinesis), particularly involving the suboccipital muscles (Komendatov, 1945).

MUSCLE TYPES AND MET

Muscle function involves postural joint stabilisation, long-lasting and repetitive activities like respiration or walking, as well as fast and generally powerful actions such as jumping or kicking (Schiaffino & Reggiani, 2011). Muscles have been distinguished/categorised in a variety of ways, for example, based on their:

1. Functional abilities: postural (tonic)/phasic and/or stabiliser/mobiliser. See further explanations below (Liebenson, 2006).
2. Reaction capacity: tight/overactive/hypertonic or weak/inhibited (Bullock-Saxton et al., 1993; Arab et al., 2011; Schuermans et al., 2017).
3. Structural locality: local/global (Bergmark, 1989; Norris, 1999). Local muscles do not typically produce movement. Instead, they create a stable joint situation that allows movement, and are therefore usually located close to joints (Bogduk, 1997; Retchford et al., 2013; Mahato, 2019). Global muscles are larger, more superficial and are mainly responsible for motion and the transfer of load between somatic regions.
4. Multijoint or monoarticular muscles: Richardson et al. (1999, 2000) have argued for the use of the terms multijoint muscles and monoarticular muscles characterisation.
5. Fibre type distribution: slow twitch/type I or fast twitch/type II – and variations on these (Liebenson, 2006). Muscles that contract slowly ('slow twitch fibres' or 'slow white fibres') are classified as type I. These have very low stores of energy-supplying glycogen but carry high concentrations of myoglobulin and mitochondria. These fibres fatigue slowly and

are mainly involved in postural and stabilising tasks (Engel, 1986; Woo, 1987). There are also several phasic/active type II fibre forms, notably:

- Type IIa fibres ('fast twitch' or 'fast red' fibres), which contract more speedily than type I and are moderately resistant to fatigue, with relatively high concentrations of mitochondria and myoglobulin.
- Type IIb fibres ('fast twitch/glycolytic fibres' or 'fast white fibres'), which are less fatigue-resistant and depend more on glycolytic sources of energy, with low levels of mitochondria and myoglobulin.
- Type IIm ('superfast' fibres), found mainly in the jaw muscles, which depend on a unique myosin structure that, along with a high glycogen content, differentiates this from the other type II fibres (Rowlerson et al., 1981).

Change of Muscle Type

Fibre type is not totally fixed. Evidence has shown the potential for adaptability of muscles, so that committed muscle fibres can be transformed from slow-twitch to fast-twitch and vice versa (Lin et al., 1994; Mukund & Subramaniam, 2019).

Apparently, by changing the frequency of stimulation to a motor unit, the biochemical properties can change, that is, slow-twitch muscle fibre that is rapidly stimulated converts to fast-twitch fibre and vice versa (Clark, 2001). An example of this potential, of clinical significance, involves the scalene muscles. Lewit (1999) confirms the scalene group can be classified as either postural or phasic. If the largely phasic scalene muscles, which are dedicated to movement, have postural functions thrust upon them – as in an asthmatic condition in which they will attempt to maintain the upper ribs in elevation to enhance lung capacity – and if, owing to the laboured breathing of such an individual, they are thoroughly and regularly stressed, their fibre type will alter and they will become postural muscles, and will shorten (Lin et al., 1994; Lin & Nardocci, 2016). This type of response has also been noted in the transversus abdominis (Richardson et al., 1992; Lynders, 2019).

A list of postural (also known as 'tonic') and phasic muscles is given below.

Stress Implications for Different Muscle Types

For practical purposes the descriptors 'postural' and 'phasic' (Janda, 1996; Lewit, 1999; Liebenson, 2006) are used in this text, despite other categorisations being available when discussing muscles. The implications of the effects of prolonged stress on different muscle types/categories cannot be emphasised too strongly. For example, long-term stress involving type I muscles results in shortening (also with global, and mobiliser muscles) (Szeto et al., 2009).

In contrast, type II fibres undergoing similar stress will weaken (as will local and stabiliser muscles), without shortening over their whole length (they may, however, develop shortened areas within the muscle) (Liebenson, 2006; Kozlovskaya et al., 2007).

It is important to emphasise that shortness or tightness of a postural (tonic) muscle does not imply strength. Such muscles may test as strong or weak; however, a weak phasic muscle will not shorten overall, and will always test as weak (Liebenson, 2006).

Which Muscles Belong in Which Groupings?

- According to Norris (2000), research has shown that muscles that are inhibited or weak may lengthen, adding to the instability of the region in which they operate. It is the 'stabiliser' muscles that have this tendency: if they are inhibited because of deconditioning they become unable to adequately perform the role of stabilising joints in their 'neutral posture'. They therefore, to a large extent, equate with '*phasic*' muscles in the descriptions used in this book. 'Stabiliser' muscles, which are deeply situated, slow-twitch and tend to weaken and lengthen if deconditioned, include: transversus abdominis, multifidus, internal obliques, medial fibres of external oblique, quadratus lumborum, deep neck flexors, serratus anterior, lower trapezius, gluteus maximus and medius. These muscles can be correlated to a large extent (apart from quadratus lumborum) with muscles designated by Lewit (1999) and Janda (1983) as 'phasic'.
- The more superficial, fast-twitch muscles which tend to shorten (i.e. 'mobilisers' in Norris's terminology)

include: suboccipital group, sternocleidomastoid, upper trapezius, levator scapulae, iliopsoas and hamstrings. These fall into the category of 'postural' muscles as described by Lewit (1999) and Liebenson (2006). Norris calls these 'mobilisers' because they cross more than one joint. They are also described in numerous texts as 'tonic' (Schleip et al., 2006).

This redefining of 'postural' (or 'tonic') as 'mobiliser' can be confusing, and many clinicians therefore prefer to refer to those muscles to which this descriptor applies, as 'having a tendency to shorten' whatever label is applied (Liebenson, 1989). Examples of patterns of imbalance that emerge as some muscles weaken and lengthen as their synergists become overworked, while their antagonists shorten, are summarised in Table 2.1.

As stated previously: to minimise confusion, this book will follow the Janda/Lewit/Liebenson categorisations of *postural* and *phasic* muscles.

Postural and phasic muscle lists. Type I postural (tonic) muscles are prone to loss of endurance capabilities when disused or subject to pathological influences and become shortened or tighter, whereas type II phasic muscles, when abused or disused, become weak (Lewit, 1999; Liebenson, 2006).

Postural muscles that become hypertonic and shorten in response to dysfunction include:
- Trapezius (upper), sternocleidomastoid, levator scapulae and upper aspects of pectoralis major, in the upper trunk; and the flexors of the arms. Quadratus lumborum, erector spinae, oblique abdominals and iliopsoas, in the lower trunk. Tensor fascia lata, rectus femoris, biceps femoris, adductors (longus brevis and magnus) piriformis, hamstrings, semitendinosus.

Phasic muscles, which weaken (i.e. are inhibited), and may lengthen, in response to dysfunction, include:
- The paravertebral muscles (not erector spinae) and scaleni, the extensors of the upper extremity (flexors are primarily postural), the abdominal aspects of

TABLE 2.1 Patterns of Imbalance		
Underactive Stabiliser	**Overactive Synergist**	**Shortened Antagonist**
Gluteus medius	Tensor fascia lata, quadratus lumborum, piriformis	Thigh adductors
Gluteus maximus	Iliocostalis lumborum, hamstrings	Iliopsoas, rectus femoris
Transversus abdominis	Rectus abdominis	Iliocostalis lumborum
Lower trapezius	Levator scapulae, upper trapezius	Pectoralis major
Deep neck flexors	Sternocleidomastoid	Suboccipitals
Serratus anterior	Pectoralis major/minor	Rhomboids
Diaphragm	Scalenes, pectoralis major	

pectoralis major; middle and inferior aspects of trapezius; the rhomboids, serratus anterior, rectus abdominis; the internal and external obliques, gluteals, the peroneal muscles and the extensors of the arms.

Muscle groups such as the scaleni are equivocal: they start out as phasic muscles but can end up as postural.

It has been suggested (Schleip et al., 2006) that differences in quantities of intramuscular connective tissue, particularly the perimysium, in relation to postural (tonic) muscles and phasic muscles has a bearing on degrees of stiffness and possible functional features of these muscles. This is discussed further in Box 2.2: *Why Fascia Matters*.

BOX 2.2   Why Fascia Matters

A state of structural and functional continuity exists between all of the body's hard and soft tissues, with fascia being the ubiquitous elastic–plastic, gluey and fluid component that invests, supports and separates, connects and divides, wraps and gives cohesion and shape to the rest of the body – the fascial, connective tissue network (Ingber, 2008; Myers, 2021). Various models for conceptualising this fascial network exist, including biotensegrity, fascintegrity and myofascial chains. Biotensegrity is a mechanical model focused on solid fascia; Fascintegrity includes both solid and the liquid fascia. Myofascial chains encompass movement and transmission of force in the soft tissue continuum (Wilke et al., 2018; Bordoni & Myers, 2020; Ajimsha et al., 2020a, 2020b).

Any tendency to think of a local dysfunction as existing in isolation should be discouraged as we try to visualise a complex, interrelated, symbiotically functioning assortment of tissues, comprising skin, muscles, ligaments, tendons and bone, as well as the neural structures, blood and lymph channels and vessels that bisect and invest these tissues – all given shape, form and functional ability by the fascia (Schleip et al., 2006; Ingber, 2008; Solomonow, 2009; Adstrum et al., 2017; Bordoni et al., 2018; Bordoni et al., 2019). Evaluation and clinical reasoning related to soft tissue dysfunction therefore needs to consider the role, features and interaction of the fascia (Chaitow, 2018).

Fascial continuity and connectivity as a multidimensional contiguous network can be supported by the structure and function of the interstitium. The interstitium's body-wide network of fluid-filled interstitial spaces is organised as a lattice or mesh across tissue layers. The fibre lattice creates the interconnected spaces that are filled with moving fluid. The interstitium expands the understanding of organisation of fascia as interconnect but also as layers with siding capacity. The interstitium may act as a body-wide communication network (Benias et al., 2018; Cenaj et al., 2021).

To understand the fascial network and function it is necessary to review the mechanical properties, especially the relationship of stiffness to loads and deformation related to the forces exerted on tissues and the resulting changes in their shape (Guimarães et al., 2020; Kozyrina et al., 2020). Fascia alters its stiffness (the resistance to external deformation) via two mechanisms: cellular contraction and the modification of the fluid characteristics. The connective tissue surrounding the muscles stretched (i.e. fascia) is the candidate component for explaining the increase in joint resistance to stretch after a stretching intervention (Freitas, 2018; Wilke et al., 2018).

When fascia is excessively mechanically stressed, inflamed or immobile, collagen and matrix deposition tends to become disorganised, potentially resulting in fibrosis, adhesions and fascial 'thickening' (Langevin, 2011) also described as 'densification', (Stecco & Stecco, 2009), involving distortion of myofascial relationships, altering muscle balance and proprioception feedback. Increased amount of myofibroblasts has been observed in pathological fascia that might create tissue contractures (Wall et al., 2017; Blottner et al., 2019; Weig, 2020).

Consequent binding among layers that should stretch, glide and/or shift on each other, potentially impairs motor function (Fourie, 2009), while chronic tissue loading may form 'global soft tissue holding patterns' (Myers, 2009; Freitas, 2018). Distribution of hyaluronan is necessary for ease of movement among structures. Viscoelastic deformation is possible due to the high concentration of Glycosaminoglycans (GAG) and hyaluronan (Fede et al., 2018).

During passive stretching, the fascia is the first tissue that limits the elongation and would be an element that contributes to bind and the region where MET contractions begin.

Epimysial fascia is a type of deep fascia that ensheaths muscles and helps to define their shape and structure. It is continuous with the tendon, allowing it to transmit forces (Stecco et al., 2013; Stecco, 2015; Stecco et al., 2021). There are three layers: internal, middle and external, each with distinct arrangements of collagen fibres. Each layer of the fascia is comprised of types I and III collagen and elastic fibres. Between each layer is areolar connective tissue rich in hyaluronan (HA) (Bhattacharya et al., 2010). HA is a polysaccharide in the extracellular matrix that provides

BOX 2.2   Why Fascia Matters—cont'd

both lubrication and resistance to compression. Under normal physiological conditions, HA is responsible for normal gliding motion between components of fascia, muscle, nerves, lymphatics and blood vessels (Dowthwaite et al., 1998; Alberts et al., 2002; Stecco et al., 2008). Fasciacytes are specialised fibroblast-like cells that secrete the HA-rich matrix in fascial tissue (Stecco et al., 2017).

Fibrotic changes in muscle may have a substantial impact on tissue dynamics and force generation capacity on other most important performance properties such as myofascial force transmission and changes of fascia properties (stiffness vs elasticity). Myofascial force transmission to neighbouring muscles represents a mechanism protecting the target muscle against overload. Stretching, so far, has been used primarily to alter the neurophysiological and biomechanical function of the lengthened muscle. However, due to the morphological connections, it might as well affect synergists and antagonists, thereby modifying sports performance (Schleip et al., 2006; Wilke et al., 2018; Schleip et al., 2019).

Mechanotransduction describes a multimodal cellular and molecular process of how cells can sense and respond to mechanical stimulation from outside, generate intracellular molecules that are eventually released into the extracellular matrix (ECM) by stimulated cells, targeted to variable receptors to regulate morphology and functions in a given tissue (Zügel et al., 2018; Ajimsha et al., 2020b).

The implications of these observations are that 'short' postural (tonic) muscles need to be considered from this fascial perspective, that is, that at least some of the stiffness/tightness relates to fascia and not muscle, and that treatment should therefore take account of this.

Treatment Options

Loose connective tissue responds to light tissue stretch, which 'may be key to the therapeutic mechanism of treatments using mechanical stimulation of connective tissue' (Langevin, 2005, 2010b).

Myers (2010) suggests that stretching can be applied not only to fascial 'length' problems, but also to 'stuck layer' problems, using shear stress to allow the restoration of increased relative movement between the adjacent planes of fascia (Schwind, 2006).

Fourie (2009) and Langevin (2009) both suggest that their animal and human studies indicate that the ideal degree of stretch required to lengthen *loose connective tissue* should not exceed 20% of the available elasticity, with 5%–6% being adequate in many instances. Light (significantly less than 20% of available elasticity), sustained stretching is more effective in affecting fascia than more vigorous approaches (Langevin, 2010a). In other words, strong stretching is not recommended where fascia is concerned, and this fits well with the protocols recommended for use of stretching during muscle energy technique (MET) usage (see Chapters 5 and 6 for more details on this). In addition, breathing retraining is likely to assist in reducing excessive contractility in myofibroblasts in fascia (Chaitow, 2007, 2018; Jensen et al., 2008).

As noted in the discussion of viscoelastic features of PNF/MET, intramuscular fascia (the series elastic component, for example) appear responsive to isometric contractions and stretching. Fryer and Fossum (2010) suggest that apart from the influence of mechanoreceptors on pain (via both ascending and descending pathways), MET induces in vivo mechanical stretching of fibroblasts that alters interstitial osmotic pressure and increases blood flow, thus reducing concentrations of pro-inflammatory cytokines and reducing sensitisation of peripheral nociceptors.

Franklyn-Miller has added a further consideration to the effects of stretching. He has evaluated the remarkable degree in which muscular effort depends on the multiple links that muscles have with each other and with connective tissue structures. These connections mean that, for example, a hamstring stretch will produce 240% of the resulting hamstring strain in the iliotibial tract and 145% in the ipsilateral lumbar fascia, compared with the strain imparted in the hamstrings. This process of strain transmission during stretching involves many other tissues beyond the muscle that is being targeted, largely due to fascial connections, making the use of the word 'isolated', together with 'stretching, difficult to justify (Franklyn-Miller et al., 2009).

Imbalances between postural and phasic muscles are features of many musculoskeletal dysfunctional patterns, amongst which some of the most obvious are the so-called 'crossed syndromes' (Janda et al., 2006; in Liebenson, 2006). For details of these see Box 6.2, Chapter 6.

Joints, Muscles and MET: Identifying Sources of Pain

Identification of the ideal target tissues for treatment can be confusing, although guidelines can help in providing answers (Kaltenborn, 1985; Kuchera & Kuchera, 1992; Clarkson, 2020).

This information is of particular relevance in MET settings where soft tissue dysfunction might attract stretching following an isometric contraction, whereas a joint problem would not.

- Does passive stretching (traction) of a painful area increase the level of pain? If so, it is probably of soft-tissue origin (extra-articular).
- Does compression of the painful area increase the pain? If so, it is probably of joint origin (intra-articular), involving tissues belonging to that joint.
- If active movement (controlled by the patient) in one direction produces pain (and/or is restricted), and passive movement (controlled by the therapist) in the opposite direction also produces pain (and/or is restricted), contractile tissues (muscle, ligament, etc.) are involved. This can be confirmed by resisted tests.
- If active and passive movements in the same direction produce pain (and/or restriction), joint dysfunction is likely to be a cause. This can be confirmed by use of traction and compression (and gliding) tests of the joint.
- As a rule, active movements test all anatomical structures as well as the psychological willingness of the patient to move the area. Passive movements, in contrast, test only non-contractile tissues, with such movements being compared with accepted norms, as well as the corresponding contralateral joint.
- Resisted tests can be used to assess both strength and painful responses to muscle contraction, either from the muscle or its tendinous attachment. This involves production of a strong contraction of the suspected muscle, while the joint is kept immobile, starting somewhere near the midrange position. No joint motion should be allowed to occur. This is done to confirm a soft tissue dysfunction rather than a joint involvement. Before performing a resisted test, it is wise to perform a compression test to clear any suspicion of joint involvement. In many instances, soft tissue dysfunction will accompany (precede, or follow on from) joint dysfunction, and there are few joint conditions, acute or chronic, without some soft tissue involvement.
- A Norwegian study involving more than 3000 people demonstrated that localised musculoskeletal pain is relatively rare and usually coexists with pain in other parts of the body (Kamaleri et al., 2008). Knowledge of the patterns of distribution of trigger-point pain symptoms allows for a swift focusing on suitable sites in which to search for an offending trigger (if the pain is indeed coming from a myofascial trigger point)

(Affaitati et al., 2020; Vulfsons & Minerbi, 2020). Alternatively, the discomfort could be a radicular symptom emanating from the spine. The functional limitations caused by trigger points include muscle weakness, poor coordination of movement, fatigue with activity, decreased work tolerance, lack of endurance and joint stiffness, as well as limitations in active and passive ROM (Dommerholt & Issa, 2009; Fernández-de-Las-Peñas & Dommerholt, 2018).

- End-feel, painful arcs, shortened muscles and restricted or exaggerated joint function should all be assessed to determine the *source of dysfunction* and not just its location.

Muscles and Joints: Causes and Effects – Janda's View

Janda (1988) has pointed out that since clinical evidence abounds that joint mobilisation (high velocity thrust or gentle articulation) influences those muscles that are in anatomic or functional relationships with a joint, it may well be that normalisation of excessive muscle tone is what provides the benefit noted, for example, in increased range of motion. By implication, normalisation of muscle tone by other means (such as MET) would produce a beneficial outcome and, potentially, joint normalisation. Since reduction in muscle spasm/contraction commonly results in a reduction in joint pain, one part of the answer to many joint problems would seem to lie in appropriate soft-tissue attention, as in MET (Gillani et al., 2020).

Mitchell's 'Short Muscle Paradigm' View

Treating motion restriction of a joint as if the cause were tight muscle(s) is one approach that makes possible restoration of normal joint motion. Regardless of the cause of restriction, MET treatment, based on a 'short muscle' paradigm, is usually completely effective in eliminating blockage, and restoring normal range of motion, even when the blockage is due to non-muscular factors.

Mitchell (1998)

(See also Chapter 7 for additional views on this perspective.)

Greenman's View

Greenman (1996) has suggested that any articulation that can be moved by voluntary muscle action can be influenced by MET. Use of Ruddy's pulsed MET, as outlined above, and more fully in Chapter 6, suggests that joints (even individual spinal articulations), can be mobilised by MET approaches.

Mense's View

Mense et al. (2001) offer guidelines to practitioners who may be seeking the source of pain:

> Since muscle pain and tenderness can be referred from trigger points, articular dysfunctions, and enthesitis (irritability of soft tissues (muscles, tendons or ligaments) where it enter into the bones), the examiner must examine these sites for evidence of a condition that would cause referred muscle pain and tenderness. Local pain and tenderness in muscle is commonly caused by trigger points, and muscles crossing involved [blocked] joints are likely to develop trigger points producing secondary muscle-induced pain because of the joint problem.

It is likely that passive joint mobilisation has the ability to immediately alter muscle function although the specific mechanisms of action are not confirmed (Pfluegler et al., 2020).

Whether a joint is treated using MET (or other modalities) depends entirely on the clinical context and whether or not it is appropriate to do so. It is assumed in this discussion that a clinical decision has been made that it is appropriate to treat a particular joint restriction using MET.

End-feel. The end of a joint's ROM may be described as having a certain quality known as 'end-feel'. When a joint is taken actively or passively to its physiological barrier there is normally a firm but not harsh end-feel. When the joint is taken to its anatomical barrier, a harder end-feel is noted, beyond which any movement is likely to produce damage. However, if there is a restriction in the normal ROM, then a pathological (or 'dysfunctional') barrier would be apparent on active or passive movement. End-feel, in cases of interosseous changes (arthritis, for example), are sudden or hard. However, if the restriction involves soft tissue dysfunction the end-feel would be of a more malleable nature. Clarkson (2020) summarises normal end-feel variations as follows:

- Normal soft end-feel is due to soft tissue approximation (such as in knee flexion) or soft-tissue stretching (as in ankle dorsiflexion).

- Normal firm end-feel results from capsular or ligamentous stretching (internal rotation of the femur, for example).
- Normal hard end-feel occurs when bone meets bone, as in elbow extension.
- Pathological end-feel can involve a number of variations such as: a firmer, less elastic feel, when scar tissue restricts movement or when shortened connective tissue exists; an elastic, less soft end-feel is noted when increased muscle tonus restricts movement; an empty end-feel occurs when the patient stops the movement (or asks for it to be stopped) before a true end-feel is reached as a result of extreme pain (fracture or active inflammation) or psychogenic factors.

Joint-play ('slack'). Joint-play refers to the particular movements between bones, associated with either separation of the surfaces (as in traction) or parallel movement of joint surfaces (also known as translation, or translatoric gliding, or 'shunt'). Some degree of such movement is possible between most joints, restricted only by the degree of soft tissue elasticity. Any change in length of such soft tissues, therefore, automatically alters the range of joint-play mobility, also known as the degree of available 'slack'.

Note: Chapter 8 describes the use of MET in cases of acute spinal dysfunction, while descriptions of MET usage in Chapter 11 reflect on rehabilitation strategies following acute low back pain.

As explained above, joint restrictions are usually treated in the same way as acute soft tissue problems, that is, isometric contractions are light and there is no stretching following isometric contractions, whether these are sustained or pulsed. Following a very light isometric contraction towards or away from the restriction barrier, or in another direction, a non-forceful attempt is made to move the joint to a new barrier (to an easy, first sign of resistance).

Note: Following the contraction, usually on an exhalation, and after the patient has consciously relaxed, the joint would be assessed to evaluate whether the barrier has retreated, or the end-feel has modified. There is no stretching, no force and no need to delay before repeating the process. In many instances having the patient actively assist the (previously restricted) movement can be helpful.

The joint restriction either releases, partially or totally, or it does not release. Isometric contractions in a variety of directions are commonly employed to test possibilities as to what the restraining features might be.

Viscoelasticity in Relation to MET/PNF Contractions and Stretching

The viscoelastic (mechanical) properties of connective tissues (fascia) are thought to relate to their fluid or gel (viscous) components, as well as to their elastic properties (Magnusson et al., 1996c; Herbert & Gandevia, 2019). During compression, these tissues tend to absorb or release fluid during loading and release or absorb it again when compressive force is removed (Böl et al., 2020).

It is suggested that the strain induced in a muscle when it is being isometrically contracted produces stretching of the series elastic component (Lederman, 2005); however, when it is additionally being actively or passively stretched, there will be elongation of muscle, as well as intramuscular connective tissue (De Deyne, 2001; Herbert et al., 2002; Andrade et al., 2020).

When a constant stretching force is loaded on a tissue (muscle, fascia), it responds with slow elongation or 'creep'. This results in loss of energy from the tissue, and repetition of loading results in greater elastic deformation. Additional loading may cause more permanent 'plastic' changes (Gajdosik, 2001; Nordez et al., 2009; Blazevich, 2019; Böl et al., 2020).

- Sarcomeres – the smallest functional (contractile) unit of a myofibril – appear as repeating units along the length of a myofibril, which is itself a slender striated strand within muscle fibres, composed of bundles of myofilaments. The thin and thick filaments of muscle sarcomeres are interconnected by the giant protein titin, which is a scaffolding filament, signalling platform, and provider of passive tension and elasticity in myocytes (Linke, 2018). When skeletal muscles are stretched without activation, there is an increase in passive forces that is developed mostly by titin molecule (Lemke & Schnorrer, 2017; Rassier, 2017). Myofibrils occur in groups of branching threads running parallel to the cellular long-axis of the muscle fibre (Fig. 2.6).
- The *series elastic components* of sarcomeres store energy when stretched and contribute to elasticity. They comprise non-contractile (fascia/connective tissue) components of muscle that lie in series with muscle fibres.
- Tendons are examples of the series elastic component, as are the cross bridges between actin and myosin, the sliding elements of muscle that allow shortening to occur (Huxley & Niedergerke, 1954; Marcucci et al., 2019).
- The *parallel elastic component* of sarcomeres provides resistive tension when a muscle is passively stretched. These are non-contractile and consist of the muscle

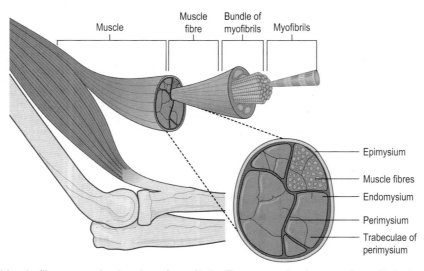

Fig. 2.6 Muscle fibres comprise bundles of myofibrils. The contractile element of myofibrils (sarcomeres) contains both series elastic and parallel elastic components, which behave differently when a contraction occurs and during stretching – (see Fig. 2.7).

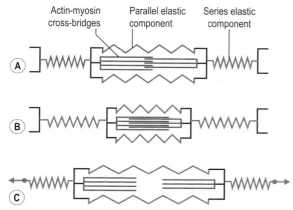

Fig. 2.7 (A) The sarcomere at rest showing parallel and series elastic components as well as actin-myosin cross bridges. (B) During an isometric contraction (as used in MET) the connective tissues in the muscle, such as the series elastic component will lengthen, while the parallel elastic component shortens, as actin-myosin cross-bridges slide across each other. (C) When stretched, following an isometric contraction, or passively, both the parallel and series elastic components lengthen, however the less stiff parallel fibres will lengthen most. (Note the separation shown in C of actin and myosin is exaggerated in this schematic representation.) (Adapted, with permission, from Lederman 1997.)

membranes (fascia), which lie parallel to the muscle fibres (Fig. 2.7).

An isometric contraction therefore introduces a lengthening of the series elastic component (fascial, tendinous structures), while the parallel elastic component of the sarcomere shortens, as actin and myosin slide across each other so that the muscle does not change overall length. Repeated isometric contractions effectively lengthen the *series elastic* structures, particularly if additional active or passive stretching is subsequently added (Lederman, 1997, 2005, 2017). In this way, both the active and passive phases of MET can be seen to contribute to muscle elongation (Milliken, 2003).

The questions arise as to whether any such biomechanical, adaptive lengthening effect on the series elastic component of muscle fibres is anything other than temporary and whether it is clinically significant (Lederman, 2005).

- Magnusson et al. (1996b), Ballantyne et al. (2003) and Park & Lim (2020) have shown that while MET does indeed produce immediate viscoelastic change in hamstring muscles, these are short-lived.

- In studies that measured passive knee extension and passive torque following MET contractions of the hamstrings, the effects of three consecutive 45-second stretches, separated by 30 seconds of viscoelastic stress relaxation of the hamstrings produced viscoelastic change, but this did not affect the resistance to the subsequent stretch 30 seconds later. In other words, viscoelastic stress relaxation was short-lived, and the energy loss was recovered within 30 seconds (Magnusson et al., 1996b; Mukund & Subramaniam, 2020). More current studies indicate change for up to 10 minutes. Although the functional changes last for at least 10 minutes, changes in muscle stiffness were only observed up to 5 minutes after the stretching exercise (Mizuno & Umemura, 2016; Konrad et al., 2019). Nevertheless, this hiatus could offer sufficient time for the brief greater degree of mobility to be exploited in settings where mobilisation or articulation are involved.

Viscoelastic changes in connective tissues within muscles can therefore be presumed to be real phenomena, but to not be able to account for all the therapeutic effects of MET. And if not due to viscoelastic changes, could the benefits of the MET process be neurologically explained?

These issues are explored further in Chapter 4, where there is evaluation of research evidence. For a summary of other reasons for giving the necessary attention to fascial features when managing somatic dysfunction, see Box 2.2.

Possible Neurological Effects of MET

Azevedo et al. (2011) observe that a variety of different explanations have been used to justify the effectiveness of PNF (and by implication, MET) in producing both analgesia and increased ROM.

Postisometric relaxation (PIR): They note that one common explanation suggests that a voluntary target muscle contraction, before muscle stretching, has the effect of reducing reflexive components of that contraction (e.g. involving the Golgi tendon organs), encouraging relaxation, increased muscle length and joint ROM, in other words, inducing PIR (Ferber et al., 2002; Rowlands et al., 2003).

However, Chalmers (2004), Mitchell et al. (2007, 2009) and many others have questioned whether the short period of inhibition that follows a target muscle contraction is sufficient to result in a clinically meaningful duration of target-muscle relaxation (Olivo & Magee, 2006).

The validity of PIR as a mechanism is also questioned by evidence from studies that demonstrate that surface electromyography (sEMG) in the previously isometrically contracted muscle may not decrease, but that it might actually increase after a PNF, or MET, contraction (Mitchell et al., 2009).

Reciprocal inhibition (RI): This physiological feature describes the reflex response in which muscles on one side of a joint relax in order to accommodate contraction of their antagonists. An isometric contraction of an antagonist muscle has been proposed as a means of inhibiting a muscle prior to stretching. As an example, excitation of the hamstring alpha-motoneurons by group Ia afferent fibres is accompanied by inhibition of quadriceps alpha-motoneurons (Burns, 2006). The arguments against RI being responsible for the changes that follow isometric contractions are similar to those discussed above in relation to PIR. In short, the effects of RI, while real, are brief and do not appear sufficient to be clinically meaningful (Fryer, 2006).

Despite lack of support for these being the actual mechanisms involved, Drysdale and Wright (2008) ascribe the equally successful outcomes from use of MET, involving either agonist (PIR) or antagonist (RI) of piriformis, to those mechanisms.

If MET/PNF effects do not stem from viscoelastic or reflexive effects (PIR/RI), all of which appear transient – and are ascribed to unexplained processes which have been labelled '*increased tolerance to stretch*' – what are those processes that may be contributing to this *increased tolerance*?

Distraction as a Means of Increasing Stretch Tolerance

Magnusson et al. (1996a) concluded that an increased level of stretch tolerance followed isometric muscle contraction. These findings have been supported by Mitchell (2007). However, as noted, the mechanism(s) whereby increased tolerance emerges in this setting remains elusively unexplained.

A suggestion by Azevedo et al. (2011) is that isometric muscle contraction might act as a *distraction* to any subsequent stretch since their study suggests that it may not be necessary to contract the actual target muscle in order to achieve increased stretch tolerance. In fact, they found that contraction of another muscle altogether appeared to be just as effective. They note that:

The purpose of [our] study was to compare the acute effect of the … PNF stretching technique, on

knee range of motion (ROM) using target muscle (hamstring muscles) contraction, or an uninvolved muscle (contralateral elbow flexors) contraction.

Their findings indicated that enhanced knee ROM following a PNF procedure would be the same whether the muscle targeted to be stretched is contracted or an uninvolved muscle group on the other side of the body is contracted, during the PNF procedure. In the study, the muscles that were stretched were the hamstrings, irrespective of whether the contraction was of those muscles, or the elbow flexors. It seems that the isometric contraction of either muscle group increased the level of comfort with which subsequent stretching of the hamstrings might be achieved.

Since isometric contractions are used as a precursor to stretching in both PNF and MET, just how this alters pain perception is of interest, if we are to come closer to understanding MET's mode of action. The focus of attention appears to be turning towards the effects of the isometric contraction itself, rather than subsequent stretching, as being able to offer possible explanations. We may be able to learn something of the mechanisms involved by a brief examination of a very different, sustained, use of isometric contraction.

Analgesia Following Sustained Isometric Contractions

Hoeger Bement et al. (2011) have compared pain ratings and thresholds in men and women with fibromyalgia syndrome (FMS), before and after isometric contractions of varying intensities and durations, performed with the elbow flexor muscles:

1. Maximal voluntary contractions (MVCs)
2. 25% MVCs sustained until task failure
3. 25% MVCs for 2 minutes
4. 80% MVCs sustained until task failure

The outcomes showed that analgesic responses were noted in some, but not all, FMS patients, with the greatest change noted after the long-duration, low-intensity isometric contraction, sustained until failure. The greatest benefits were experienced by younger women (average age 39) who had the lowest pain thresholds at the outset.

Additional Studies Also Show Analgesic Responses to Isometric and Isotonic Contractions

Hypoalgesia that follows stimulation of muscle and joint mechanoreceptors during an isometric contraction might result from activation of centrally mediated pain modulating pathways, for example, by the periaqueductal grey in the midbrain region, together with non-opioid serotonergic and noradrenergic descending inhibitory pathways. At the same time nociceptive inhibition may occur at the dorsal horn of the cord due to ('gating') impulses resulting from mechanoreceptor stimulation (Fryer & Fossum, 2010; Parmar et al., 2011; Muhsen et al., 2019). The most commonly proposed mechanism involves enhanced descending inhibition by activation of the opioid and cannabinoid systems. The contraction of skeletal muscle increases the discharge of A-delta and C-fibres, which in turn activates central descending opioid pain pathways. Exercise also increases the release of endogenous cannabinoids. These opioid and cannabinoid pathways have receptors throughout the peripheral and central nervous systems that can produce analgesia (Dietrich & McDaniel, 2004; Vaegter & Jones, 2020; Wewege & Jones, 2020).

MET may also produce hypoalgesia via peripheral mechanisms associated with increased fluid drainage, since muscle contraction, parsticularly if these are rhythmic as in pulsed MET, increases muscle blood and lymph flowrates (Havas et al., 1997). The mechanisms that lead to analgesia in these studies remain elusive. Also unknown at this stage is whether repeated mild isometric contractions, as used in pulsed MET (see Chapter 7), or those employed in MET (as described above) might have similar effects by activating descending inhibitory pathways, resulting in systemic hypoalgesia as occurs with exercise (Alsouhibani et al., 2019).

The isometric contractions used in MET and PNF tend to be brief, with a 5- to 10-second range the commonest. However as outlined above, lengthier, more sustained, isometric contractions can produce analgesia in (some) healthy adults – and in cases where chronic pain is a feature – involving both high- and low-intensity isometric contractions (Hoeger Bement et al., 2008).

Additionally, mechanical forces may affect fibroblast mechanical signal transduction processes (Langevin et al., 2004), changing interstitial pressure and increasing trans-capillary blood flow (Langevin et al., 2005; Parmar et al., 2011).

The endocannabinoid (eCB) system, similar to endorphin or enkephalin influences, offers 'resilience to allostatic load', dampening nociception and pain. Endocannabanoids are anxiolytic, decrease inflammation and play a role in fibroblast reorganisation. Two eCB receptors have been identified: CB1 in the nervous system, and CB2 associated with the immune system (and gut). There are several clinical tools that are known to upregulate eCB activity, including manual therapy modalities such as PNF and MET, stretching and exercise (Degenhardt et al., 2007; McPartland, 2008; Fede et al., 2016; Onifer et al., 2019; Buscemi et al., 2020).

Klingler et al. (2004) measured wet and dry fresh human fascia and found that during an isometric stretch, water is extruded, refilling afterwards in a sponge-like manner. As water extrudes, temporary relaxation occurs in the longitudinal arrangement of the collagen fibres and the tissues become more pliable. They found that with moderate strain there are no micro-injuries, and water eventually (minutes or hours, not seconds) soaks back into the tissue until it swells ('*matrix hydration*'), becoming stiff once more. It is hypothesised that some tissue responses to manual therapy, such as stretching, compression and contraction, may relate to this sponge-like squeezing and refilling of the semi-liquid ground substance (superficial fascia), with its water binding glycosaminoglycans and proteoglycans (Schleip et al., 2012). While this 'hydraulic' mechanism might be implicated in increased range of movement following an isometric contraction (of the tissues involved in the contraction), it could not account for hypoalgesia or increased ROM of distant structures, as discussed above in relation to the Hoeger Bement et al. (2011) study.

It is not yet possible to say which of these potential influences on hypoalgesia and/or increased flexibility are operating in response to isometric contractions as used in MET (and PNF). A mix of neurological, biochemical and hydraulic influences appear to follow contractions, reducing the mystery of the observed effects (hypoalgesia and increased ROM) to some extent, but without offering clear answers (Zügel et al., 2018; Naweed et al., 2020). Further research is undoubtedly required to clarify the relative influences on pain perception, following isometric contraction or stretch of factors such as:

- Neurologically induced hypoalgesia (Fryer & Fossum, 2010; Parmar et al., 2011, Phadke et al., 2016).
- Improved drainage of inflammatory substances (Havas et al., 1997; Stenersen & Bordoni, 2020; Bordoni et al., 2018).
- Altered fibroblast function involving mechanotransduction (Langevin et al., 2004).
- The release of endorphins and/or endocannabinoids (McPartland, 2008; Fede et al., 2020).

- A hydraulic effect involving connective tissue structures that temporarily allows increased freedom of movement following stretching or isometric contractions (Klingler et al., 2004).
- Changes in both the series elastic and parallel elastic elements of sarcomeres (as discussed earlier in this chapter), occurring during the active and passive phases of MET, can be seen to potentially contribute to muscle elongation and increased ROM (Milliken, 2003; Nugraha et al., 2020).

Stretching Increases Stretch Tolerance

Of passing interest in considering 'increased tolerance' mechanisms is the outcome of a randomised controlled trial that demonstrated what might be summarised as: *'stretching increases tolerance to stretching'* (Law et al., 2009; Kisilewicz et al., 2018).

If regular stretching increases tolerance but not extensibility, and isometric contractions increase tolerance and potentially, extensibility (see viscoelasticity discussion above), a combination of isometric contractions and stretching would seem to offer dual benefits.

A further influence, mechanotransduction occurring on a cellular level, also deserves consideration and explanation.

MET in Tissue Remodelling and Mechanotransduction

Khan and Scott (2009) succinctly summarise mechanotransduction as a process where cells sense and respond to mechanical loads. They elaborate:

> *Mechanotransduction refers to the process by which the body converts mechanical loading into cellular responses. These cellular responses, in turn, promote structural change. A classic example of mechanotransduction in action is bone adapting to load.*

It is therefore a process in which load (possibly involving isometric contractions or stretching) could be used therapeutically to stimulate tissue repair and remodelling, for example, of tendon, muscle, cartilage and bone (LaStayo et al., 2014; Berrueta et al., 2016; Csapo et al., 2020; Wang et al., 2020).

Mechanotransduction can be encouraged by numerous means, including exercise. In animal studies Heinemeier et al. (2007) demonstrated that short-term imposition of load – for example, involving isometric or

isotonic contractions – results in collagen expression in both skeletal muscle and tendons. A key in this process appears to be the upregulation of *Cytokine Transforming Growth Factor-beta-1* (TGF-β-1). This response has major implications in management of scar tissue (Fourie & Robb, 2009) and fibrosis (Altomare & Monte-Alto-Costa, 2018). Heinemeier et al. (2007) have observed that eccentric training appears to have a larger potential than concentric training for increasing the expression of collagen-inducing growth factor in muscle.

THE ROLE OF STRUCTURED TOUCH IN THE THERAPEUTIC SETTING

Manual therapy, including MET, is a form of touch interaction in the context of therapeutic intervention. The biological and physiological impacts of touch include analgesic, affective and somatoperceptual effects. Recent breakthroughs have impacted the scientific understanding of mechanotransduction. These include new work exploring the mechanism of action of Piezo ion channels signalling mechanical sensation to cells to produce chemical responses. In time, this may provide significant insight as to the mechanisms underlying the documented effects of touch in manual therapy and in relation to proprioception (Ranade et al., 2014; Woo et al., 2015; Murthy et al., 2018a, 2018b; Choi et al., 2020). In due course, these may better explain many modalities already in use, and lead to their refinement and evolution.

While research into mechanisms continues, the beneficial effects of structured touch such as MET, massage and other modalities on pain, anxiety and proprioception, as well as their role in patient well-being, are well-established. People expect to be touched when seeking manual therapy and until fairly recently, the role of patient expectation on clinical outcomes has not been given sufficient attention in the research or clinical context with regard to those suffering from musculoskeletal pain conditions (Bialosky et al., 2010).

It seems, however, that when visiting a practitioner known to provide manual therapy (physical therapist, osteopath, chiropractor, massage therapist etc.), the inclusion of manual therapy interventions and exercise ranks highly for a majority of patients seeking such care for low back pain (Bishop et al., 2011; Verbeek et al., 2004), and for neck pain (Bishop et al., 2013). Though research into patient preference in relation to manual

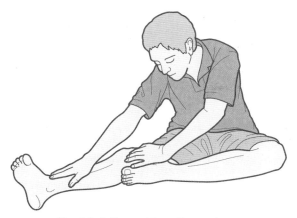

Fig. 2.8 Self-stretching of hamstrings.

therapy and other bodywork modalities is a fairly recent development, a few studies highlight the degree and impact of patient expectation. A 2021 Australian study of patients seeking osteopathic treatment found that 85.7% of the 161 patients interviewed expected between 50% and 75% of their consultation to consist of manual treatment. Only 49% stated that they were likely or extremely likely to attend a consultation without manual therapy involved, as long as they understood that it was 'best practice for their condition' (Tripodi et al., 2021).

Further comparative studies also suggest that the inclusion of touch, whether this is modified by expectations or other variables, remains significant to patient satisfaction. Comparison between patient education programmes with and without manual therapy with a minimal control intervention group looked at the outcomes among unilateral hip osteoarthritis patients. The combined manual therapy and patient education strategy proved more effective than either of the other interventions, with the beneficial results maintained over a 12-month follow-up period (Poulsen et al., 2013). See Fig. 2.8 for an example of self-treatment. In addition, as discussed in more depth in Chapter 7, the process of dialogue and shared decision-making (SDM) between patient and practitioner is especially significant for positive outcomes (Bernhardsson et al., 2019; Grenfell & Soundy, 2022). Worryingly, however, some studies suggest that few therapists are comfortable with fully collaborative therapeutic relationships (Dierckx et al., 2013).

Robust literature across a variety of specialties now demonstrates support for the connection between physical health and mental well-being (Langevin, 2020). Touch from an empathetic practitioner is capable of reducing pain perception and modulating biomarkers related to stress, negative emotions and mechanisms related to the perception of threats (Viceconti et al., 2019; Baroni et al., 2021; Bizzarri & Foglia, 2020). Structured touch in the form of OMT and a form of deep-touch treatment described in osteopathic literature (Cerritelli et al., 2015; Edwards et al., 2018; Licciardone et al., 2020) have been shown to regulate the parasympathetic nervous system and assist in balancing stress and mental health (Giles et al., 2013; Fornari et al., 2017). Moderation of heart rate variability (HRV) and interoceptive accuracy (IAc) have a positive influence on behavioural self-regulation and ROM through neural feedback mechanisms (Edwards et al., 2018). This work highlights the importance of the interoceptive system and the need to address it more thoroughly (D'Alessandro et al., 2016).

Thus, as MET application involves skilled therapeutic contact between the practitioner and the patient, and the statistics suggest that patients overall do expect manual treatment when visiting a practitioner traditionally associated with such methods, given the impact of patient expectations on treatment outcome, it is crucial to implement shared decision-making (SDM) as part of the clinical encounter, and maintain professional equipoise (neutrality as to practitioner preference) in discussing the outcome-based options (Bishop et al., 2017; Fryer, 2017).

SUMMARY

The key features in this chapter that it is hoped the reader will note include:

- MET methods are gentle, involving light, brief isometric contractions from 'easy' barriers of resistance.
- MET differs markedly from PNF where barriers are harder, contractions stronger (often full strength) and longer; and the focus is different, with MET more particularly occupied with enhancing joint function.
- MET is applicable in treatment of both acute and chronic soft tissue dysfunction, as well as in treatment involving joint restriction.
- MET appears to safely and beneficially influence pain, inflammation, viscoelastic features and ROM of previously restricted structures, including joints.
- A variety of MET procedures exist, ranging from isotonic eccentric to rhythmic pulsing protocols, thus making it clinically flexible.

- A variety of mechanisms have been proposed to explain METs analgesic and other effects, including neurological, reflexive, viscoelastic/fascial, hydraulic, lymphatic and biochemical, as well as the, as yet, unexplained phenomenon of *'increased tolerance to stretch'*. See Chapters 4 and 10 for more discussion of this phenomenon.
- A great deal of clinical research has validated MET usage both in regard to safety and efficacy.
- Recent understanding of mechanotransduction and other fascial functions, offers increased awareness of MET's potential role in tissue remodelling contexts.
- MET is a form of touch used in a client centred therapeutic environment by trained practitioners, within the biopsychosocial model of care, that can effectively address interoceptive as well as exteroceptive phenomena.

REFERENCES

Adstrum, S., Hedley, G., Schleip, R., Stecco, C., Yucesoy, C.A., 2017. Defining the fascial system. J. Bodyw. Mov. Ther. 21 (1), 173–177.

Affaitati, G., Costantini, R., Tana, C., Cipollone, F., Giamberardino, M.A., 2020. Co-occurrence of pain syndromes. J Neural Transm (Vienna) 127 (4), 625–646. doi:10.1007/s00702-019-02107-8.

Ajimsha, M.S., Shenoy, P.D., Gampawar, N., 2020a. Role of fascial connectivity in musculoskeletal dysfunctions: a narrative review. J. Bodyw. Mov. Ther. 24 (4), 423–431. doi:10.1016/j.jbmt.2020.07.020.

Ajimsha, M., Surendran, P., Jacob, P., Shenoy, P., Bilal, M., 2020b. Myofascial force transmission in the humans: a systematic scoping review of in-vivo studies. Preprints, 2020110212. doi:10.20944/preprints202011.0212.v1.

Alberts, B., Johnson, A., Lewis, J., Raff, M., Roberts, K., Walter, P., 2002. The extracellular matrix of animals. In *Molecular Biology of the Cell*, 4th edition. Garland Science, New York.

Alghadir, A.H., Iqbal, A., Anwer, S., Iqbal, Z.A., Ahmed, H., 2020. 2020. Efficacy of combination therapies on neck pain and muscle tenderness in male patients with upper trapezius active myofascial trigger points. Biomed. Res. Int., 9361405. doi:10.1155/2020/9361405.

Al-Najjar, H.M.M., Mohammed, A.H., Mosaad, D.M., 2020. Effect of ice massage with integrated neuromuscular inhibition technique on pain and function in subjects with mechanical neck pain: randomised controlled trial. Bull Fac. Phys. Ther. 25, 10. https://doi.org/10.1186/s43161-020-00011-x.

Alsouhibani, A., Vaegter, H.B., Hoeger Bement, M., 2019. Systemic exercise-induced hypoalgesia following isometric exercise reduces conditioned pain modulation. Pain Med 20 (1), 180–190. doi:10.1093/pm/pny057.

Altomare, M., Monte-Alto-Costa, A., 2018. Manual mobilization of subcutaneous fibrosis in mice. J. Manipul. Physiol. Ther. 41 (5), 359–362.

Andrade, R.J., Freitas, S.R., Hug, F., Le Sant, G., Lacourpaille, L., Gross, R., et al., 2020. Chronic effects of muscle and nerve-directed stretching on tissue mechanics. J. Appl. Physiol. 129 (5), 1011–1023. doi:10.1152/japplphysiol.00239.2019.

Arab, A.M., Ghamkhar, L., Emami, M., Nourbakhsh, M.R., 2011. Altered muscular activation during prone hip extension in women with and without low back pain. Chiropr. Man. Therap. 19, 18. doi:10.1186/2045-709X-19-18.

Azeim, A.S.A.E., Ahmed, S.E.B., Draz, A.H., Elhafez, H.M., Kattabei, O.M., 2018. Integrated neuromuscular inhibition technique versus kinesiotape on upper trapezius myofascial trigger points a randomised clinical trial. Int. J. Physiother. 5 (3), 105–112. https://doi.org/10.15621/ijphy/2018/v5i3/173934.

Azevedo, D.C., Melo, R.M., Alves Corrêa, R.V., Chalmers, G., 2011. Uninvolved versus target muscle contraction during contract: relax proprioceptive neuromuscular facilitation stretching. Phys. Ther. Sport. 12 (3), 117–121. doi:10.1016/j.ptsp.2011.04.003.

Ballantyne, F., Fryer, G., McLaughlin, P., 2003. Effect of MET on hamstring extensibility: the mechanism of altered flexibility. J. Osteopath. Med. 6 (2), 59–63.

Baroni, F., Ruffini, N., D'Alessandro, G., Consorti, G., Lunghi, C., 2021. The role of touch in osteopathic practice: a narrative review and integrative hypothesis. Complem. Ther. Clin. Pract. 42, 101277. doi:10.1016/j.ctcp.2020.101277.

Benias, P.C., Wells, R.G., Sackey-Aboagye, B., Klavan, H., Reidy, J., Buonocore, D., et al., 2018. Structure and distribution of an unrecognised interstitium in human tissues. Sci. Rep. 8, 4947. https://doi.org/10.1038/s41598-018-23062-6.

Bergmark, A., 1989. Stability of the lumbar spine. A study in mechanical engineering. Acta Orthop. Scand. Suppl. 230, 1–54. doi:10.3109/17453678909154177.

Bernhardsson, S., Samsson, K.S., Johansson, K., Öberg, B., Larsson, M.E., 2019. A preference for dialogue: exploring the influence of patient preferences on clinical decision making and treatment in primary care physiotherapy. Eu. J. Physiother. 21 (2), 107–114. doi:10.1080/21679169.2018.1496474.

Berrueta, L., Muskaj, I., Olenich, S., Butler, T., Badger, G.J., Colas, R.A., et al., 2016. Stretching impacts inflammation resolution in connective tissue. J. Cell. Physiol. 231 (7), 1621–1627. https://doi.org/10.1002/jcp.25263.

Bhattacharya, V., Barooah, P.S., Nag, T.C., Chaudhuri, G.R., Bhattacharya, S., 2010. Detail microscopic analysis of deep fascia of lower limb and its surgical implication. Indian J. Plast. Surg. 43 (2), 135–140.

Bialosky, J.E., Bishop, M.D., Cleland, J.A., 2010. Individual expectation: an overlooked, but pertinent, factor in the treatment of individuals experiencing musculoskeletal pain. Phys. Ther. 90 (9), 1345–1355. https://doi.org/10.2522/ptj.20090306.

Bishop, M.D., Bialosky, J.E., Cleland, J.A., 2011. Patient expectations of benefit from common interventions for low back pain and effects on outcome: secondary analysis of a clinical trial of manual therapy interventions. J. Man. Manip. Ther. 19 (1), 20–25. doi:10.1179/1066981 10X12804993426929.

Bishop, M.D., Bialosky, J.E., Penza, C.W., Beneciuk, J.M., Alappattu, M.J., 2017. The influence of clinical equipoise and patient preferences on outcomes of conservative manual interventions for spinal pain: an experimental study. J. Pain. Res. 10, 965–972. https://doi.org/10.2147/JPR.S130931.

Bishop, M.D., Mintken, P.E., Bialosky, J.E., Cleland, J.A., 2013. Patient expectations of benefit from interventions for neck pain and resulting influence on outcomes. J. Orthop. Sports Phys. Ther. 43 (7), 457–465. doi:10.2519/jospt.2013.4492.

Bizzarri, P., Foglia, A., 2020. Manual therapy: art or science? In: Bernardo-Filho, M. et al. (Ed.), Physical Therapy Effectiveness. IntechOpen. doi:10.5772/intechopen.90730.

Blazevich, A.J., 2019. Adaptations in the passive mechanical properties of skeletal muscle to altered patterns of use. J. Appl. Physiol. 126 (5), 1483–1491. doi:10.1152/japplphysiol.00700.2018.

Blottner, D., Huang, Y., Trautmann, G., Sun, L, 2019. The fascia: continuum linking bone and myofascial bag for global and local body movement control on Earth and in Space. A scoping review. REACH 14. https://doi.org/10.1016/j.reach.2019.100030.

Böl, M., Iyer, R., Garcés-Schröder, M., Kohn, S., Dietzel, A., 2020. Mechano-geometrical skeletal muscle fibre characterisation under cyclic and relaxation loading. J. Mech. Behav. Biomed. Mat. 110, 104001.

Bordoni, B., Myers, T., 2020. A review of the theoretical fascial models: biotensegrity, fascintegrity, and myofascial chains. Cureus 12 (2), e7092.

Bordoni, B., Marelli, F., Morabito, B., Castagna, R., 2018. A new concept of biotensegrity incorporating liquid tissues: blood and lymph. J. Evid. Based. Integr. Med. 23. doi:10.1177/2515690X18792838.

Bordoni, B., Varacallo, M.A., Morabito, B., Simonelli, M., 2019. Biotensegrity or fascintegrity? Cureus 11 (6), e4819.

Bove, G.M., Delany, S.P., Hobson, L., Cruz, G.E., Harris, M.Y., Amin, M., Chapelle, S.L., Barbe, M.F., 2019. Manual therapy prevents onset of nociceptor activity, sensorimotor dysfunction, and neural fibrosis induced by a volitional repetitive task. Pain 160 (3), 632–644. https://doi.org/10.1097/j.pain.0000000000001443.

Bullock-Saxton, J., Janda, V., Bullock, M., 1993. Reflex activation of gluteal muscles in walking. Spine 18, 704.

Burns, D.K., 2006. Gross range of motion in the cervical spine: the effects of osteopathic muscle energy technique in asymptomatic subjects. J. Am. Osteopath. Assoc. 106 (3), 137–142.

Buscemi, A., Martino, S., Scirè Campisi, S., Rapisarda, A., Coco, M., 2020. Endocannabinoids release after osteopathic manipulative treatment. A brief review. J. Complem. Integr. Med. 18 (1), 1–7. doi:10.1515/jcim-2020-0013.

Carnevali, L., Lombardi, L., Fornari, M., Sgoifo, A., 2020. Exploring the effects of osteopathic manipulative treatment on autonomic function through the lens of heart rate variability. Front. Neurosci. 14, 579365. https://doi.org/10.3389/fnins.2020.579365.

Cenaj, O., Allison, D.H., Imam, R., Zeck, B., Drohan, L.M., Chiriboga, L., et al., 2021. Evidence for continuity of interstitial spaces across tissue and organ boundaries in humans. Commun. Biol. 4, 436. https://doi.org/10.1038/s42003-021-01962-0.

Cerritelli, F., Chiacchiaretta, P., Gambi, F., Perrucci, M.G., Barassi, G., Visciano, C., et al., 2020. Effect of manual approaches with osteopathic modality on brain correlates of interoception: an fMRI study. Sci. Rep. 10 (1), 3214. https://doi.org/10.1038/s41598-020-60253-6.

Cerritelli, F., Ginevri, L., Messi, G., Caprari, E., Di Vincenzo, M., Renzetti, C., et al., 2015. Clinical effectiveness of osteopathic treatment in chronic migraine: 3-armed randomized controlled trial. Complement. Ther. Med. 23, 149–156.

Chaitow, L., 1994. Integrated neuromuscular inhibition technique. Mass. Ther. J. 33, 60–68.

Chaitow, L., 2007. Chronic pelvic pain: pelvic floor problems, sacroiliac dysfunction and the trigger point connection. J. Bodyw. Mov. Ther. 11, 327–339.

Chaitow, L., 2008. Naturopathic Physical Medicine: Theory and Practice for Manual Therapists and Naturopaths. Churchill Livingstone, Edinburgh.

Chaitow, L., 2018. Fascial Dysfunction: Manual Therapy Approaches. Handspring, East Lothian.

Chalmers, G., 2004. Re-examination of the possible role of Golgi tendon organ and muscle spindle reflexes in proprioceptive neuromuscular facilitation muscle stretching. Sports Biomech 3, 159–183.

Chavan, S.E., Shinde, S., 2019. Effect of integrated neuromuscular inhibition technique on iliotibial band tightness in osteoarthritis of knee. Int. J. Health Sci. Res. 9 (6), 125.

Choi, S., Hachisuka, J., Brett, M.A., Magee, A.R., Omori, Y., Iqbal, N.U.A., et al., 2020. Parallel ascending spinal pathways for affective touch and pain. Nature. 587 (7833), 258–263. doi:10.1038/s41586-020-2860-1.

Cifu, D.X., 2020. Braddom's physical medicine and rehabilitation E-book. Elsevier Health Sciences.

Clark, M.A., 2001. A Scientific Approach to Understanding Kinetic Chain Dysfunction. The National Academy of Sports Medicine, Thousand Oaks, CA.

Clarkson, H., 2020. Musculoskeletal Assessment: Joint Range of Motion, Muscle Testing, and Function. Wolters Kluwer, Philadelphia.

Coke, S.V., Silva, A.J., Quiñinao, F.R., Zambra, R.F., Reyes, J.T., 2020. Evaluation of short-term effectiveness of orthopedic manual therapy in signs and symptoms of myofascial pain: a controlled clinical trial. J. Oral Res. 9 (2), 121–128.

Csapo, R., Gumpenberger, M., Wessner, B., 2020. Skeletal muscle extracellular matrix – what do we know about its composition, regulation, and physiological Roles? A narrative review. Front. Physiol. 11, 253. doi:10.3389/fphys.2020.00253.

Curcio, J.E., Grana, M.J., England, S., Banyas, P.M., Palmer, B.D., Placke, A.E., et al., 2017. Use of the spencer technique on collegiate baseball players: effect on physical performance and self-report measures. J. Am. Osteopath. Assoc. 117 (3), 166–175. doi:10.7556/jaoa.2017.031.

D'alessandro, G., Cerritelli, F., Cortelli, P., 2016. Sensitization and interoception as key neurological concepts in osteopathy and other manual medicines. Front. Neurosci. 10, 100. doi:10.3389/fnins.2016.00100.

Dal Farra, F., Risio, R.G., Vismara, L., Bergna, A., 2021. Effectiveness of osteopathic interventions in chronic non-specific low back pain: a systematic review and meta-analysis. Complement Ther. Med. 56, 102616. doi:10.1016/j.ctim.2020.102616.

De Deyne, P.G., 2001. Application of passive stretch and its implications for muscle fibers. Phys. Ther. 81, 819–827.

Degenhardt, B.F., Darmani, N.A., Johnson, J.C., Towns, L.C., Rhodes, D.C., Trinh, C., et al., 2007. Role of osteopathic manipulative treatment in altering pain biomarkers: a pilot study. J. Am. Osteop. Assoc. 107, 387–394.

Degenhardt, B.F., Johnson, J.C., Brooks, W.J., Norman, L., 2018. Characterising adverse events reported immediately after osteopathic manipulative treatment. J. Am. Osteopath. Assoc. 118 (3), 141–149.

Dierckx, K., Deveugele, M., Roosen, P., Devisch, I., 2013. Implementation of shared decision making in physical therapy: observed level of involvement and patient preference. Phys. Ther. 93 (10), 1321–1330. https://doi.org/10.2522/ptj.20120286.

Dietrich, A., McDaniel, W.F., 2004. Endocannabinoids and exercise. Br. J. Sports Med. 38 (5), 536–541.

Dommerholt, J., Issa, T., 2009. Differential diagnosis of fibromyalgia. In: Chaitow, L. (Ed.), Fibromyalgia Syndrome: A Practitioner's Guide To Treatment, third ed. Churchill Livingstone, Edinburgh.

Dowling, D., 1998. S.T.A.R.: a more viable alternative descriptor system of somatic dysfunction. Am. Acad. Appl. Osteop. J. 8 (2), 34–37.

Dowthwaite, G.P., Edwards, J.C., Pitsillides, A.A., 1998. An essential role for the interaction between hyaluronan and hyaluronan binding proteins during joint development. J. Histochem. Cytochem. 46 (5), 641–651.

Drysdale, I., Wright, P., 2008. A comparison of post-isometric relaxation (PIR) and reciprocal inhibition (RI) muscle energy techniques applied to piriformis. Int. J. Osteopath. Med. 11 (4), P158–P159.

Edwards, D.J., Young, H., Cutis, A., Johnston, R., 2018. The immediate effect of therapeutic touch and deep touch pressure on range of motion, interoceptive accuracy and heart rate variability: a randomized controlled trial with moderation analysis [published correction appears in Front. Integr. Neurosci. 14, 28]. Front. Integr. Neurosci 12, 41. Published 21 September 2018. doi:10.3389/fnint.2018.00041.

Ehrenfeuchter, C., William, A., Kappler, D., Kimberly, F.P., 2011. Glossary of osteopathic terminology. Prin. Palpat. Diagn. Manip. Tech. 1.

Engel, A., 1986. Skeletal Muscle Types in Myology. McGraw-Hill, New York.

Faulkner, J.A., 2003. Terminology for contractions of muscles during shortening, while isometric, and during lengthening. J. Appl. Physiol. 95 (2), 455–459.

Fede, C., Albertin, G., Petrelli, L., Sfriso, M.M., Biz, C., De Caro, R., et al., 2016. Expression of the endocannabinoid receptors in human fascial tissue. Eu. J. Histochem. 60 (2), 2643. https://doi.org/10.4081/ejh.2016.2643.

Fede, C., Angelini, A., Stern, R., Macchi, V., Porzionato, A., Ruggieri, P., De Caro, R., 2018. Quantification of hyaluronan in human fasciae: variations with function and anatomical site. J. Anat. 233 (4), 552–556.

Fede, C., Pirri, C., Petrelli, L., Guidolin, D., Fan, C., De Caro, R., et al., 2020. Sensitivity of the fasciae to the endocannabinoid system: production of hyaluronan-rich vesicles and potential peripheral effects of cannabinoids in fascial tissue. Int. J. Mol. Sci. 21 (8), 2936. doi:10.3390/ijms21082936.

Ferber, R., Osternig, L., Gravelle, D., 2002. Effect of PNF stretch techniques on knee flexor muscle EMG activity in older adults. J. Electromyograp. Kinesiol. 12, 391–397.

Fernández-de-Las-Peñas, C., Dommerholt, J., 2018. International consensus on diagnostic criteria and clinical considerations of myofascial trigger points: a delphi study. Pain Med 19 (1), 142–150. doi:10.1093/pm/pnx207.

Fornari, M., Carnevali, L., Sgoifo, A., 2017. Single osteopathic manipulative therapy session dampens acute autonomic and neuroendocrine responses to mental stress in healthy male participants. J. Am. Osteopath. Assoc. 117, 559–567. doi:10.7556/jaoa.2017.110.

Fourie, W., 2009. Fascial Research II: Basic Science and Implications for Conventional and Complementary Health Care. Elsevier GmbH, Munich.

Fourie, W.J., Robb, K., 2009. Physiotherapy management of axillary web syndrome following breast cancer treatment: discussing the use of soft tissue techniques. Physiotherapy 95, 314–320.

Franklyn-Miller, A., Falvey, E., Clark, R., 2009. Fascial Research II: Basic Science and Implications for Conventional and Complementary Health Care. Elsevier GmbH, Munich.

Freitas, S.R., 2018. Does the fascia stiffness increase after stretching also occurs in human individuals? J. Appl. Physiol. 125 (2), 683. doi:10.1152/japplphysiol.00281.2018.

Fryer, G., 2006. Muscle energy. In: Chaitow, L. (Ed.), Techniques, edition 2. Churchill Livingstone, Edinburgh.

Fryer, G., 2017. Integrating osteopathic approaches based on biopsychosocial therapeutic mechanisms. Part 1: the mechanisms. Int. J. Osteopa. Med. 25, 30–41.

Fryer, G., Ruszkowski, W., 2004. The influence of contraction duration in muscle energy technique applied to the atlanto-axial joint. J. Osteopath. Med. 7 (2), 79–84.

Fryer, G., Fossum, C., 2010. Therapeutic mechanisms underlying muscle energy approaches. In: Fernández-de-las-Peñas, C., Arendt-Nielsen, L., Gerwin, R. (Eds.), Tension-type and Cervicogenic Headache: Pathophysiology, Diagnosis, and Management. Jones and Bartlett Publishers, Sudbury, MA, pp. 221–229.

Fryer, G., Morris, T., Gibbons, P., 2004. The relationship between palpation of thoracic paraspinal tissues and pressure sensitivity measured by a digital algometer. J. Osteopath. Med. 7, 64–69.

Fryer, G., Morris, T., Gibbons, P., 2005. The relationship between palpation of thoracic tissues and deep paraspinal muscle thickness. Int. J. Osteopath. Med. 8, 22–28.

Fryer, G., Morris, T., Gibbons, P., Briggs, A., 2006. The electromyographic activity of thoracic paraspinal muscles identified as abnormal with palpation. J. Manipulative Physiol. Ther. 29 (6), 437–447.

Fryer, G., Bird, M., Robbins, B., Fossum, C., Johnson, J.C., 2010. Resting electromyographic activity of deep thoracic transversospinalis muscles identified as abnormal with palpation. J. Am. Osteopath. Assoc. 110 (2), 61–68. doi:10.7556/jaoa.2010.110.2.61.

Fung, D.T., Wang, V.M., Laudier, D.M., Shine, J.H., Basta-Pljakic, J., Jepsen, K.J., et al., 2009. Subrupture tendon fatigue damage. J. Orthop. Res. 27 (2), 264–273.

Gajdosik, R.L., 2001. Passive extensibility of skeletal muscle: review of the literature with clinical implications. Clin. Biomech. 16, 85–101.

Giles, P.D., Hensel, K.L., Pacchia, C.F., Smith, M.L., 2013. Suboccipital decompression enhances heart rate variability indices of cardiac control in healthy subjects. J. Alternat. Complement. Med. 19, 92–96. doi:10.1089/acm.2011.0031.

Gillani, S.N., Ain, Q., Rehman, S.U., Masood, T., 2020. Effects of eccentric muscle energy technique versus static stretching exercises in the management of cervical dysfunction in upper cross syndrome: a randomised control trial. J. Pak. Med. Assoc. 70 (3), 394–398. doi:10.5455/JPMA.300417.

Glynn, A., Fiddler, H., 2009. The Physiotherapist's Pocket Guide to Exercise. Churchill Livingstone.

Goossens, N., Janssens, L., Caeyenberghs, K., Albouy, G., Brumagne, S., 2019. Differences in brain processing of proprioception related to postural control in patients with recurrent non-specific low back pain and healthy controls. Neuroimage Clin 23, 101881. doi:10.1016/j.nicl.2019.101881.

Greenman, P., 1996. Principles of Manual Medicine, second ed. Williams and Wilkins, Baltimore.

Greenman, P.E., 2003. Principles of Manual Medicine, third ed. Williams & Wilkins, Lippincott.

Grenfell, J., Soundy, A., 2022. 2022. People's experience of shared decision making in musculoskeletal physiotherapy: a systematic review and thematic synthesis. Behav. Sci, (Basel). 12 (1), 12. doi:10.3390/bs12010012.

Grieve, G., 1986. Modern Manual Therapy. Churchill Livingstone, London.

Guimarães, C.F., Gasperini, L., Marques, A.P., Reis, R.L., 2020. The stiffness of living tissues and its implications for tissue engineering. Nat. Rev. Mater. 5, 351–370. https://doi.org/10.1038/s41578-019-0169-1.

Havas, E., Parviainen, T., Vuorela, J., Toivanen, J., Nikula, T., Vihko, V., 1997. Lymph flow dynamics in exercising human skeletal muscle as detected by scintography. J. Physiol. 504, 233–239.

Heinemeier, K.M., Olesen, J.L., Haddad, F., 2007. Expression of collagen and related growth factors in rat tendon and skeletal muscle in response to specific contraction types. J. Physiol. 582 (3), 1303–1316.

Herbert, R.D., Gandevia, S.C., 2019. The passive mechanical properties of muscle. J. Appl. Physiol. 126 (5), 1442–1444.

Herbert, R.D., Moseley, A.M., Butler, J.E., Gandevia, S.C., 2002. Change in length of relaxed muscle fascicles and tendons with knee and ankle movement in humans. J. Physiol. (Lond) 539, 637–645.

Hidalgo, B., Hall, T., Bossert, J., Dugeny, A., Cagnie, B., Pitance, L., 2017. The efficacy of manual therapy and exercise for treating non-specific neck pain: a systematic review. J. Back Musculoskelet. Rehabil. 30 (6), 1149–1169.

Hlaing, S.S., Puntumetakul, R., Wanpen, S., Boucaut, R., 2020. Balance control in patients with subacute non-specific low back pain, with and without lumbar instability: a cross-sectional study. J. Pain Res. 13, 795–803. https://doi.org/10.2147/JPR.S232080.

Hodges, P.W., Danneels, L., 2019. Changes in structure and function of the back muscles in low back pain: different time points, observations, and mechanisms. J. Orthop. Sports. Phys. Ther. 49 (6), 464–476. doi:10.2519/jospt.2019.8827.

Hoeger Bement, M.K., Weyer, A., Hartley, S., Hunter, S.K., 2008. Dose response of isometric contractions on pain perception in healthy adults. Med. Sci. Sports Exerc. 40 (11), 1880–1889.

Hoeger Bement, M.K., Weyer, A., Hartley, S., Drewek, B., Harkins, A.L., Hunter, S.K., 2011. Pain perception after isometric exercise in women with fibromyalgia. Arch. Phys. Med. Rehabil. 92, 89–95.

Hunt, G., Legal, L., 2010. Comparative study on the efficacy of thrust and muscle energy techniques in the piriformis muscle. Osteopatía. Scientífica. 5 (2), 47–55.

Huxley, A.F., Niedergerke, R., 1954. Structural changes in muscle during contraction: interference microscopy of living muscle fibres. Nature 173 (4412), 971–973.

Ingber, D., 2008. Tensegrity and mechanotransduction. J. Bodyw. Mov. Ther. 12 (3), 198–200.

Iqbal, M., Riaz, H., Ghous, M., Masood, K., 2020. Comparison of spencer muscle energy technique and passive stretching in adhesive capsulitis: a single blind randomised control trial. J. Pak. Med. Assoc. 70 (12(A)), 2113–2118. doi:10.5455/JPMA.23971.

Janda, V., 1983. Muscle Function Testing. Butterworths, London.

Janda, V., 1988. Muscles and cervicogenic pain syndromes. In: Grant, R. (Ed.), Physical Therapy in the Cervical and Thoracic Spine. Churchill Livingstone, New York.

Janda, V., 1993. Presentation to Physical Medicine Research Foundation, Montreal, Oct 9–11.

Janda, V., 1996. Evaluation of muscular imbalances. In: Liebenson, C. (Ed.), Rehabilitation of the Spine. Williams and Wilkins, Baltimore.

Janda, V., Frank, C., Liebenson, C., 2006. Evaluation of muscular imbalance. In: Liebenson, C. (Ed.), Rehabilitation of the Spine, second ed. Lippincott Williams and Wilkins, Baltimore.

Jensen, D., Duffinc, J., Lamd, Y.M., et al., 2008. Physiological mechanisms of hyperventilation during human pregnancy. Respir. Physiol. Neurobiol. 161, 76–86.

Jones, R., 2001. Pelvic Floor Muscle Rehabilitation. Urology News 5 (5), 2–4.

Joshi, T.M., Wani, S.K., Ashok, S., 2017. Immediate effects of two different types of muscle energy techniques (MET) on hamstring muscle flexibility in young healthy females: a comparative study. Int. J. Health Sci. Res. 7 (5).

Kaltenborn, F., 1985. Mobilization of the Extremity Joints. Olaf Norlis Bokhandel, Oslo.

Kamaleri, Y., Natvig, B., Ihlebaek, C.M., Benth, J.S., Bruusgaard, D., 2008. Number of pain sites is associated with demographic, lifestyle, and health-related factors in the general population. Eur. J. Pain. 12 (6), 742–748.

Kansagara, P.R., Patel, J.K., 2019. Muscle energy technique for sacroiliac joint dysfunction–an evidence based practice. Exec. Ed 13 (2), 122.

Kappler, R.E., Jones, J.M., 2003. Thrust (High-Velocity/Low-Amplitude) techniques. In: Ward, R.C. (Ed.), Foundations for Osteopathic Medicine, second ed. Lippincott, Williams & Wilkins, Philadelphia, pp. 852–880.

Khan, K.M., Scott, A., 2009. Mechanotherapy: how physical therapists' prescription of exercise promotes tissue repair. Br. J. Sports Med. 43, 247–251.

Kisilewicz, A., Urbaniak, M., Kawczyński, A., 2018. Effect of muscle energy technique on increased calf muscle stiffness after eccentric exercise in athletes. Antropomotoryka. J. Kinesiol. Exer. Sci. 81 (28), 21–29. doi:10.5604/01.3001.0012.7985.

Klingler, W., Schleip, R., Zorn, A., 2004. European Fascia Research Project Report. 5th World Congress Low Back and Pelvic Pain. Melbourne November 2004.

Knebl, J., 2002. Improving functional ability in the elderly via the Spencer technique, an osteopathic manipulative treatment: a randomised, clinical trial. J. Am. Osteopath. Assoc. 102 (7), 387–400.

Komendatov, G., 1945. Proprioceptivije refl exi glaza i golovy u krolikov. Fiziologiceskij Zurnal 31, 62.

Konrad, A., Reiner, M.M., Thaller, S., Tilp, M., 2019. The time course of muscle-tendon properties and function responses of a five-minute static stretching exercise. Eur. J. Sport Sci. 19 (9), 1195–1203. doi:10.1080/17461391.2019.1580319.

Kozlovskaya, I., Sayenko, I., Sayenko, D., 2007. Role of support afferentation in control of the tonic muscle activity. Acta Astronautica 60, 285–294.

Kozyrina, A.N., Piskova, T., Di Russo, J., 2020. Mechanobiology of epithelia from the perspective of extracellular matrix heterogeneity. Front. Bioeng, Biotechnol. doi:10.3389/fbioe.2020.596599.

Kuchera, W.A., Kuchera, M.L., 1992. Osteopathic Principles in Practice, second ed. KCOM Press, Kirksville, MO.

Küçükşen, S., Yilmaz, H., Sallı, A., Uğurlu, H., 2013. Muscle energy technique versus corticosteroid injection for management of chronic lateral epicondylitis: randomised controlled trial with 1-year follow-up. Arch. Phys. Med. Rehab. 94 (11), 2068–2074.

Langevin, H., 2009. Fascial Research II: Basic Science and Implications for Conventional and Complementary Health Care. Elsevier GmbH, Munich.

Langevin, H., 2010a. Tissue stretch induces nuclear remodeling in connective tissue fibroblasts Histochem. Cell Biol 133 (4), 405–415.

Langevin, H., 2010b, Presentation: Ultrasound Imaging of Connective Tissue Pathology Associated With Chronic Low Back Pain. 7th Interdisciplinary Congress on Low Back & Pelvic Pain Los Angeles, 11 November 2010.

Langevin, H., 2011. Integrative pain medicine. In: Audette, J.F., Bailey, A. (Eds.), The Science and Practice of Complementary and Alternative Medicine in Pain Management (Contemporary Pain Medicine). Humana Press, New York.

Langevin, H., Bouffard, N., Badger, G., et al., 2005. Dynamic fibroblast cytoskeletal response to subcutaneous tissue stretch ex vivo and in vivo. Am. J. Physiol. Cell Physiol. 288, C747–C756.

Langevin, H., Cornbrooks, C., Taatjes, D., 2004. Fibroblasts form a body-wide cellular network. Histochem. Cell Biol. 122 (1), 7–15.

Langevin, H.M., Bouffard, N.A., Badger, G.J., Iatridis, J.C., Howe, A.K., 2005. Dynamic fibroblast cytoskeletal response to subcutaneous tissue stretch ex vivo and in vivo. Am. J. Phys. Cell Physiol. 288, C747–C756.

Langevin, H.M., 2020. Reconnecting the brain with the rest of the body in musculoskeletal pain research. J. Pain. 22 (1), 1–8.

Larson, D.J., Menezes, P.G., Brown, S.H.M., 2020. Influence of creep deformation on sub-regional lumbar spine motion during manual lifting. Ergonomics 63 (10), 1304–1311. doi:10.1080/00140139.2020.1774666.

LaStayo, P., Marcus, R., Dibble, L., Frajacomo, F., Lindstedt, S., 2014. Eccentric exercise in rehabilitation: safety, feasibility, and application. J. Appl. Physiol. 116 (11), 1426–1434.

Law, R.Y., Harvey, L.A., Nicholas, M.K., Tonkin, L., De Sousa, M., Finniss, D.G., 2009. Stretch exercises increase tolerance to stretch in patients with chronic musculoskeletal pain: a randomised controlled trial. Phys. Ther. 89, 1016–1026.

Lederman, E., 1997. Fundamentals of Manual Therapy. Churchill Livingstone, London.

Lederman, E., 2017. A process approach in osteopathy: beyond the structural model. Int. J. Osteopath. Med. 23, 22–35.

Lederman, I., 2005. The Science and Practice of Manual Therapy, second ed. Churchill Livingstone, Edinburgh.

Lemke, S.B., Schnorrer, F., 2017. Mechanical forces during muscle development. Mech. Develop. 144, 92–101.

Lenehan, K., Fryer, G., McLaughlin, P., 2003. Effect of MET on gross trunk range of motion. J. Osteopath. Med. 6 (1), 13–18.

Lewit, K., 1986. Postisometric relaxation in combination with other methods of muscular facilitation and inhibition. Man. Med. 2, 101–104.

Lewit, K., 1999. Manipulation in Rehabilitation of the Locomotor System, third ed. Butterworths, London.

Li, L., Patel, N., Solomonow, D., Le, P., Hoops, H., Gerhardt, D., et al., 2007. Neuromuscular response to cyclic lumbar twisting. Hum. Fact. 49 (5), 820–829.

Licciardone, J.C., Buchanan, S., Hensel, K.L., King, H.H., Fulda, K.G., Stoll, S.T., 2010. Osteopathic manipulative treatment of back pain and related symptoms during pregnancy: a randomised controlled trial. Am. J. Obstetr. Gynecol. 202, 43.e1–43.e8.

Licciardone, J.C., Schultz, M.J., Amen, B., 2020. Osteopathic manipulation in the management of chronic pain: current perspectives. J. Pain Res. 20 (13), 1839–1847. doi:10.2147/JPR.S183170.

Liebenson, C., 1989. Active muscular relaxation methods. J. Manip. Physiol. Ther. 12 (6), 446–451.

Liebenson, C., 2006. Rehabilitation of the Spine, second ed. Williams and Wilkins, Baltimore.

Lin, J.P., Brown, J.K., Walsh, E.G., 1994. Physiological maturation of muscles in childhood. Lancet, 1386–1389.

Lin, J.P., Nardocci, N., 2016. Recognising the common origins of dystonia and the development of human movement: a manifesto of unmet needs in isolated childhood dystonias. Front. Neurol. 7, 226.

Linke, W.A., 2018. Titin gene and protein functions in passive and active muscle. Ann. Rev. Physiol. 80, 389–411.

Lisberger, S., Pavelko, T.A., Broussard, D.M., 1994. Responses during eye movement of brain stem neurons that receive monosynaptic inhibition from the flocculus and ventral paraflocculus in monkeys. J. Neurophysiol. 72 (2), 909–927.

Lynders, C., 2019. The critical role of development of the transversus abdominis in the prevention and treatment of low back pain. HSS J 15 (3), 214–220.

Magnusson, S., Simonsen, E.B., Aagaard, P., Dyhre-Poulsen, P., McHugh, M.P., Kjaer, M., 1996a. Mechanical and physiological responses to stretching with and without pre-isometric contraction in human skeletal muscle. Arch. Phys. Med. Rehab. 77, 373–377.

Magnusson, S.P., Simonsen, E.B., Aagaard, P., 1996b. Biomechanical responses to repeated stretches in human hamstring muscle in vivo. Am. J. Sports Med. 24, 622–628.

Magnusson, S.P., Simonsen, E.B., Aagaard, P., Sorensen, H., Kjaer, M., 1996c. A mechanism for altered flexibility in human skeletal muscle. J. Physiol. 497 (1), 291–298.

Mahato, N.K., 2019. Reviewing complex static-dynamic concepts of spine stability: does the spine care only to be stiff to be stable? J. Morphol. Sci. 36 (4), 309–316.

Marcucci, L., Washio, T., Yanagida, T., 2019. Proposed mechanism for the length dependence of the force developed in maximally activated muscles. Sci. Rep. 9 (1), 1–13.

McPartland, J.B., 2008. Expression of the endocannabinoid system in fibroblasts and myofascial tissues. J. Bodyw. Mov. Ther. 12 (2), 169.

Mense, S., Simons, D., Russell, I.J., 2001. Muscle Pain 6. Williams and Wilkins, Philadelphia.

Milliken, K., 2003. The Effects pf Muscle Energy Technique on Psoas Major Length. Unpublished Thesis, Unitec New Zealand, Auckland, New Zealand.

Mitchell Jr., F., 1998. The Muscle Energy Manual Vol. 2. MET Press, East Lansing, Michigan, p. 1.

Mitchell Jr., F., 2009. Interview. In: Franke, H. (Ed.), The History of MET. Muscle Energy Technique History-Model-Research. Verband der Osteopathen Deutschland, Wiesbaden.

Mitchell, U.H., Myrer, J.W., Hopkins, J.T., Hunter, I., Feland, J.B., Hilton, S.C., 2007. Acute stretch perception alteration contributes to the success of the PNF 'contract-relax' stretch. J. Sport Rehab 16, 85–92.

Mitchell, U.H., Myrer, J.W., Hopkins, J.T., Hunter, I., Feland, J.B., Hilton, S.C., 2009. Neurophysiological reflex mechanisms' lack of contribution to the success of PNF stretches. J. Sport Rehab. 18, 343–357.

Mizuno, T., Umemura, Y., 2016. Dynamic stretching does not change the stiffness of the muscle-tendon unit. Int. J. Sports Med. 37 (13), 1044–1050.

Moore, S., Laudner, K., Mcloda, T., Shaffer, M.A., 2011. The immediate effects of muscle energy technique on posterior shoulder tightness: a randomised controlled trial. J. Orthop Sports Phys. Ther. 41 (6), 400–407.

Muhsen, A., Moss, P., Gibson, W., Walker, B., Jacques, A., Schug, S., Wright, A., 2019. The association between conditioned pain modulation and manipulation-induced analgesia in people with lateral epicondylalgia. Clin. J. Pain. 35 (5), 435–442. doi:10.1097/AJP.0000000000000696.

Mukund, K., Subramaniam, S., 2019. Skeletal muscle: a review of molecular structure and function, in health and disease. Wiley Interdiscip. Rev. Syst. Biol. Med. 12 (1), e1462. doi:10.1002/wsbm.1462.

Mukund, K., Subramaniam, S., 2020. Skeletal muscle: a review of molecular structure and function, in health and disease. Wiley Interdiscip. Rev. Syst. Biol. Med. 12 (1), e1462. doi:10.1002/wsbm.1462.

Murphy, D., Hurwitz, E., Gregory, A., 2006. Nonsurgical approach to the management of patients with cervical radiculopathy. J. Manipulative Physiol. Ther. 29, 279–287.

Murphy, D., Hurwitz, E., McGovern, E., 2009. A nonsurgical approach to the management of patients with lumbar radiculopathy secondary to herniated disk: a prospective observational cohort study with follow-up. J. Manipulative Physiol. Ther. 32, 723–733.

Murthy, S.E., Dubin, A.E., Whitwam, T., Jojoa-Cruz, S., Cahalan, S.M., Mousavi, S.A.R., et al., 2018a. OSCA/TMEM63 are an evolutionarily conserved family of mechanically activated ion channels. Elife 7, e41844. doi:10.7554/eLife.41844.

Murthy, S.E., Loud, M.C., Daou, I., Marshall, K.L., Schwaller, F., Kühnemund, J., et al., 2018b. The mechanosensitive ion channel Piezo2 mediates sensitivity to mechanical pain in mice. Sci. Transl. Med. 10 (462), aat9897. doi:10.1126/scitranslmed.aat9897.

Myers, T., 2009. Anatomy Trains, second ed. Elsevier, Churchill Livingstone, Edinburgh.

Nagrale, A., Glynn, P., Joshi, A., Ramteke, G., 2010. Efficacy of an integrated neuromuscular inhibition technique on upper trapezius trigger points in subjects with non-specific neck pain: a randomised controlled trial. J. Man. Manip. Ther. 18 (1), 38.

Naweed, J., Razzaq, M., Sheraz, S., Anwar, N., Sadiq, N., Naweed, S., 2020. Comparison of active isolated stretch and post isometric relaxation for improving hamstring flexibility in young healthy adults. PAFMJ 70 (3), 770–775. https://www.pafmj.org/index.php/PAFMJ/article/view/4658.

Nordez, A., Guevel, A., Casari, P., Catheline, S., Cornu, C., 2009. Assessment of muscle hardness changes induced by a submaximal fatiguing isometric contraction. J. Electromyogr. Kinesiol. 19, 484–491.

Norris, C., 1999. Functional load abdominal training. J. Bodyw. Mov. Ther. 3, 150–158.

Norris, C., 2000. The muscle designation debate: the experts respond. Response from Chris Norris. J. Bodyw. Mov. Ther. 4 (4), 225–241.

Nugraha, M.H.S., Antari, N.K.A.J., Saraswati, N.L.P.G.K., 2020. The efficacy of muscle energy technique in individuals with mechanical neck pain: a systematic review. Sport Fit. J. 8 (2), 91–98.

Olivo, S.A., Magee, D.J., 2006. Electromyographic assessment of the activity of the masticatory using the agonist contract-antagonist relax technique (AC) and contracterelax technique (CR). Man. Ther. 11, 136e145.

Onifer, S.M., Sozio, R.S., Long, C.R., 2019. Role for endocannabinoids in spinal manipulative therapy analgesia? Evid. Based Complement. Alternat. Med. 2019.

Park, S., Lim, W., 2020. Effects of proprioceptive neuromuscular facilitation stretching at low-intensities with standing toe touch on developing and maintaining hamstring flexibility. J. Bodyw. Mov. Ther. 24 (4), 561–567.

Parmar, S., Shyam, A., Sabnis, S., Sancheti, P., 2011. The effect of isolytic contraction and passive manual stretching on pain and knee range of motion after hip surgery: a prospective, double-blinded, randomised study. Hong Kong Physiother. J. 29, 25–30.

Parsons, J., Marcer, N., 2005. Osteopathy: Models for Diagnosis, Treatment an Practice. Churchill Livingstone, Edinburgh.

Pfluegler, G., Kasper, J., Luedtke, K., 2020. The immediate effects of passive joint mobilisation on local muscle function. A systematic review of the literature. Musculoskel. Sci. Pract. 45, 102106.

Phadke, A., Bedekar, N., Shyam, A., Sancheti, P., 2016. Effect of muscle energy technique and static stretching on pain and functional disability in patients with mechanical neck pain: a randomised controlled trial. Hong Kong Physiother. J. 35, 5–11.

Poulsen, E., Hartvigsen, J., Christensen, H.W., Roos, E.M., Vach, W., Overgaard, S., 2013. Patient education with or without manual therapy compared to a control group in patients with osteoarthritis of the hip. A proof-of-principle three-arm parallel group randomised clinical trial. Osteoarthritis Cartilage 21 (10). 1494e1503. https://doi.org/10.1016/j.joca.2013.06.009.

Rabia, K., Nasir, R.H., Hassan, D., 2019. Immediate effect of muscle energy technique in comparison with passive stretching on hamstring flexibility of healthy individuals: a randomised clinical trial. Isra Med. J. 11 (4)-Part B, 310–313.

Rajadurai, V., 2011. The effect of muscle energy technique on temporomandibular joint dysfunction: a randomised clinical trial. Asian J. Sci. Res. 4, 71–77.

Ranade, S.S., Woo, S.-H., Dubin, A.E., Moshourab, R.A., Wetzel, C., Petrus, M., et al., 2014. Piezo2 is the major transducer of mechanical forces for touch sensation in mice. Nature 516 (7529), 121–125. doi:10.1038/nature13980.

Rassier, D.E., 2017. Sarcomere mechanics in striated muscles: from molecules to sarcomeres to cells. Am. J. Physiol.-Cell Physiol. 313 (2), C134–C145.

Retchford, T.H., Crossley, K.M., Grimaldi, A., Kemp, J.L., Cowan, S.M., 2013. Can local muscles augment stability in the hip? A narrative literature review. J. Musculoskelet. Neuronal. Interact. 13 (1), 1–12.

Richardson, C., 2000. The muscle designation debate: the experts respond. J. Bodyw. Mov. Ther. 4 (4), 235–236.

Richardson, C., Jull, G., Toppenberg, R., Comeford, M., 1992. Techniques for active lumbar stabilization for spinal protection. Aust. J Phys. 38, 105–112.

Richardson, C., Jull, G., Hodges, P., Hides, J., 1999. Therapeutic Exercise for Spinal Segmental Stabilization in Low Back Pain. Churchill Livingstone, Edinburgh.

Rowlands, A.V., Marginson, V.F., Lee, J., 2003. Chronic flexibility gains: effect of isometric contraction duration during proprioceptive neuromuscular facilitation stretching techniques. Res. Quart. Exer. Sport 74, 47e51.

Rowlerson, A., Pope, B., Murray, J., Whalen, R.B., Weeds, A.G., 1981. A novel myosin present in cat jaw-closing muscles. J. Muscle. Res. Cell. Motil. 2 (4), 415–438.

Ruddy, T., 1962. Osteopathic rapid rhythmic resistive technic. Acad. Appl. Osteopath Yearbook. Carmel, CA.

Sánchez-Zuriaga, D., Adams, M.A., Dolan, P., 2010. Is activation of the back muscles impaired by creep or muscle fatigue? Spine 35 (5), 517–525.

Sandhouse, M., 2011. Glossary of Osteopathic Terminology. American Association of Colleges of Osteopathic Medicine.

Schiaffino, S., Reggiani, C., 2011. Fiber types in mammalian skeletal muscles. Physiol. Rev. 91 (4), 1447–1531.

Schleip, R., Naylor, I.L., Ursu, D., Melzer, W., Zorn, A., Wilke, H.J., et al., 2006. Passive muscle stiffness may be influenced by active contractility of intramuscular connective tissue. Med. Hypoth. 66, 66–71.

Schleip, R., Gabbiani, G., Wilke, J., Naylor, I., Hinz, B., Zorn, A., et al., 2019. Fascia is able to actively contract and may thereby influence musculoskeletal dynamics: a histochemical and mechanographic investigation. Front. Physiol. 10, 336.

Schleip, R., Duerselen, L., Vleeming, A., Naylor, I.L., Lehmann-Horn, F., Zorn, A., et al., 2012. Strain hardening of fascia: static stretching of dense fibrous connective tissues can induce a temporary stiffness increase accompanied by enhanced matrix hydration. J. Bodyw. Mov. Ther. 16 (1), 94–100.

Schuermans, J., Van Tiggelen, D., Witvrouw, E., 2017. Prone hip extension muscle recruitment is associated with hamstring injury risk in amateur soccer. Int. J. Sports Med. 38 (9), 696–706.

Schwerla, F., Hinse, T., Klosterkamp, M., Schmitt, T., Rütz, M., Resch, K.L., 2020. Osteopathic treatment of patients with shoulder pain. A pragmatic randomised controlled trial. J. Bodyw. Mov. Ther. 24 (3), 21–28.

Schwind, P., 2006. Fascial and Membrane Technique. Churchill Livingstone, Edinburgh.

Sewani, R., Shinde, S., 2017. Effect of hot moist pack and muscle energy technique in subjects with sacro-iliac joint dysfunction. Int. J. Sci. Res. 6 (2), 669–672.

Shadmehr, A., Hadian, M.R., Naiemi, S.S., Jalaie, S., 2009. Hamstring flexibility in young women following passive stretch and muscle energy technique. J. Back Musculoskelet. Rehabil. 22 (3), 143–148.

Sheard, P., Smith, P., Paine, T., 2009. Athlete compliance to therapist requested contraction intensity during proprioceptive neuromuscular facilitation. Man. Ther. 14 (5), 539–543.

Shoup, D., 2006. An osteopathic approach to performing arts medicine. Phys. Med. Rehabil. Clin. N. Am. 17, 853–864.

Simons, D., 2002. Understanding effective treatments of myofascial trigger points. J. Bodyw. Mov. Ther. 6 (2), 81–88.

Singh, S., Kaushal, K., 2020. Change in hamstrings flexibility: a comparison between three different manual therapeutic techniques in normal individuals. Adesh Uni. J. Med. Sci. Res. 2 (1), 49–51.

Smith, M., Fryer, G., 2008. Comparison of two MET techniques for increasing flexibility of the hamstring muscle group. J. Bodyw. Mov. Ther. 12 (4), 312–317.

Smith, M.S., Olivas, J., Smith, K., 2019. Manipulative therapies: what works. Am. Fam. Phys. 99 (4), 248–252.

Solomonow, M., 2009. Ligaments: a source of musculoskeletal disorders. J. Bodyw. Mov. Ther. 13 (2), 136–154.

Solomonow, M., 2011. Time dependent spine stability. Clin. Biomech. 26 (3), 219–228.

Solomonow, M., Baratta, R.V., Banks, A., Freudenberger, C., Zhou, B.H., 2003. Flexion-relaxation response to static lumbar flexion in males and females. Clin. Biomech. (Bristol, Avon) 18 (4), 273–279.

Solomonow, M., Bing He Zhou, E.E., Yun, L., King, K.B., 2011. Acute repetitive lumbar syndrome. J. Bodyw. Mov. Ther. 16 (2), 134–147.

Stecco, A., Busoni, F., Stecco, C., Mattioli-Belmonte, M., Soldani, P., Condino, S., Ermolao, A., Zaccaria, M., Gesi, M., 2015. Comparative ultrasonographic evaluation of the Achilles paratenon in symptomatic and asymptomatic subjects: an imaging study. Surg. Radiol. Anat. 37, 281–285.

Stecco, A., Gesi, M., Stecco, C., Stern, R., 2013. Fascial components of the myofascial pain syndrome. Curr. Pain Headache Rep. 17, 1–10.

Stecco, C., Fede, C., Petrelli, L., Biz, C., Macchi, V., Stern, R., et al., 2017. Fasciacytes: specialised fibroblast-like cells that secrete the hyaluronan-rich matrix in fascial tissue. Ital. J. Anat. Embryol. 122 (1), 206.

Stecco, C., Pirri, C., Fede, C., Yucesoy, C.A., Caro, R.D., Stecco, A., 2021. Fascial or muscle stretching? A narrative review. Appl. Sci. 11 (1), 307.

Stecco, C., Porzionato, A., Lancerotto, L., Stecco, A., Macchi, V., Day, J.A., et al., 2008. Histological study of the deep fasciae of the limbs. J. Bodyw. Mov. Ther. 12, 225–230.

Stecco, L., Stecco, C., 2009. Fascial Manipulation: Practical Part. Piccin, Italy.

Stenersen, B., Bordoni, B., 2022. Osteopathic Manipulative Treatment: Muscle Energy Procedure - Cervical Vertebrae. In: StatPearls. StatPearls Publishing. Treasure Island, FL.

Stiles, E., 2009. The origin of muscle energy techniques. In: Franke, H. (Ed.), Muscle Energy Technique History-Model-Research. Verband der Osteopathen Deutschland, Wiesbaden.

Surbeck, U., Pfeiffer, F., Hotz-Boendermaker, S., 2020. How Do Pain-Response Patterns Influence the Course of Acute Low Back Pain? A Longitudinal Cohort Study.

Szeto, G.P.Y., Straker, L.M., O'Sullivan, P.B., 2009. During computing tasks symptomatic female office workers demonstrate a trend towards higher cervical postural muscle load than asymptomatic office workers: an experimental study. Aust. J. Physiother. 55, 257–262.

Thomas, E., Cavallaro, A.R., Mani, D., Bianco, A., Palma, A., 2019. The efficacy of muscle energy techniques in symptomatic and asymptomatic subjects: a systematic review. Chiropr. Man. Ther. 27 (1), 35.

Tousignant-Laflamme, Y., Martel, M.O., Joshi, A.B., Cook, C.E., 2017. Cook. Rehabilitation management of low back pain–it's time to pull it all together! J. Pain Res. 10, 2373.

Tramontano, M., Cerritelli, F., Piras, F., Spanò, B., Tamburella, F., Piras, F., et al., 2020. Brain connectivity changes after osteopathic manipulative treatment: a randomised manual placebo-controlled trial. Brain Sci. 10 (12), 969. https://doi.org/10.3390/brainsci10120969.

Tripodi, N., Garrett., A., Savic., D., Sadrani, K., Robertson, L., Volarich, S., et al., 2021. Patient expectations of manual and non-manual therapy within an osteopathic consultation: a cross-sectional study. Int. J. Osteop. Med. 39, 41–46. https://doi.org/10.1016/j.ijosm.2020.08.002.

Vaegter, H.B., Jones, M.D., 2020. Exercise-induced hypoalgesia after acute and regular exercise: experimental and clinical manifestations and possible mechanisms in individuals with and without pain. Pain Rep 5 (5).

Verbeek, J., Sengers, M.J., Riemens, L., Haafkens, J., 2004. Patient expectations of treatment for back pain: a systematic review of qualitative and quantitative studies. Spine (Phila Pa 1976) 29 (20), 2309–2318.

Viceconti, Geri, T., A., Minacci, M., Testa, M., Rossettini, G., 2019. Manual therapy: exploiting the role of human touch. Musculoskelet. Sci. Pract. 44, 102044.

Voss, D.E., Marjorie, K.I., Beverly, J.M., Margaret, K., 1985. Proprioceptive Neuromuscular Facilitation: Patterns and Techniques. Harper & Row, Philadelphia, PA.

Vulfsons, S., Minerbi, A., 2020. The case for comorbid myofascial pain – a qualitative review. Int. J. Environ. Res. Public Health. 17 (14), 5188.

Waddell, G., Burton, A.K., 2005. Concepts of rehabilitation for the management of low back pain. Best Pract. Res. Clin. Rheumatol. 19 (4), 655–670.

Wagh, S.D., W., Kadam, N., 2020. Effect of eccentric training and isolytic contraction to improve flexibility of quadriceps in recreational marathoners. Int. J. Life Sci. Pharma Res. 10(3), 1–5.

Wall, M., Butler, D., El Haj, A., Bodle, J.C., Loboa, E.G., Banes, A.J., 2017. Key developments that impacted the field of mechanobiology and mechanotransduction. J. Orthop. Res. 36 (2), 605–619.

Wang, H.N., Huang, Y.C., Ni, G.X., 2020. Mechanotransduction of stem cells for tendon repair. World J. Stem Cells. 12 (9), 952.

Weig, D., 2020. Fascias: methodological propositions and ontologies that stretch and slide. Body Soc 26 (3), 94–109.

Wells, M.R., Giantinoto, S., D'agate, D., Areman, R.D., Fazzini, E.A., Dowling, D., et al., 1999. Standard osteopathic manipulative treatment acutely improves gait performance in patients with Parkinson's disease. JAOA February 99 (2), 92–98.

Wendt, M., Małgorzata, W., 2020. Evaluation of the combination of muscle energy technique and trigger point therapy in asymptomatic individuals with a latent trigger point. Int. J. Environ. Res. Public Health. 17 (22), 8430.

Weng, M., Lee, C., Chen, C., Hsu, J.J., Lee, W.D., Huang, M.H., et al., 2009. Effects of different stretching techniques on the outcome of isokinetic exercise in patients with knee arthritis. Kaohsiung J. Med. Sci. 25 (6), 306–315.

Weppler, C.H., Magnusson, S.P., 2010. Increasing muscle extensibility: a matter of increasing length or modifying sensation? Phys. Ther. 90 (3), 438–449.

Wewege, M.A., Jones, M.D., 2020. Exercise-induced hypo-algesia in healthy individuals and people with chronic musculoskeletal pain: a systematic review and meta-analysis. J. Pain 22 (1), 21–31.

Wilke, J., Schleip, R., Yucesoy, C.A., Banzer, W., 2018. Not merely a protective packing organ? A review of fascia and its force transmission capacity. J. Appl. Physiol. 124 (1), 234–244.

Wilson, E., Payton, O., Donegan-Shoaf, L., Dec, K., 2003. Muscle energy technique in patients with acute low back pain: a pilot clinical trial. J. Orthop. Sports Phys. Ther. 33 (9), 502–512.

Woo, S.-H., Lukacs, V., de Nooij, J.C., Zaytseva, D., Criddle, C.R., Francisco, A., et al., 2015. Piezo2 is the principal mechanotransduction channel for proprioception. Nat. Neurosci. 18 (12), 1756–1762. doi:10.1038/nn.4162.

Woo, S.L. -Y., 1987. Injury and repair of musculoskeletal soft tissues. American Academy of Orthopedic Surgeons Symposium, Savannah, Georgia.

Wright, P., Drysdale, I., 2008. A comparison of post-isometric relaxation (PIR) and reciprocal inhibition (RI) muscle energy techniques applied to piriformis. Int. J. Med. 11 (4), 158–159.

Yao, S.C., Hart, A.D., Terzella, M.J., 2013. An evidence-based osteopathic approach to Parkinson disease. Osteopath. Fam. Phys. 5 (3), 96–101.

Zügel, M., Maganaris, C.N., Wilke, J., Jurkat-Rott, K., Klingler, W., Wearing, S.C., et al., 2018. Fascial tissue research in sports medicine: from molecules to tissue adaptation, injury and diagnostics: consensus statement. Br. J Sports Med. 52 (23), 1497 –1497.

Zuil Escobar, J., Garcia del Pozo, M., Propin, G., 2010. Changes in pain threshold in myofascial trigger point after muscle energy technique. Rev. Soc. Esp. Dolor 17 (7), 313–319.

The History and Context of Muscle Energy Technique

Sasha Chaitow, Helge Franke[*]

CHAPTER CONTENTS

INTRODUCTION: WHY A HISTORY?

A history chapter in a book on technique application may seem extraneous. Some perspectives even consider that past approaches are best forgotten, their valuable, scientifically verified elements subsumed into modern evidence-based guidelines. After all, the historical conceptual frameworks of health and disease are considered outdated. Osteopathy grew out of vitalism and some of its practices have still deeper esoteric roots (Chaitow, 2020). Given its long path and achievement of validation by a large part of the medical establishment, these early origins are considered by some to be intensely important, but by others to be altogether embarrassing (indicatively McGrath, 2013; Vogel, 2021) or perceived as 'skeletons in the closet,' as termed in the recent (May 2022) history panel of the International Consortium of Manual Therapies inaugural conference. Sometimes this is due to their occasional use as justification for the continuation of outdated practices, historical misperceptions of what these professionals actually do, or for emphasising

tradition or even hagiographical personality cults over science – a point addressed at the end of this chapter.

This perspective is itself based on key mistaken impressions within the sciences regarding the role of histories in clinical practice. Firstly, there is an impression that explanations across disciplines (including the humanities) ought to follow the same deductive form as that of the natural sciences. Since they do not, they are considered either problematic or irrelevant. Secondly, they originate in a misconception that is over a century old, drawing on the ideas of William Osler (d. 1919), a Canadian doctor considered to be the father of modern medical practice. The Oslerian view, taken up by physicians with an interest in the history of medicine, saw the history of medicine as a source of models and guidance based on great physicians of the past, stripped of its wider context. Academic historians, in contrast, took the view that medical history is an ongoing process of inquiry that critically evaluates past and present medical approaches within their broader context. This divide led to two forms of medical history: internalist histories that look at medical progress in isolation from wider culture and society, frequently written by physicians without training in historical research, whereas academic histories by trained, specialised historians holistically investigate the many

---

[*] *The previous version of this chapter integrated here on pages 58–68 was contributed by Dr Helge Franke.*

factors that impact health, disease, patient narratives and the clinical encounter (Kushner, 2008).

In the case of manual therapies, an internalist history looks specifically at the development of a particular set of techniques, or profession, with only cursory outlines of the broader context of their evolution and impact. An academic history, on the other hand, takes a bird's eye view, factoring in the sociological, intellectual, cultural and political parameters, to explain not only the main highlights of the evolution of a technique but also the reasons and the forces impacting that evolution. In that sense, academic histories are the equivalent of holistic reasoning, whereas internalist ones are more closely comparable to focusing on the point of pain, and not the biopsychosocial whole. The crucial implication of internalist histories is that they overlook and dismiss the well-established direct value of holistic academic ones to clinical practice (Batistatou et al., 2010; Kollmer Horton, 2019; Wald et al., 2019).

With regard to muscle energy technique (MET), academic histories of medicine explain the driving forces motivating historical individuals such as Mitchell, Ruddy and the others mentioned in this chapter; how and why change occurs in practice, attitudes and methods, the relationship between medicine and society, and how principles impact actual events (Arabatzis, 2019). They also crucially support the understanding of what is practised, how, and why, raise critical awareness and recover neglected themes (Chang, 2017).

In modern medical education, histories of science and medicine alongside other Humanities disciplines are being integrated into standard curricula worldwide as part of the overall development of the Medical Humanities discussed in Chapter 1 (indicatively Gurtoo et al., 2013; Pentecost et al., 2018; Howick et al., 2022; Mi et al., 2022; Stouffer et al., 2021), though this has been impeded by these conflicting understandings of history (Kushner, 2008). Their significance is not solely academic, nor do they represent some misplaced reverence for specific forefathers or philosophies. A history of any given science, and especially of healthcare, is not a linear story of transmission of a practice in a vacuum. It shows us the messy, slow, human, interpersonal context in which ideas emerge, are forged, succeed or fail and the many complex layers of society and reality that shape such developments. It places health and disease back in society, where it originates. Acknowledging contributions and expertise should not be interpreted as undue

deference to an outdated tradition; rather, they show how dependent the present is on the past, including the fact that what we consider truth today, depended on a complex series of contingencies that might have turned out differently. The academic historian is able to weigh the significance of these contingencies and summarise them in a way that can inform current practice, rather than focusing on anecdotal, or event-specific detail that risks overshadowing the whole. This expands our understanding, rather than narrowing it (Chang, 2017), offers explanations and insight into why practice takes the shapes it does, and crucially, reveals ways to avoid old errors or find new paths.

When we scorn practices that research has correctly dropped by the wayside with an overly simplistic understanding by valuing presentist thinking over a more careful evaluation (see Box 3.1), we reduce our capacity for critical thinking, because learning such histories forces us to weigh multiple factors and develop higher reasoning skills. Awareness of uncertainty principles and the human efforts that underpin the development of any healing approach allows optimal application of such skills in a clinical setting, where we encounter equally complex people and their conditions. It is excellent training for the clinical reasoning process because the inquiry process for investigating history mirrors that of the patient narrative (Kollmer Horton, 2019), and also encourages humility as well as therapeutic scepticism (Batistatou et al., 2010). Thus, it becomes especially valuable for applying the whole-person approach and viewing people as narratives in all their complexity. Adapted academic historical training is therefore a valuable adjunct tool for manual therapy, as recent curriculum developments demonstrate.

The only thing separating social science from historical studies is time. Sociology, which considers the complexity of current human interactions, is a discipline

---

BOX 3.1   Presentism and Progressivism

In the terminology of historical studies, 'presentism' refers to an attitude that we are more enlightened in the present day than in the past and that anything past an undefined sell-by date is to be scorned. This grows out of 'progressivism' (not to be confused with its political connotations, here it is used as part of the philosophy of history), according to which human society is always evolving towards a more refined state, so the past is perceived as an imperfect version of the present (Chang, 2021).

without which the biopsychosocial model would never have developed. Interdisciplinary applications of both history and sociology, and indeed elements of literary studies, gave us Narrative Medicine as outlined in Chapter 1. Phenomena such as evidence nihilism also mentioned in that chapter, the character of debates such as those seen in social media contexts, and ideologically or commercially driven positions that create barriers to exchange and evolution may all be mitigated with the improved integration of such skills. More urgently, considering histories also allows us to see where severe errors have sometimes been made – albeit with good intent – and thus avoid or mitigate them when we encounter them (Wootton, 2006; Batistatou et al., 2010). These appear to be among the considerations driving a fresh appreciation of the role played by history both in osteopathy, and in numerous medical disciplines (Kollmer Horton, 2019; Zegarra-Parodi et al., 2021; Vogel & Zegarra-Parodi, 2022).

These are among the reasons that the original version of this chapter was commissioned for the fourth edition of this book. Originally intended to give credit where it is due for the evolution of MET and to provide insight into the development of its variations, it comprised a classic internalist history with its own value. Though there is little to add to the basic facts regarding the origins and development of MET, the past decade has seen growth in the evidence base and considerable interest in understanding the profile of osteopathic practice, which includes the frequency of application of the array of techniques available to osteopaths and regional differences in treatment preference. These are presented in Box 3.2. To interpret this data, we need today's sociology, and tomorrow's history, in a clear example of the value of these perspectives; thus in this revision, both this and Chapter 1 have been infused with elements of the academic historical perspective, to demonstrate the degree to which these approaches complement each other, and clinical application by extension. Further additions to this chapter include remarks on current debates and recent developments regarding manual therapy application in regard to their impact on this evolving field.

THE HISTORY OF MET

Thirty-five years ago, in a retrospective on the history of MET, Viola Fryman described one of its important characteristics:

Muscle energy technic was a combination of operator force and patient force. This you see began to give the idea that maybe the patient might be able to make a contribution to the treatment with a minimum of activity on the part of the operator.

Fryman also wrote that 'this took another few years to really penetrate our consciousness' (Fryman, 1987). Today this understanding is as important as 60 years ago when the history of MET began. In the context of whole-person healthcare, and ethical considerations discussed in Chapter 1, and throughout this book, the concept of patient contribution to treatment acquire far-reaching implications. Although the osteopathic approach to somatic dysfunction – a whole-body approach defined as 'an altered regulative function associated with inflammatory signs palpable in the body framework in different body regions that can be remote from the symptomatic area' (Tramontano et al., 2021) – has inhered elements of patient empowerment since its early inception, this takes on fresh importance in light of the renewed emphasis on whole-person care.

The Glossary of Osteopathic Terminology defines MET as follows:

A direct treatment method in which the patient's muscles are employed upon request, from a precisely controlled position, in a specific direction, and against a distinctly executed physician counterforce.
Educational Council on Osteopathic Principles and the American Association of Colleges of Osteopathic Medicine (2017, p. 37).

This short definition describes a technique which is widely recognised today in the world of manual therapy and which can look back on a 60-year history. Its philosophical principle is elegantly summarised as follows:

The aim of treatment, whether functional technique or structural technique is applied, is to re-establish motion that is consistent with the associated structure. The goal of manipulative therapy is harmonious motion. Motion is the added dimension to the structure.

Fred Mitchell Sr. (1967)

The published history of MET commenced with a short five-page article entitled 'The Balanced Pelvis

BOX 3.2 **Usage and Awareness of METs in Manual Therapy Professions**

Muscle energy techniques are used and applied by a wide variety of healthcare professionals, including osteopaths, physiotherapists, chiropractors, and massage therapists. In recent years several national and international surveys explored the profile of osteopathic practice and the degree to which MET is used in comparison to other osteopathic manipulation techniques (OMTs) and other approaches. Similar information is lacking for other professions, although the profile of the evidence base as cited throughout this book suggests that METs are widely known across these professions; however, data on their uptake and application is unknown.

A major systematic review investigated the international profile of osteopathic practice over the past decade (Ellwood & Carnes, 2021). Fourteen surveys met the inclusion criteria, representing Australia (Adams et al., 2018), Belgium/Luxembourg (van Dun et al., 2019b), Netherlands (van Dun et al., 2016), Italy, Spain (Alvarez et al., 2020; Alvarez-Bustins et al., 2018), Switzerland (Bill et al., 2020; Dubois et al., 2019; Vaucher et al., 2018), Canada, Germany (Dornieden, 2019) and the United Kingdom (Plunkett et al., 2020). Surveys of American osteopathic practice were not included in the study. The review reports a tendency towards gentler techniques (including OCF, visceral and functional methods) in Germany, Spain, the Benelux area and Switzerland. In these regions, MET use was respectively reported as 61% (Germany), 10% (very often); 90% (often) (Spain), and an average of approximately 36% (Benelux and Switzerland). In contrast, British and Australian osteopaths appear to prefer soft tissue and spinal manipulation/high velocity thrust (HVT) techniques. Frequent use of MET was reported by 79.5% of Australian osteopaths and 29% of British ones in the reviewed studies, the latter showing a marked preference for other soft tissue and mobilisation techniques. This figure is in line with a 2001 'snapshot survey' commissioned by the General Osteopathic Council (GOsC) in the UK that reported 26% of osteopaths used MET, but it diverges significantly from Fryer's 2010 survey of British osteopaths reporting that MET was always/frequently employed in the treatment of spinal, pelvic or sacroiliac dysfunctions in 60% of the treatments provided (Fryer et al., 2010). The reasons for this divergence are due to survey design: the GOsC survey asked for data on the number of patients in a given year who had received a given treatment, whereas Fryer's survey asked for respondents to self-report on the frequency with which they tend to employ one or other technique.

With regard to MET application in the United States, a 2003 study showed MET to be one of the three most commonly used techniques clinically applied by American osteopaths (Johnson & Kurtz, 2003). A web-based survey 6 years later (Fryer et al., 2009) involving members of the American Academy of Osteopathy reported that muscle energy technique was most commonly used in treatments of the pelvis and sacroiliac joint and that 70% of respondents stated their frequent use of the technique. In general, musculoskeletal/spinal complaints and back pain formed the majority of cases seen in these clinics, though within a study focusing on treatment choices within the osteopathic conceptual framework of somatic dysfunction (SD), MET seems to find application in 55.6% of cases where OMT techniques were implemented (Tramontano, 2020).

The search strategy used to investigate the usage of MET among osteopaths was replicated for other health professionals (physiotherapists, chiropractors, massage therapists) but these yielded a single preprint from Nigeria (Ahmed et al., 2019) investigating the knowledge of physiotherapists on MET use for non-specific low back pain. The study found that only 16.7% of the professionals surveyed had knowledge of MET application for non-specific low back pain, while similar studies profiling technique usage in other countries are lacking.

MET is integrated into the curricula of osteopathic colleges and reputable textbooks on osteopathy describe MET as one of its fundamental treatment methods (Ehrenfeuchter & Sandhouse, 2002). Though METs are known and applied by a variety of professionals and taught widely in the context of continuing professional development courses, data on their formal curricular inclusion are unknown as this and the question of actual clinical application do not appear to have been researched outside the osteopathic profession. In a recent (2022) development, one Greek university textbook (Fousekis, 2022) is known to include MET as a formal part of undergraduate physiotherapy training, but wider data on uptake and from other regions remains unknown.

and its Relationship to Reflexes' (Mitchell Sr., 1948) that appeared in the American Academy of Osteopathy (AAO) yearbook in 1948. It discussed the impact of pelvic dysfunction on human health:

That pelvic imbalance will prevent the normal function of the body in both directions; (toward the feet and toward the head) is, I believe, an accepted fact among us. Reflexes, the movement of lymph, the physiological movements of the spine, all depend on Pelvic Balance.

Mitchell Sr. (1948, p. 146)

The author was Fred Mitchell Sr, according to whom a reflex therapy could only be successfully applied after correcting any existing pelvic dysfunction (Greenman, 2003). Mitchell quoted Charles Owens' concept which he expanded with his own observations (Mitchell Jr. & Mitchell, 1999). Mitchell defined five pelvic and sacral dysfunctions, described the biomechanics and diagnoses and explained two thrust techniques for the treatment of these dysfunctions. The article caused a lot of controversy, especially with respect to the enormous importance Mitchell allocated to pelvic balance. For example, for him, even asthma was a pathological sign suggesting pelvic dysfunction (Mitchell Sr., 1948).

FRED L. MITCHELL SR'S APPROACH TO OSTEOPATHY

Frederic Lockwood Mitchell was 39 years old at that time. He had graduated 8 years earlier from the Chicago College of Osteopathy. Since then he had been working in his own practice in Tennessee. He had been influenced by the remarkable benefit to his son (Fred Jr) of the treatment offered by osteopathic physician, Charles Owen, 14 years previously (Stiles, 2009).

Prior to his entry into medicine, Mitchell was a businessman with a 5-year-old son who had been badly burned in a fire and was under medical care. The little boy experienced increasingly poor health until his kidneys started to fail and he was expected to die. His parents heard about Dr Owens who worked with Dr Chapman— the osteopath who developed 'Chapman's Reflexes'. Dr Owens employed the use of Chapman's Reflexes for Fred Jr's kidneys, adrenal glands and liver, with the result that the boy rapidly recovered (Magoun Jr., 2003).

Mitchell was convinced that this method had saved his son's life. He sold his business and became a student of Charles Owens. In 1937, Mitchell enrolled in the Chicago College of Osteopathic Medicine, where he successfully graduated in 1941.

The Origin of the Development of MET

The techniques, described in Mitchell's 1948 article, were conventional and complied with the repertoire of most osteopaths.

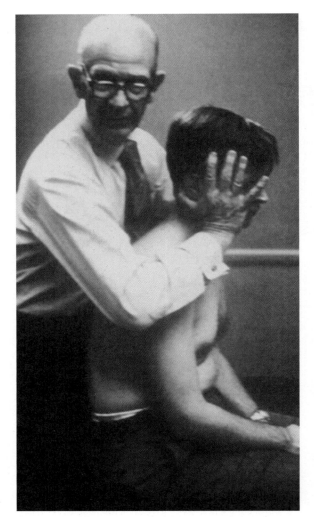

Fig. 3.1 Fred Mitchell Sr demonstrating treatment of acute torticollis, 1973.

According to Mitchell's 1948 paper, the techniques he had used previously to treat the pelvis were passive, mainly thrust (high velocity, low amplitude) procedures – the style of osteopathic manipulation learned in medical school for the treatment of vertebral, costovertebral, and extremity joints.

Soon, however, Mitchell's pelvic thrust techniques were replaced by techniques requiring the active participation of the patient, influenced by the work of osteopaths Ruddy and Kettler.

Mitchell Jr. (1993)

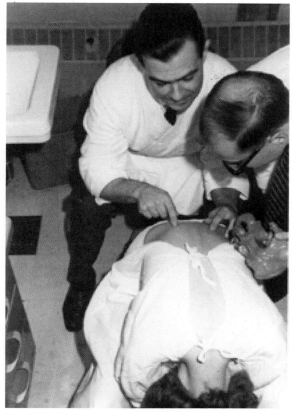

Fig. 3.2 Fred Mitchell Jr instructing a Kansas City student on physical examination of the pelvis, 1965.

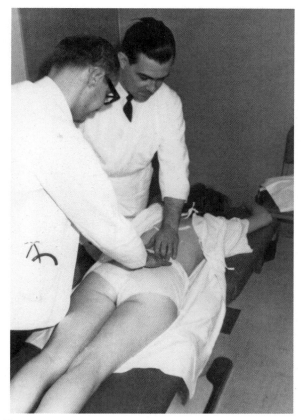

Fig. 3.3 Fred Mitchell Jr instructing a Kansas City student on physical examination of the pelvis, 1965.

Ruddy's Influence

Thomas Jefferson Ruddy was born in 1874 in Iowa. He graduated in 1902 from the Still College of Osteopathic Medicine, in Des Moines. After working for several years as an osteopath in California, he specialised as an 'ear, nose and throat' (ENT) physician, and became quite famous in his field. In the 1950s, Ruddy developed a method called 'rapid resistive duction'. In this procedure, he carefully positioned the patient's muscles requiring correction and had the patient contract those muscles against the resistance offered by the therapist. Ruddy described his technique as follows:

1. *Resist the levers to which the correcting muscle is attached.*
2. *Patient contracts the muscle repeatedly, synchronous with the pulse rate and faster, to double the pulse rate or higher, counting one-two, two-two, three-two, up to ten-two, the frequency at*

the close to be five-two in five seconds, if not an acute painful movement.
3. *Press the part to be moved aiding the contracting muscle.*
4. *Counter pressure on the part articulating with the restricted unit.*
5. *Employ skeletal muscle contraction to pump visceral circulation.*

Ruddy (1961)

Ruddy used the surrounding muscle tissue to affect the motion and circulation of blood, lymph and tissue fluids into dysfunctional areas.

The purpose of rapid rhythmic resistive duction is:
1. *to increase the speed and strength of blood and tissue fluid flow, in skeletal, visceral and nerve structures ensuring nutrient substances to each cell, and the removal of extrinsic toxins and wastes from the tissues,*

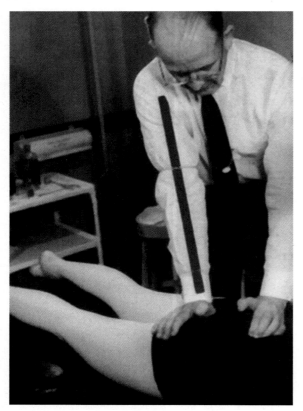

Fig. 3.4 Fred Mitchell Sr demonstrates a muscle energy technique, 1970.

2. *to create homeostasis between the fasciculi of all muscles by correcting fixations, and reconditioning through muscle contraction,*
3. *to engender normal afferent impulses to all nerve centres particularly the pre-motor cortical area for re-establishing normal tone.*

Ruddy (1961)

Ruddy taught this method to his patients and assigned self-treatment as homework. He often used this technique in eye treatment, but also used it for the treatment of spinal injuries (Ruddy, 1961, 1962; Wolf, 1987). Lawrence Jones, the developer of 'Strain and Counterstrain' described Ruddy's technique as a very effective method of treating joint disorders (Jones, 1995).

Mitchell eventually learned about Ruddy's methods and became excited about this approach, having realised the potential of using the patients' '*muscle energy*'

for treatment. In 1951, Nelson described a method, used by osteopath Carl Kettler, for the treatment of '*pelvic blocks*' (sacroiliac joint restriction). Kettler had observed that specific treatment of the supporting structures of the pelvis were more successful and lasting than the use of direct impulse (high velocity) manipulation (Nelson, 1951). In 1952, Pratt mentioned a technique, used by Kettler for the treatment of the 'lumbo pelvic torsion syndrome' in the *Journal of the American Osteopathic Association*. Pratt claims that this technique had an extraordinary effect and became euphoric as he wrote that:

> *with the use of this technic the sacral torsion is corrected, lumbar realignment is accomplished, and fascial, ligamentous and muscular tensions are normalized so that when the patient again assumes the upright position all factors are realigned and true physiologic balance of the pelvis and spine is achieved*
>
> *Pratt (1952)*

Unfortunately, he failed to describe his technique in depth; however, years later, Fred Mitchell Sr observed Kettler demonstrating his techniques. In this process, Carl Kettler used the formulation: 'the patient presses against a precisely executed counterforce'. This left a lasting impression on Mitchell, who became preoccupied with Kettler's and Ruddy's approaches (Mitchell Jr., 1987). Years later, he named Ruddy as an important source in the development of MET (Jones, 1995). He also wrote that Kettler was the person who directed his

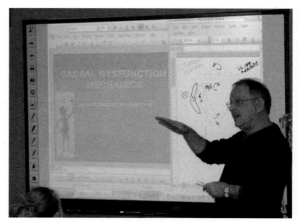

Fig. 3.5 Ed Stiles teaching the MET concept at Virginia Tech College of Osteopathic Medicine, 2007.

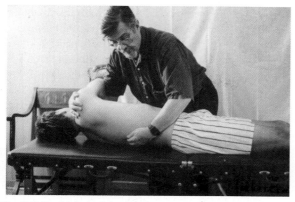

Fig. 3.6 Fred Mitchell Jr showing a muscle energy technique to treat a rib for restricted inhalation, 2004.

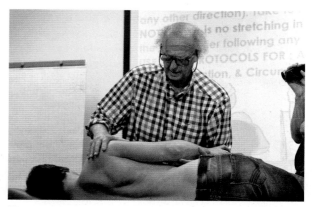

Fig. 3.7 Leon Chaitow demonstrating a muscle energy technique, 2017.

attention to the huge significance of muscles and fasciae that are affected by dysfunction (Mitchell Sr., 1958).

> *The high velocity, low amplitude (thrust) techniques which Fred had used so effectively during the 1940s were already giving way to the development of combinations using Kettler's 'distinctively executed counterforce' and Ruddy's 'resistive duction' ideas, which evolved into the term 'muscle energy', and to mean the patient contraction of muscle against the physician counterforce.*
>
> **Kimberly (2009, p. 18).**

FURTHER DEVELOPMENT OF MET

Fred Mitchell Sr was a member of a teaching faculty for the AAO. At a course in New York in the spring of 1955, which he presented together with Paul Kimberly, members of the AAO executive committee commented negatively about the quality of the workshop. The discussion became heated and a new date for the recommencing of talks was set. Kimberly, who was the moderator, wrote nearly 30 years later:

> *For reasons that are not clear at this late date, I sensed that Fred had a 'very short fuse' and that it might be for the good of all present if he 'kept his mouth shut' for the evening. He did at my request. It was probably one of my few strokes of genius for I sincerely believe that we would have had a physical skirmish that night if he had participated in the discussion.*

> *The 'adrenalin flow' resulting from the often heated discussion going around him was so great that it took Fred an even twelve months to work it off. He went back to Chattanooga and read everything he could get his hands on regarding the low back. This included medical as well as osteopathic literature... He had been aware of multiple axes around which the pelvic girdle moved for several years but had not been motivated to put it together into a comprehensible package. The argument of April 1955 proved to be the motivator. He spent the year putting his thoughts together and returned to St. Petersburg in the Spring of 1956 for the annual meeting of the Anthropometric Society for Medicine and Nutrition. At this meeting, he invited me to his hotel room, offered me a chair and stated that 'it was my turn to keep my mouth shut'. His demeanour raised my adrenalin levels to full attention because I had no idea of what was coming. My first thought, probably due to a guilty feeling over last year, made me fearful of a deserved verbal lashing. Instead, he very carefully and meticulously described to me his 'motion cycle of walking' concept. Eventually, I was permitted to ask questions and finally was 'ordered' to go home and put it on paper for him. It was a pleasure to do so.*
>
> **Kimberly (2009, p. 18)**

In 1958, Mitchell published the article 'Structural Pelvic Function' (Mitchell Sr., 1958). In this he wrote:

> *The subject, I realize, is controversial and there are probably as many different opinions as there are*

authors, and even more. These facts notwithstanding, my purpose here is to present an explanation of sacroiliac, iliosacral and symphyseal motion that will stand the scrutiny of the anatomist as well as the clinician and technician.

Mitchell Sr. (1958, p. 71)

Fred Mitchell's article is based on his contribution, published 10 years previously in the yearbook of the AAO. This time his explanations were more accurate.

He postulated six axes for the mobility of the pelvis and sacrum: one axis through the symphysis for pelvic rotation, one upper transverse axis for Sutherland's craniosacral movement, one middle transverse axis for the movement of the sacrum in flexion and extension, and one lower transverse axis for the movement of the pelvis while walking. Finally, one right and left diagonal axis for the torsion of the sacrum. He explained how an increased number of sacroiliac joint dysfunctions can occur, which in turn are caused by the increased number of axes. His focus on the pelvic area as a central region for therapeutic efforts remained unchanged.

When the osteopathic physician appreciates the relationship of the bony structures of the pelvic girdle to good body mechanics, circulation to the pelvic organs and lower extremities, reflex disturbances to remote parts of the organism through endocrine or neurogenic perverted physiology, and can master the diagnosis and manipulative correction, he has the basic tool from which all therapy can begin.

Mitchell Sr. (1958, p. 71)

The real quantum leap in Mitchell's work consisted not of biomechanical details and the resulting pathological situations but related to the technique of his treatments. It was only one method, of which he showed seven variations for seven different lesions – the well-dosed and targeted exertion of certain muscles against the resistance of the therapist. Mitchell called this action *'muscular cooperation technique'* (years later Fred Mitchell Jr. changed the name of the procedure to *'muscle energy technique'*, used to the present).

PNF and MET

In the 1940s and 1950s Herman Kabat, a neurophysiologist, together with Dorothy Voss and Margaret Knott,

two physical therapists, observed functional movement patterns that were important for the rehabilitation process of patients with neurological disorders. They developed specific contract/relax techniques based on clinical experience and neurophysiological principles (Sherrington's first (relaxation after contraction) and second (reciprocal inhibition) laws). In 1956 Voss and Knott published their concept entitled 'Proprioceptive Neuromuscular Facilitation' (Knott & Voss, 1956).

Kabat described PNF exercises 9 years later (Kabat, 1965). PNF techniques were used to improve muscle strength, range of movement and neuromuscular functions. The PNF procedures were similar to the isometric and isotonic variations of MET although they differed, for example, in the degree of force requested of the patient. The concepts behind the technique were also different. In the beginning, PNF focused on neurological aspects of movement patterns, while MET emphasised the biomechanical aspects of movement restriction. Nevertheless:

The similarities between MET and PNF are difficult to ignore, especially as they have both evolved over many years. Both systems depend on the spinal cord and brain anatomy and physiology, and the organisation of locomotor control systems. My own development of MET has certainly been influenced by the neurophysiologic concepts and mechanisms of PNF as well as Cranial Osteopathy and other emerging science… I do not know if my father was aware of PNF before he taught his tutorial courses in the 1970s. If my father had ever heard of PNF, he never mentioned it to me. As far as I know, he had no exposure to PNF.

F. L. Mitchell Jr. (2011, personal communication)

He [Mitchell Sr.] was focused on using muscles to [treat] restricted joint function. His main focus was not relaxing muscles but re-establishing joint mechanics. He never mentioned PNF and its principles as influencing his MET conceptual development.

Ed Stiles (2011, personal communication)

Ehrenfeuchter assumed that Mitchell Sr and Kettler were both unaware of PNF techniques because they were not widely known at the time (Ehrenfeuchter & Sandhouse, 2002). Other authors including Stiles

(Fig. 3.5), Sutton, Kimberly and Greenman do not mention PNF as influencing MET.

Kimberly and Mitchell Sr

Mitchell Sr continued to develop MET, refining variations and variables in the treatment of different forms of pelvic dysfunction. From 1960 to 1964, (Figs. 3.2, 3.3, 3.6) he worked together with his son, Fred Mitchell Jr, who had graduated from the Chicago College of Osteopathy in 1959. Those were years of observation and clinical experience. During this period of common work, Mitchell Jr investigated the possibility that the early MET principles that his father had described, or similar techniques, could be applied to all joints of the body. Mitchell Sr thought that this was possible in principle.

In 1964, Fred Mitchell Jr became a member of the faculty at the Kansas City College of Osteopathy and Surgery which became the first osteopathic college in the USA to teach MET – alongside standard osteopathic methods. During this period Mitchell Sr was close friends with Paul Kimberly DO, who was known as an extremely capable and versatile osteopath. Kimberley's influence on the thoughts on MET cannot be determined precisely.

> *In some way, the extent to which Dr Kimberly influenced the development of MET may possibly be better understood and judged by understanding his way of classifying manual therapies, as presented in a talk titled 'The Manipulative Prescription' (Kimberly, 1992). Kimberly was someone Mitchell Sr. communicated with, and received feedback from, while he was developing his theories and concepts, and who probably therefore influenced Mitchell Sr.'s concepts.*
>
> **F. L. Mitchell Jr. and P.K.G. Mitchell (2005, personal communication)**

THE MEANING AND RECOGNITION OF MET

During this period, in the early 1960s, few osteopaths were aware of or interested in MET. The only teachers were Fred Mitchell Sr and Jr and Paul Kimberly. Osteopathy at that time was dominated by practitioners who worked manually but to a large extent did not have explanations for what they did. There was no mutual language, rather an unclear nomenclature and an abundance of techniques, with multiple explanations and interpretations as to the mechanisms involved. Communication amongst osteopaths was difficult, as characterised by Edward Stiles' description of his meeting with G.A. Laughlin, the grandson of A.T. Still (founder of osteopathy):

> *I believe George had the best hands of anybody I'd ever met. Unfortunately, he had difficulty verbalizing what he did...this was in the early '60s [and] this is about where the profession was at that time.*
>
> **Stiles (1987)**

Fred Mitchell Jr ironically commented in his book *Muscle Energy Technique*:

> *I have always suspected that my father developed what I chose to call (ungrammatically) Muscle Energy Technique after he realized that I, like most of my classmates, had learned few OMT skills in my four years of osteopathic education and that he needed something simple and safe to teach to me.*
>
> **Mitchell Jr. and Mitchell (1999, p. XVII)**

It seems that it was difficult to understand new ideas. Thrust techniques constituted the dominating element of osteopathic treatment and methods that were based on different principles were viewed suspiciously.

> *The resistance that we found globally throughout the profession to using this approach was political, because at the time what any group or school was doing was satisfactory; they were getting good results. They perceived us as trying to be an elite, exclusive group; that what we were doing was somehow inferior to the current state of the art.*
>
> **Blood (2009, p. 25)**

The search for alternatives took place in small groups rather than in larger, organisational ones.

> *Now the significance of muscle energy technic, in that era, was that it formed a bridge, as it were, between the forceful technics which we had been taught in school and the very mellow technics which used the patient's own motive forces that Dr Hoover was teaching in his functional technic.*
>
> **Fryman (1987, p. 27)**

First Tutorial

At a congress in New York, in 1970, Edward Stiles and Fred Mitchell Sr were introduced to each other. Stiles told Mitchell that he had read his articles but did not understand them completely and asked him to explain the details:

> *That was all Fred needed, I remember he went and got Freddy Jr. and we went up to Fred's room. About 4 hours later I got out of there, after 4 hours of lecture, demonstration and being treated. I knew that I had had a different experience.*
>
> **Stiles (1987, p. 78)**

Two months later, in March 1970, Stiles was part of the small circle of six osteopaths (Sarah Sutton, Edward Stiles, Philip Greenman, Devota Nowland, John Goodridge and Rolland Miller) who received a personal introduction to MET by Mitchell. 'It was a very intense week, which started with breakfast at 7 a.m. and often lasted into the evening hours (Sutton, 2009: 16).

Besides the cognitive understanding of MET, the participants were taught to improve their palpation techniques. The workload was immense. Mitchell Sr was even unsure if MET could be taught which is why the first tutorial was just a test. Edward Stiles describes experiences from this period as being very impressive:

> *Having been initially trained to use HV/LA techniques, I challenged Fred on how a gentle MET effort could cause both the remarkable local as well as distant changes we were observing as he demonstrated the MET treatment of various mechanical problems. He illustrated the MET truth by a quick, low amplitude kick to a rolling stool. It moved about 3–4 feet. He brought the stool back to the original starting point, put one finger on the stool and pushed it 6–7 feet with minimal effort by using a longer, yet gentler, force. My paradigm concerning the forces required to effectively treat patients was permanently altered.*
>
> **Stiles (2009, p. 45)**

> *Fred had tremendous faith in osteopathy in its value in treating people with chronic health problems. This was probably best illustrated by an answer that Fred once gave to a question during a tutorial. The question came from one of the students [who]*

> *said, 'You know Dr Mitchell I've been sitting here for several days and I hear you talk about treating this condition and that condition. Exactly what do you treat with osteopathic manipulation?' Fred said I treat, falling hair, falling arches and everything in between. That again would pretty well characterize Fred.*
>
> **Stiles (1987, p. 79)**

MET After the Death of Fred Mitchell Sr

On 2nd March 1974, Fred Mitchell Sr died from a heart attack on his farm at the age of 64. After Mitchell Sr's death, a task group led by Sara Sutton gathered to work on the development of a curriculum for MET.

> *From 1970–1975 I served as the Secretary to the Academy of Applied Osteopathy (AAO). At the end of that time, I was asked by the Board of the AAO, to chair a committee to document what was unique about Dr Mitchell's Muscle Energy work. Over the next five years, the committee met at Michigan State University, three or four times a year over long weekends. The end result was the development of a curriculum for three forty-hour courses: Basic, Above the Diaphragm, and Below the Diaphragm. Paul Kimberly, D.O. served as a consultant to the committee.*
>
> **Sutton (2009, p. 16)**

Supported by the AAO, the first MET course, after Fred Mitchell Senior's death, took place in December 1974. In the beginning, only a few osteopaths showed interest in MET, but their numbers were steadily increasing. In 1973, the students Neil Pruzzo and Peter Moran collected notes from Mitchell Jr's class and published the notes under the title 'An Evaluation and Treatment Manual of Osteopathic Manipulative Procedures' together with him. Later on, the records were revised by Mitchell and were now completely focused on the field of MET. They were published in 1979, in the first MET textbook entitled *An Evaluation and Treatment Manual of Osteopathic Muscle Energy Procedures* (Mitchell Jr. et al., 1979). In the following years, different authors published articles about MET (Goodridge, 1981; Graham, 1985; Neumann 1985, 1988). In 1980, on the initiative of Paul Kimberly, the concept of MET was incorporated into the osteopathic catalogue of therapies of the Kirksville College of Osteopathic Medicine, the college founded by A.T. Still. Fred Mitchell Jr was the driving force in developing and advancing his father's original concept over the years. As early as the first half of the 1960s he extended the concentric isotonic techniques of his father by isometric methods.

> *Parenthetically, the first MET procedures developed by my father to treat vertebral segmental dysfunction were techniques that used concentric isotonic contractions of the muscles assumed to be the antagonists of the presumed tight/short muscles (applying Sherrington's second principle). Later, before I went to Kansas City, I developed the isometric techniques that are widely used these days because they require less force and are more specific. Lewit's PIR techniques were modelled on these.*
>
> **Mitchell Jr. (2009b)**

Lewit confirmed this statement when he wrote that post isometric relaxation was pioneered by Mitchell Sr and clearly described by Mitchell Jr (Lewit & Simons, 1984). Over the years the MET procedures became more precise and gentle.

> *Muscle energy technique is not a wrestling match… A small amount of force should be used at first, with increases as necessary. This is much more productive than beginning with too much force… Localization of force is more important than intensity of force.*
>
> **Goodridge (1981, p. 253)**

Lewit and MET

In 1977 the physician and manual therapist Karel Lewit visited Michigan State University and met Mitchell Jr for the first time. Lewit had developed a therapeutic procedure that he called postisometric relaxation (PIR), some years after Fred Mitchell Sr published his article in the AAO Journal. Over the years, PIR was more and more popular among manual therapists in Europe.

> *When he first came to visit me at Michigan State University's College of Osteopathic Medicine, he brought his (diapositive) slides with him to show*

> *my department the PIR techniques he had developed. When I first saw those slides, I thought I could probably give a lecture with them. They seemed to be illustrating procedures I used myself. As Lewit and I got to know each other, we learned from each other at that meeting, and subsequent departmental meetings, and in the ensuing correspondence. He was not shy about pointing out some of the errors in what I was teaching, as well as some good things I was doing. I owe many important insights to him.*
>
> **Mitchell Jr. (2009a, p. 37)**

In MET, the restrictive barrier must be located precisely. If using an isometric technique, the therapist uses the first palpated barrier as the starting position. For many years, Mitchell taught that the blocked joint must be directed to this movement barrier on all three planes, followed by a guided contraction at this point. It was the exchange of ideas with Lewit, which led Mitchell Jr to the conviction that a precisely carried out localisation on one plane – in most cases side-bending – is sufficient for a successful treatment (Mitchell Jr & Mitchell, 1999). The correspondence between Mitchell Jr and Lewit over the following years provided the basis for the further development and a significant step forward in bringing the two models closer together. Today PIR is similar to MET, however, some significant differences exist regarding the diagnostic orientation (Franke, 2009)(Table 3.1).

> *MET and PIR differ mainly in how they view the indications. PIR sees its primary application in muscle tightness, spasms, and myofascial trigger points, with joint mobilisation the consequence of muscle relaxation. MET sees its primary application in the mobilisation of both … joints, and regards muscle spasm and tightness, when they occur, as neurological consequences of postural and locomotor adaptation to articular dysfunction usually located elsewhere in the body.*
>
> **Mitchell Jr. and Mitchell (2004, p. 12)**

Karel Lewit saw the fixation of MET on the joints as critical. For him, the blockage was a functional disorder, which was only to be understood in connection within the framework of functional pathology of the entire locomotor system. He did not favour or commit himself to one determined functional chain, because he was of the opinion that there was insufficient knowledge

TABLE 3.1 MET and PIR Compared

	MET	PIR
Variants	• Isometric contraction using RI (Reciprocal Inhibition) with/without post-contraction stretching • Ruddy's Rapid Resistive Duction (Isometric intermittent) • Isotonic concentric • Eccentric isotonic (Isolytic) • Vibratory Isolytic • Isokinetic contraction (isotonic and isometric combined)	• Isometric contraction using AI (Autogenic Inhibition) with/without post-contraction stretching • Isometric towards barrier • Isotonic intermittent
Barrier definition	Easy restriction barrier (feather edge)	Restriction barrier
Contraction begins	Slightly before the barrier	At the barrier
Direction	Away from barrier	Away from barrier
Force applied by the patient		
• Isometric	20–30%	20%
• Isotonic	30–100%	50%
Contraction duration	3–5 seconds	7–10 seconds
Repetitions	3–5 times	3–5 times
Other elements	Visual and/or respiratory synkinesis	Visual and/or respiratory synkinesis
Resistance	Practitioner, self-administered (ball, pillow, etc)	Practitioner, gravity, visual synkinesis (self-administered)
Concepts and assessment approaches	Somatic dysfunction; Mitchell's pelvic model; Fryette's laws of spinal motion; restricted ROM.	Multidisciplinary mobility assessments of soft tissue and joints; muscular imbalance.

Note: See Chapters 2 and 5 for details on barriers. See Chapter 5 for more detailed descriptions of assessment, variations, and protocols (Chaitow, 2013; Liebenson, 1989, 2006).

and that clinical pathology was an area of study that remained to be more fully explored (Lewit, 1998, 2009).

Janda and Mitchell

Through Lewit, Mitchell Jr met Vladimir Janda, a Czech who fell ill with polio in his teens. Perhaps because he had developed a post-polio syndrome, Janda was very interested in pain, and by the age of 21 had written a book about muscle function and testing. Janda was convinced that muscular balance was the deciding factor for the quality of movement. He identified two groups of muscles based on their phylogenetic development and classified them as 'tonic' and 'phasic'. He discovered that tonic muscles have a tendency to shortness, whereas phasic muscles have a tendency to weakness, and that muscular asymmetry was frequently the result of an imbalance between 'tonic' and 'phasic' muscles (Janda, 1983). In the late 1970s, he defined different patterns of

muscular imbalance which he called 'upper crossed syndrome', 'lower crossed syndrome' and 'layer syndrome' (see notes on these patterns in Chapter 5, Box 5.2). Janda shifted the focus from the joint to the muscle as a common source of disorders in the locomotor system (Janda, 1987) and influenced many manual therapists with his theories. Mitchell wrote later that Janda rather neglected the application of post isometric techniques to arthrokinematic range-of-motion dysfunctions, but that he (Mitchell Jr) had learned important lessons about the rehabilitation of the motor system from him (Mitchell Jr., 2009a).

In 1992, Fred Mitchell Jr retired as a professor of biomechanics at Michigan State University. However, he continued to practise and give MET seminars. Between 1995 and 1999, Mitchell published three textbooks on MET, together with his son Kai Galen Mitchell (Mitchell Jr. & Mitchell, 1999, 2001a, 2001b).

Fred Mitchell Jr suffered a stroke in March 2005, however he overcame most of the post-stroke neurological deficits. In the same month, he was awarded the Andrew Taylor Still Medallion of Honor. He could not take part in the award ceremony due to his health problems but 4 months later his state of health improved and he held a seminar, together with Greenman and Edward Stiles for the AAO in Chicago, entitled 'Muscle Energy: Three Visions'.

THE MODEL OF MET AND RESEARCH FINDINGS IN RECENT YEARS

Fred Mitchell Sr and Jr have both expanded the osteopathic framework of therapies. Sixty years ago Fred Mitchell Sr and his son started to improve the diagnostic foundation of osteopathy, systematised it with the help of treatment protocols and made dysfunction treatable through MET.

To understand the concept of muscle energy technique it is necessary to think beyond the isometric treatment principle. The classical concept of MET is embedded in the framework of osteopathic diagnosis and clinical reasoning (Graham, 1985; Mitchell Jr. & Mitchell, 1999, 2001a, 2001b; Ehrenfeuchter & Sandhouse, 2002; DiGiovanna et al., 2004; Stiles, 2009), whereas the isolated isometric principle has a great compatibility to several diagnostic and therapeutic concepts. This is often overlooked but easy to see when the diagnostic procedure of (Mitchell's model of) MET is considered in more detail. For Mitchell, the muscle only serves the purpose of treating the malfunction of the joint. He emphasises that MET includes a diagnostic procedure and a therapeutic treatment, which are inseparable from each other. For the diagnostic orientation, Mitchell Jr refers to the spinal kinematics by Fryette (Fryette, 1954) and the pelvi-sacral model which was developed by his father and modified by himself (Mitchell Sr., 1958; Mitchell Jr. & Mitchell, 1999). At the beginning of the last century, Fryette examined the biomechanical behaviour of the vertebral column, where he detected a coupled movement behaviour in the three-dimensional mobility of the vertebral body. Extension and flexion of segments were possible as isolated movements, but side-bending or rotary movements behaved differently when freely moving, compared with when blocked. In connection with mobility levels, Fryette explained the neutral position as well as a variety of pathological positions. This is similar to the pelvi-sacral axes model of mobility by Mitchell Sr Clearly defined descriptions of the positioning around clearly defined axes allow for a complete physiology-pathology scheme of sacrum and ilium joint.

> *Many practitioners utilizing MET use these laws of coupled motion, as a predictive model, to both formulate a mechanical diagnosis and to select the precisely controlled position required in the application of the technique. Current literature challenges the validity of Fryette's laws.*
>
> ***Gibbons and Tehan (1998, p. 1)***

There is growing evidence that the recording of the joint position or rather a categorised definition of a coupled movement for the determination of the (dys-) functionality, especially for the area of the lumbar spine, is insufficient (Pearcy & Tibrewal, 1984; Vincenzino & Twomey, 1993), and that the physiological position of the associated joints and their coupled movements can vary (Krid, 1993; Chopin, 2001; Vogt, 1996).

Muscle tension, irritated ligaments, weight, back pain and inherent or acquired changes of the facets are all factors that can be responsible for altered movement patterns. Coupled movements of the lumbar spine are far more complex than generally assumed and the specific effect that the muscular system (for example) has on coupled movement, is still unknown (Panjabi et al., 1989).

By contrast, an isometric contraction is a technique-procedure that (among other things) releases muscular contractions, and which does not in itself constitute a concept. The features that are required to ensure successful use of MET include a precise positioning to the barrier; an active and appropriately formulated (strength, timing) muscle contraction, by the patient against a defined resistance of the therapist, in a precise direction; the number of repetitions, and finally an accurate assessment of the therapeutic outcome.

Isometric contractions form part of various procedures, appropriate to different indications, but all are based on the same physiological principles, whereas the concepts behind them may all be different (MET, PIR, PNF, neuromuscular technique (NMT)).

Chaitow

Leon Chaitow's (Fig. 3.7) MET approach is largely based on a synthesis of different concepts. We not only see

Mitchell's influence, but also the theories and methods of Lewit, Janda, Kabat and others. Chaitow has also rediscovered Ruddy's rapid resistive duction technique (now termed 'pulsed MET') which had unfortunately become almost completely forgotten. He taught the pulsed technique as a major part of MET, finding it to be one of the most useful of MET's tools since it also encourages proprioceptive rehabilitation and enhanced motor control (L. Chaitow 2011, personal communication with H. Franke).

In his earliest work presenting MET, writing in 1980 Chaitow described it as 'a revolution taking place in manipulative therapy', which he saw as a valuable alternative to the more commonly practised HVLA techniques. Crucially for him, MET considered more subtle soft tissue elements. In this early iteration, he acknowledged the similarity of PNF techniques used in physiotherapy, sought evidence and expert opinion from both sides of the Atlantic, and though he used different terms, emphasised the value of a multimodal approach, foreshadowing the research that has confirmed its value. In the same book, Chaitow queried early perspectives on potential mechanisms of action for MET, then in their infancy, and cited early connective tissue research (Scott, 1983) to highlight his belief in the significance of its influence on dysfunction and the role of MET in restoring functionality. This too has been borne out by current fascia research.

The same chapter presents variations of MET application that have changed little in the intervening years; as noted by the co-editor of the present volume, 'what we do has not really changed, but we understand it better'. (Sandy Fritz, personal communication to S. Chaitow, 2019). Of the four main variations of MET (isometric, isotonic, Ruddy's rapid resistive duction (pulsed MET), and isolytic) the isometric version is the most widely utilised form. Thus all clinical studies regarding MET, for example, involving subjects with back pain, or subjects without nonspecific back pain, but with restriction in their active range of motion, are based on postisometric procedures (Franke, 2010).

In the early chapter, Chaitow notes the value of the unlimited variables and the potential for individualised care that they provide. Following the success of this early work and its development into standalone textbooks, he repeatedly collected and critically appraised the sparse evidence that was available, until the mid-1990s when, through founding and editing the Journal of Bodywork and Movement Therapies (1996), he actively began fostering interprofessional collaboration on the development of the evidence base, for MET as well as numerous other modalities, initiating and hosting professional scientific debates on the many areas yet to acquire satisfactory evidence [including the trigger point debate, on which more in Chapter 4, and questions on structural/biomechanical frameworks (Chaitow, 2011; Franke, 2011)]. His emphasis on the importance of interprofessional exchange and the danger of professional, disciplinary, or ideological silos is reflected in all his books, including this one, as well as his teaching and practice records, his contribution to the establishment of the Fascia Research Congress, and the work of the Ida P. Rolf Institute. These techniques and principles were built into his curriculum when he was Senior Lecturer at the University of Westminster and formed part of his interdisciplinary practice as the first osteopath appointed to the British National Health Service (NHS) in 1996. His direct influence launched the careers of many of the next generation of bodywork researchers and teachers, allowing for the evolution of evidence and practice as described in Chapter 4 and elsewhere in this book. After retiring from the University of Westminster, he made a point of teaching MET alongside other techniques within this interdisciplinary context across the spectrum of professions, in several European countries as well as the United States, aiming for better understanding across borders. The information in Box 3.2 demonstrates the variation in application and uptake of MET and the sources cited there also reflect practitioner preference for other therapeutic methods.

Chaitow's original contribution to MET application was typical of his tendency for synthesis, in the form of integrated neuromuscular inhibition technique (INIT), presented and discussed in Chapter 14, along with the supporting evidence.

FUTURE SYNERGIES

This is a chapter on history, and as these lines are being written in May 2022, history is being made at the inaugural conference of the International Consortium on Manual Therapies (ICMT) bringing together working groups from across the bodywork professions and soliciting clinician input through open discussion fora in order to resolve ongoing issues in matters of nomenclature and promote interprofessional communication. Its core themes are the nomenclature issue, technique descriptions in both education and research, and the all-important question regarding mechanisms of action. The professions' histories are also being explored, though the academic historical approach remains to be integrated. Held online, the virtual, month-long conference is the first of its kind to allow input and real-time discussion among stakeholders of all levels, from vocationally trained therapists to lab scientists, educators and funding body representatives.

Chaired by Brian Degenhardt DO, Director of the A.T. Still Institute and Assistant Vice President for Osteopathic Research at A.T. Still University, the consortium is the product of long deliberations among professionals over many years, to which Leon Chaitow contributed with his concerns regarding the need for translational research, improved validation and education, the bridging of boundaries between professions and across the hierarchy of stakeholders (Degenhardt, personal communication to S. Chaitow, 2021). This last element will allow researchers to understand what it is that diverse practitioners actually practice, and to direct research towards those areas, thus allowing the development of useful, clinically applicable research of better quality.

Key guidelines developed through the consortium's working groups, resting on vast evidence reviews, include the necessity of focusing on techniques that are widely used across manual therapy professions, grouping them into the essence of what the techniques represent so as to avoid the fragmentation observed through branding and commercially-driven technique presentations, and the avoidance of eponym-based techniques (Still, Maitland, Sutherland, Rolf, etc). With regard to the last point, we have elected to maintain some eponym usage in this edition to avoid reader confusion, but it is expected that in future, these will have consolidated, scientific names based on broad, grounded consensus, and it will be for chapters such as this one to ensure the preservation of legacies.

This represents a major step in the evolution of manual therapies, which can only result in positive outcomes, that, it is hoped, will be reflected in future editions of this book. The following chapter provides a comprehensive review of the evidence to date, highlighting key areas where improvement is needed and the role of clinicians in achieving it. The contingencies presented in the present chapter may form a valuable substrate in which to consider future directions.

REFERENCES

Adams, J., Sibbritt, D., Steel, A., Peng, W., 2018. A workforce survey of Australian osteopathy: analysis of a nationally-representative sample of osteopaths from the Osteopathy Research and Innovation Network (ORION) project. BMC Health Serv. Res. 18 (1), 352.

Ahmed, U.A., Maharaj, S.S., Thaya, N., Kaka, B., Akodu, A.K., 2019. Knowledge of physiotherapists on the use of muscle energy technique in the management of non-specific low back pain, preprint (version 1). https://doi.org/10.21203/rs.2.17864/v1.

Alvarez, G., Roura, S., Cerritelli, F., Esteves, J.E., Verbeeck, J., van Dun, P.L.S., 2020. The Spanish Osteopathic Practitioners Estimates and RAtes (OPERA) study: a cross-sectional survey. PloS One 15 (6), Article e0234713.

Alvarez Bustins, G., López Plaza, P.-V., Carvajal, S.R., 2018. Profile of osteopathic practice in Spain: results from a standardized data collection study. BMC Compl. Altern. Med. 18, 129.

Arabatzis, T., 2019. Explaining science historically. Isis 110 (2). doi:10.1086/703513.

Batistatou, A., Doulis, E.A., Tiniakos, D., Anogiannaki, A., Charalabopoulos, K., 2010. The introduction of medical humanities in the undergraduate curriculum of Greek medical schools: challenge and necessity. Hippokratia 14 (4), 241–243.

Bill, A.S., Dubois, J., Pasquier, J., Burnand, B., Rodondi, P.Y., 2020. Osteopathy in the French-speaking part of Switzerland: practitioners' profile and scope of back pain management. PloS One 15 (5), Article e0232607.

Blood, S.D., 2009. Passing on the tradition. In: Franke, H. (Ed.), Muscle Energy Technique. History – Model – Research. Marixverlag, Wiesbaden.

Chaitow, L., 2011. Is a postural-structural-biomechanical model, within manual therapies, viable? A JBMT debate. J. Bodyw. Mov. Therap. 15 (2), 130–152. doi:10.1016/j.jbmt.2011.01.004.

Chaitow, L., 2013. Muscle Energy Techniques, fourth ed. Edinburgh, Elsevier.

Chaitow, S., 2020. Intelligent fascia? Massage and Bodywork, 44–49, November/December 2020.

Chang, H., 2017. Who cares about the history of science? Notes and Records 71, 91–107. http://doi.org/10.1098/rsnr.2016.0042.

Chang, H., 2021. Presentist history for pluralist science. J. Gen. Philos. Sci. 52, 97–114. doi:10.1007/s10838-020-09512-8.

Chopin, V., 2001. Etude du comportement des vertèbres lombaires in vivo lors de la latéroflexion. Mémoire DEA en Kinésithérapie Ostéopathique. Dir. Klein P. Université Libre de Bruxelles.

DiGiovanna, E.L., Schiowitz, S., Dowling, S., 2004. An Osteopathic Approach to Diagnosis and Treatment, third ed. Lippincott Williams & Wilkins, Philadelphia.

Dornieden, R., 2019. Exploration of the Characteristics of German Osteopaths and Osteopathic Physicians: Survey Development and Implementation. University of Bedfordshire.

Dubois, J., Bill, A.S., Pasquier, J., Keberle, S., Burnand, B., Rodondi, P.Y., 2019. Characteristics of complementary medicine therapists in Switzerland: a cross-sectional study. PloS One 14 (10), Article e0224098.

Ehrenfeuchter, W.C., Sandhouse, M., 2002. Muscle energy techniques. In: Ward, R.C. (Ed.), Foundations for Osteopathic Medicine, second ed. Lippincott Williams & Wilkins, Philadelphia.

Ellwood, J., Carnes, D., 2021. An international profile of the practice of osteopaths: a systematic review of surveys. Int. J. Osteopath. Med 40, 14–21.

Fousekis, K. (Ed.), 2022. Soft Tissue Techniques in Physiotherapy. Broken Hill Publishing, Nicosia, Cyprus.

Franke, H., 2009. The muscle energy model. In: Franke, H. (Ed.), Muscle Energy Technique. History – Model – Research. Marixverlag, Wiesbaden.

Franke, H., 2010. Clinical effects of muscle energy technique (MET) for nonspecific back pain. A systematic review and meta-analysis. Thesis for Master of Science in Osteopathic Clinical Research, A.T. Still University, Kirksville.

Franke, H., 2011. Re: Is a postural-structural-biomechanical model, within manual therapy, viable? A JBMT debate. J. Bodyw. Mov. Ther. 15 (3), 259–261. doi:10.1016/j.jbmt.2011.03.002.

Fryer, G., Johnson, J.C., Fossum, C., 2010. The use of spinal and sacroiliac joint procedures within the British osteopathic profession. Part 2: treatment. Int. J. Osteopath. Med. 13, 152–159.

Fryer, G., Morse, C.M., Johnson, J.C., 2009. Spinal and sacroiliac assessment and treatment techniques used by osteopathic physicians in the United States. Osteopath. Med. Prim. Care 3, 4.

Fryette, H., 1954. Principles of Osteopathic Technique. American Academy of Osteopathy, Newark, Ohio.

Fryman, V.M., 1987. Cranial Concept. Its Impact on the Profession. AAO Yearbook: American Academy of Osteopathy, Indianapolis, IN, pp. 26–29.

Gibbons, P., Tehan, P., 1998. Muscle energy concepts and coupled motion of the spine. Man. Ther. 3 (2), 95–101.

Giusti, R., (Ed.), 2017. Glossary of Osteopathic Terminology, third ed., Educational Council on Osteopathic Principles and the American Association of Colleges of Osteopathic Medicine. https://www.aacom.org/docs/default-source/insideome/got2011ed.pdf

Goodridge, J., 1981. Muscle energy technique: definition, explanation, methods of procedure. JAOA 81, 249–254.

Graham, K.E., 1985. Outline of Muscle Energy Techniques. Oklahoma College of Osteopathic Medicine and Surgery, Tulsa, Oklahoma.

Greenman, P.E., 2003. Principles of Manual Medicine, third ed. Lippincott Williams & Wilkins, Philadelphia.

Gurtoo, A., Ranjan, P., Sud, R., Kumari, A., 2013. A study of acceptability & feasibility of integrating humanities based study modules in undergraduate curriculum. Indian J. Med. Res. 137 (1), 197–202.

Howick, J., Zhao, L., McKaig, B., Rosa, A., Campaner, R., Oke, J., et al., 2022. Do medical schools teach medical humanities? Review of curricula in the United States, Canada and the United Kingdom. J. Eval. Clin. Pract. 28 (1), 86–92. doi:10.1111/jep.13589.

Janda, V., 1983. Muscle Function Testing Butterworth, London.

Janda, V., 1987. Muscles and motor control in low back pain. Assessment and management. In: Twomey, L.T. (Ed.), Physical therapy of the low back. Churchill Livingstone, New York.

Johnson, S.M., Kurtz, M.E., 2003. Osteopathic manipulative treatment techniques preferred by contemporary osteopathic physicians. JAOA 103 (5), 219–224.

Jones, L.H., 1995. Strain-Counterstrain. Jones Strain-Counterstrain Inc, Tyrell Lane.

Kabat, H., 1965. Proprioceptive facilitation in therapeutic exercise. In: Light, S. (Ed.), Therapeutic Exercise. Waverly Press, Baltimore.

Kimberly, P.E., 1992. Formulating a Prescription for Osteopathic Manipulative Treatment. AAO Yearbook: American Academy of Osteopathy, Indianapolis, IN, pp. 146–152.

Kimberly, P.E., 2009. The origin of muscle energy technique. In: Franke, H. (Ed.), Muscle Energy Technique. History – Model – Research. Marixverlag, Wiesbaden.

Knott, M., Voss, D.E., 1956. Proprioceptive Neuromuscular Facilitation: Patterns and Techniques. Paul B Haeber, New York.

Kollmer Horton, M.E., 2019. The orphan child: humanities in modern medical education. Philos. Ethics Humanit. Med. 14 (1). doi:10.1186/s13010-018-0067-y.

Krid, M.A., 1993. Etude radiologique de la rotation associeé à l'inclinaison latérale au niveau lombaire. Mémoire de Diplôme en Ostéopathie. Dir. P Klein, C Dethier. Jury National Belge d'Ostéopathie.

Kushner, H.I., 2008. Medical historians and the history of medicine. Perspectives: the art of medicine. Lancet 372 (9640), 710–711.

Liebenson, C., 1989. Active muscular relaxation methods. J. Manip. Physiol. Ther. 12 (6), 446–451.

Liebenson, C., 2006. Rehabilitation of the Spine, second ed. Williams and Wilkins, Baltimore.

Lewit, K., 1998. Artikuläre Funktionsstörungen. Manuelle Medizin 36, 100–105.

Lewit, K., 2009. Manipulative Therapy: Musculoskeletal Medicine. Edinburgh; New York. Elsevier/Churchill Livingstone.

Lewit, K., Simons, D.G., 1984. Myofascial pain. Relief by post-isometric relaxation. Arch. Med. Phys. Rehabil. 65, 452–456.

Magoun Jr., H., 2003. Passing on the tradition. AAO Newsletter. August, p. 12.

McGrath, M.C., 2013. From distinct to indistinct, the life cycle of a medical heresy. Is osteopathic distinctiveness an anachronism? Int. J. Osteopath. Med. 16 (1), 54–61.

Mi, M., Wu, L., Zhang, Y., Wu, W., 2022. Integration of arts and humanities in medicine to develop well-rounded physicians: the roles of health sciences librarians. J. Med. Libr. Assoc. 110 (2), 247–252. doi:10.5195/jmla.2022.1368.

Mitchell Jr., F.L., 1987. The History of the Development of Muscle Energy Concepts. AAO Yearbook: American Academy of Osteopathy, Indianapolis, IN, pp. 62–68.

Mitchell Jr., F.L., 1993. Elements of muscle energy technique. In: Basmajian, J.V., Nyberg, R. (Eds.), Rational Manual Therapies. Williams & Wilkins, Baltimore.

Mitchell Jr., F.L., 2009a. Influences, inspirations, and decision points. In: Franke, H. (Ed.), Muscle Energy Technique. History – Model – Research. Marixverlag, Wiesbaden.

Mitchell Jr., F.L., 2009b. Forty-eight years living with MET. In: Franke, H. (Ed.), Muscle Energy Technique. History – Model – Research. Marixverlag, Wiesbaden.

Mitchell Jr., F.L., Mitchell, P.K.G., 1999. The Muscle Energy Manual. MET Press, East Lansing, vol. 3.

Mitchell Jr., F.L., Mitchell, P.K.G., 2001a. The Muscle Energy Manual, second ed. MET Press, East Lansing, Michigan, vol. 1.

Mitchell Jr., F.L., Mitchell, P.K.G., 2001b. The Muscle Energy Manual, second ed. MET Press, East Lansing, Michigan, vol. 2.

Mitchell Jr., F.L., Mitchell, P.K.G., 2004. Handbuch der MuskelEnergieTechniken. Hippokrates Verlag, Stuttgart Band 1.

Mitchell Jr., F.L., Moran, P.S., Pruzzo, N.A., 1979. An Evaluation and Treatment Manual of Osteopathic Muscle Energy Procedures. Institute for Continuing Education in Osteopathic Principles, Valley Park, Missouri.

Mitchell Sr., F.L., 1948. The Balanced Pelvis and its Relationship to Reflexes. AAO Yearbook: American Academy of Osteopathy, Indianapolis, IN, pp. 146–151.

Mitchell Sr., F.L., 1958. Structural Pelvic Function. AAO Yearbook: American Academy of Osteopathy, Indianapolis, IN, pp. 71–89, reprint 1965, pp. 178–199.

Mitchell Sr., F.L., 1967. Motion discordance. Academy Lecture 1966. AAO Yearbook: American Academy of Osteopathy, Indianapolis, IN, pp. 1–5.

Morin, C., Aubin, A., 2014. Primary reasons for osteopathic consultation: a prospective survey in Quebec. PloS One 9 (9), Article e106259.

Nelson, C.R., 1951. The Postural Factor. AAO Yearbook, pp. 116–120.

Neumann, H.D., 1985. Manuelle Diagnostik und Therapie von Blockierungen der Kreuzdarmbeingelenke nach F. Mitchell. Manuelle Medizin 23, 116–126.

Neumann, H.D., 1988. Die Behandlung der HWS mit der Muskelenergietechnik nach Mitchell. Manuelle Medizin 26, 17–25.

Panjabi, M., Yamamoto, I., Oxland, T., Crisco, J., 1989. How does posture affect coupling in the lumbar spine? Spine 14, 1002–1011.

Pearcy, M.J., Tibrewal, S.B., 1984. Axial rotation and lateral bending in the normal lumbar spine measured by three-dimensional radiography. Spine 9 (6), 582–587.

Pentecost M, Gerber B, Wainwright M, et al., 2018. Critical orientations for humanising health sciences education in South Africa. Med. Humanit. 44, 221–229.

Plunkett, A., Fawkes, C.A., Carnes, D., 2020. UK osteopathic practice in 2019: a retrospective analysis of practice data. https://www.medrxiv.org/content/10.1101/2021.01.28.21250601v1.

Pratt, W., 1952. The lumbopelvic torsion syndrome. J. Am. Osteopath. Assoc. 51 (7), 335–340.

Ruddy, T.J., 1961. Osteopathic Rhythmic Resistive Duction Therapy. AAO Yearbook, pp. 58–68.

Ruddy, T.J., 1962. Osteopathic Rapid Rhythmic Resistive Technic. AAO Yearbook, pp. 23–31.

Scott, J.E., 1983. Connective tissues: the natural fibre-reinforced composite material. J. R. Soc. Med. 76 (12), 993–994. doi:10.1177/014107688307601201.

Stiles, E.G., 1987. Bridging the Generations. AAO Yearbook, pp. 73–78.

Stiles, E.G., 2009. Muscle energy technique. In: Franke, H. (Ed.), Muscle Energy Technique. History – Model – Research. Marixverlag, Wiesbaden.

Stouffer, K., Kagan, H.J., Kelly-Hedrick, M, See, J., Benskin, E., Wolffe, S., et al., 2021. The role of online arts and humanities in medical student education: mixed methods study of feasibility and perceived impact of a 1-week online course. JMIR Med. Educ. 7 (3), e27923. doi:10.2196/27923.

Sutton, S., 2009. The Mitchell Tutorials from, 1970 to 1975. In: Franke, H. (Ed.), Muscle Energy Technique. History – Model – Research. Marixverlag, Wiesbaden.

Tramontano, M., Pagnotta, S., Lunghi, C., Manzo, C., Manzo, F., Consolo, S., Manzo, V., 2020. Assessment and management of somatic dysfunctions in patients with patellofemoral pain syndrome. J. Am. Osteopath. Assoc. 120, 165–173. doi:10.7556/jaoa.2020.029.

Tramontano, M., Tamburella, F., Dal Farra, F., Bergna, A., Lunghi, C., Innocenti, M., et al., 2021. International overview of somatic dysfunction assessment and treatment in osteopathic research: a scoping review. Healthcare (Basel) 10 (1), 28. doi:10.3390/healthcare10010028.

van Dun, P.L.S., Nicolaie, M.A., Van Messem, A., 2016. State of affairs of osteopathy in the Benelux: Benelux osteosurvey 2013. Int. J. Osteopath. Med. 20, 3–17.

van Dun, P., Verbeeck, J., Esteves, J.E., Cerritelli, F., 2019a. Osteopathic practitioners estimates and rates (OPERA) study Belgium – Luxemburg: part I. https://www.opera-project.org/

van Dun, P., Verbeeck, J., Esteves, J., Cerritelli, F., 2019b. Osteopathic practitioners estimates and rates (OPERA) study Belgium – Luxemburg: part II. https://www.opera-project.org/

Vaucher, P., Macdonald, M., Carnes, D., 2018. The role of osteopathy in the Swiss primary health care system: a practice review. BMJ Open 8, e023770. doi:10.1136/bmjopen-2018-023770.

Vincenzino, G., Twomey, L., 1993. Sideflexion induced lumbar spine conjunct rotation and its influencing factors. Aust. Physiother. 39 (4), 299–306.

Vogt, F., 1996. Electrogoniométrie du rachis lombaire. Etude approfondie et application clinique. Mémoire de Licence en Kinésithérapie et Réadaptation. Dir Feipel V, Rooze M. Université Libre des Bruxelles.

Vogel, S., 2021. W(h)ither osteopathy: a call for reflection; a call for submissions for a special issue. Int. J. Osteopath. Med. 41, 1–3.

Vogel, S., Zegarra-Parodi, R., 2022. Relevance of historical osteopathic principles and practices in contemporary care: another perspective from traditional/complementary and alternative medicine. Int. J. Osteopath. Med. doi:10.1016/j.ijosm.2022.04.008.

Wald, H.S., McFarland, J., Markovina, I., 2019. Medical humanities in medical education and practice. Med. Teach. 41 (5), 492–496. doi:10.1080/0142159X.2018.1497151.

Wolf, A.H., 1987. Contributions of T. J. Ruddy, D.O., Osteopathic Pioneer. AAO Yearbook, pp. 30–33.

Wootton, D., 2006. Bad Medicine: Doctors Doing Harm Since Hippocrates Oxford.

Zegarra-Parodi, R., Esteves, J.E., Lunghi, C., Baroni, F., Draper-Rodi, J., Cerritelli, F., 2021. The legacy and implications of the body-mind-spirit osteopathic tenet: a discussion paper evaluating its clinical relevance in contemporary osteopathic care. Int. J. Osteopath. Med. 41, 57–65.

MET: Efficacy and Research

Gary Fryer

INTRODUCTION

The importance of research evidence to guide clinical decision-making in manual therapy practice is widely accepted and advocated. Manual therapy practitioners from different professions are generally supportive of evidence-based practice (EBP) – integrating the best available research evidence with clinical expertise and the patient's values and circumstances (Sackett et al., 1996) – even though their EBP skills may vary (Sundberg et al., 2018; Leach et al., 2019, 2021). Aspects of the EBP movement have attracted justified criticism, as discussed in Chapter 1, and its detractors have argued that the focus should be on providing useable evidence that can be combined with patient context and professional expertise for the best care of the patient (Greenhalgh et al., 2014).

The political, economic and academic environments of the allied health professions have changed substantially in recent decades. First and foremost, research is required to validate the efficacy of manual treatment: increasingly, we are asked by governments, health authorities and insurers to *prove* that what we

do works. Second, there is an academic quest to understand the nature of dysfunction and *why* (or *if*) manual treatment works. Third, and most importantly for practitioners, clinical research should guide us towards the most effective ways to manage our patients.

Like many manual techniques, robust, high-quality research investigating the clinical effectiveness of muscle energy technique (MET) is lacking (Fryer, 2011). MET was developed through clinical observation, experimentation and creative innovation, and was based on a rationale that was consistent with knowledge at the time. Rarely has scientific discovery been the primary instigator for a new manual approach. Research typically follows creative innovation to explain physiological mechanisms, verify effectiveness and test the relative superiority of variations or different approaches. Fred Mitchell Sr and Jr developed an innovative, gentle manual approach that is practised by the osteopathic profession and practitioners from other disciplines around the world. The contributions of Mitchell Sr and Jr should be acknowledged, but critical appraisal of concepts and practices and – where necessary – revision in response to evolving scientific research will ensure the approach does not become dissociated from research and best practice (Fryer, 2000, 2011).

More research, and particularly better-quality research, is needed to guide clinician use of MET for patients with spinal pain and disability. A number of small randomised controlled trials (RCTs) offer low-quality evidential support for the effectiveness of MET for acute and chronic low back pain (LBP) as well as for neck pain. Evidence also supports short-term increases in spinal range of motion (ROM) and muscle extensibility after MET although there is a need for more research in symptomatic individuals. Research relevant to the use of MET for stretching muscles typically comes from the study of related techniques, such as proprioceptive neuromuscular facilitation (PNF) stretching (as discussed in Chapter 9), and mostly involves the hamstring muscles. MET is not commonly employed as a stand-alone technique (for instance, in the treatment of LBP) but is combined with other manual approaches (Burke et al., 2013; Adams et al., 2018; Bill et al., 2020), which may partially explain the paucity of clinical research for this technique.

This chapter provides an overview of the evidence of the clinical effectiveness of MET for spinal pain and for increasing ROM and muscle extensibility. It will also explore the evidence underpinning the possible therapeutic mechanisms of the technique and highlight concerns and issues with common diagnostic approaches associated with the application of MET.

EFFICACY AND EFFECTIVENESS

The number and scope of studies investigating the efficacy of MET in experimental conditions and its effectiveness in real-world pragmatic conditions are growing. What seems to be lacking is a concurrent growth in the size of the studies. Most studies examining MET as a stand-alone intervention have generally suffered from very small sample sizes. This leads to low statistical power to detect changes, overestimation of the effect sizes of the intervention, greater heterogeneity when included in meta-analyses and poorer generalisability to clinical practice. When compared with manual interventions such as spinal manipulation, MET studies are fewer and considerably smaller. Furthermore, there is a lack of standardised MET

treatment protocols and controls and comparison interventions between studies, which makes pooling and comparisons difficult.

Some pragmatic clinical trials have investigated spinal pain using an intervention that included MET as a component of the treatment protocol (Chown et al., 2008; Schwerla et al., 2008; Licciardone et al., 2010), which represents the common practice of osteopaths and other practitioners of combining MET with other manual therapy techniques (Burke et al., 2013; Adams et al., 2018; Bill et al., 2020). Given that MET is rarely used as a stand-alone intervention, it is therefore understandable why there are limited clinical studies on MET only. Nevertheless, there are a growing number of clinical trials that have examined MET as the primary treatment for spinal pain, ROM and increasing muscle extensibility, and reported effectiveness of the technique, but these studies are often limited by low participant numbers, differing methods and lack of long-term follow-up.

Many aspects of the evidence-based medicine movement have attracted criticism, including the unmanageable volume of evidence, inflexible rules and guidelines that map poorly to patient complexity. EBP should involve ethical and expert judgement, evidence summaries based on clinically meaningful outcomes and a patient-centred, shared decision-making process during the consultation (Greenhalgh et al., 2014). Given the growing volume of evidence for many topics and the limited time and critical appraisal skills of most practitioners, practice guidelines and systematic reviews can provide meaningful summaries of treatment outcomes with an analysis of the methodological quality and believability of the reviewed studies, which may provide clinicians with more easily translatable and usable evidence. The focus of the following overview will therefore be on available systematic reviews rather than on individual clinical studies.

Back Pain

Even though many texts (Mitchell & Mitchell 1995; Ehrenfeuchter, 2011; DeStefano, 2016) have emphasised the application of MET for the treatment of spinal pain and dysfunction, rigorous research demonstrating clinical benefits of this treatment is still emerging. The number of studies in this area continues to grow and support the effectiveness of MET for the treatment of back pain, but – as previously noted – most are limited by low participant numbers, differing methods, incomplete reporting and lack of long-term follow-up.

In a 2015 Cochrane systematic review, Franke et al. (2015) examined the effectiveness of MET compared with control interventions in the treatment of people with non-specific LBP. Studies were required to use MET as a primary intervention (involving diagnosis of restricted joint or shortened muscle and application using isometric contraction) and only RCTs were included. The review identified 12 RCTs with 14 comparison interventions, with a total sample of 500 participants across all comparisons. The studies typically had very small participant numbers (20 to 72), and all but one study was deemed to have high risk of bias, indicating potential issues with the methodology of the studies. A lack of adequate blinding, baseline equivalence between groups, use of co-interventions and lack of concealment of random allocation were common issues.

The included studies used a wide variety of MET approaches, outcome measures and comparison interventions, which made pooling of the studies for meta-analysis difficult. Seven comparison groups were assessed using meta-analyses, but most of these had few studies in each group. The comparison with the most studies (MET plus any intervention vs other therapies plus that intervention for chronic non-specific LBP) demonstrated low-quality evidence for a non-significant effect regarding pain and functional status.

Although many studies reported beneficial effects from MET, the heterogeneity and lack of common outcomes and comparisons prevented clear conclusions. There was variation between the studies for the type of MET intervention delivered, and most studies focused on treatment limited to specific findings or dysfunctions rather than a pragmatic approach to treatment. The included studies were generally of low quality with small sample sizes, high risk of bias and inadequate standard treatment protocols and follow-up periods. The review concluded that there is a need for larger, higher-quality studies with more robust methodology, clearer reporting of methods and results as well as treatment protocols that can be generalised to clinical practice (Franke et al., 2015).

In a 2019 systematic review, Thomas et al. (2019) reported more positive findings regarding the efficacy of MET for LBP and neck pain. This review examined the effect of MET in both symptomatic and asymptomatic individuals, included 26 studies, and was not limited to either LBP or RCT designs. The risk of bias in the studies was assessed using the PEDro scale and the authors reported that 10 of the 14 RCTs achieved 'moderate to high quality' scores. This differed substantially from Franke et al. (2015) and may be attributed to including studies only on LBP in the Franke et al. (2015) review and their use of the Cochrane Risk of Bias instrument, which involves a qualitative judgement of each criterion.

Thomas et al. (2019) identified two studies on chronic LBP and two studies on acute LBP, considerably fewer than the Franke et al. (2015) review. One of these included studies (Wilson et al., 2003) was excluded from the Franke et al. (2015) review because it did not use a strictly randomised allocation, and another study (Ulger et al., 2017) used MET as part of a manual therapy protocol. Thomas et al., (2019) did not undertake a meta-analysis but reported evidence of effectiveness for MET as a treatment for both acute and chronic LBP. Additionally, the Thomas et al. (2019) review included three studies on chronic neck pain. Each of the three studies had different comparison treatments (exercise, stretching and mobilisation), but MET was reported as being more effective for reduction of pain and disability. Again, no meta-analysis was undertaken, and given the heterogeneity of the studies, Thomas et al. (2019) also acknowledged that further studies on MET are required.

In the only systematic review found on MET for neck pain, Sbardella et al. (2021) concluded that MET was useful for the treatment of acute and chronic neck pain. The review identified 21 clinical studies of acute and chronic neck pain that included MET as part of a rehabilitative programme. Again, the sample sizes of the studies were small (28 to 90) and a variety of comparison interventions were used, including forms of physical therapy and neck flexor exercises. No meta-analysis was performed. Risk of bias was judged to be low for only five studies, and the majority being assessed as high risk of bias.

Most of the studies in the Sbardella et al. (2021) review reported that MET, or the addition of MET to physical therapy, reduced neck pain and disability. The results appeared more favourable for acute neck pain than for chronic neck pain, where the key findings were improvement in ROM. Although the findings are favourable, they are limited by the different interventions and comparisons among studies, small sample sizes, risk of bias and lack of long-term follow-up.

Although more research is needed on the benefit of MET for patients with back and neck pain as well as disability, a substantial number of studies support the effectiveness of MET approaches. Many of these studies did not report on adverse effects or harms; of those that did report adverse effects, none reported any serious adverse effects. Additional studies with larger sample sizes, standard MET protocols, similar comparison interventions and controls as well as longer follow-up are required to be more confident about the effect of MET. Given the evidence of benefit and likely small risk of harm, MET should be considered in back and neck pain, either as a stand-alone technique or as part of a combination of approaches. Most of the studies used three to five contraction phases and light to moderate isometric contractions (20% to 75% of maximal). Because of widely differing techniques used in the studies – sometimes aimed at the lumbar spine, pelvis, sacroiliac joint or hip musculature – and different co-interventions, it is not possible to provide guidance about the most effective method for treating spinal pain.

Muscle Pain

A small number of studies have examined the effect of MET or similar isometric techniques on muscle pain and tenderness. Most of these studies have examined the application of MET, sometimes in combination with other techniques, to myofascial trigger points (MTrPs). MTrPs are tender spots on taut bands of skeletal muscle that produce local and/or referred pain (Travell & Simons, 1983). The aetiology and clinical significance of MTrPs are subject to debate (Chaitow, 2015; Dommerholt & Gerwin, 2015; Quintner et al., 2015), but these tender spots appear to be common and respond to manual therapy (Fryer & Hodgson, 2005).

In an early study, Lewit and Simons (1984) performed a contract–relax (CR) technique on 244 patients with MTrPs. The problematic muscle was passively stretched, and a gentle 10-second isometric contraction was executed followed by relaxation and further stretching, performed three to five times. Treatment resulted in immediate pain relief in 94% of patients and lasting relief in 63%, but pain was measured by a non-blinded assessment of palpation for tenderness. Other studies have demonstrated similar results using more

quantifiable and reliable measures. Dearing and Hamilton (2008) examined 50 asymptomatic participants with trapezius MTrPs and found both MET and ischaemic compression significantly reduced MTrP sensitivity (using pressure pain thresholds (PPT) measured with a pressure algometer). Sadria et al. (2017) also reported that MET reduced the symptoms of MTrPs in the upper trapezius of asymptomatic participants as measured by a visual analogue scale.

A number of studies have found that the benefits of MET approaches for pain and tenderness of MTrPs increase when applied in combination with soft tissue techniques. Trampas et al. (2010) examined the effect of CR (6-second maximum voluntary isometric contraction (MVIC) and 10-second stretch, repeated three times) with and without MTrP massage therapy in 30 males with tight hamstrings and MTrPs. One group received CR and the other group received cross-fibre massage to the MTrP followed by the same CR. The addition of the cross-fibre therapy produced significant improvements in pressure pain sensitivity and, although the sample was small, large between-group effect sizes suggested a real difference between the treatments.

Alghadir et al. (2020) examined the individual and combined effect of MET and ischaemic compression in 60 participants with neck pain and upper trapezius MTrPs. The combination of MET (5-second contraction and 3-second relaxation) and ischaemic compression (90 seconds of sustained manual pressure) showed greater immediate and short-term (2-week follow-up) improvements in neck pain and muscle tenderness than either of the single interventions. Similarly, Wendt and Waszak (2020) reported that MET combined with trigger point therapy (2 minutes of manual compression) was more effective than the single interventions alone and caused changes in PPT and cervical ROM in 60 asymptomatic participants with upper trapezius MTrPs.

Given the findings of these studies (Trampas et al., 2010; Alghadir et al., 2020, Wendt & Waszak, 2020), combining soft tissue techniques with MET is recommended for the treatment of MTrP sensitivity. Interestingly, Yeganeh Lari et al. (2016) found that combining MET with dry needling for participants with upper trapezius MTrPs was also more effective for pain, PPT and neck ROM than the individual interventions alone and may be considered in the treatment of muscle pain and MTrPs.

Improvement in Range of Motion

Improving ROM in a dysfunctional, restricted joint is one of the primary goals in the application of MET (Mitchell & Mitchell, 1995). A small number of 'proof of principle' studies have reported that MET increases ROM in the cervical, thoracic and lumbar regions (Table 4.1). These results support the rationale of applying MET to spinal dysfunction to improve segmental ROM, as described in texts. However, these studies examined asymptomatic participants, which makes generalisation to clinical outcomes unclear.

In the cervical spine, Schenk et al. (1994) examined 18 asymptomatic participants with limitations of cervical active motion (10 degrees or more) during seven sessions of MET over a 4-week period. Those in the MET group achieved significant gains in rotation (approximately 8 degrees) and smaller non-significant gains in all other planes, whereas the control group had little change. Similarly, Burns and Wells (2006) treated 18 asymptomatic participants with MET according to diagnosed motion restrictions and measured active cervical ROM using a three-dimensional motion analysis system. MET produced a significant increase in side bending and rotation (4 degrees) when compared with a sham control group.

To study the effect of different contraction durations on a single spinal segment, Fryer and Ruszkowski (2004) examined the application of MET directed at the rotational restriction of the C1 to C2 motion segment, which was isolated using cervical flexion and rotation. Fifty-two asymptomatic volunteers with at least 4 degrees of asymmetry in active C1 to C2 rotation were randomly allocated to an MET (a 5- or 20-second isometric contraction phase) or sham control treatment. The authors found that MET with a 5-second contraction phase produced a significant increase in the restricted direction (6.7 degrees), but not the unrestricted range, when compared with the control group. The increase in ROM was not at the expense of the unrestricted direction, which also had small mean increases. The 20-second isometric contraction phase MET also had increased ROM, but appeared to be less effective than the 5-second contraction phase.

In the lumbar spine, Schenk et al. (1997) treated 26 asymptomatic subjects having limited active lumbar extension (<25 degrees), measured with a bubble goniometer, with MET. These subjects assigned to the treatment group received an application of MET, consisting of four repetitions of a light 5-second isometric contraction with the joint positioned against the restrictive

TABLE 4.1 Overview of Studies That Have Investigated Muscle Energy for Increasing Spinal Range of Motion

Study	Treatment Duration	Technique	Measurement	Findings
Schenk et al. (1994)	4 weeks	MET	Cervical goniometer: rotation, side bend, flexion, extension	MET > baseline rotation; MET > control
Schenk et al. (1997)	4 weeks	MET	Bubble goniometer: lumbar extension	MET > baseline; MET > control
Lenehan et al. (2003)	Single application	MET	Trunk goniometer: seated trunk rotation	MET > baseline; MET > control
Fryer and Ruszkowski (2004)	Single application	MET (5- and 20-s contraction duration)	Compass goniometer: cervical (C0–C1) rotation	MET 5 s > MET 20 s > sham control
Burns and Wells (2006)	Single application	MET	Three-dimensional motion analysis system	MET > baseline; MET > sham control; significant rotation and side bending

MET, Muscle energy technique (contract–relax form); >, produced greater changes.

barriers in extension, rotation and side bending twice a week for 4 weeks. The MET significantly increased lumbar extension (7 degrees), but there was no increase in the control group.

Increases in thoracic ROM following MET have been reported by Lenehan et al. (2003). Fifty-nine asymptomatic subjects were randomly assigned to either an MET or control group, and blinded pre-intervention and post-intervention measurements of trunk rotation were performed using a custom-made goniometer. The MET group had significantly greater trunk rotation (10.7 degrees), but not to the unrestricted side, and there was no change in the control group.

In a systematic review, Thomas et al. (2019) found the quality of studies for pain and ROM was 'moderate to high' and concluded that MET could be applied to increase ROM of a joint with a functional restriction. These studies support the use of MET to increase spinal ROM, but additional investigation of the lasting duration of increased motion and the clinical benefit to symptomatic individuals is needed. The studies used three to four contraction phases, typically with light contractile forces (25% to 50% of maximal), and relaxation phases of a few seconds. Given the findings of Fryer and Ruszkowski (2004), a shorter duration isometric contraction (5 seconds) is recommended since longer durations appear to produce no greater benefit.

Myofascial Extensibility

Most researchers who have studied isometric-assisted stretching – MET, PNF, postisometric relaxation – have examined the effect of these techniques for increasing the extensibility of the hamstring muscles. The most common forms of isometric stretching in the literature are CR, where the muscle being stretched is contracted and then relaxed; agonist contract–relax (ACR),[1] where contraction of the agonist (rather than the muscle being stretched) actively moves the joint into increased ROM; and contract–relax agonist contract (CRAC), a combination of these two methods (Table 4.2). These techniques are commonly referred to as PNF stretching, but the similarity to MET procedures for lengthening

muscles, particularly CR, is obvious. Another variant is hold–relax (HR). In HR, the contraction is isometric, and no movement or shortening should occur, which is most similar to the common application of MET (DeStefano, 2016). In CR, the muscle may be allowed to shorten, but descriptions from studies have not always specified this and at times the terms CR and HR have been used interchangeably.

Numerous studies have reported that MET and PNF stretching methods produce greater improvements in joint ROM and muscle extensibility than passive, static stretching (SS), both in the short and long term (Sady et al., 1982; Wallin et al., 1985; Osternig et al., 1990; Magnusson et al., 1996b; Feland et al., 2001; Ferber et al., 2002b), but there are conflicting results. Further, researchers have used different treatment protocols (varying the force and duration of contraction and stretching, number of repetitions, direction of contraction) and different methods of measuring hamstring length (active knee extension (AKE), passive knee extension (PKE), measurement of passive torque) to assess the effect of techniques on immediate changes to hamstring length. Studies have reported immediate hamstring length and ROM increases from 3 degrees (Ballantyne et al., 2003) to 33 degrees (Magnusson et al., 1996b) after MET or similar treatments.

In a systematic review of CR and HR, Cayco et al. (2019) identified 39 RCTs that met their inclusion criteria. The methodological quality of the studies assessed using the PEDro scale ranged from 2 to 7, with a median of 4/10, indicating relatively low quality and potentially high risk of bias.

Cayco et al. (2019) found significant effects from a meta-analysis of CR and HR for increasing hamstring flexibility measured with either AKE or PKE, both immediately after a single session and immediately after multiple sessions. When comparing CR and HR with SS, the conclusions from the five relevant studies were inconsistent. A meta-analysis of these studies revealed a small significant advantage of CR and HR when hamstring length was measured with AKE, but not when measured with PKE. The authors concluded that CR and

---

[1]The term 'agonist contract–relax' may be confusing to many because 'agonist' refers to the motion produced, not the relationship of the contracting muscle to the one being stretched. When using this technique to stretch the hamstring muscles (i.e. to increase knee extension), the contracting muscle is the quadriceps femoris. The quadriceps is the 'agonist' muscle for knee extension (the movement being increased) – hence the name ACR – but is the 'antagonist' of the muscle being stretched (hamstrings). This terminology is confusing for those who believe this technique has effect by producing hamstring relaxation through reciprocal inhibition.

TABLE 4.2 MET and PNF Isometric Contraction-Assisted Stretching Techniques	
Manual Procedure	**Procedure Applied to Increase Hamstring Muscle Extensibility**
Hold–relax (HR)	Hamstring muscles are passively stretched, active isometric contraction of the hamstrings against operator resistance, relaxation followed by additional passive stretching; sometimes used interchangeably with CR
Contract–relax (CR)	Hamstring muscles are passively stretched, active contraction (isometric or eccentric) of the hamstrings against operator resistance, relaxation followed by additional passive stretching; sometimes used interchangeably with HR
Agonist contract–relax (ACR)	Hamstring muscles are passively stretched, active contraction of the quadriceps muscles to further increase range of motion and hamstring stretching, relaxation followed by additional passive stretching
Contract–relax agonist contract (CRAC)	Hamstring muscles are passively stretched, active isometric contraction of the hamstrings against operator resistance, relaxation followed by additional passive stretching, active contraction of the quadriceps muscles to further increase range of motion and hamstring stretching, relaxation followed by additional passive stretching

MET, Muscle energy technique; *PNF*, proprioceptive neuromuscular facilitation.

HR were better than control for improving hamstring flexibility, the effects of which lasted for at least 24 hours, but the superiority of these techniques over other forms of stretching are unclear (Cayco et al., 2019).

CR and HR methods, which reflect the typical application of MET for stretching muscles, are effective treatments for stretching. There may be some advantage over SS, but the evidence is still unclear. Most studies have examined the immediate effects of these techniques, but there has been little investigation of long-term changes, which requires additional research.

Variations of Application

MET and related isometric stretching techniques can be varied by changes to the different components of the technique: direction of contraction, duration of contraction and post-contraction stretch, intensity of contraction, number of repetitions and frequency of application. Because of differences in measurement methodology, it is difficult to determine the most efficacious elements of the various treatment protocols, but ACR and CRAC methods seem more effective at increasing extensibility than CR and HR methods.

Agonist Contract–Relax Versus Contract–Relax

Several researchers have compared the effectiveness of ACR, CR and CRAC (a combination of ACR and CR) and found that ACR and CRAC produce more ROM gain than CR. However, some researchers noted that ACR and CRAC appeared less comfortable for subjects and may not be effective for older adults.

Osternig et al. (1990) found that ACR produced 9% to 13% more knee joint ROM than CR and SS. These researchers examined the impact of the three techniques in 10 endurance athletes (distance runners), 10 high-intensity athletes (volleyball players and sprinters) and 10 control subjects (not involved in competitive sports). The CR group received five applications (5-second MVIC, 5-second stretch, performed twice) to the hamstrings; the ACR group received a similar procedure except the quadriceps musculature was contracted to extend the knee. The SS group received an 80-second stretch. The ACR group had significantly greater ROM (approximately 20 degrees) than the CR and SS groups.

ACR techniques are also more effective at increasing hamstring extensibility in older adults. Ferber et al. (2002b) examined the effects of ACR, CR and SS of the hamstrings on PKE in adults aged 50 to 75 years. The mean change produced by the ACR was 15.7 degrees and was significantly greater than CR (12.1 degrees) and SS (11.7 degrees). Interestingly, 77% of subjects thought the ACR was the most uncomfortable procedure. In another investigation of PNF stretching in older adults, Ferber et al. (2002a) found that ACR produced 4 to 6 degrees more knee ROM than CR and SS in trained subjects (master level endurance runners) aged 45 to 75 years and in untrained subjects aged 45 to 50 years, but not in untrained subjects aged 65 to 75 years. The researchers suggested the lack of effect in the older untrained group was possibly due to a lack of neuromuscular control or strength.

Etnyre and Abraham (1986a) found that CRAC was more effective than CR at increasing the range of ankle dorsiflexion. Twelve subjects performed CRAC, CR and SS on separate days. The CRAC produced significantly greater increases in ROM than the CR method, which was significantly better than the SS method. Similarly, Youdas et al. (2010) performed CR or CRAC, randomly assigned to opposite lower extremities, on 35 subjects with reduced hamstring length and found that CRAC produced greater PKE increases than CR (15 vs 11 degrees).

Some researchers have suggested that the muscle performing the contraction and the direction of contraction may be unimportant. Azevedo et al. (2011) compared the effect of hamstring CR, the CR of an uninvolved muscle (elbow flexors), and no treatment (control) on AKE in 60 healthy males. They found that the hamstring CR and the elbow flexor CR increased AKE (9 degrees), whereas the control did not change. In contrast, Moore et al. (2011) found MET of the glenohumeral joint horizontal abductors produced greater ROM in abduction and internal rotation than those treated with MET in external rotation, suggesting that direction has a specific effect.

Osama (2021) compared a reciprocal inhibition (ACR) MET applied to muscles of the cervical spine (scalenes, sternocleidomastoid, levator scapulae, upper trapezius) with an autogenic (CR) MET. For both techniques, three to five repetitions of a 30% to 50% isometric contraction for 7 to 10 seconds were followed by 5 seconds of rest and a stretch of 10 to 60 seconds. Osama (2021) found that the autogenic CR technique was more effective than the ACR reciprocal inhibition technique and SS for reducing pain and increasing ROM. The participants had moderate intensity neck pain, and it is possible that the ACR contraction may have been provocative, thereby causing dissimilar results from studies meant to increase flexibility in asymptomatic participants.

Given the evidence that ACR produces greater increases than CR, the direction of contraction most likely plays an important role in the efficacy of treatment. For increasing muscle extensibility where the muscles or joints are not painful or are recovering from injury, it is recommended that isometric stretching techniques use a contraction towards the restricted barrier, as in ACR and CRAC.

Duration of Contraction

Different durations for the muscular contraction for MET and similar techniques have been recommended, but few have investigated the optimal durations. Many have advocated 3 to 7 seconds of resisted contraction for therapeutic effect (Mitchell & Mitchell, 1995; DeStefano, 2016). Others have suggested 5-second (Ballantyne et al., 2003), 5- and 20-second (Mehta & Hatton, 2002), 6- and 12-second (Schmitt et al., 1999) and 20-second (Ferber et al., 2002b) contraction durations. The value of longer isometric contraction durations is uncertain because of conflicting results in the few studies that have examined this variable and lack of sufficient statistical power due to low number of subjects.

Schmitt et al. (1999) examined the relationship between durations of sub-maximal isometric contraction on hamstring flexibility using an ACR technique and compared the effects of 6- and 12-second isometric contraction durations in 10 subjects. Both groups individually produced significant increases in ROM, measured by an active sit-and-reach test, but there were no significant differences between groups. The 12-second contraction group had greater ROM than the 6-second group, but given the small group sizes (five in each group), this study may have lacked power to detect differences between the contraction durations. Mehta and Hatton (2002) performed a hamstring CR in 24 subjects using a 5-second sub-maximal contraction and, after a 14-day washout period, used a 20-second contraction MET. The authors found a significant increase in passive ROM after both contraction durations, but no significant difference between the two treatments.

Bonnar et al. (2004) examined the immediate effect of a CR performed three times using a 3-, 6- or 10-second MVIC on passive straight leg raise (SLR) in 60 subjects. A significant increase in SLR was found for all groups, and slightly greater increases in ROM were found for the longer contraction durations, but these between-group differences were not significant. Similarly, Nelson and Cornelius (1991) examined the effect of the same contraction durations for a CRAC stretching procedure on the range of internal rotation of the shoulder joint in 60 subjects. The shoulders were passively internally rotated just short of end range followed by an MVIC external rotation effort, an internal rotation isometric effort (3, 6 or 10 seconds), and relaxation and passive stretching for an unspecified duration, performed three times. The researchers found all treatments produced significantly greater ROM than baseline measures, but there were no differences among the various contraction durations.

In contrast to these studies, Rowlands et al. (2003) reported that longer contraction durations in CRAC resulted in greater increases in hamstring flexibility. Forty-three women were assigned to a 5- or 10-second isometric contraction group or to a no-treatment control group, and ROM was measured by SLR to pain tolerance. The treatment groups followed a CRAC stretching programme twice a week for 6 weeks. The hamstrings were passively stretched, and the subject performed an MVIC of the hamstrings for 5 or 10 seconds followed by 5 seconds of relaxation, contraction of the agonist (quadriceps) and 10 seconds of passive stretch. Both treatment groups had significant increases over the control group, and the 10-second group had significantly greater gains than the 5-second group at 3 weeks (20 vs 16 degrees) and 6 weeks (33 vs 28 degrees).

Given these conflicting results and reported ROM gains irrespective of contraction duration, the shorter duration of 3 to 5 seconds is recommended until benefits of longer durations are confirmed.

Intensity of Contraction

Different intensities of contraction force have been used in different studies and recommended by different authors. Many researchers investigating isometric stretching have used moderate or MVIC intensities, but because of different treatment and ROM measurement methods, comparisons among these studies are difficult. However, four studies were found that examined the optimal intensity of contraction for increasing ROM.

Sheard and Paine (2010) studied 56 athletes using CR (5-second contraction, three repetitions) for the hamstrings with contraction intensities of 20%, 50% and 100% MVIC and ROM measured with an SLR. They found the change in ROM was 8.4, 12.9 and 11.6 degrees, respectively, and recommended that intensities of approximately 65% MVIC were optimal for increasing ROM. Similarly, Lim (2018) examined the hamstring flexibility of 68 participants with AKE and used a 10%, 40%, 70% or 100% MVIC HR technique (10-second contraction, three repetitions). The 70% and 100% MVIC techniques produced more ROM than the 10% and 40% techniques, but the post-stretch pain level was significantly greater for the 100% MVIC. Therefore, the author recommended a moderate stretching intensity for effectiveness and safety. Kwak and Ryu (2015) examined prone knee flexion ROM in 60 participants using a CR (8-second contraction, three repetitions) with

quadriceps contraction intensities of 20%, 60% or 100% MVIC. They found that changes were larger in the 60% and 100% MVIC groups than the 20% MVIC group.

In contrast, Feland and Marin (2004) found no differences when varying the intensity of isometric contraction. These researchers assigned 72 volunteers with tight hamstrings to one of three CR treatment groups using 20%, 60% or 100% MVIC for a stretching session once a day for 5 days. All groups achieved greater PKE than the control group, but there was no difference between three groups.

Additional research is warranted to determine the effect of isometric contraction intensity in MET, but there is evidence that using at least a moderate contraction intensity (60% MVIC) is more effective than gentle intensities in healthy adults for increasing ROM. Using lower intensities is recommended to minimise the risk of injury to target muscles that are smaller, painful or recovering from injury. It is worth noting that athletes have shown a poor level of accuracy and consistency for instructed targets of 20%, 50% and 100% MIVC (Sheard et al., 2009), so patients may have difficulty performing muscle contractions at specific intensities.

Number of Contraction Phases

Even though application of one contraction and stretch phase produces increased ROM, little evidence is available to guide the practitioner on the number of contraction–relaxation phases to use for optimal ROM gain. Magnusson et al. (1996b) achieved a large hamstring ROM gain (33 degrees) following one 6-second CR isometric contraction phase. However, it seems that additional repetitions of contraction and stretch produce diminishing gains. Osternig et al. (1990) found that 64% to 84% of ROM gain was produced in the first phase (one 5-second contraction followed by 5-second relaxation and stretch) of each trial for passive stretching, CR and ACR, suggesting little benefit from additional repetitions of isometric contraction.

In contrast, Mitchell et al. (2007) reported that four contraction applications produced the greatest ROM gains. Four applications of a 6-second MVIC with a 10-second stretch phase were performed, with 20 seconds between each application, and were measured with PKE. Progressive increases in ROM and tolerance to increasing force of stretch were found after each application. The researchers did not investigate more repetitions of the contractions, so it is unknown whether additional benefit would be gained using additional contraction applications.

Clearly, the number of contraction and relaxation applications for optimal ROM gain deserves further investigation. Although there is uncertainty whether more than one contraction produces additional ROM gains, one to three applications are recommended because the additional applications require little additional effort or time and more gains may be possible.

Duration of Post-Contraction Stretch

In the osteopathic literature, two applications of MET for increasing muscle extensibility have been advocated by Chaitow (2006) and DeStefano (2016), but with differences in the number of repetitions three to five, and three repetitions, respectively) and the period of passive stretching between isometric contractions. Chaitow (2006) suggests a stretch duration after isometric contraction for 30 seconds up to 60 seconds for chronically shortened muscles. American authors, such as DeStefano (2016) and Mitchell et al. (1979), recommend only enough time (several seconds) for patient relaxation and tension to be taken up in the affected tissue. The stretching literature suggests that a 30-second SS may be optimal (Bandy & Irion, 1994; Bandy et al., 1997), and considering the Greenman procedure (DeStefano, 2016) places the muscle in a position of stretch in excess of 30 seconds when the application is repeated several times as recommended, longer stretch phase durations may have no benefit.

Only one study has compared the effectiveness of these MET variations for stretching muscles. Smith and Fryer (2008) randomly allocated 40 asymptomatic subjects with short hamstrings to one of two groups: CR with a 30-second postisometric stretch phase or CR with a 3-second postisometric stretch phase. Two applications, 1 week apart, were performed and hamstring length was measured with AKE. Both techniques produced significant immediate increases in hamstring extensibility relative to baseline. Improvement was partially sustained 1 week after the initial treatment, but there were no significant differences between the interventions.

Given that no benefit of a longer stretch duration was found, a shorter stretch duration is recommended. However, the optimal duration of the passive stretch phase in MET requires additional investigation.

Frequency of Application

The frequency of isometric stretching for optimal and long-lasting gains in ROM has received little investigation. Although some studies have reported only short-term gains in muscle extensibility after a session of isometric stretching (Spernoga et al., 2001), others have reported longer lasting gains. Wallin et al. (1985) found that after a 30-day stretching programme (three sessions of CR or ballistic stretching per week) volunteers who performed CR once a week maintained their improved flexibility and those who performed CR two or five times a week gained additional increases in ROM.

Based on these findings, applying MET at least twice a week is suggested for increased ROM; however, the effect of frequency of isometric stretching also deserves further investigation.

Post-Exercise

CR has produced increased hamstring extensibility immediately after exercise. Funk et al. (2003) examined hamstring extensibility using AKE in 40 elite athletes following SS or CR, either without exercise or immediately after a 60-minute cycling and upper body conditioning programme. The hamstring CR technique consisted of a 30-second MVIC repeated for 5 minutes. No significant differences in AKE were found between the two treatment groups, but there was a significant increase in the CR group after exercise compared with baseline (9.6 degrees) and with CR without exercise (7.8 degrees). Therefore MET may be more effective when performed after exercise.

Heat and Cold

The application of cryotherapy may facilitate PNF stretching because cold increases the threshold stimulus of the muscle spindles and attenuates the stretch reflex, which may result in a more relaxed muscle and increased ROM. However, Cornelius et al. (1992) examined the effect of cold (ice cubes in a plastic bag placed on the posterior thigh for 10 minutes) or no cold on the hamstring extensibility of 120 male subjects immediately before the application of SS, CR, ACR or CRAC and found that the cold application did not influence the effectiveness of the techniques even though all PNF techniques produced significantly greater increases in ROM than SS. Similarly, Burke et al. (2001) investigated the effect of 10 minutes of hot-water or cold-water immersion with the application of ACR over a 5-day stretching period. They found that all ACR groups (ACR + heat, ACR + cold, ACR alone) produced significant increases in hamstring length compared with baseline active SLR, but application of neither hot nor cold influenced post-treatment flexibility. Applications of heat or cold are therefore not recommended.

Conclusion

MET and other isometric stretching techniques appear to be more effective for muscle extensibility than SS, but the most efficacious application remains unclear. CRAC and ACR appear to be more effective applications than CR methods, but given that they involve the patient actively pushing into the restricted ROM, they may only be suitable to increase flexibility in healthy individuals and not when the restriction involves pain or discomfort. There is evidence that moderate to maximal contraction intensities (60% to 100% MVIC) are more effective than light intensities for increasing ROM, but MVIC intensities produce more post-stretching pain and the risk of injury, so moderate (approximately 60% MVIC) forces are recommended. The most efficacious passive torque for stretching, duration of isometric contraction and number of repetitions for MET need additional research to be determined. Based on the limited evidence available, short contraction durations of 3 to 5 seconds, moderate contraction intensities to minimise the risk of injury and one to three applications of the procedures applied at least twice a week are recommended. Combining soft tissue techniques with MET is also recommended for the treatment of MTrPs. It should also be noted that MET, like any stretching protocol, will produce temporary energy loss from the tissue and reduce subsequent performance, so these treatments should not be applied before sporting activities (Sá et al., 2016).

RESEARCH INTO THE MECHANISMS OF THERAPEUTIC EFFECT

When examining the mechanisms responsible for the therapeutic effect of a manual therapy intervention, it is tempting to attribute all effects to biological and biomechanical mechanisms. In recent decades, there has been a growing awareness of the powerful contribution of psychosocial factors to an individual's experience of pain and associated disability. Similarly, there is growing recognition that psychosocial factors play an important role in the therapeutic effect of many interactions. The language and messages that the therapist uses can reassure, educate and empower the patient or, alternatively, encourage the patient to catastrophise, engage in fear avoidance behaviour and become more disabled and reliant on short-term passive treatments (Darlow et al., 2015).

It has been argued that any manual therapy encounter is a complex intervention and therapeutic effect may result from a combination of biological (encompassing biomechanical, tissue changes and neurologically mediated mechanisms) and psychosocial mechanisms (Fryer, 2017a). The relative influence of these different mechanisms varies between people. Careful choice of language and messages can provide a positive and empowering psychological context that reinforces the positive gains from tissue and neurological mechanisms (Fryer, 2017b). The focus of the following examination of therapeutic mechanisms will be on the biological mechanisms, but all practitioners should be cognisant that the language used and the intentional and unintentional messages delivered to the patient may have a greater influence than the specific effects of the treatment intervention itself.

Mechanisms for Improving Function
Increase in Range of Motion

Studies reporting increases in spinal ROM after MET have measured active ROM without measuring passive torque, so conclusions about the mechanism behind the increased ROM are limited. Changes to the viscoelasticity of segmental muscles or peri-articular tissues are unlikely given the lack of long-term changes evidenced for hamstring extensibility. Further, the light stretching loads applied to spinal tissues mean that viscoelastic or plastic changes in tissues are unlikely.

Some authors have postulated that reflex muscle relaxation after MET produces ROM gains (Mitchell & Mitchell, 1995), but this mechanism seems unsupported by evidence from PNF studies (discussed below). Changes in paraspinal muscle electromyographic (EMG) activity or reflex muscle relaxation after spinal MET have not been examined, but there is evidence of decreased corticospinal and spinal reflex excitability (Fryer & Pearce, 2013), suggesting overall decreased motor excitability following MET. Since only changes to active spinal ROM have been investigated, a change in stretch tolerance (as is the case for stretching muscles) may largely be responsible for spinal ROM gains.

Although evidence of inflammation in acute spinal pain using MRI is lacking (Fryer & Adams, 2011), acute spinal pain may involve zygapophysial capsule sprain, joint effusion and tissue inflammation, which would disturb active and passive motion at the segment (Fryer, 2016). If acute spinal pain involves effusion and inflammation of surrounding tissues, MET may play a role in fluid drainage (discussed below) for improved motion. This mechanism is speculative but appears plausible in cases of minor trauma to the spinal complex.

Reduction in Pain

The exact mechanisms for hypoalgesia following MET are unknown, but possible mechanisms include neurological and tissue factors. Neurological mechanisms include the stimulation of low threshold mechanoreceptors on centrally mediated pain inhibitory mechanisms and on neuronal populations in the dorsal horn with possible gating effects, and tissue mechanisms may include the effect of rhythmic muscle contractions on interstitial and tissue fluid flow (Vigotsky & Bruhns, 2015; Fryer, 2017a).

Low threshold mechanoreceptors from joints and muscles project to the periaqueductal grey (PAG) in the midbrain region (Yezierski, 1991). Evidence from animal and human studies suggests that induced or voluntary muscle contraction results in sympathoexcitation and localised activation of the lateral and dorsolateral PAG (Li & Mitchell, 2003; Seseke et al., 2006). Further, stimulation of the lateral PAG through spinal manipulative therapy may result in a non-opioid form of analgesia accompanied by sympathoexcitation (Souvlis et al., 2004). Activation of non-opioid descending inhibitory pathways (serotonergic and noradrenergic) following peripheral joint mobilisation has been demonstrated in an animal model (Skyba et al., 2003). Spinal blockade of serotonin receptors and noradrenalin receptors prevented the hypoalgesic effect of joint mobilisation (Skyba et al., 2003; Hoeger Bement & Sluka, 2007), suggesting involvement of serotonergic and noradrenergic receptors and pathways.

Rhythmic muscle contractions increase muscle blood and lymph flow rates (Schmid-Schonbein, 1990; Coates et al., 1993; Havas et al., 1997). Mechanical forces (loading and stretching) acting on connective tissues have the potential to change the interstitial pressure and increase transcapillary blood flow (Langevin et al., 2005). These factors may influence the tissue response to injury and inflammation. Furthermore, MET may support these processes by reducing the concentrations of pro-inflammatory cytokines, resulting in decreased sensitisation of peripheral nociceptors.

Therefore, MET may produce hypoalgesia centrally and peripherally through the activation of muscle and joint mechanoreceptors, involving centrally mediated pathways, such as the PAG and non-opioid serotonergic and noradrenergic descending inhibitory pathways, and producing peripheral effects associated with increased fluid drainage.

Improvement of Proprioception and Motor Control

Spinal pain produces disturbances in proprioception and motor control. Patients with pain have decreased awareness of spinal motion and position (Gill & Callaghan, 1998; Grip et al., 2007; Stanton et al., 2016) and of cutaneous touch perception (Voerman et al., 2000; Stohler et al., 2001). Spinal pain also appears to disturb the contraction of deep paraspinal musculature, while causing superficial spinal muscles to overreact to stimuli (Fryer et al., 2004).

Although there is some evidence of benefit from spinal manipulative therapy for proprioception and motor control in pain patients (Karlberg et al., 1991; Rogers, 1997; Heikkila et al., 2000; Sterling et al., 2001; Palmgren et al., 2006), little research has been conducted on MET or related techniques. Joseph et al. (2010) examined 40 subjects with chronic recurrent ankle sprains and found that both high-velocity thrust and MET improved balance, ROM and function, while decreasing short-term pain. Ryan et al. (2010) examined the effect of CRAC to the hamstrings, plantar flexors and hip flexors on postural stability. They found that CRAC improved medial and lateral postural stability, with or without a warm-up. Additionally, Malmstrom et al. (2010) found that a prolonged unilateral neck contraction task (30% MVIC for 5 minutes) increased the accuracy of head repositioning, which is a test of cervical proprioception.

Although these studies have not directly investigated MET, they support the likelihood that MET may improve proprioception in patients with pain. Given that other manipulative techniques appear useful for proprioception and that active approaches are likely to be superior to passive techniques for motor learning, more study of the use of MET for proprioception, motor control and motor learning is recommended.

Tissue Fluid Drainage

Authors of MET texts have proposed that MET can improve lymphatic flow and reduce oedema (Mitchell et al., 1979), and this suggestion is consistent with evidence that muscle contraction influences interstitial tissue fluid collection and lymphatic flow (Schmid-Schonbein, 1990). For example, physical activity increased lymph flow peripherally in the collecting ducts, centrally in the thoracic duct and within the muscle during concentric and isometric muscle contractions (Coates et al., 1993; Havas et al., 1997). Although speculative, MET may have a role in reducing pain and increasing ROM by promoting drainage of injured and inflamed joints and tissues (Fryer, 2017a).

Mechanisms for Increasing Myofascial Extensibility

The physiological mechanisms behind the changes in muscle extensibility produced by MET are still being investigated. Of the three most studied mechanisms proposed to account for short-term and medium-term changes in muscle extensibility – stretch tolerance changes, reflex muscle relaxation, viscoelastic or muscle property change – stretch tolerance change is most supported by the scientific literature.

Stretch Tolerance

Despite lack of evidence of lasting viscoelastic change in human muscle after SS, many clinical studies have reported ROM gains after SS and isometric stretching of the hamstring muscles. The ROM gains may be best explained by an increase in tolerance to stretching force. PKE (when passive torque is not measured) and AKE are usually performed to the point of hamstring tension or pain. Studies have demonstrated that the increase in extensibility after SS or MET is caused by a tolerance of greater stretching force when extended the muscle.

Magnusson et al. (1996a, 1998) measured the passive torque of the hamstring muscle during PKE to the point of pain before and after 90 seconds of SS and found that ROM and passive torque were increased following the stretch. Magnusson et al. (1996b) also compared the effect of a 90-second SS with the addition of a 6-second CR contraction and found that ROM and passive torque increased, indicating an increase in stretch tolerance.

Ballantyne et al. (2003) found that MET (5-second moderate force contraction, 3-second stretch and relaxation, performed four times) applied to the hamstrings produced no evidence of viscoelastic change, but when the PKE was taken to pain tolerance (pre-MET and post-MET), a greater passive torque was tolerated post-MET that allowed a subsequent increase in ROM. Mitchell et al. (2007) also found that increased force of stretch of the hamstrings could be tolerated with successive trials of CR.

In studies by Magnusson et al. (1996b) and Mitchell et al. (2007), CR produced greater ROM than SS, which suggests that MET produces a greater change in stretch tolerance than SS. Stretching and isometric contraction stimulate muscle and joint mechanoreceptors and may attenuate the sensation of pain. Although MET and SS do not have obvious lasting effects on the viscoelastic properties of muscle tissue, there still may be clinically relevant changes for enhanced stretching and performance. A change in stretch tolerance may condition and prepare the muscle for athletic activity. Further, if MET influences neurological pain mechanisms, it may have a role in the improvement of joint and muscle proprioception for better coordination and performance. Future studies should examine the effect of isometric techniques on sporting performance and injury prevention.

Reflex Muscle Relaxation

Many authors have proposed that MET and PNF techniques facilitate stretching by producing neurological reflex muscle relaxation after isometric muscle contraction (Osternig et al. 1987; Mitchell & Mitchell, 1995). Reflex muscle relaxation after contraction theoretically occurs through activation of Golgi tendon organs and their inhibitory influence on the α-motor neuron pool or through reciprocal inhibition produced by contraction of a muscle antagonist. Although it is accepted that these reflex pathways exist, Golgi tendon organ inhibition is not evident after SS (Miller & Burne, 2014), and its role in postisometric relaxation has not been established.

Several studies support the concept of neurological muscle relaxation in MET through demonstration of a strong, brief neuromuscular inhibition after isometric muscle contraction. Moore and Kukulka (1991) examined H-reflexes (an indicator of α-motor neuron pool excitability) of the soleus muscle in 16 subjects who performed isometric 65% to 75% MVIC in plantar flexion. They found a strong brief depression of the soleus H-reflex in all subjects that lasted for about 10 seconds with maximal depression between 0.1 and 1 second post-contraction. Similarly, Etnyre and Abraham (1986b) found that SS of the soleus muscle reduced the H-reflex slightly, whereas CR and CRAC markedly reduced the reflex. Other researchers have reported decreases in EMG activity in response to a sudden stretch (Carter et al., 2000) and reductions of motor cortex activity following isometric contractions (Gandevia et al., 1999). Fryer and Pearce (2013) reported decreased corticospinal and H-reflex excitability following application of a lumbar MET. Although these studies support the potential of MET to produce reflex muscle relaxation, evidence of a decrease in EMG activity following the use of MET is lacking.

Implicit in the suggestion that MET acts by producing reflex muscle relaxation is the assumption that low-level motor activity is elevated in dysfunctional muscle and plays a role in limiting passive stretch. Active motor activity, however, appears to have a limited role in producing resistance to passive stretch. The hamstring muscles have shown a very low-level EMG response when undergoing SS (Magnusson et al., 1995, 1996a, 1996c) and, therefore, this activity probably does not contribute to passive resistance to stretch. Furthermore, studies have demonstrated that increases in muscle length after 90 seconds of SS occur without any changes to the low-level EMG activity of that muscle (Magnusson et al., 1996a, 1996c; Youdas et al., 2010).

Not only does neurological motor activity appear to have no role in passive resistance to stretch, but researchers have found that isometric stretching techniques do not decrease the low-level EMG activity associated with muscle stretching. Magnusson et al. (1995) found that the low-level EMG response of the hamstrings was unchanged in the 60 seconds after 40 maximal-effort, repetitive hamstring contractions (concentric or eccentric) before a second stretch. In a later study, Magnusson et al. (1996b) compared the effects of passive stretching (80 seconds) and a 6-second forceful isometric contraction of the hamstrings (in a position of stretch followed by 80 seconds of stretch) on ROM and hamstring electromyography. They found that low-level EMG activity was unchanged after both stretching procedures.

Contrary to the proposal that MET and PNF produce reflex muscle relaxation, several studies have reported *increased* electromyography after these techniques.

Osternig et al. (1987) examined the effect of CR, ACR and SS on hamstring extensibility and EMG activity in 10 subjects. SS produced a small decrease (11%) in hamstring EMG response between a first and second stretch, whereas CR and ACR produced increases in hamstring EMG activity, which was recorded during the stretch (relaxation) phase of the techniques. In a later study, Osternig et al. (1990) found the same pattern of EMG activity in several athlete populations, where ACR produced greater ROM and EMG activity than CR or SS. Similarly, Ferber et al. (2002b) examined the effects of CR, ACR and SS to the hamstrings in a population of older adults and found that ACR produced greater EMG activity, as well as ROM, than CR and SS. Youdas et al. (2010) performed CR and CRAC on the hamstrings of 35 healthy subjects and found that, despite gains in ROM, electromyography was increased following application of the techniques. Mitchell et al. (2009) used surface and indwelling wire electrodes and also found that EMG activity in the hamstrings increased after CR and CRAC techniques. These results confirm that motor tone in a muscle increases during contraction of its antagonist and do not support reflex or reciprocal inhibition as a mechanism for these techniques. Olivo and Magee (2006) reported similar findings for the masticatory muscles, where CR and ACR increased EMG activity rather than reflex muscle relaxation.

Clearly, evidence suggests that neurological EMG activity in hamstring muscles does not contribute to resistance to passive stretching, and although MET and PNF techniques produce greater ROM changes than SS, these techniques paradoxically produce greater EMG activity in the muscle undergoing the stretch. Thus, increased extensibility must occur because of other factors, such as viscoelastic change or increased stretch tolerance.

Viscoelastic or Muscle Property Change

Connective tissues have mechanical properties related to their fluid or gel components (viscous) and their elastic properties; this phenomenon is called viscoelasticity. Connective tissue elongation is time- and history-dependent, and if a constant stretching force is loaded on a tissue, the tissue will respond with slow elongation or 'creep'. Tissue creep results in loss of energy (hysteresis), and repetition of loading before the tissue has recovered results in greater deformation (Norkin & Levangie, 1992). Additional loading may cause permanent 'plastic' change, which is caused by micro-tearing of collagen fibres (resulting in an immediate change in the stiffness of the tissue) and subsequent remodelling of the fibres to a longer length (Lederman, 2005).

The addition of an isometric contraction to a passive stretch may be more effective for viscoelastic change than passive stretching alone. Taylor et al. (1997) found that muscle contraction and muscle stretching in a rabbit model resulted in passive tension reductions of similar magnitude, indicating viscoelastic stress relaxation of the muscle-tendon unit. For a muscle to maintain the same length during an isometric contraction, the connective tissues must undergo lengthening to compensate for contractile element shortening, which suggests that isometric stretching more effectively loads these connective tissues than passive stretching alone.

Kay et al. (2015) found that CR produced reductions in both tendon and muscle stiffness, when compared with SS and isometric contraction alone, and even though all interventions produced similar increases in stretch tolerance, the authors speculated that stiffness changes may explain the superior efficacy of CR. Lederman (2005) proposed that passive stretching elongates the parallel fibres but has little effect on the 'in-series' fibres; however, the addition of an isometric contraction may cause loading on these fibres that produces viscoelastic or plastic changes greater than that achieved by passive stretching alone (Figs. 4.1 and 4.2).

Thixotropy refers to resistance of a muscle to motion in relation to its immediate history of contraction and length (Proske & Morgan, 1999), and may provide another explanation for the tension and length changes in muscles following MET. A property shown by some gels, thixotropy causes a temporary reduction in viscosity as a result of stirring, where the stirring forces disrupt bonds between molecules that are subsequently reformed when the stirring forces cease (Izumizaki et al., 2006). Thixotropy causes muscle stiffness or slackness, depending on the history of the muscle and whether the muscle was previously contracted at a longer or shorter length. Similar to the process used in MET, slack can be introduced at a specific length by contracting the muscle at a longer length, letting it relax completely and then returning it to the previous length. This phenomenon may be explained by long-lasting, stable cross-bridges between actin and myosin filaments in the muscle (Proske & Morgan, 1999; Izumizaki et al., 2006). When a muscle is contracted and relaxes, stable cross-bridges

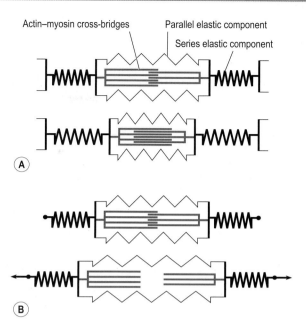

Fig. 4.1 Changes in the connective tissue of the muscle during muscle contraction and passive stretching. (A) During contraction, the series elastic components are under tension and elongate, while the tension in the parallel elastic components is reduced. (B) During passive stretching, both the elastic and parallel components are under tension. However, the less stiff parallel fibres will elongate more than the series component. (The separation between the actin and myosin has been exaggerated.)

form in the fibres at that length. When the muscle is passively shortened, the fibres do not fully take up the shorter length without falling slack, and this slack may last for long periods if the muscle is left undisturbed (Proske & Morgan, 1999). However, this intriguing phenomenon has not been investigated in relation to MET.

Stretch and isometric contractions may affect water content of the tissue and cause alterations in the length and stiffness of connective tissues. Lanir et al. (1988) investigated rat collagen fibre bundles under high-strain loads and found an initial reduction in fibre diameter due to loss of water and glycosaminoglycan molecules, which was followed by swelling of the fibre beyond its initial diameter. Similarly, Yahia et al. (1993) found human lumbodorsal fascia tissue stiffness increased after successive stretching (initial, 30 minutes, 1 hour later) and greater loads were required to deform (lengthen) the tissue on subsequent stretch applications. Schleip et al. (2004) proposed that this hydration effect may have a

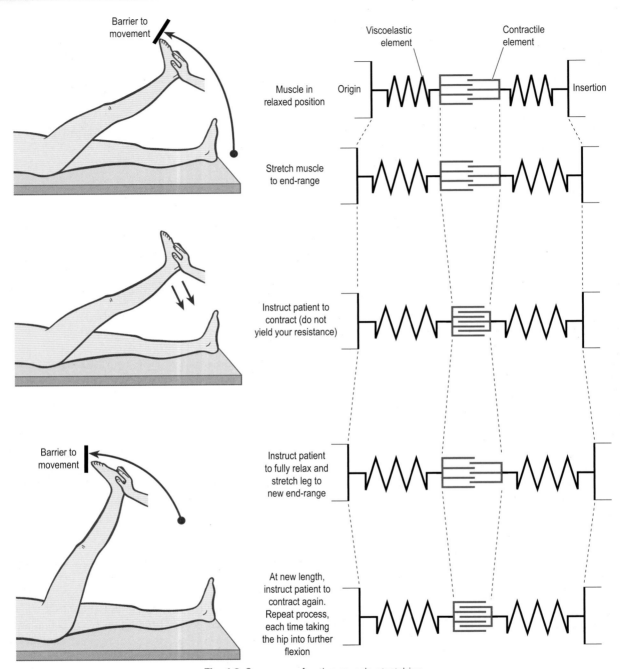

Fig. 4.2 Sequence of active muscle stretching.

role in the therapeutic action of stretching and connective tissue manipulation through increases in the water content and alterations in the stiffness of the tissue. This 'sponge effect' may have a role in tissue texture change following MET or connective tissue manipulation and warrants additional investigation.

Most researchers who have reported ROM gains following passive stretching of the hamstring muscles have monitored hamstring length using PKE and have not measured passive torque (force applied to produce the stretch). Similarly, researchers who have reported ROM gains following CR or AKE have used methods such as AKE, sit-and-reach, PKE and SLR without measurement of passive torque. Measurement of ROM without passive torque does not represent a change in muscle property (change in the biomechanical structure of the muscle) because there is no way of determining whether the same torque was used in subsequent measurements. For example, when using PKE to the point of discomfort or knee buckling, there is no way to be certain that the force used to stretch and measure the hamstrings was the same as before the treatment intervention. When using AKE, there is no certainty that the subject did not use greater active muscle effort during the post-treatment measure. Only with a measurement of torque can the passive stretching force be consistently maintained pre-intervention and post-intervention as well as information gained about any change to the properties of muscle tissues.

Evidence of lasting viscoelastic change has been difficult to demonstrate in human muscle. Researchers who have investigated the effect of SS on hamstring extensibility using torque-controlled PKE have found little evidence of any lasting change to tissue properties (Magnusson et al., 1996a, 1998). Further, isometric stretching may produce little immediate viscoelastic change in the hamstring muscles. Magnusson et al. (1996b) and Ballantyne et al. (2003) measured PKE and passive torque following isometric stretching to the hamstrings and found little evidence of viscoelastic change. Both studies reported significant ROM gains, but only when the passive torque was increased to stretch the hamstrings to the point of discomfort, which indicated that this increase was not caused by a change in muscle properties.

Little is known about the benefit of SS or MET for the extensibility of injured and healing muscle, so this area is a fertile ground for research. Furthermore, anecdotal reports and observations of dancers, martial artists and athletes with above average flexibility because of dedicated stretching programmes suggest that stretching can influence long-term muscle extensibility, therefore, the type and duration of stretching required to produce lasting changes should be investigated.

DIAGNOSTIC ISSUES

Diagnosis of Spinal Dysfunction

Mitchell Sr and Jr based their approach to treatment of the spine on Fryette's physiological spinal coupling model (Fryette, 1954). Many MET texts still use this model of spinal coupled motion for predictive diagnosis and treatment applications (Mitchell & Mitchell, 1995; DiGiovanna et al., 2005; DeStefano, 2016). Although studies have refuted the predictability of spinal coupled motion (Malmstrom et al., 2006, Legaspi & Edmond, 2007; Sizer et al., 2007), they raise questions about the validity and reproducibility of the reommended diagnostic tests (Gibbons & Tehan, 1998; Fryer, 2011).

The traditional paradigm for diagnosis and treatment has been biomechanical, where multiple planes of motion loss are identified and each restrictive barrier is engaged to increase motion in all restricted planes. The model proposed by Fryette (1954) describes two types of coupled motion restrictions: Type 1, also known as contralateral coupling, is based on spinal asymmetry in neutral; and Type 2, also known as ipsilateral coupling, is based on non-neutral spinal postures. Fryette's model has been criticised for its prescriptive diagnostic labelling and invalid inferences from static positional assessment (Gibbons & Tehan, 1998; Fryer, 2000, 2011). Further, only three combinations of multiple plane motion restrictions are allowed – a neutral Type 1, a non-neutral Type 2 with flexion or a non-neutral Type 2 with extension. The model does not allow for other combinations, such as Type 1 with extension.

Osteopathic texts advocate detection of dysfunctional spinal segments by using the diagnostic criteria of segmental tenderness, asymmetry, restricted ROM and altered tissue texture (Mitchell & Mitchell, 1995; DeStefano, 2016). However, the validity, reliability and specificity of detecting these clinical signs have been questioned (Chaitow, 2001; Seffinger et al., 2004). For instance, only palpation for tenderness and pain provocation have acceptable interexaminer reliability, while motion palpation and static spinal asymmetry have poor reliability (Spring et al., 2001; Seffinger et al., 2004).

MET texts commonly advocate for the comparison of static positional asymmetry of the spinal transverse process or sacral base with the spine in neutral, flexion and extension. Based on these findings, specific motion restriction combinations are diagnosed and treated with MET. With this approach, there is an assumption that a transverse process posterior or resistant to posterior–anterior springing represents a restriction of rotation on the opposite side. Although muscle and anatomical vertebral asymmetries are common in healthy individuals, normal variation is a complicating factor typically not considered. Additionally, assessment of segmental static asymmetry has not been reliable (Spring et al., 2001), and spinal coupled motion in the lumbar, thoracic and cervical regions is inconsistent, as evidenced by variability between spinal levels and individuals (Edmondston et al., 2005; Cook et al., 2006; Ishii et al., 2006; Malmstrom et al., 2006; Legaspi & Edmond, 2007; Sizer et al., 2007). Even though one study suggested that coupled motion in the upper cervical region is more consistent (Ishii et al., 2004), inconsistencies of coupled motion in the lumbar and thoracic regions invalidate the Fryette model as a means of predicting triplanar motion restrictions based on static asymmetry, which is recommended in many texts (Mitchell & Mitchell, 1995; DiGiovanna et al., 2005; DeStefano, 2016).

Because of the unpredictability of coupled motions in the spine, practitioners should address motion restrictions present on palpation (despite the issues of reliability of motion palpation) rather than follow assumptions based on biomechanical models and static palpatory findings. This author suggests that, if corrective motion is introduced in the primary planes of restriction, spinal coupling (in whatever direction) will occur automatically – because of the nature of conjunct motion – and without being intentionally introduced by the practitioner (Fryer, 2009, 2011). Therefore, the pragmatic approach is to address the primary motion restriction(s) as observed and palpated without consciously introducing coupled motions.

REFERENCES

Adams, J., Sibbritt, D., Steel, A., Peng, W., 2018. A workforce survey of Australian osteopathy: analysis of a nationally-representative sample of osteopaths from the Osteopathy Research and Innovation Network (ORION) project. BMC Health Serv. Res. 18, 352.

Alghadir, A.H., Iqbal, A., Anwer, S., Iqbal, Z.A., Ahmed, H., 2020. Efficacy of combination therapies on neck pain and muscle tenderness in male patients with upper trapezius active myofascial trigger points. BioMed Res. Int. 10, 9361405.

Azevedo, D.C., Melo, R.M., Alves Correa, R.V., Chalmers, G., 2011. Uninvolved versus target muscle contraction during contract: relax proprioceptive neuromuscular facilitation stretching. Phys. Ther. Sport 12 (3), 117–121.

Ballantyne, F., Fryer, G., McLaughlin, P., 2003. The effect of muscle energy technique on hamstring extensibility: the mechanism of altered flexibility. J. Osteopath. Med. 6 (2), 59–63.

Bandy, W.D., Irion, J.M., 1994. The effect of time on static stretch on the flexibility of the hamstring muscles. Phys. Ther. 74 (9), 845–850.

Bandy, W.D., Irion, J.M., Briggler, M., 1997. The effect of time and frequency of static stretching on flexibility of the hamstring muscles. Phys. Ther. 77, 1090–1096.

Bill, A.-S., Dubois, J., Pasquier, J., Burnand, B., Rodondi, P.Y., 2020. Osteopathy in the French-speaking part of Switzerland: practitioners' profile and scope of back pain management. PLoS One 15, e0232607.

Bonnar, B.P., Deivert, R.G., Gould, T.E., 2004. The relationship between isometric contraction durations during hold-relax stretching and improvement of hamstring flexibility. J. Sports Med. Phys. Fitness 44 (3), 258–261.

Burke, D.G., Holt, L.E., Rasmussen, R., MacKinnon, N.C., Vossen, J.F., Pelham, T.W., 2001. Effects of hot or cold water immersion and modified proprioceptive neuromuscular facilitation flexibility exercise on hamstring length. J. Athl. Train. 36 (1), 16–19.

Burke, S.R., Myers, R., Zhang, A.L., 2013. A profile of osteopathic practice in Australia 2010–2011: a cross sectional survey. BMC Musculoskelet. Disord. 14, 227.

Burns, D.K., Wells, M.R., 2006. Gross range of motion in the cervical spine: the effects of osteopathic muscle energy technique in asymptomatic subjects. J. Am. Osteopath. Assoc. 106 (3), 137–142.

Carter, A., Kinzey, S.J., Chitwood, L.F., 2000. Proprioceptive neuromuscular facilitation decreases muscle activity during the stretch reflex in selected posterior thigh muscles. J. Sport Rehabil. 9, 269–278.

Cayco, C.S., Labro, A.V., Gorgon, E.J.R., 2019. Hold-relax and contract-relax stretching for hamstrings flexibility: a systematic review with meta-analysis. Phys. Ther. Sport 35, 42–55.

Chaitow, L., 2001. Palpatory accuracy: time to reflect. J. Bodyw. Mov. Ther. 5 (4), 223–226.

Chaitow, L., 2006. Muscle Energy Techniques, third ed. Churchill Livingstone, Edinburgh.

Chaitow, L., 2015. Contrasting views of myofascial pain. J. Bodyw. Mov. Ther. 19 (2), 191–192.

Chown, M., Whittamore, L., Rush, M., Allan, S., Stott, D., Archer, M., 2008. A prospective study of patients with chronic back pain randomised to group exercise, physiotherapy or osteopathy. Physiotherapy 94 (1), 21–28.

Coates, G., O'Brodovich, H., Goeree, G., 1993. Hindlimb and lung lymph flows during prolonged exercise. J. Appl. Physiol. 75, 633–638.

Cook, C., Hegedus, E., Showalter, C., Sizer Jr., P.S., 2006. Coupling behavior of the cervical spine: a systematic review of the literature. J. Manipulative Physiol. Ther. 29 (7), 570–575.

Cornelius, W.L., Ebrahim, K., Watson, J., Hill, D.W., 1992. The effects of cold application and modified PNF stretching techniques on hip joint flexibility in college males. Res. Q. Exerc. Sport 63 (3), 311–314.

Darlow, B., Dean, S., Perry, M., Mathieson, F., Baxter, G.D., Dowell, A., 2015. Easy to harm, hard to heal: patient views about the back. Spine (Phila Pa 1976) 40, 842–850.

Dearing, J., Hamilton, F., 2008. An examination of pressure-pain thresholds (PPT's) at myofascial trigger points (MTrP's), following muscle energy technique or ischaemic compression treatment. Man. Ther. 13 (1), 87–88.

DeStefano, L., 2016. Greenman's Principles of Manual Medicine, fifth ed. Lippincott Williams & Wilkins, Philadelphia.

DiGiovanna, E.L., Schiowitz, S., Dowling, D.J., 2005. An Osteopathic Approach to Diagnosis & Treatment, third ed. Lippincott William & Wilkins, Philadelphia.

Dommerholt, J., Gerwin, R.D., 2015. A critical evaluation of Quinter et al.: missing the point. J. Bodyw. Mov. Ther. 19 (2), 193–204.

Edmondston, S.J., Henne, S.E., Loh, W., Ostvold, E., 2005. Influence of cranio-cervical posture on three-dimensional motion of the cervical spine. Man. Ther. 10, 44–51.

Ehrenfeuchter, W.C., 2011. Muscle energy approach. In: Chila, A.G. (Ed.), Foundations for Osteopathic Medicine, third ed. Lippincott William & Wilkins, Philadelphia, pp. 682–697.

Etnyre, B.R., Abraham, L.D., 1986a. Gains in range of ankle dorsiflexion using three popular stretching techniques. Am. J. Phys. Med. 65 (4), 189–196.

Etnyre, B.R., Abraham, L.D., 1986b. H-reflex changes during static stretching and two variations of proprioceptive neuromuscular facilitation techniques. Electroencephalogr. Clin. Neurophysiol. 63 (2), 174–179.

Feland, J.B., Marin, H.N., 2004. Effect of submaximal contraction intensity in contract–relax proprioceptive neuromuscular facilitation stretching. Br. J. Sports Med. 38 (4), E18.

Feland, J.B., Myrer, J.W., Merrill, R.M., 2001. Acute changes in hamstring flexibility: PNF versus static stretch in senior athletes. Phys. Ther. Sport 2 (4), 186–193.

Ferber, R., Gravelle, D.C., Osternig, L.R., 2002a. Effect of proprioceptive neuromuscular facilitation stretch techniques on trained and untrained older adults. J. Aging Phys. Act. 1, 132–142.

Ferber, R., Osternig, L.R., Gravelle, D.C., 2002b. Effect of PNF stretch techniques on knee flexor muscle EMG activity in older adults. J. Electromyogr. Kinesiol. 12, 391–397.

Franke, H., Fryer, G., Ostelo, R.W., Kamper, S.J., 2015. Muscle energy technique for non-specific low-back pain. Cochrane Database Syst. Rev. 2, CD009852.

Fryer, G., 2000. Muscle energy concepts: a need for change. J. Osteopath. Med. 3 (2), 54–59.

Fryer, G., 2009. Research-informed muscle energy concepts and practice. In: Franke, H. (Ed.), Muscle Energy Technique: History – Model – Research (Monograph). Jolandos, Ammersestr, Germany, pp. 57–62.

Fryer, G., 2011. Muscle energy technique: an evidence-informed approach. International J. Osteopath. Med. 14 (1), 3–9.

Fryer, G., 2016. Somatic dysfunction: an osteopathic conundrum. Int. J. Osteopath. Med. 22, 52–63.

Fryer, G., 2017a. Integrating osteopathic approaches based on biopsychosocial therapeutic mechanisms. Part 1: the mechanisms. Int. J. Osteopath. Med. 25, 30–41.

Fryer, G., 2017b. Integrating osteopathic approaches based on biopsychosocial therapeutic mechanisms. Part 2: clinical approach. Int. J. Osteopath. Med. 26, 36–43.

Fryer, G., Adams, J.H., 2011. Magnetic resonance imaging of subjects with acute unilateral neck pain and restricted motion: a prospective case series. J. Spine 11 (3), 171–176.

Fryer, G., Hodgson, L., 2005. The effect of manual pressure release on myofascial trigger points in the upper trapezius muscle. J. Bodyw. Mov. Ther. 9, 248–255.

Fryer, G., Pearce, A.J., 2013. The effect of muscle energy technique on corticospinal and spinal reflex excitability in asymptomatic participants. J. Bodyw. Mov. Ther. 17, 440–447.

Fryer, G., Ruszkowski, W., 2004. The influence of contraction duration in muscle energy technique applied to the atlanto-axial joint. J. Osteopath. Med. 7 (2), 79–84.

Fryer, G., Morris, T., Gibbons, P., 2004. Paraspinal muscles and intervertebral dysfunction, part 2. J. Manipulative Physiol. Ther. 27 (5), 348–357.

Fryette, H.H., 1954. Principles of Osteopathic Technic. American Academy of Osteopathy, Newark, OH.

Funk, D.C., Swank, A.M., Mikla, B.M., Fagan, T.A., Farr, B.K., 2003. Impact of prior exercise on hamstring flexibility: a comparison of proprioceptive neuromuscular facilitation and static stretching. J. Strength Cond. Res. 17 (3), 489–492.

Gandevia, S.C., Peterson, N., Butler, J.E., Taylor, J.L., 1999. Impaired response of human motoneurones to corticospinal stimulation after voluntary exercise. J. Physiol. 521 (3), 749–759.

Gibbons, P., Tehan, P., 1998. Muscle energy concepts and coupled motion of the spine. Man. Ther. 3 (2), 95–101.

Gill, K.P., Callaghan, M.J., 1998. The measurement of lumbar proprioception in individuals with and without low back pain. Spine 23 (3), 371–377.

Greenhalgh, T., Howick, J., Maskrey, N., 2014. Evidence based medicine: a movement in crisis? BMJ 348, g3725.

Grip, H., Sundelin, G., Gerdle, B., Karlsson, J.S., 2007. Variations in the axis of motion during head repositioning: a comparison of subjects with whiplash-associated disorders or non-specific neck pain and healthy controls. Clinical Biomechanics 22 (8), 865–873.

Havas, E., Parviainen, T., Vuorela, J., Toivanen, J., Nikula, T., Vihko, V., 1997. Lymph flow dynamics in exercising human skeletal muscle as detected by scintography. J. Physiol. 504 (Pt 1), 233–239.

Heikkila, H., Johansson, M., Wenngren, B.I., 2000. Effects of acupuncture, cervical manipulation and NSAID therapy on dizziness and impaired head positioning of suspected cervical origin: a pilot study. Man. Ther. 5 (3), 151–157.

Hoeger Bement, M.K., Sluka, K.A., 2007. Pain: perception and mechanisms. In: Magee, D.J., Zachazewski, J.E., Quillen, W.S. (Eds.), Scientific Foundations and Principles of Practice in Musculoskeletal Rehabilitation. Saunders Elsevier, St Louis, pp. 217–237.

Ishii, T., Mukai, Y., Hosono, N., Sakaura, H., Nakajima, Y., Sato, Y., et al., 2004. Kinematics of the upper cervical spine in rotation. In vivo three-dimensional analysis. Spine 29 (7), E139–E144.

Ishii, T., Mukai, Y., Hosono, N., Sakaura, H., Fujii, R., Nakajima, Y., et al., 2006. Kinematics of the cervical spine in lateral bending: in vivo three-dimensional analysis. Spine 31 (2), 155–160.

Izumizaki, M., Iwase, M., Ohshima, Y., Homma, I., 2006. Acute effects of thixotropy conditioning of inspiratory muscles on end-expiratory chest wall and lung volumes in normal humans. J. Appl. Physiol. 101 (1), 298–306.

Joseph, L.C., De Buser, N., Brantingham, J.W., Globe, G.A., Cassa, T.K., Korporaal, C., et al., 2010. The comparative effect of muscle energy technique vs. manipulation for the treatment of chronic recurrent ankle sprain. J. Am. Chiropractic Assoc. 47 (5), 8–22.

Karlberg, M., Magnusson, M., Malmstrom, E.M., Melander, A., Moritz, U., 1991. Postural and symptomatic improvement after physiotherapy in patients with dizziness of suspected cervical origin. Arch. Phys. Med. Rehabil. 72, 288–291.

Kay, A.D., Husbands-Beasley, J., Blazevich, A.J., 2015. Effects of contract-relax, static stretching, and isometric contractions on muscle-tendon mechanics. Med. Sci. Sports Exerc. 47 (10), 2181–2190.

Kwak, D.H., Ryu, Y.U., 2015. Applying proprioceptive neuromuscular facilitation stretching: optimal contraction intensity to attain the maximum increase in range of motion in young males. J. Phys. Ther. Sci. 27 (7), 2129–2132.

Langevin, H., Boulfard, N.A., Badger, G.J., Iatridis, J.C., Howe, A.K., 2005. Dynamic fibroblast cytoskeletal response to subcutaneous tissue stretch ex vivo and in vivo. Am. J. Physiol. Cell Physiol. 288 (3), C747–C756.

Lanir, Y., Salant, E.L., Foux, A., 1988. Physio-chemical and microstructural changes in collagen fibre bundles following stretching in-vitro. Biorheology 25, 591–603.

Leach, M.J., Palmgren, P.J., Thomson, O.P., Fryer, G., Eklund, A., Lilje, S., et al., 2021. Skills, attitudes and uptake of evidence-based practice: a cross-sectional study of chiropractors in the Swedish Chiropractic Association. Chiropr. Man. Ther. 29 (1), 2.

Leach, M.J., Sundberg, T., Fryer, G., Austin, P., Thomson, O.P., Adams, J., 2019. An investigation of Australian osteopaths' attitudes, skills and utilisation of evidence-based practice: a national cross-sectional survey. BMC Health Serv. Res. 19 (1), 498.

Lederman, E., 2005. The Science and Practice of Manual Therapy, second ed. Elsevier Churchill Livingstone, Edinburgh.

Legaspi, O., Edmond, S.L., 2007. Does the evidence support the existence of lumbar spine coupled motion? A critical review of the literature. J. Orthop. Sports Phys. Ther. 37 (4), 169–178.

Lenehan, K.L., Fryer, G., McLaughlin, P., 2003. The effect of muscle energy technique on gross trunk range of motion. J. Osteopath. Med. 6 (1), 13–18.

Lewit, K., Simons, D.G., 1984. Myofascial pain: relief by postisometric relaxation. Arch. Phys. Med. Rehabil. 65, 452–456.

Li, J., Mitchell, J.H., 2003. Glutamate release in midbrain periaqueductal grey by activation of skeletal muscle receptors and arterial baroreceptors. Am. J. Physiol. Heart Circ. 285 (1), H137–H144.

Licciardone, J.C., Buchanan, S., Hensel, K.L., King, H.H., Fulda, K.G., Stoll, S.T., 2010. Osteopathic manipulative treatment of back pain and related symptoms during pregnancy: a randomised controlled trial. Am. J. Obstet. Gynecol. 202 (1) 43e1-8.

Lim, W., 2018. Optimal intensity of PNF stretching: maintaining the efficacy of stretching while ensuring its safety. J. Phys. Ther. Sci. 30 (8), 1108–1111.

Magnusson, M., Simonsen, E.B., Aagaard, P., Moritz, U., Kjaer, M., 1995. Contraction specific changes in passive torque in human skeletal muscle. Acta Physiol. Scand. 155 (4), 377–386.

Magnusson, M., Simonsen, E.B., Aagaard, P., Sørensen, H., Kjaer, M., 1996a. A mechanism for altered flexibility in human skeletal muscle. J. Physiol. 497 (Pt 1), 293–298.

Magnusson, S.P., Simonsen, E.B., Aagaard, P., Dyhre-Poulsen, P., McHugh, M.P., Kjaer, M., 1996b. Mechanical and physiological responses to stretching with and without preisometric contraction in human skeletal muscle. Arch. Phys. Med. Rehabil. 77, 373–377.

Magnusson, M., Simonsen, E.B., Dyhre-Poulsen, P., Aagaard, P., Mohr, T., Kjaer, M., 1996c. Viscoelastic stress relaxation during static stretch in human skeletal muscle in the absence of EMG activity. Scand. J. Med. Sci. Sports 6 (6), 323–328.

Magnusson, M., Aagaard, P., Simonsen, E.B., Bojsen-Møller, F., 1998. A biomechanical evaluation of cyclic and static stretch in human skeletal muscle. Int. J. Sports Med. 19, 310–316.

Malmstrom, E., Karlberg, M., Fransson, P.A., Melander, A., Magnusson, M., 2006. Primary and coupled cervical movements: the effect of age, gender, and body mass index. A 3-dimensional movement analysis of a population without symptoms of neck disorders. Spine 31 (2), E44–E50.

Malmstrom, E.M., Karlberg, M., Holmstrom, E., Fransson, P.A., Hansson, G.A., Magnusson, M., 2010. Influence of prolonged unilateral cervical muscle contraction on head repositioning: decreased overshoot after a 5-min static muscle contraction task. Man. Ther. 15 (3), 229–234.

Mehta, M., Hatton, P., 2002. The relationship between the duration of sub-maximal isometric contraction (MET) and improvement in the range of passive knee extension (abstract). In: Abstracts from 3rd International Conference for the Advancement of Osteopathic Research, Melbourne, Australia, 2002. J. Osteopath. Med. 5 (1), 40.

Miller, K.C., Burne, J.A., 2014. Golgi tendon organ reflex inhibition following manually applied acute static stretching. J. Sports Sci. 32, 1491–1497.

Mitchell Jr., F.L., Mitchell, P.K.G., 1995. The Muscle Energy Manual, vol. 1. MET Press, Michigan.

Mitchell Jr., F.L., Moran, P.S., Pruzzo, N.A., 1979. An Evaluation and Treatment Manual of Osteopathic Muscle Energy Procedures. Mitchell, Moran and Pruzzo Associates, Missouri.

Mitchell, U.H., Myrer, J.W., Hopkins, J.T., Hunter, I., Feland, J.B., Hilton, S.C., 2007. Acute stretch perception alteration contributes to the success of the PNF "contract-relax" stretch. J. Sport Rehabil. 16 (2), 85–92.

Mitchell, U.H., Myrer, J.W., Hopkins, J.T., Hunter, I., Feland, J.B., Hilton, S.C., 2009. Neurophysiological reflex mechanisms' lack of contribution to the success of PNF stretches. J. Sport Rehabil. 18 (3), 343–357.

Moore, M., Kukulka, C., 1991. Depression of Hoffman reflexes following voluntary contraction and implications for proprioceptive neuromuscular facilitation therapy. Phys. Ther. 71 (4), 321–329.

Moore, S.D., Laudner, K.G., McLoda, T.A., Shaffer, MA., 2011. The immediate effects of muscle energy technique on posterior shoulder tightness: a randomised controlled trial. J. Orthop. Sports Phys. Ther. 41 (6), 400–407.

Nelson, K.C., Cornelius, W.L., 1991. The relationship between isometric contraction durations and improvement in shoulder joint range of motion. J. Sports Med. Phys. Fitness 31 (3), 385–388.

Norkin, C.C., Levangie, P.K., 1992. In: Davis, F.A. (Ed.), Joint Structure and Function: A Comprehensive Analysis, second ed. F.A. Davis, Philadelphia.

Olivo, S.A., Magee, D.J., 2006. Electromyographic assessment of the activity of the masticatory using the agonist contract-antagonist relax technique (AC) and contract-relax technique (CR). Man. Ther. 11 (2), 136–145.

Osama, M., 2021. Effects of autogenic and reciprocal inhibition muscle energy techniques on isometric muscle strength in neck pain: a randomised controlled trial. J. Back Musculoskelet. Rehabil. 34 (4), 555–564.

Osternig, L.R., Robertson, R., Troxel, R.K., Hansen, P., 1987. Muscle activation during proprioceptive neuromuscular facilitation (PNF) stretching techniques. Am. J. Phys. Med. 66 (5), 298–307.

Osternig, L.R., Robertson, R.N., Troxel, R.K., Hansen, P., 1990. Differential responses to proprioceptive neuromuscular facilitation (PNF) stretch techniques. Med. Sci. Sports Exerc. 22 (1), 106–111.

Palmgren, P.J., Sandstrom, P.J., Lundqvist, F.J., Heikkilä, H., 2006. Improvement after chiropractic care in cervicocephalic kinesthetic sensibility and subjective pain intensity in patients with nontraumatic chronic neck pain. J. Manipulative. Physiol. Ther. 29 (2), 100–106.

Proske, U., Morgan, D.L., 1999. Do cross-bridges contribute to the tension during stretch of passive muscle? J. Muscle Res. Cell. Motil. 20 (5), 433–442.

Quintner, J.L., Bove, G.M., Cohen, M.L., 2015. A critical evaluation of the trigger point phenomenon. Rheumatology (Oxford) 54, 392–399.

Rogers, R.G., 1997. The effects of spinal manipulation on cervical kinesthesia in patients with chronic neck pain: a pilot study. J. Manipulative Physiol. Ther. 20 (2), 80–85.

Rowlands, A.V., Marginson, V.F., Lee, J., 2003. Chronic flexibility gains: effect of isometric contraction duration during proprioceptive neuromuscular facilitation stretching techniques. Res. Q. Exerc. Sport 74 (1), 47–51.

Ryan, E.E., Rossi, M.D., Lopez, R., 2010. The effects of the contract-relax-antagonist-contract form of proprioceptive neuromuscular facilitation stretching on postural stability. J. Strength Cond. Res. 24 (7), 1888–1894.

Sá, M.A., Matta, T.T., Carneiro, S.P., Araujo, C.O., Novaes, J.S., Oliveira, L.F., 2016. Acute effects of different methods of stretching and specific warm-ups on muscle architecture and strength performance. J. Strength Cond. Res. 30 (8), 2324–2329.

Sackett, D.L., Rosenberg, W.M., Gray, J.A., Haynes, R.B., Richardson, W.S., 1996. Evidence based medicine: what it is and what it isn't. BMJ 312 (7023), 71–72.

Sadria, G., Hosseini, M., Rezasoltani, A., Akbarzadeh Baghe-ban, A., Davari, A., Seifolahi, A., 2017. A comparison of the effect of the active release and muscle energy techniques on the latent trigger points of the upper trapezius. J. Bodyw. Mov. Ther. 21 (4), 920–925.

Sady, S.P., Wortman, M., Blanke, D., 1982. Flexibility training: ballistic, static or proprioceptive neuromuscular facilitation? Arch. Phys. Med. Rehabil. 63 (6), 261–263.

Sbardella, S., La Russa, C., Bernetti, A., Mangone, M., Guarnera, A., Pezzi, L., et al., 2021. Muscle energy technique in the rehabilitative treatment for acute and chronic non-specific neck pain: a systematic review. Healthcare 9 (6), 746.

Schenk, R.J., Adelman, K., Rousselle, J., 1994. The effects of muscle energy technique on cervical range of motion. J. Man. Manip. Ther. 2 (4), 149–155.

Schenk, R.J., MacDiarmid, A., Rousselle, J., 1997. The effects of muscle energy technique on lumbar range of motion. J. Man. Manip. Ther. 5 (4), 179–183.

Schleip, R., Klingler, W., Lehman-Horn, F., 2004. Active contraction of the thoracolumbar fascia (abstract), 5th Interdisciplinary World Congress on Low Back and Pelvic Pain. Melbourne, Australia.

Schmid-Schonbein, G.W., 1990. Microlymphatics and lymph flow. Physiol. Rev. 70, 987–1028.

Schmitt, G. D., Pelham, T. W., & Holt, L. E, 1999. From the field. A comparison of selected protocols during proprioceptive neuromuscular facilitation stretching. Clinical Kinesiology 53 (1), 16–21.

Schwerla, F., Bischoff, A., Nurnberger, A., Genter, P., Guillaume, J.-P., Resch, K.-L., 2008. Osteopathic treatment of patients with chronic non-specific neck pain: a randomised controlled trial of efficacy. Forsch. Komplementmed. 15, 138–145.

Seffinger, M.A., Najm, W.I., Mishra, S.I., Adams, A., Dickerson, V.M., Murphy, L.S., et al., 2004. Reliability of spinal palpation for diagnosis of back and neck pain: a systematic review of the literature. Spine 29 (19), E413–E425.

Seseke, S., Baudewig, H., Kallenberg, K., Ringert, R.H., Seseke, F., Dechent, P., 2006. Voluntary pelvic flow muscle control: an fMRI study. Neuroimage 31 (4), 399–407.

Sheard, P.W., Paine, T.J., 2010. Optimal contraction intensity during proprioceptive neuromuscular facilitation for maximal increase of range of motion. J. Strength Cond. Res. 24 (2), 416–421.

Sheard, P.W., Smith, P.M., Paine, T.J., 2009. Athlete compliance to therapist requested contraction intensity during proprioceptive neuromuscular facilitation. Man. Ther. 14 (5), 539–543.

Sizer, P.S., Brismee, J.M., Cook, C., 2007. Coupling behavior of the thoracic spine: a systematic review of the literature. J. Manipulative Physiol. Ther. 30 (5), 390–399.

Skyba, D.A., Radhakrishnan, R., Rohlwing, J.J., Wright, A., Sluka, K.A., 2003. Joint manipulation reduces hyperalgesia by activation of monoamine receptors but not opioid or GABA receptors in the spinal cord. Pain 106 (1–2), 159–168.

Smith, M., Fryer, G., 2008. A comparison of two muscle energy techniques for increasing flexibility of the hamstring muscle group. J. Bodyw. Mov. Ther. 12 (4), 312–317.

Souvlis, T., Vicenzino, B., Wright, A., 2004. Neurophysiological effects of spinal manual therapy. In: Boyling, J.D., Jull, G.A. (Eds.), Grieve's Modern Manual Therapy: The Vertebral Column, third ed. Elsevier Churchill Livingstone, Edinburgh, pp. 367–380.

Spernoga, S.G., Uhl, T.L., Arnold, B.L., Gansneder, B.M., 2001. Duration of maintained hamstring flexibility after a one-time, modified hold-relax stretching protocol. J. Athl. Train. 36 (1), 44–48.

Spring, F., Gibbons, P., Tehan, P., 2001. Intra-examiner and inter-examiner reliability of a positional diagnostic screen for the lumbar spine. J. Osteopath. Med. 4 (2), 47–55.

Stanton, T.R., Leake, H.B., Chalmers, K.J., Moseley, G.L., 2016. Evidence of impaired proprioception in chronic, idiopathic neck pain: systematic review & meta-analysis. Phys. Ther. 96 (6), 876–887.

Sterling, M., Jull, G.A., Wright, A., 2001. Cervical mobilisation: concurrent effects on pain, sympathetic nervous system activity and motor activity. Man. Ther. 6 (2), 72–81.

Stohler, C.S., Kowalski, C.J., Lund, J.P., 2001. Muscle pain inhibits cutaneous touch perception. Pain 92, 327–333.

Sundberg, T., Leach, M.J., Thomson, O.P., Austin, P., Fryer, G., Adams, J., 2018. Attitudes, skills and use of evidence-based practice among UK osteopaths: a national cross-sectional survey. BMC Musculoskelet. Disord. 19 (1), 439.

Taylor, D.C., Brooks, D.E., Ryan, J.B., 1997. Visco-elastic characteristics of muscle: passive stretching versus muscular contractions. Med. Sci. Sports Exerc. 29 (12), 1619–1624.

Thomas, E., Cavallaro, A.R., Mani, D., Bianco, A., Palma, A., 2019. The efficacy of muscle energy techniques in symptomatic and asymptomatic subjects: a systematic review. Chiropr. Man. Ther. 27, 35.

Trampas, A., Kitsios, A., Sykaras, E., Symeonidis, S., Lazarou, L., 2010. Clinical massage and modified proprioceptive neuromuscular facilitation stretching in males with latent myofascial trigger points. Phys. Ther. Sport 11 (3), 91–98.

Travell, J.G., Simons, D.G., 1983. Myofascial Pain and Dysfunction, vol 1. William & Wilkins, Baltimore.

Ulger, O., Demirel, A., Oz, M., Tamer, S., 2017. The effect of manual therapy and exercise in patients with chronic low back pain: double blind randomised controlled trial. J. Back Musculoskelet. Rehabil. 30, 1303–1309.

Vigotsky, A.D., Bruhns, R.P., 2015. The role of descending modulation in manual therapy and its analgesic implications: a narrative review. Pain Res. Manag. 2015, 292805.

Voerman, V.F., Van Egmond, J., Crul, B.J.P, 2000. Elevated detection thresholds for mechanical stimuli in chronic pain patients: support for a central mechanism. Arch. Phys. Med. Rehabil. 81, 430–435.

Wallin, D., Ekblam, B., Grahn, R., Nordenborg, T., 1985. Improvement of muscle flexibility. A comparison between two techniques. Am. J. Sports Med. 13 (4), 263–268.

Wendt, M., Waszak, M., 2020. Evaluation of the combination of muscle energy technique and trigger point therapy in asymptomatic individuals with a latent trigger point. Int. J. Environ. Res. Public Health 17 (22), 8430.

Wilson, E., Payton, O., Donegan-Shoaf, L., & Dec, K., 2003. Muscle energy technique in patients with acute low back pain: a pilot clinical trial. J. Orthop. Sports Phys. Ther. 33, 502–512.

Yahia, L.H., Pigeon, P., DesRosiers, E.A., 1993. Viscoelastic properties of the human lumbodorsal fascia. J. Biomed. Eng. 15, 425–429.

Yeganeh Lari, A., Okhovatian, F., Naimi, S.S., Baghban, A.A., 2016. The effect of the combination of dry needling and MET on latent trigger point upper trapezius in females. Man. Ther. 21, 204–209.

Yezierski, R.P., 1991. Somatosensory input to the periaqueductal grey: a spinal relay to a descending control center. In: Depaulis, A., Bandler, R. (Eds.), The Midbrain Periaqueductal Grey Matter. Plenum Press, New York, pp. 365–386.

Youdas, J.W., Haeflinger, K.M., Kreun, M.K., Holloway, A.M., Kramer, C.M., Hollman, J.H., 2010. The efficacy of two modified proprioceptive neuromuscular facilitation stretching techniques in subjects with reduced hamstring muscle length. Physiother. Theory Pract. 26 (4), 240–250.

5

How to Use MET

Leon Chaitow, Sandy Fritz

CHAPTER CONTENTS

Chapter 2 described a number of variations on the theme of MET (and stretching) as well as the need to identify 'easy' restriction barriers for the efficient and safe application of Muscle Energy Technique (MET).

In this chapter, suggestions are given as to how to begin to learn the application of MET treatment methods, both for muscles and for joints (specific muscle by muscle and particular joint descriptions of MET

treatment can be found in Chapters 6 and 7, respectively). This includes 'barrier' palpation exercises. Chapter 6 describes a suggested sequence for the evaluation/assessment of the major postural (or *mobiliser*) muscles of the body – for relative shortness – along with details of suggested MET approaches for normalising, stretching and relaxing those muscles. See Chapter 2 for discussion of muscle types and the relevance to MET.

Additionally, there will be examples of the use of pulsed MET (repetitive mini-contractions based on the work of T. J. Ruddy, 1962) in facilitating proprioceptive re-education of weak and shortened structures, particularly in Chapter 7.

Some of the guidelines and many of the suggestions for MET protocols derive from a mix of clinical experience and expert opinion. As discussed in Chapters 1, 2 and 4, the fact remains that despite the growth of the evidence base, at this time there remain areas of MET methodology that are only partially supported by research validation. Where this exists, it is provided. The reader therefore needs to decide whether to wait for future evidence as to just why and how MET produces its apparent benefits – and how to harness these most effectively – or whether, based on clinical and anecdotal reporting, together with the body of evidence that already exists, to trust the quoted authorities.

Whichever option is chosen, a primary requirement for the practitioner is the assessment and thereby identification of a need for the use of MET – or an alternative method of manual therapy and what adaptations may be required. Based on the study conducted by Sharan (2018), the most common presenting symptoms leading patients to a manual practitioner are regional pain (78%), stiffness (58%) and generalised pain (40%). As these are also common symptoms of both hypermobility and hypomobility syndromes (Ali et al., 2020), differential diagnosis may sometimes be called for and the practitioner should be mindful of this possibility.

The experience and description of muscle tightness and stiffness can be difficult to explain. Bhimani et al. (2020) determine a key feature of muscle tightness is limited range of motion. However, other factors are involved, such as loss of function, changes in muscle texture, change in sensation, asymmetry, pain and contracted muscle state. Understanding these can be complicated because these sensations are largely subjective and interrelated, and may be experienced or described as stiffness. Stiffness is often related to elastic properties in soft tissues, tissue density and resistance to deformation. Simply put, tightness involves contraction/shortening and is more neuro-driven, while stiffness involves mechanical changes in soft tissue structural components related to connective tissue fluid and fibre (Pruyn et al., 2016). Regardless, MET has the potential to address both tightness and stiffness, but caution is needed when symptoms are related to adaptation to hypermobility, since tightness may relate to compensation, and therefore attempts to 'loosen' contractions may do more harm than good; thus, other approaches may be called for.

Lewit (2009) observed that pain is also often noted in the loose rather than in the tight areas of the body, possibly involving hypermobility and ligamentous laxity. Hypermobility spectrum disorder (HSD) and hypermobile Ehlers-Danlos syndrome (hEDS) can cause widespread or chronic pain, fatigue and proprioceptive and coordination deficits, and these conditions affect multiple body systems rather than just joints (Reuter & Fichthorn, 2019; Russek et al., 2019).

These (lax, loose) areas appear to be vulnerable to injury and prone to recurrent dysfunctional episodes, for example, affecting the low back or sacroiliac joint or other areas such as the knee (Muller et al., 2003; Zaidi & Ishaq, 2020; Zhong et al., 2021). Careful assessment is necessary to determine the causal factors in order to implement the most appropriate treatment.

PALPATION SKILLS

The concept and reality of palpating hands or fingers being able to sense states of relative tension, or 'bind', in soft tissues – as opposed to states of relaxation or 'ease' – is one which the beginner needs to grasp, and that the advanced practitioner probably takes for granted. There can never be enough focus on these two characteristics – identification of 'ease' and 'bind' – two features that allow soft tissues to report on their current relative degree of comfort or distress. What's loose, what's tight, what's stiff (or 'dense'), what asymmetries are there and to what extent is malalignment a feature of this individual's dysfunction?

Robert Ward (1997) has discussed the 'loose–tight' model as a concept that may help us to appreciate three-dimensionality, as the body, or part of it, is palpated/assessed. This assessment may involve large or local areas, in which interactive asymmetry produces changes that can be described as 'tight or loose', relative to each other. Pain is more commonly associated with tight and bound/tethered structures, which may be due to local overuse/misuse/abuse factors, to scar tissue, to reflexively induced influences, or to centrally mediated neural effects. When a tight tissue is required to either contract, or lengthen, pain is often experienced. Paradoxically, underlying hypermobility can result in tightness and stiffness to counteract the laxity (see the discussions on STAR and TART palpation in Chapter 2).

Assessment of the 'tethering' of tissues, and of the subtle qualities of 'end-feel' in soft tissues and joints, are prerequisites for appropriate treatment being applied, whether this is of a direct or indirect nature, or whether it involves active or passive methods. Indeed, the awareness of end-feel, tight–loose, ease–bind features may be the determining factor as to which therapeutic approaches should best be introduced, and in what sequence. These barriers (tight and loose) can be seen to refer to the obstacles that are identified in preparation for direct methods such as MET (where the barrier of restriction is engaged and movement is towards bind, tightness) as well as for indirect methods, such as strain/counterstrain (where movement is towards ease, looseness) (Jones, 1981).

It is worth remembering that 'tight' tissues are not necessarily undesirable – as they may represent a protective guarding process. 'Tightness suggests tethering, while looseness suggests joint and/or soft tissue laxity, with or without neural inhibition' (Ward, 1997).

Three-Dimensional Patterns

Areas of dysfunction will usually involve a more complex set of associations than just 'loose–tight'. There are likely to be vertical, horizontal and 'encircling' (also described as crossover, spiral or 'wrap-around') patterns of involvement.

Ward (1997) identified a 'typical' wrap-around pattern associated with a tight left low-back area (which ends up involving the entire trunk and cervical area), as tight areas evolve to compensate for loose, inhibited areas (or vice versa):

- Tightness in the posterior left hip, SI joint, lumbar erector spinae and lower rib cage
- Looseness on the right low back
- Tightness in the lateral and anterior rib cage on the right
- Tight left thoracic inlet, posteriorly
- Tight left craniocervical attachments (involving jaw mechanics).

Janda (1986) has described a theoretical three-dimensional chain of changes that may be associated with temporomandibular joint (TMJ) problems. He points out that locally TMJ dysfunction probably involves hypertonicity of the temporal and/or masseter muscles, with reciprocal inhibition (RI) of the suprahyoid, digastric and mylohyoid muscles. The imbalance between mandibular elevators and depressors would alter condylar motion, redistributing joint stress – leading to pain and possibly to joint surface changes.

Globally, in the same individual Janda outlines a typical pattern of musculoskeletal dysfunction involving upper trapezii, levator scapulae, scaleni, sternocleidomastoidii, suprahyoids, lateral and medial pterygoids (as well as the masseter and temporalis muscles), all demonstrating a tendency to tighten and shorten. Simultaneously the scalenes may become atrophied and weak while also developing tenderness, and myofascial trigger points (TrPs).

Further postural pattern changes might involve:

- Hyperextension of the knees
- Increased anterior tilt of the pelvis
- Increased flexion of the hip joints
- Lumbar hyperlordosis
- Protracted shoulders and winged scapulae
- Cervical hyperlordosis, with a forward thrust of the head
- Compensatory overactivity of the upper trapezius and levator scapulae muscles
- Retraction of the mandible. See Box 5.2 for further discussion of this pattern.

One message to be drawn from this example is that global as well as local patterns need to be identified before the role they might be playing in the person's symptoms can be understood, and before the individual can be appropriately treated.

Part of that task lies in being able to identify which structures are too tight, too short, too loose, which too weak, and whether and how these may be negatively affecting function. We also have to identify the causes and what can be done to assist normalisation. In the TMJ example above, the causes may involve descending dysfunction sequences starting with malocclusion, or ascending dysfunctional sequences commencing in the feet, ankles, knees, hips, pelvis or spine (Liem, 2004). In other words, identifying what the 'tight/loose' features are is the easy part of the puzzle-solving exercise. That does not however make it unimportant for attention to be given to restoring balance between the restricted and the lax structures. However, without attention to aetiology, such a focus would most likely be of short-term benefit.

Clinical Possibilities

When managing dysfunctional patterns, clinical experience and evidence deriving from numerous clinicians and researchers suggest a rational sequence of management:

- Identify local and general imbalances that may be contributing to the symptoms being presented (posture, patterns of use, local dysfunction).
- Identify, relax and stretch overactive, tight muscles, using appropriate modalities. This would appear to be an ideal setting for the use of MET.
- Mobilise restricted joints – possibly using pulsed or regular MET.
- Facilitate and strengthen inhibited or weak muscles – possibly using isotonic-eccentric MET.
- Re-educate (exercises, training, etc.) functional movement patterns, posture and/or breathing function – something far more readily achieved once imbalances (e.g. short/tight/weak/loose) are improved or eliminated.
- Approaches that focus on reducing or eliminating peripheral or local areas of pain and dysfunction are seen to have the potential for major clinical benefit, even when the patient's symptoms involve central sensitisation in chronic pain settings (Niddam et al., 2008; Nijls & van Houdenhove, 2009; Affaitati et al., 2011).

This suggested sequence is therefore based on sound biomechanical and physiological principles, serving as a useful basis for care and rehabilitation of patients with musculoskeletal and more diverse health problems (Jull & Janda, 1987; Liebenson, 2006; Lewit, 2009).

Palpating Balance

Osteopathic pioneer H. V. Hoover (1969) described ease as a state of equilibrium, or 'neutral', which the practitioner senses by having at least one completely passive 'listening' contact (either the whole hand or a single or several fingers or thumb) in touch with the tissues being assessed. Bind is, of course, the opposite of ease, and can most easily be noted by lightly palpating the tissues surrounding, or associated with, a joint, as this is taken towards the end of its range of movement – its resistance barrier (see Box 5.1 for a summary of barrier characteristics; however, for a fuller explanation see Chapter 2, p. 19, and Box 2.2, p. 36).

Greenman (1996) suggests:

The examiner must be able to identify and characterise normal and abnormal ranges of movement, as well as normal and abnormal barriers to movement, in order to make an accurate assessment of tissue status. Most joints allow motion in multiple planes, but for descriptive purposes barriers to movement are described within one plane of

motion, for a single joint. The total range of motion from one extreme to the other is limited by the anatomical integrity of the joint and its supporting ligaments, muscles and fascia, and somewhere within the total range of movement is found a neutral point of balance.

This is the point of 'maximum ease' which the exercises described below attempt to identify. In order to 'read' hypertonicity (bind), and the opposite, a relaxed (ease) state, palpation skills need to be refined. As a first step, Goodridge (1981) suggested the following test, which examines medial hamstring and short adductor status. This exercise offers the opportunity for becoming comfortable with the reality of 'ease and bind' in a practical manner.[1]

Test for Palpation of Ease and Bind During Assessment of Adductors of the Thigh (Fig. 5.1A and B)

Goodridge (1981) described a basic method for familiarisation with MET. Before starting this exercise, ensure that the patient/model lies supine, so that the non-tested leg is slightly abducted, and leg to be tested close to the edge of the table. Ensure that the tested leg is in the anatomically correct position, knee in full extension and with no external rotation, which would negate the test (see Fig. 5.1A and B).

Goodridge's Ease–Bind Palpation Exercise, Part 1 (Goodridge, 1981)

1. The practitioner slowly eases the straight leg into abduction. 'After grasping the supine patient's foot and ankle, in order to abduct the lower limb, the practitioner closes his eyes during the abduction, and feels, in his own body, from his hand through his forearm, into his upper arm, the beginning of a sense of resistance'.
2. 'He stops when he feels it, opens his eyes, and notes how many degrees in an arc the patient's limb has travelled'.

---

[1]This test and its interpretation, and suggested treatment, using MET (should shortness be noted), will be fully explained in Chapter 6, but in this setting it is being used as an exercise for the purposes of the practitioner becoming familiar with the sense of 'ease and bind', and not for actually testing the muscles involved for dysfunction.

BOX 5.1   Barriers (see also Chapter 2, p. 19, and Box 2.2, p. 36)

When measuring the range of motion of a joint, the structures surrounding the joint itself – joint capsules, ligaments and physical structures of the articulation – provide resistance to the overall range of motion of the joint. In addition to this, the skin and subcutaneous connective tissue also play a part in restriction of a joint's motion (Shellock & Prentice, 1985; Gajdosik, 1991). Johns and Wright (1962) have shown that the passive torque that is required to move a joint is contributed by the joint capsule (47%), tendon (10%), muscle (41%) and skin (2%).

In discussion of the process of identifying restriction barriers in cases of carpal tunnel syndrome, Sucher (1994) notes: 'Restrictive barriers often were noted towards the middle to end of range of motion tested; however [in more severe conditions] the restriction was noted earlier throughout the range, at the initiation of movement'. Sucher suggests that this phenomenon of almost instant awareness of dysfunction may be considered as an 'immediate yes-or-no signal', indicating a change from 'ease' to 'bind'.

Kappler and Jones (2003) emphasise the soft-tissue nature of many joint restrictions:

As the joint reaches the barrier, restraints in the form of tight muscles and fascia, serve to inhibit further motion. We are pulling against restraints rather than pushing against some anatomic structure.

A variety of different terms can be used to describe what is perceived when a restriction barrier is reached or engaged. These terms frequently relate to the type of tissue providing the restriction, and to the nature of the restriction. For example:

- Normal end of range for soft tissues is felt as a progressive build-up of tension, leading to a gradually reached barrier, as all slack is removed.
- If a fluid restriction (oedema, congestion, swelling) causes reduction in the range of motion, the end-feel will be 'boggy', yielding yet spongy.
- If muscle physiology has changed (hypertonicity, spasm, contracture), the end-feel will be a tight, tugging sensation.
- If fibrotic tissue is responsible for a reduction in range, end-feel will be rapid and harsh but with a slight elasticity remaining.
- In hypermobile individuals, or structures, the end-feel will be loose and the range greater than normal.
- If bony tissue is responsible for a reduction in range (arthritis for example), end-feel will be sudden and hard without any elasticity remaining.
- Pain may also produce a restriction in range, and the end-feel resulting from sudden pain will be rapid and widespread, as surrounding tissues protect against further movement.

The barrier used in MET treatment is a 'first sign of resistance' barrier, in which the very first indication of the onset of 'bind' is noted.

This is the place at which further movement would produce stretching of *some* fibres of the muscle(s) involved.

This is where MET isometric contractions, whether these involve the agonists or antagonists, commence in acute (and joint) problems, and short of which contractions should commence in chronic problems.

What Goodridge (1981) is trying to establish is that the practitioner senses the *very beginning, the first sign,* of the end of the range of free movement, where easy, *'free-floating'* motion ceases, and effort on the part of the practitioner who is moving the limb begins. This barrier is not a pathological one, but represents the first sign of resistance, the place at which tissues require some degree of passive effort to move them. This is also the place at which the first signs of bind should be palpated (see part 2 of this exercise).

It is suggested that the process described by Goodridge be attempted several (indeed many) times, so that the practitioner gets a sense of *where resistance begins* – the *'feather-edge'* of resistance.

The exercise is then performed again – as described below.

Goodridge's Ease–Bind Palpation Exercise, Part 2

1. The patient lies close to the edge of the table on the side of the leg being tested. The practitioner stands between the patient's partially abducted leg and the table, facing the head of the table, so that all control of the tested leg is achieved by using the lateral (non-table-side) hand, which holds and supports the leg at the ankle. The other (table-side) hand rests passively on the inner thigh, palpating the muscles which are being tested (adductors and medial hamstrings).

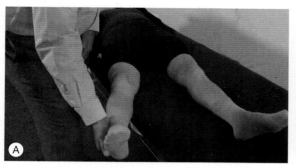 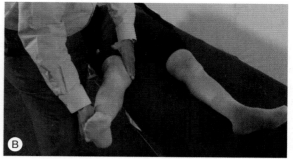

Fig. 5.1 (A) Assessment of 'bind'/restriction barrier with the first sign of resistance in the adductors (medial hamstrings) of the right leg. In this example, the practitioner's perception of the transition point, where easy movement alters to demand some degree of effort, is regarded as the barrier. (B) Assessment of 'bind'/ restriction barrier with the first sign of resistance in the adductors (medial hamstrings) of the right leg. In this example, the barrier is identified when the palpating hand notes a sense of bind in tissues which were relaxed (at ease) up to that point.

2. This palpating hand (often described as the 'listening' hand in osteopathy) must be in touch with the skin, moulded to the contours of the tissues being assessed, but should exert no pressure, and should be completely relaxed.

3. As in part 1 of this exercise, abduction of the tested leg is introduced by the non–table-side hand/arm, until the first sign of resistance is noted by the hand that is providing the motive force (i.e. the one holding the leg). As this point of resistance is approached, a tightening of the tissues ('a sense of bind') in the mid-inner thigh should be noted under the palpating hand.

4. If this sensation is not clear, then the leg should be taken back towards the table, and slowly abducted again, but this time it should be taken past the point where easy movement is lost, and effort begins, and towards its end of range. Here 'bind' will certainly be sensed.

5. As the leg is taken back towards the midline once more, a softening, a relaxation, a sensation of 'ease', will be noted, in these same tissues.

6. The same sequence should then be performed with the other leg, so that the practitioner becomes increasingly familiar with the sense of these two extremes (ease and bind). It is important to try to note the very moment at which the transition from ease to bind (and bind to ease) occurs, whether movement is into abduction or back towards the table.

7. Normal excursion of the straight leg into abduction is around 45°, and by testing both legs, as described, it is possible to evaluate whether the inner thigh muscles are tight and short on both sides, or whether one is and the other is not. Even if both are tight and short, one may be more restricted than the other. This is the one to treat first using MET.

Note: When learning to assess the first sign of resistance barrier, by applying parts 1 and 2 of this exercise, the contralateral ASIS should be observed, to see whether or not the resistance barrier has been passed. The pelvis (ASIS) will be seen to move in response to any movement that introduces a degree of stretch into the tissues being evaluated, as the assessment is being performed, that is, once the barrier has been passed, preceded by a feeling of 'effort' in part 1 of the exercise, and of 'bind' in part 2. Once the barrier is sensed it has been passed. Therefore, application of MET, starting with an isometric contraction, should commence just short of where bind was noted.

MET Exercise

Before using MET clinically, it may be helpful for you to perform palpation exercises relating to ease and bind (as described above), on many other muscles, as they are being both actively and passively moved, until skill in 'reading' changes in tone (ease and bind) has been acquired. In the example described above, once you can feel the beginnings of bind in the adductors and have decided which leg to treat, it is appropriate to attempt basic use of MET.

The point where the very first sign of bind was noted (or where the hand carrying the leg felt the first sign that effort was required, during abduction) is the resistance barrier (see Box 5.1). In subsequent chapters this barrier will be referred to many times. It is the place where an MET isometric contraction is commenced, in some applications of the methods (notably postisometric relaxation (PIR) – see below). It is also the place which is mentally/visually marked if the practitioner wishes to start a contraction from an easier mid-range position, but which it is necessary to note as the place at which resistance *became* a feature, before the isometric contraction.

Identification and appropriate use of the first sign of the barrier of resistance (i.e. where bind is first noted) is a fundamental part of the successful application of MET, along with other key features which include the degree of effort to be used by the patient, how long this should be maintained, and whether subsequently (after the contraction) the tissues should be taken to a new barrier, or through the old one, to introduce passive stretching, and most importantly how long stretches should be held for maximum benefit.

The following exercises in MET variations include the key features emphasised by some of the leading clinicians who have contributed to MET modern methodology.

Chapter 4 offers a background to current research evidence that validates some of these variables.

◉ Basic MET Exercise Using Postisometric Relaxation in an *Acute* Context

- The patient's limb is positioned at the point at which resistance was first perceived during abduction.
- The patient/model is asked to use no more than 20% of available strength to attempt to take the leg gently back towards the table (i.e. to adduct the leg) against firm, unyielding resistance offered by the practitioner.
- In this example the patient is trying to take the limb away from the barrier, while the practitioner holds the limb firmly at (towards) the barrier (this is described as a practitioner-direct method).
- The patient/model will be contracting the agonists, the muscles that require release (and which, once released, should allow greater and less restricted abduction).

- As the patient/model induces and holds the contraction they may be asked to hold an inhaled breath.
- The isometric contraction should be introduced slowly, and resisted without any jerking, wobbling or bouncing.
- Maintaining the resistance to the contraction should produce no strain for the practitioner, and no pain for the patient. This is maintained for 5 to 7 seconds, the length of time suggested for the various changes resulting from the isometric contraction to emerge, before the muscle is taken to a new resting length/resistance barrier, without effort (appropriate in an acute setting), or into stretch in a chronic setting (see below) (Scariati, 1991; Lewit, 2009).
- An instruction is given to the patient, 'Release your effort, slowly and completely', while the practitioner maintains the limb at the same resistance barrier.
- The patient/model is asked to breathe in and out, and to completely relax, and as they exhale, the limb is gently guided to the new resistance barrier, where bind is once more sensed (the range should almost always be able to be increased by a significant degree).
- Some studies suggest that following the use of the isometric contraction there exists a latency period of some 10 to 20 seconds, during which the muscle can be taken to its new resting length, or stretched more easily than would have been the case before the contraction (Moore & Kukulka,1991; Guissard et al., 1988). The possible mechanisms involved are discussed in Chapters 2, 4 and 10.

The exercise can be repeated, precisely as described above, to see whether even more release is possible, working from the new resistance barrier to whatever new range is gained following each successive contraction. This approach represents an example of Lewit's PIR method, as described in Chapter 2 (Lewit, 1999, 2009), and is ideal for releasing tone and relaxing spasm, particularly in acute conditions.

Basic MET Exercise Using Postisometric Relaxation Followed by Stretch, in a *Chronic* Context ◉

Where fibrosis is a feature, or when treating chronic conditions, a more vigorous approach is required in order to actually stretch the muscle(s), rather than simply taking them to a new barrier. Janda's (1993) approach, which he termed 'postfacilitation stretch', calls for the commencement of the contraction from a more relaxed, mid-range position, rather than at the actual barrier.

- Janda suggested stretching the tissues *immediately* following cessation of the contraction, and holding the stretch for at least 10 seconds, before allowing a rest period of up to half a minute. A lengthier holding period for the stretch may also be more appropriate in some circumstances (see below).
- Janda also suggested the procedure be repeated if necessary.

Modification of Janda's Approach

- The recommendation for use of MET for chronic fibrotic, or indurated, tissues, based on the lead author's experience, is that following a contraction of between 5 and 7 seconds, commencing from a mid-range position rather than at a barrier, using more than 20% but not more than 35% of the patient's available strength (Janda asks for full strength), a short (2 to 3 seconds) rest period is allowed for complete PIR, before stretch is introduced, which takes the tissues to a point *just beyond* the previous barrier of resistance.
- It is useful to have the patient gently assist in movement of the (now) relaxed area towards and through the barrier. Patient participation in such movement towards stretch activates the antagonists, and therefore reduces the danger of a stretch reflex (Mattes, 1990).
- The stretch is held for up to 30 seconds (Smith & Fryer, 2008). See also Chapter 4, *Duration of post-contraction stretch*.
- The procedure of contraction, relaxation, followed by patient-assisted stretch is repeated (ideally with a rest period between contractions) until no more gain in length of restricted tissues is being achieved (usually after 2 or 3 repetitions).

The Differences Between Janda's and Lewit's Use of PIR

- Lewit starts at, and Janda starts short of ('mid-range'), the restriction barrier.
- Janda utilises a longer and stronger contraction.
- Janda suggests taking the tissues beyond, rather than just to, the new barrier of resistance (with or without patient assistance).

Janda's approach is undoubtedly successful but carries with it a possibility of mildly traumatising the tissues (albeit that this is an approach only recommended for chronic

and not acute situations). The stronger contraction which he suggests, and the rapid introduction of stretching following the contraction, are the areas which it is suggested should be modified in application of MET, with no loss of benefit, and with a greater degree of comfort.

Reciprocal Inhibition

An alternative physiological mechanism, RI, is thought by some to produce a very similar latency ('refractory') period to that produced by PIR (Kuchera & Kuchera, 1992). See discussions in Chapters 2 and 4 that suggest alternative mechanisms, and that this so-called refractory period is too brief to influence the mechanisms operating following an isometric contraction.

RI is advocated for acute problems, especially where the muscle(s) requiring release have been recently traumatised, or are painful, and which cannot easily or safely be called on to produce sustained contractions such as those described in the notes on PIR above.

To use RI, the tissues requiring treatment should be placed just short of their resistance barrier (as identified by palpation) (Liebenson, 1989, 2006). This requirement relates to two factors:

1. The greater ease of initiating a contraction from a mid-range position as opposed to the relative difficulty of doing so when at an end of range.
2. Reduced risk of inducing cramp when commencing from a mid-range position, particularly in lower extremity structures such as the hamstrings, and especially if longer or stronger contractions than the norm (±20% strength, 5 to 7 seconds) are being used.

Basic Exercise in MET Using Reciprocal Inhibition in Acute and Chronic Contexts

The example involves abduction of the limb (i.e. shortened adductors), as outlined above:

- The first sense of restriction/bind is evaluated as the limb is abducted, at which point the limb is returned a fraction towards a mid-range position (by a few degrees only).
- From this position the patient/model is asked to attempt to *abduct* the leg themselves, using no more than 20% of strength, taking it towards the restriction barrier, while the practitioner resists this effort (as discussed earlier, this would be described as a patient-direct method).

- Following the end of the contraction, the patient/model is asked to 'release and relax', followed by inhalation and exhalation and further relaxation, at which time the limb is guided by the practitioner *to* (in an acute problem) or *through* (in a chronic problem) the new barrier *with* (if chronic) or *without* (if acute) the patient's/model's assistance.

MET – SOME COMMON ERRORS AND CONTRAINDICATIONS

Greenman (2003), King (2010) and others have summarised several of the important component elements of MET as follows. There is always a patient-active, operator resisted muscle contraction:

1. From a controlled position
2. In a specific direction
3. MET by practitioner-applied distinct counterforce
4. Involving a controlled intensity of contraction.

The common errors which may occur include those listed below.

Possible Patient Errors During MET

(Commonly based on inadequate instruction from the practitioner!)

1. Contraction is too strong (remedy: give specific guidelines, e.g. 'use only 20% of strength', or whatever is more appropriate).
2. Contraction is in the wrong direction (remedy: give simple but accurate instructions).
3. Contraction is not sustained for long enough (remedy: instruct the patient/model to hold the contraction until told to ease off, and give an idea ahead of time as to how long this will be).
4. The individual does not relax completely after the contraction (remedy: have them release and relax, and then inhale and exhale once or twice, with the suggestion 'now relax completely').
5. Starting and/or finishing the contraction too hastily. There should be a slow build-up of force and a slow letting go; this is easily achieved if a rehearsal is carried out first to educate the patient into the methodology.

Practitioner Errors in Application of MET

These may include:

1. Inaccurate control of the position of a joint or muscle in relation to the resistance barrier (remedy: have a clear image of what is required and apply it).

2. Inadequate counterforce to the contraction (remedy: meet and match the force in an *isometric* contraction; allow movement in an *isotonic* concentric contraction; and rapidly overcome the contraction in an *isolytic* manoeuvre, or slowly in a slow eccentric isotonic contraction – see Chapters 2 and 6).
3. Counterforce is applied in an inappropriate direction (remedy: ensure precise direction needed for best results).
4. Moving to a new position too hastily after the contraction (there is ample time to allow for muscle tone release during which time a new position can easily be adopted – haste is unnecessary and may be counterproductive) (Moore & Kukulka, 1991).
5. Inadequate patient instruction is given (remedy: get the instructions right, so that the patient can cooperate). Whenever force is applied by the patient, in a particular direction, and when it is time to release that effort, the instruction must be to do so gradually. Any rapid effort may be uncomfortable and self-defeating.
6. The coinciding of the forces at the outset (patient and practitioner), as well as at release, is important. The practitioner must be careful to use enough, but not too much, effort, and to ease off at the same time as the patient.
7. The practitioner fails to maintain the stretch position for a period of time that allows soft tissues to begin to lengthen (ideally 30 seconds for chronically shortened muscles, but certainly not just a few seconds) (Smith & Fryer, 2008).

Contraindications and Side Effects of MET

Carnes et al. (2010) have concluded that MET (and other manual therapy modalities) are safe and result in minimal side effects – when appropriately applied:

Nearly half of patients after manual therapy experience adverse events that are short-lived and minor; most will occur within 24 hours and resolve within 72 hours. The risk of major adverse events is very low, lower than that from taking medication.

Nevertheless, if pathology is suspected, MET should not be used until an accurate diagnosis has been established. Pathology (osteoporosis, arthritis, etc.) does not rule out the use of MET, but its presence needs to be established so that dosage of application can be modified accordingly (amount of effort used, number of repetitions, stretching introduced or not, etc.). See in particular the discussions regarding the safe and effective use of MET in potentially hazardous situations, in Chapters 7 and 8, for example, and such examples are extremely rare.

In the authoritative text *Contraindications in Physical Rehabilitation*, Batavia (2006) notes that:

Most concerns [relating to MET] were either procedural (e.g. overly aggressive, particularly in inexperienced practitioners) or related to musculoskeletal problems that are also a concern for joint manipulation therapy (e.g. tissue fragility, hypermobility). Myositis is contraindicated because MET involves resisted movements that may further aggravate an inflamed condition.

Greenman (2003) has explained the processes leading to post-MET-treatment discomfort:

All muscle contractions influence surrounding fascia, connective tissue ground substance and interstitial fluids, and alter muscle physiology by reflex mechanisms. Fascial length and tone are altered by muscle contraction. Alteration in fascia influences not only its biomechanical function, but also its biochemical and immunological functions. The patient's muscle effort requires energy and the metabolic process of muscle contraction results in carbon dioxide, lactic acid and other metabolic waste products that must be transported and metabolised. It is for this reason that the patient will frequently experience some increase in muscle soreness within the first 12 to 36 hours following MET treatment. Muscle energy procedures provide safety for the patient since the activating force is intrinsic and the dosage can easily be controlled by the patient, but it must be remembered that this comes at a price. It is easy for the inexperienced practitioner to overdo these procedures and in essence to overdose the patient.

DiGiovanna (1991) states that side effects are minimal with MET:

MET is quite safe. Occasionally some muscle stiffness and soreness after treatment. If the area being treated is not localised well or if too much contractive force is used pain may be increased. Sometimes the patient is in too much pain to contract a muscle or may be unable to cooperate with instructions or positioning. In such instances MET may be difficult to apply.

These clinical perspectives are supported by more recent investigations into the utility of eccentric exercise in vulnerable populations of elderly or chronically ill patients (LaStayo et al., 2014; Hoppeler, 2016), where it is found that an adaptation period and appropriate dosage makes it possible to avoid delayed onset muscle soreness (DOMS) and muscle damage even in frail or elderly patients (LaStayo et al., 2014). Despite the overwhelming evidence noting the benefits for these populations, in the absence of streamlined guidelines or recommendations (Lovering & Brooks, 2014), particular care is needed.

Side Effects Will be Limited if MET is Used in Ways That

1. Stay within the very simple guideline which states categorically *cause no pain when using MET.*
2. Stick to light (approximately 20% of strength) contractions.
3. Do not stretch over-enthusiastically, but only take muscles a short way past the restriction barrier, when stretching.
4. Have the patient assist in this stretch whenever possible.

No side effects are likely, apart from the soreness mentioned above, a common feature of most manual methods of treatment.

While Leon Chaitow advocates that the above recommendations be kept as a guideline for all therapists and practitioners exploring the MET approach, not all texts advocate a completely painless use of stretching and the contrary view needs to be reported.

- Sucher (1990), for example, suggests that discomfort is inevitable with stretching techniques, especially when self-applied at home: 'There should be some discomfort, often somewhat intense locally… however, symptoms should subside within seconds or minutes following the stretch'.
- Kottke (1982) says: 'Stretching should be past the point of pain, but there should be no residual pain when stretching is discontinued'.

Clearly what is perceived as pain for one individual will be described as discomfort by another, making this a subjective experience. It is hoped that sufficient emphasis has been given to the need to keep stretching associated with MET light, just past the restriction barrier, and any discomfort tolerable to the patient.

Breathing and MET

Many of the guidelines for application of isometric contraction call for patient participation over and above their 'muscle energy' activity, most notably involving respiratory synkinesis, the holding of a breath during the contraction/effort and the release of the breath as the new position or stretch is passively or actively adopted (Lewit et al., 1998; Lewit, 1999). Is there any valid evidence to support this apparently clinically useful element of MET methodology?

There is certainly 'common practice' evidence, for example in weight training, where the held breath is a feature of the harnessing and focusing of effort, and in yoga practice, where the released breath is the time for adoption of new positions. Fascinating as such anecdotal material might be, it is necessary to explore the literature for evidence which carries more weight, and fortunately this is available in abundance.

Cummings and Howell (1990) have looked at the influence of respiration on myofascial tension and have clearly demonstrated that there is a mechanical effect of respiration on resting myofascial tissue (using the elbow flexors as the tissue being evaluated). They also quote the work of Kisselkova and Georgiev (1976), who reported that resting electromyographic (EMG) activity of the biceps brachii, quadriceps femoris and gastrocnemius muscles 'cycled with respiration following bicycle ergonometer exercise, thus demonstrating that non-respiratory muscles receive input from the respiratory centres. The conclusion was that:

> these studies document both a mechanically and a neurologically mediated influence on the tension produced by myofascial tissues, which gives objective verification of the clinically observed influence of respiration on the musculoskeletal system, and validation of its potential role in manipulative therapy.

So, there is an influence, but what variables does it display?

Lewit helps to create subdivisions in the simplistic picture of 'inhalation enhances effort' and 'exhalation enhances movement', and a detailed reading of his book *Manipulative Therapy: Musculoskeletal Medicine*

(Lewit, 2009) is highly recommended for those who wish to understand the complexities of the mechanisms involved. Among the simpler connections which Lewit (1999) has discussed, and for which evidence is provided, are the following:

- The abdominal muscles are assisted in their action during exhalation, especially against resistance.
- Movement into flexion of the lumbar and cervical spine is assisted by exhalation.
- Movement into extension (i.e. straightening up from forward bending; bending backwards) of the lumbar and cervical spine is assisted by inhalation.
- Movement into extension of the thoracic spine is assisted by exhalation (try it and see how much more easily the thoracic spine extends as you exhale than when you inhale).
- Thoracic flexion is enhanced by inhalation.
- Rotation of the trunk in the seated position is enhanced by inhalation and inhibited by exhalation.
- Neck traction (stretching) is easier during exhalation, but lumbar traction (stretching) is eased by inhalation and retarded by exhalation.

Many individuals find controlled breathing and holding of the breath distressing, in which case these aspects of MET should be avoided altogether.

Note that breathing assistance to isometric contractions should only be employed if it proves helpful to the patient, and in specific situations. For example, in the case of the scalene muscles, a held inhalation automatically produces an isometric contraction. Therefore, in treating these muscles with MET, a held breath would seem to be potentially useful.

Degree of Effort With Isometric Contraction

Most MET contractions should be light and only rarely, when large muscle groups are involved, might it be necessary for there to be contractions involving up to 50% of a patient's strength. Among the reasons for suggesting lighter contractions are the practical ones of a lessened degree of difficulty for the practitioner in controlling the forces involved, as well as greater comfort and reduced likelihood of pain being produced when contractions are not strong.

It has also been suggested that recruitment of phasic muscle fibres occurs when an effort in excess of 30% to 35% of strength is used (Liebenson, 1996). If this is a valid position, and since in most instances it is the postural fibres that will have shortened and require stretching, little advantage would seem to be offered by inducing reduced tone, in phasic fibres. There would therefore seem to be greater advantage in using mild contractions, rather than increasing the force of a contraction.

See Box 5.2 on the topic of crossed syndromes involving imbalances between postural and phasic muscles – a particularly relevant subject in the context of MET. Postural and phasic muscles are discussed more fully in Chapter 2.

MORE ON MET VARIATIONS

Strength Testing – Mitchell's (1979) View

Mitchell et al. (1979) maintain that MET is best applied to a short, strong muscle, therefore before applying MET to an apparently shortened muscle, they suggest that the muscle, and its pair, should be assessed for relative strength. If the muscle that requires lengthening tests as weaker than its pair, it is suggested that the reasons for this relative weakness be identified and treated. For example, an overactive antagonist, or a myofascial TrP, might be producing inhibition (Lucas et al., 2004), and either of these factors should be dealt with so that the muscle that ultimately receives MET attention is strengthened – before being stretched. Goodridge (1981) concurs with this view:

When a left–right asymmetry in range of motion exists, in the extremities that asymmetry may be due to either a hypertonic or hypotonic condition. Differentiation is made by testing for strength, comparing left and right muscle groups. If findings suggest weakness is the cause of asymmetry in range of motion, the appropriate muscle group is treated to bring it to equal strength with its opposite number, before range of motion is retested to determine whether shortness in a muscle group may also contribute to the restriction.

One common reason for a muscle testing as 'weak' (compared with norms, or with its pair) involves increased tone in its antagonist, which would automatically inhibit the weakened muscle. One approach to restoring relative balance might therefore involve the antagonists to any muscle which tests as weak receiving attention first – possibly using an appropriate form of MET on the antagonists – to reduce excessive tone and/or to initiate stretching. Following MET treatment of the muscles found

to be short and/or hypertonic, subsequent assessment may show that previously weak or hypotonic antagonists will have strengthened – but still require further toning. This can be achieved using isotonic eccentric contractions, or Ruddy's methods (see below), or some other form of rehabilitation.

Reference to strength testing will be made periodically in descriptions of MET application to particular muscles in Chapter 6, whenever this factor seems important clinically.

Janda's Contrary View on the Accuracy of Muscle Testing

Janda (1993) provides evidence for the relative lack of accuracy involved in strength testing, preferring instead functional assessments, including tests for relative shortness in particular muscles, considered in the context of overall musculoskeletal function, as a means of deciding what needs attention. This seems to be close to the 'loose–tight' concept discussed earlier in this chapter (Ward, 1997). Janda effectively dismisses the idea of using strength tests to any degree in evaluating functional imbalances (Kraus, 1970; Janda, 1993;), when he states:

Individual muscle strength testing is unsuitable because it is insufficiently sensitive and does not take into account evaluation of coordinated activity between different muscle groups. In addition, in patients with musculoskeletal syndromes, weakness in individual muscles may be indistinct, thus rendering classical muscle testing systems unsatisfactory. This is probably one of the reasons why conflicting results have been reported in studies of patients with back pain.

Janda is also clear in his opinion that weak, shortened muscles will regain tone if stretched appropriately.

Janda is accurate in his scepticism regarding manual muscle testing accuracy unless dynamometers are used, and even then, very precise protocols are required to counter the numerous variables that can affect findings, including among other factors: gender, the particular muscle group involved, position of associated joints, time of day and age (Li et al., 2006; Abizanda et al., 2012).

Strain-Transmission and Stretching

Falvey et al. (2010), Clark et al. (2009) and Franklyn-Miller et al. (2009) – using embedded strain-gauges in

BOX 5.2   Crossed Syndromes

Upper Crossed Syndrome

Postural adaptation frequently involves a series of changes to the relative positions of the head, neck and shoulders, in which the extensor muscles of the head shorten and tighten as the flexors (deep neck flexors in particular), weaken:

1. The occiput and C1/2 hyperextend, with the head being pushed forward.
2. The lower cervical to fourth thoracic vertebrae become posturally stressed.
3. Rotation, abduction and 'winging' of the scapulae occurs.
4. The shoulders protract creating an altered direction of the axis of the glenoid fossa, resulting in the humerus requiring stabilisation by means of additional levator scapula and upper trapezius activity, with additional activity from supraspinatus and general rotator-cuff imbalance.

The result of these changes – commonly dubbed 'upper crossed syndrome' – is greater cervical segment strain, commonly associated with referred pain to the chest, shoulders and arms, together with a decline in respiratory efficiency.

Part of the solution, according to Janda (Liebenson, 1996), is to be able to identify the shortened structures and to release (stretch and relax) them, followed by re-education towards more appropriate function.

Lower Crossed Syndrome

Commonly the pelvis tips forward on the frontal plane, flexing the hip joints and producing lumbar lordosis, and stress at L5-S1 accompanied by pain and irritation. In the sagittal plane quadratus lumborum tightens and gluteus maximus and medius weakens.

When this 'lateral corset' becomes unstable, the pelvis is held in increased elevation, accentuated when walking, resulting in L5-S1 stress in the sagittal plane as well, resulting in low back pain. The combined stresses described produce instability at the lumbodorsal junction, an unstable transition point at best.

Also commonly involved are the piriformis muscles which in 20% of individuals are penetrated by the sciatic nerve, allowing piriformis to produce direct sciatic pressure and pain. Arterial involvement resulting from piriformis shortness produces ischaemia of the lower extremity, as well as sacroiliac dysfunction and pain in the hip through a relative fixation of the sacrum.

Part of the solution for this all too common pattern is to identify the shortened structures and to release them, ideally using variations on the theme of MET, followed by re-education of posture and use.

Chain Reaction Leading to Facial and Jaw Pain

Such imbalances are not merely of academic interest. A practical example of the negative effects of the chain reactions, as described above, is given by Janda (1986) in an article entitled 'Some aspects of extracranial causes of facial pain'. Janda's premise is that temporomandibular joint (TMJ) problems and facial pain can be analysed in relation to the patient's whole posture. He hypothesised that the muscular pattern associated with TMJ problems may be considered as locally involving hyperactivity and tension in the temporal and masseter muscles which reciprocally inhibits the suprahyoid, digastric and mylohyoid muscles. The external pterygoid may develop spasm. This imbalance between jaw adductors and jaw openers alters the ideal position of the condyle leading to a consequent redistribution of stress on the joint and degenerative changes.

Janda describes the typical pattern of muscular dysfunction of an individual with TMJ problems as involving upper trapezius, levator scapula, scaleni, sternomastoid, suprahyoid, lateral and medial pterygoid, masseter and temporal muscles, all of which show a tendency to tighten and to develop spasm.

He notes that while the scalenes are unpredictable, and while commonly, under overload conditions, they become atrophied and weak, they may also develop spasm, tenderness and trigger points.

The postural pattern in a TMJ patient might involve:

1. Hyperextension of knee joints
2. Increased anterior tilt of pelvis
3. Pronounced flexion of hip joints
4. Hyperlordosis of lumbar spine
5. Rounded shoulders and winged (rotated and abducted) scapulae
6. Cervical hyperlordosis
7. Forward thrust of head
8. Compensatory overactivity of upper trapezius and levator scapulae
9. Forward thrust of head resulting in opening of mouth and retraction of mandible.

This series of changes provokes increased activity of the jaw adductor and protractor muscles, creating a vicious cycle of dysfunctional activity. Inter-vertebral joint stress in the cervical spine follows.

Training in observation, palpation and assessment skills is clearly an essential foundation, since the sort of evidence

BOX 5.2   Crossed Syndromes—cont'd

Janda offers makes it clear that such patterns first need to be identified before they can be assessed for the role they might be playing in the patient's pain and restriction conditions, and certainly before these can be successfully and appropriately treated. (Liebenson discusses a number of Janda's observation assessment methods in Chapter 9.)

Additional Models of Crossed Syndrome

Key (2008) has expanded on Janda's original work in describing variations on the theme of crossed syndromes (Fig. 5.2A, B and C). In this readily recognised clinically familiar model, not only are overactive and underactive

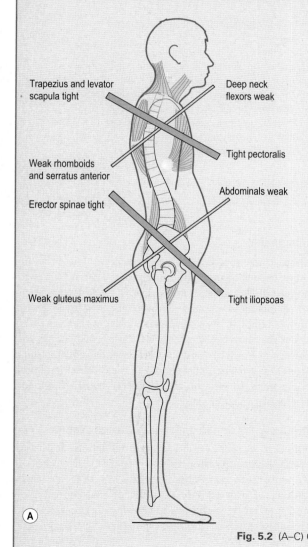

Trapezius and levator scapula tight

Deep neck flexors weak

Weak rhomboids and serratus anterior

Tight pectoralis

Erector spinae tight

Abdominals weak

Weak gluteus maximus

Tight iliopsoas

(A)

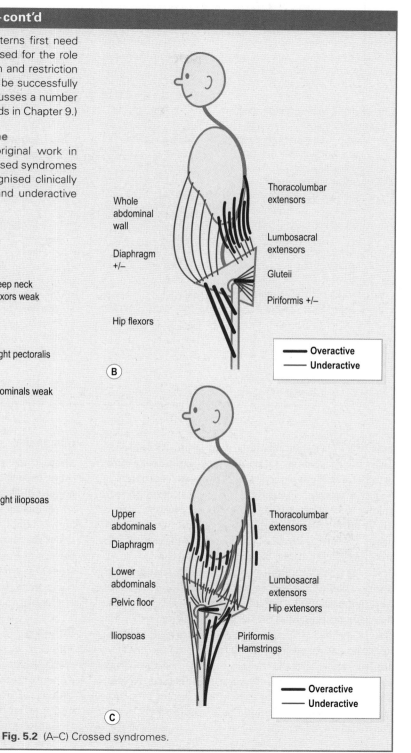

Whole abdominal wall

Diaphragm +/–

Hip flexors

Thoracolumbar extensors

Lumbosacral extensors

Gluteii

Piriformis +/–

—— Overactive
—— Underactive

(B)

Upper abdominals

Diaphragm

Lower abdominals

Pelvic floor

Iliopsoas

Thoracolumbar extensors

Lumbosacral extensors

Hip extensors

Piriformis Hamstrings

—— Overactive
—— Underactive

(C)

Fig. 5.2 (A–C) Crossed syndromes.

(Continued)

BOX 5.2   Crossed Syndromes—cont'd

muscles identified, but the functional patterns that follow can be predicted – ranging from back pain to head/neck/shoulder dysfunction, breathing pattern disorders and pelvic pain and dysfunction.

Posterior Crossed Pelvic Pattern
Characterised by:
- Pelvis – posterior shift + increased anterior sagittal tilt
- Trunk – anterior translation of thorax
- Increased lordosis at the thoracolumbar junction.

Hypoactivity/lengthened muscles:
- Entire abdominal wall and pelvic floor
- Lumbosacral multifidus
- Inefficient diaphragm activity.

Hyperactivity/adaptive shortened muscles:
- Thoracolumbar erector spinae
- Anterior hip flexor groups, primarily psoas
- Piriformis
- Hip internal rotators and external rotators.

Trunk extension will be reduced and the thoracolumbar region will be hyperstabilised, leading to:
- Poor pelvic control
- Decreased hip extension
- Abnormal axial rotation
- Dysfunctional breathing patterns
- Pelvic floor dysfunction.

Anterior Crossed Pelvic Pattern
Characterised by:
- Pelvis – anterior shift + increased posterior tilt
- Trunk (thorax) backward loaded, lumbar spine flexed
- Hips in extension – tight posterior hip structures
- Atrophied buttocks, head forward, kyphosis, knees extended.

Hypoactivity/lengthened muscles:
- Lower abdominal group and pelvic floor
- Lumbar multifidus – particularly over lower levels
- Diaphragm – reduced excursion ++
- Iliacus; psoas
- Glutei.

Hyperactivity/adaptive shortened muscles:
- Hamstrings
- Piriformis
- Upper abdominal group + lateral internal oblique
- Hip external rotators > internal rotators

Flexor muscles tend to dominate leading to:
- Loss of extension through spine
- Thoracolumbar junction hyperstabilised in flexion
- Poor pelvic control
- Dysfunctional breathing patterns.

---

cadavers – have demonstrated that strain-transmission, involving musculofascial connections, produces a range of unpredictable and unexpected effects during stretching.

For example, Franklyn-Miller et al. (2009) were able to show that a hamstring stretch creates 240% of the resulting strain in the iliotibial tract – and 145% in the ipsilateral lumbar fascia – as compared with the strain registered in the hamstrings themselves.

The implication of this phenomenon, in relation to any muscle assessed as 'short' or 'tight', is that the relative shortness/tightness might actually be due to influences other than features present in that muscle itself. Therefore, in the case of the hamstrings, the assessed 'shortness/tightness' might be – to a large extent – deriving from the ipsilateral lumbar fascia. Equally, thoracolumbar fascial tightness might be the direct result of hamstring influences. Not only does any apparently local stretch have distant influences, but the reason for stretching ('tight/short') might also be due to distant influences.

Conclusion

Strain-transmission, during stretching, affects many other tissues beyond the muscle that is being targeted, largely due to fascial connections, suggesting that, in some instances, apparent muscular restrictions, shortening, might in fact be fascial in origin. Fascial influences may have relevance to MET usage in general, and the use of isometric and isotonic eccentric contractions/stretches in particular, as noted in the discussion on viscoelasticity, in relation to MET/PNF contractions and stretching, in Chapters 2 and 6.

Mitchell and Janda and 'the Weakness Factor'

Mitchell et al.'s (1979) recommendation regarding strength testing prior to use of MET adds another dimension to assessment approaches that use indications of over-activity or signs of mal-coordination and imbalance as clues as to whether or not a postural (mobiliser) muscle should be considered as short.

'Functional' tests, such as those devised by Janda, and described by Liebenson and Rigney in Chapter 9, or objective evidence of dysfunction (using one of the many tests for shortness described in Chapter 6) can be used to provide such evidence.

Put simply (and keeping in mind the potential influence on muscles via strain-transmission of fascial connections):

- If a postural (mobiliser, see Chapter 2) muscle is over-used, misused, abused (traumatised) or disused, it is likely to modify by shortening. Evidence of over-activity, or of being involved in inappropriate firing sequences (see Janda's functional tests in Chapters 6 and 9), and/or demonstrating excessive tone, are all suggestive of such a muscle (i.e. postural) being dysfunctional and probably short (Janda, 1990; Tunnell, 1997; Hammer, 1999).
- If such a distressed muscle falls within one of the groups described in Chapter 2 as postural or as a mobiliser, then it may be considered to have shortened.
- The degree of such shortening may then be assessed using palpation and basic tests, as described in Chapters 6 or 9.

Additional evidence of a need to use MET-induced stretching can be derived from palpatory or assessment evidence of the presence of fibrosis and/or myofascial TrP activity, or of inappropriate EMG activity (should such technology be available).

Ideally, therefore, some observable and/or palpable evidence of functional imbalance will be available which can guide the therapist/practitioner as to the need for MET use, or other interventions, in particular muscles.[2] For example, in testing for overactivity, and by implication shortness, in quadratus lumborum (QL), an attempt may be made to assess the muscle firing sequence involved in raising the leg laterally in a side-lying position. There is a 'correct' and an 'incorrect' (or balanced and unbalanced) sequence according to Jull and Janda (1987). If the latter is noted, stress is proved and, since this is a postural muscle (or at least the lateral aspect of it is, see discussion of QL in Box 6.8, Chapter 6), shortness can be assumed and stretching indicated.

---

[2]This topic is discussed further in Chapter 9, which is devoted to Liebenson and Rigney's views on rehabilitation and which further discusses aspects of Janda's functional tests. Some of Janda's, as well as Lewit's, functional assessments are also included in the specific muscle evaluations described in Chapter 6.

Whether or not to introduce Mitchell's (1979) recommendation for strength testing into any assessment protocol is an individual clinical choice. The recommendation that muscle strength be taken into account before MET is used will not be detailed in each paired muscle discussed in the text and is highlighted here (and in a few specific muscles where these noted authors and clinicians place great emphasis on its importance) in order to remind the reader of the possible value of this approach.

Leon Chaitow did not find that application of strength/weakness testing (as part of the work-up before deciding on the suitability or otherwise of MET use for particular muscles) significantly improves results. He did, however, recognise that in individual cases it might be a useful approach, but considered that systematic weakness testing may be left until later in a treatment programme, after dealing with muscles which show evidence of shortness.

Fig. 5.3 shows EMG readings of specific muscle activity, possibly relevant to SIJ, low-back and/or pelvic dysfunction, during right hip extension in an individual representative of someone with a lower-crossed syndrome, as described earlier in this chapter (Janda, 1978; Lewit, 1991; Key, 2008):

- Gluteus maximus right side – showing virtually no firing activity
- Biceps femoris and semimembranosus right side – showing excessive activity
- Erector spinae left and right – both showing excessive activity.

Should You Stretch Short/Tight Muscles Before Facilitating Tone in Inhibited Antagonists?

Janda's experience – and therefore recommendation – suggests (in this example) that attention should initially be given to the overactive hamstrings and low back muscles before consideration of toning, facilitating the apparent gluteal weakness.

He offers additional evidence in Fig. 5.4 that shows the behaviour (via EMG readings) before and after stretching of hypertonic low-back muscles (three: erector spinae on the left, upper and lower rectus abdominis on the left) during the performance of three exercises:

- Sit-up – arms extended: Before treatment this resulted in overactivity of erector spinae group which should be silent during a sit-up, as well as relatively poor recruitment of the abdominal muscles. Following treatment

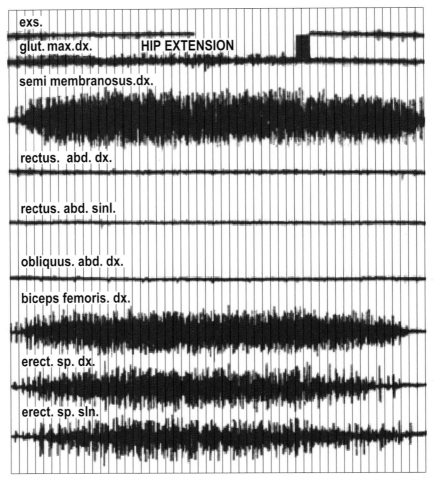

exs.

glut. max.dx.   HIP EXTENSION

semi membranosus.dx.

rectus. abd. dx.

rectus. abd. sinl.

obliquus. abd. dx.

biceps femoris. dx.

erect. sp. dx.

erect. sp. sln.

Fig. 5.3 Electromyographic readings of gluteus maximus (silent), semimembranosus, biceps femoris, right and left erector spinae (all overactive) during right hip extension. This is typical of a crossed syndrome pattern.

(stretching of the erector spinae group) these were silent during sit-ups and the previously inhibited abdominal muscles showed appropriately enhanced activity.

- Rolling back to the floor from a sit-up, with hands behind the neck: This exercise resulted in a very similar pattern to that shown in the sit-up exercise before treatment. After erector spinae stretching the abdominals produced a strong response, appropriately, and the low-back muscles were silent, as they should have been.
- Lying prone and extending the lumbar spine: This activity produced silent abdominals (as expected) and an excessively strong erector spinae response

before treatment. After stretching of the low-back muscles these produced the extension movement with far less force.

The implications deriving from this evidence is that by removing inhibiting influences (from the overactive erector spinae in this case) strength was restored to the abdominal muscles, and all the muscles assessed produced more appropriate levels of effort.

Strength Testing Methodology

In order to test a muscle for strength a standard procedure is carried out as follows:

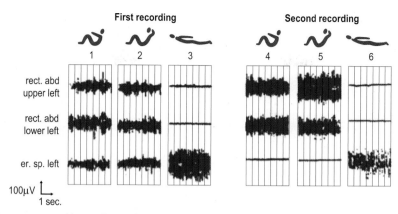

Fig. 5.4 Electromyographic readings of listed muscles, during performance of illustrated exercises, before and then following stretching of hypertonic lumbar erector spinae group.

- The area should be relaxed and not influenced by gravity.
- The area/muscle/joint should be positioned so that whatever movement is to be used can be comfortably performed.
- The patient should be asked to perform a concentric contraction that is evaluated against a scale, as outlined in Box 5.3.

The degree of resistance required to prevent movement is a subjective judgement, unless mechanical resistance and/or electronic measurement is available. For more detailed understanding of muscle strength evaluation, texts such as Janda's *Muscle Function Testing* (Janda, 1983) are recommended.

Ruddy's Methods – 'Pulsed MET'

In the 1940s and 1950s, osteopathic physician T. J. Ruddy developed a method which utilised a series of rapid pulsating contractions against resistance, which he termed 'rapid rhythmic resistive duction'. As described in Chapters 2, 3 and 6, it was in part this work that Fred Mitchell Sr used as his base for the development of MET. Ruddy's method (Ruddy, 1962) called for a series of muscle contractions against resistance, at a rhythm a little faster than the pulse rate. This approach can be applied in all areas where isometric contractions are suitable and is particularly useful for self-treatment following instruction from a skilled practitioner.

According to Greenman (1996), who studied with him, 'He [Ruddy] used these techniques in the cervical

BOX 5.3   **Scale for Evaluation of Concentric Contractions (Janda, 1983)**
Grade 0   No contraction/paralysis
Grade 1   No motion noted but contraction felt by palpating hand
Grade 2   Some movement possible on contraction, if gravity influence eliminated ('poor')
Grade 3   Motion possible against gravity's influence ('fair')
Grade 4   Movement possible during contraction against resistance ('good')

spine and around the orbit in his practice as an [osteopathic] ophthalmologist'.

For the sake of convenience, the lead author has abbreviated the title of Ruddy's work from 'rapid rhythmic resistive duction', to 'pulsed MET'. The simplest use of this approach involves the dysfunctional tissue/joint being held at its resistance barrier, at which time the patient, ideally (or the practitioner if the patient cannot adequately cooperate with the instructions), against the resistance of the practitioner, introduces a series of rapid (2 per second), very small contraction efforts towards the barrier.

The barest initiation of effort is called for with, to use Ruddy's words, 'no wobble and no bounce'. The use of this 'conditioning' approach involves contractions that are 'short, rapid and rhythmic, gradually increasing the amplitude and degree of resistance, thus conditioning the proprioceptive system by rapid movements'.

In describing application of pulsed MET to the neck (in a case of vertigo) Ruddy gave instruction as to the directions in which the series of resisted efforts should be made. These, he said, should include:

movements... in a line of each major direction, forwards, backwards, right forward and right backwards or along an antero-posterior line in four directions along the multiplication 'X' sign, also a half circle, or rotation right and left.

If reducing joint restriction, or elongation of a soft tissue, is the objective, then, following each series of 20 mini-contractions, the slack should be taken out of the tissues, and another series of contractions should be commenced from the new barrier, possibly in a different direction – which can and should be varied according to Ruddy's guidelines, to take account of all the different elements in any restriction. Despite Ruddy's suggestion that the amplitude of the contractions be increased over time, the effort itself must never exceed the barest initiation (and then ceasing) of an isometric contraction.

The benefits are likely, Ruddy suggests, to include enhanced oxygenation and improved venous and lymphatic circulation through the area being treated. Furthermore, he believed that the method influences both static and kinetic posture because of the effects on proprioceptive and interoceptive afferent pathways, and that this can assist in maintenance of 'dynamic equilibrium', which involves 'a balance in chemical, physical, thermal, electrical and tissue fluid homeostasis'.

In a setting in which tense, hypertonic, possibly shortened musculature has been treated by stretching, it may prove useful to begin facilitating and strengthening the inhibited, weakened antagonists by means of Ruddy's methods. Additionally, it would appear logical to use these methods where underlying hypermobility exists. This is true whether the hypertonic muscles have been treated for reasons of shortness/hypertonicity alone, or because they accommodate active TrPs within their fibres, or because of clear evidence of joint restriction of soft tissue origin, or because there is a change in tone and stiffness related to hypermobility.

The introduction of a pulsating muscle energy procedure such as Ruddy's, involving these weak antagonists, therefore offers the opportunity for:

- Proprioceptive re-education

- Strengthening facilitation of weak antagonists
- Further inhibition of tense agonists (possibly in preparation for stretching)
- Enhanced local circulation and drainage
- In Liebenson's words (2006), '*re-education of movement patterns on a reflex, subcortical basis*'.

Ruddy's work was a part of the base on which Mitchell Sr, and others, constructed MET, and his work is worthy of study and application since it offers, at the very least, a useful means of modifying the employment of sustained isometric contraction, and has particular relevance to acute problems and safe self-treatment settings. Examples of Ruddy's method will be described in later chapters.

Isotonic Concentric Strengthening MET Methods

Contractions that occur against a resistance that is then overcome allow toning and strengthening of the muscle(s) involved in the contraction. For example:

- The practitioner positions the limb, or area, so that a muscle group will be at a comfortable resting length, and thus will develop a strong contraction.
- The practitioner explains the direction of movement required, as well as the intensity and duration of that effort. The patient contracts the muscle with the objective of moving the muscle through a complete range, rapidly (in about 2 seconds).
- The practitioner offers counterforce that is slightly less than that of the patient's contraction and maintains this throughout the contraction. This is repeated several times, with a progressive increase in the practitioner's counterforce (the patient's effort in the strengthening mode builds towards maximal).
- Where weak muscles are being toned using these isotonic methods, the practitioner allows the concentric contraction of the muscles (i.e. offers only partial resistance to the contractile effort).
- Such exercises should always involve practitioner effort which is less than that applied by the patient. The subsequent isotonic concentric contraction of the weakened muscles should allow approximation of the origins and insertions to be achieved under some degree of control by the practitioner.
- Isotonic concentric efforts are usually suggested as being of short duration, ultimately employing maximal effort on the part of the patient.

- The use of concentric isotonic contractions to tone a muscle or muscle group can be expanded to become an isokinetic, whole joint movement (see below).

Isotonic Eccentric Alternatives

Norris (1999) suggests that there is evidence that when rapid movement is used in isotonic concentric activities it is largely phasic, type II, fibres that are being recruited. In order to tone postural (type I) muscles that may have lost their endurance potential, *eccentric isotonic exercises, performed slowly,* are more effective. Norris states: 'Low resistance, slow movements should be used… eccentric actions have been shown to be better suited for reversal of serial sarcomere adaptation'.

Note: Rapidly applied isometric *eccentric* manoeuvres ('isolytic') are described later in this chapter. Confusingly, slow isometric stretches have sometimes been labelled as *isolytic* in books (Kuchera & Kuchera, 1992) and journal articles (Parmar et al., 2011). It is suggested that this tendency be avoided, since *lysis* implies damage, something that is not likely during slow stretches, but which is almost certain, during rapid eccentric isotonic stretching.

Example of a Slow Eccentric Isotonic Stretch

Rationale: In the case of an individual with hamstring hypertonicity accompanied by inhibited quadriceps, a slow eccentric isotonic stretch (SEIS) of the quadriceps would both tone these and reciprocally inhibit the hamstrings, allowing subsequent stretching of the hamstrings to be more easily achieved.

- The patient is supine with hip and knee of the leg to be treated, flexed to 90°. (*Note:* It is sometimes easier to perform this manoeuvre with the patient prone.)
- The practitioner extends the flexed knee to its first barrier of resistance, palpating the hamstring tissues proximal to the knee crease for a first sign of 'bind'.
- The patient is then asked to resist, using a little more than half available strength, the attempt the practitioner will make to slowly flex the knee fully.
- An instruction should be given which makes clear the objective, 'I am going to slowly bend your knee, and I want you to partially resist this, but to let it happen slowly'.

After performing the slow isotonic stretch of the quadriceps, the hamstring should be retested for length and ease of straight leg raising, and if necessary, the hamstrings should be taken into a lightly stretched position and held for up to 30 seconds before repeating the procedure.

Strengthening a Joint Complex With Isokinetic MET

A variation on the use of simple isotonic concentric contractions, as described above, is to use isokinetic contraction (also known as progressive resisted exercise). In this method the patient, starting with a weak effort but rapidly progressing to a maximal contraction of the affected muscle(s), introduces a degree of resistance to the *practitioner's* effort to put a joint, or area, through a full range of motion. An alternative or subsequent exercise involves the practitioner partially resisting the patient's active movement of a joint through a rapid series of as full a range of movements as possible.

Mitchell et al. (1979) describe an isokinetic exercise as follows: 'The counterforce is increased during the contraction to meet changing contractile force as the muscle shortens and its force increases'. This approach is considered to be especially valuable in improving efficient and coordinated use of muscles, and in enhancing the tonus of the resting muscle. 'In dealing with paretic muscles, isotonics (in the form of progressive resistance exercise) and isokinetics, are the quickest and most efficient road to rehabilitation' (Mitchell et al., 1979).

The use of isokinetic contraction is reported to be a most effective method of building strength, and to be superior to high repetition, lower resistance exercises (Blood, 1980). It is also felt that a limited range of motion, with good muscle tone, is preferable (to the patient) to normal range with limited power. Thus, the strengthening of weak musculature in areas of limited mobility is seen as an important contribution, towards which isokinetic contractions may assist.

Isokinetic contractions not only strengthen (largely phasic, type II) fibres, but have a training effect which enables them to subsequently operate in a more coordinated manner. There is often a very rapid increase in strength. Because of neuromuscular recruitment, there is a progressively stronger muscular effort as this method is repeated. Contractions and accompanying mobilisation of the region should take no more than 4 seconds for each repetition, in order to achieve maximum benefit with as little fatiguing as possible of either the patient or the practitioner. Prolonged contractions should be avoided (DiGiovanna, 1991).

The simplest and safest applications of isokinetic methods involve small joints such as those in the extremities, largely because they are more easily controlled by the practitioner's hands. Spinal joints are more difficult to mobilise and to control when muscular resistance is being utilised at close to full strength.

The options for achieving increased tone and strength via these methods therefore involves a choice between a partially resisted isotonic concentric contraction, or the overcoming of such a contraction (i.e. eccentric), at the same time as the full range of movement is being introduced. Both of these options can involve close to maximum strength contraction of the muscles by the patient. Home treatment of such conditions is possible via self-treatment, as in other MET methods.[3]

DiGiovanna (1991) suggests that isokinetic exercise increases the work which a muscle can subsequently perform more efficiently and rapidly than either isometric or isotonic exercises.

To summarise:

- To tone weak phasic (stabiliser, see Chapter 2) muscles, perform concentric isotonic exercises using up to full strength, rapidly (4 seconds maximum).
- To tone weak postural (mobiliser, see Chapter 2) muscles, slowly perform eccentric isotonic (i.e. SEIS above) exercises using increasing degrees of effort (Norris, 1999).

Reduction of Fibrotic Changes With Isolytic (Rapid Isotonic Eccentric) MET

As discussed above, when a patient initiates a contraction, and it is overcome by the practitioner, this is termed an 'isotonic *eccentric* contraction' (e.g. when a patient tries to flex the arm and the practitioner overrides this effort and straightens it during the contraction of the flexor muscles). In such a contraction the origins and insertions of the muscles are separated, despite the patient's effort to approximate them, while the joint angle increases.

When such a procedure is performed rapidly this is termed an isolytic contraction, in that it involves the stretching and to an extent the breaking down (sometimes called 'controlled microtrauma') of fibrotic tissue present in the affected muscles.

Microtrauma is inevitable, and this form of 'controlled' injury is seen to be useful especially in relation to altering the interface between elastic and non-elastic tissues between fibrous and non-fibrous tissues. Mitchell (Mitchell et al., 1979) states that: 'Advanced myofascial

fibrosis sometimes requires this 'drastic' measure, for it is a powerful stretching technique'.

'Adhesions' of this type are broken down by the application of force by the practitioner which is just a little greater than that of the patient. Such procedures can be uncomfortable, and patients should be advised of this, as well as of the fact that they need only apply sufficient effort to ensure that they remain comfortable. Limited degrees of effort are therefore called for at the outset of isolytic contractions.

However, in order to achieve the greatest degree of stretch (in the condition of myofascial fibrosis for example), it is necessary for the largest number of fibres possible to be involved in the isotonic eccentric contraction. There is an apparent contradiction to usual practice in that, in order to achieve as large an involvement as possible, the degree of contraction force should be strong, likely to produce pain which, while undesirable in most manual treatment, may be deemed necessary in instances where fibrosis is being targeted.

In many situations the procedure involving a strong contraction might be impossible to achieve if a large muscle group (e.g. hamstrings) is involved, especially if the patient is strong and the practitioner slight, or at least inadequate to the task of overcoming the force of the contracting muscle(s). In such a situation, less than optimal contraction is called for, repeated several times perhaps, but confined to specific muscles where fibrotic change is greatest (e.g. tensor fascia lata), and to patients who are not frail, pain-sensitive or in other ways unsuitable for what is a vigorous MET method.

Unlike SEISs, in which the aim is to strengthen weak postural (mobiliser) muscles, and which are performed slowly (as discussed earlier in this chapter), isolytic contractions aimed at stretching fibrotic tissues are performed rapidly.

Summary of Choices for MET in Treating Muscle Problems

To return to Goodridge's introduction to MET (see earlier in this chapter), using the adductors as our target tissues we can now see that a number of choices are open to the practitioner once the objective has been identified, for example, to lengthen shortened adductor muscles.

If the objective is to lengthen shortened adductors, on the right, several methods could be used:

- With the right leg of the supine patient abducted to its first barrier of resistance, the patient could contract

---

[3]Both isotonic concentric and eccentric contractions take place during the isokinetic movement of a joint.

the *right abductors,* against equal practitioner counterforce, in order to relax the adductors by RI. This would be followed by stretching of the adductors.

- Instead of this the patient could contract the *right adductors,* against equal practitioner counterforce, in order to achieve 'increased tolerance to stretch'. This would be followed by stretching of the adductors.
- In another alternative, if chronic fibrosis is a feature, the patient, with the leg at the abduction barrier, could contract the *right adductors* while the practitioner offered greater counterforce, thus *rapidly* overcoming the isotonic contraction (producing a fast eccentric isotonic, or isolytic, contraction), introducing microtrauma to fibrotic tissues in the adductors. This could be followed by further stretching of the adductors. (*Note:* This isolytic approach is not recommended as a procedure unless the patient is robust and prepared for a degree of microtrauma and soreness for some days following treatment.) See Chapter 10 for details of the use of these methods post-surgically.
- To use the methodology of SEIS the leg would be taken to its abduction barrier, with the patient instructed to attempt to maintain it in that position as the practitioner slowly returns it to the midline. This would tone the inhibited abductors and inhibit the overtight adductors. This would be followed by stretching of the adductors past their restriction barrier. OR: with the leg in neutral, the practitioner could slowly abduct it towards the restriction barrier against patient resistance, thus both stretching and toning the adductors simultaneously, if this were thought appropriate.
- Or the limb could be abducted to the restriction barrier where Ruddy's 'pulsed MET' could be introduced, with the practitioner offering counterforce as the patient 'pulses' towards the barrier 20 times in 10 seconds.

In most of these methods the shortened muscles would have been taken to an appropriate barrier before commencing the contraction – either at the first sign of resistance if PIR and movement to a new barrier was the objective, or in a mid-range (just short of the first sense of 'bind') position if RI or a degree of post-facilitation stretching was considered more appropriate.

For an isolytic stretch, the contraction commences from the resistance barrier, as do all isokinetic and 'Ruddy' activities.

The essence of muscle energy methods then is the harnessing of the patient's own muscle power.

The next prerequisite is the application of counterforce, in an appropriate and predetermined manner. In isometric methods this counterforce must be unyielding. No contest of strength must ever be attempted. Thus, the patient should never be asked to 'try as hard as possible' to move in this or that direction. It is important before commencing that all instructions be carefully explained, so that the patient has a clear idea of their role.

The direction, degree of effort required, and duration, must all be clear, as must any associated instructions regarding respiratory or visual synkinesis (breathing patterns and eye movements) methods, if these are being used (see self-treatment examples of this below).

Joints and MET

MET uses muscles and soft tissues for its effects; nevertheless, the impact of these methods on joints is clearly profound since it is impossible to consider joints independently of the muscles which support and move them. For practical purposes, however, an artificial division is made in the text of this book, and in Chapter 7 there will be specific focus given to topics such as MET in treatment of joint restriction and dysfunction; preparing joints for manipulation with MET; as well as the vexed question of the primacy of muscles or joints in dysfunctional settings.

The opinions of experts such as Hartman, Stiles, Evjenth, Lewit, Janda, Goodridge and Harakal will be outlined in relation to these and other joint-related topics.

A chiropractic view is provided in Chapter 9, which includes rehabilitation implications, but which also touches on the treatment protocol which chiropractic experts Craig Liebenson and Curtis Rigney suggest in relation to dysfunctional imbalances which involve joint restriction/blockage.

In Chapters 9, 10, 11, 12 and 13 a variety of other professional variations are described, including the use of MET in post-surgical, physical therapy, massage therapy and athletic training contexts.

Self-Treatment

Lewit (1991) is keen to involve patients in home treatment, using MET. He describes this aspect thus:

Receptive patients are taught how to apply this treatment to themselves, as autotherapy, in a home programme. They passively stretched the tight muscle with their own hand. This hand next provided counter pressure to voluntary contraction of the tight muscle (during inhalation) and then held the muscle from shortening, during the relaxation phase. Finally, it supplied the increment in range of motion (during exhalation) by taking up any slack that had developed.

How Often Should Self-Treatment be Prescribed?

Gunnari and Evjenth (1983) recommend frequent applications of mild stretching or, if this is not possible, more intense but less frequent self-stretching at home. They state that: 'Therapy is more effective if it is supplemented by more frequent self-stretching. In general, the more frequent the stretching, the more moderate the intensity; less frequent stretching, such as that done every other day, may be of greater intensity'.

Self-treatment methods are not suitable for all regions (or for all patients) but there are a large number of areas which lend themselves to such methods. Use of gravity as a counterpressure source is often possible in self-treatment. For example, in order to stretch QL (Fig. 5.5A–C), the patient stands, legs apart and side-bending, in order to impose a degree of stretch to the shortened muscle. By inhaling and slightly easing the trunk towards an upright position, against the

weight of the body, which gravity is pulling towards the floor, and then releasing the breath at the same time as trying to side-bend further towards the floor, a lengthening of quadratus will have been achieved.

Lewit (1999) suggests, in such a procedure, that the movement against gravity be accompanied by movement of the eyes in the direction away from which bending is taking place, while the attempt to bend further – after the contraction – should be enhanced by looking in the direction towards which bending is occurring. Use of eye movements in this way facilitates the effects. Several attempts by the patient to induce greater freedom of movement in any restricted direction by means of such simple measures should achieve good results. This approach should also be considered when addressing areas of hypermobility since it engages whole body movement mechanisms and is less likely to result in overstretching.

The use of eye movements relates to the increase in tone that occurs in muscles as they prepare for movement when the eyes move in a given direction. Thus, if the eyes look down there will be a general increase in tone (slight, but measurable) in the flexors of the neck and trunk. In order to appreciate the influence of eye movement on muscle tone the reader might experiment by fixing their gaze to the left as an attempt is made to

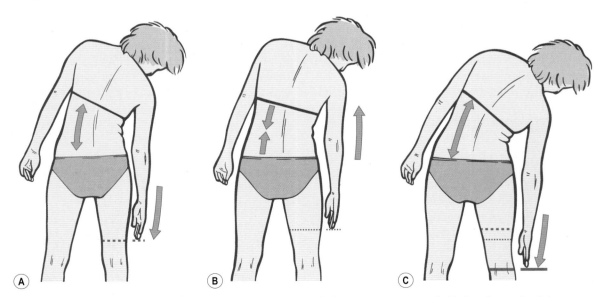

Fig. 5.5 (A) MET self-treatment for quadratus lumborum. Patient assesses range of side-bending to the right. (B) Patient contracts quadratus lumborum by straightening slightly, thereby introducing an isometric contraction against gravity. (C) After 7 to 10 seconds, the contraction is released and the patient will be able to side-bend further, stretching quadratus lumborum towards its normal resting length.

turn the head to the right. This should be followed by gazing right and simultaneously turning the head to the right. The evidence from this simple self-applied example should be convincing enough to create an awareness of what the patient's eyes are doing during subsequent stretching procedures!

It is hoped that the principles of MET are now clearer, and the methods seen to be applicable to a large range of problems.

Rehabilitation, as well as first-aid, and some degree of normalisation of both acute and chronic soft tissue and joint problems are all possible, given correct application. Combined with NMT, this offers the practitioner additional tools for achieving safe and effective therapeutic interventions.

When Should MET be Applied to a Muscle?

When should MET (PIR, RI or post-facilitation stretch) be applied to a muscle to relax and/or stretch it?

1. When it is demonstrably shortened – unless the shortening is attributable to associated joint restriction or stabilising adaptation in case of hypermobility in which the underlying cause should receive primary attention, possibly also involving MET (see Chapter 7).

2. When it contains areas of shortening, such as are associated with myofascial TrPs or palpable fibrosis. It is important to note that TrPs evolve within stressed (hypertonic) areas of phasic, as well as postural, muscles, and that these tissues will require stretching, based on evidence which shows that TrPs reactivate unless shortened fibres in which they are housed are stretched to a normal resting length as part of a therapeutic intervention (Simons et al., 1999). (See also Chapter 14.)

3. When periosteal pain points are palpable, indicating stress at the associated muscle's origin and/or insertion (Lewit, 1999).

4. In cases of muscular imbalance, in order to reduce hypertonicity when weakness in a muscle is attributable, in part or totally, to inhibition deriving from a hypertonic antagonist muscle (group).

Caution is needed when the underlying reason for shortening, stiffening and TrP development is part of an adaptive process such as found in hypermobility syndromes. In these instances, any interventions need to be minimal to avoid destabilising stability.

Evaluation

It is seldom possible to totally isolate one muscle in an assessment, and reasons other than muscle shortness can account for apparent restriction (intrinsic joint dysfunction for example). Other methods of evaluation as to relative muscle shortness are also called for, including direct palpation.

The 'normal' range of movements of particular muscles should be taken as guidelines only, since individual factors will often determine that what is 'normal' for one person is not so for another.

Wherever possible, an understanding is called for of functional patterns which are observable, for example in the case of the upper fixators of the shoulder/accessory breathing muscles. If a pattern of breathing is observed which indicates a predominance of upper chest involvement, as opposed to diaphragmatic, this in itself would indicate that this muscle group was being 'stressed' by overuse. Since stressed postural (mobiliser) muscles will shorten, an automatic assumption of shortness can be made in such a case regarding the scalenes, levator scapulae, etc.

Once again let it be clear that the various tests and assessment methods suggested in Chapter 6, even when utilising evidence of an abnormally short range of motion, are meant as indicators, rather than proof, of shortness. As Gunnari and Evjenth (1983) observe:

> If the preliminary analysis identifies shortened muscles, then a provisional trial treatment is performed. If the provisional treatment reduces pain and improves the affected movement pattern, the preliminary analysis is confirmed, and treatment may proceed.

Evidence would then be clinical rather than research-based (Box 5.4).

MUSCLE MAPS

This chapter contains descriptions of the MET approaches to individual muscles. It is assumed that before using MET methods, a sound grounding will have been achieved in understanding both the anatomy and physiology of the musculoskeletal system.

In almost all instances, lengthening/stretching strategies involve following fibre direction. To assist in application of MET, Figs 5.6 to 5.16 may enhance awareness of fibre direction.

BOX 5.4 MET Summary of Variations

1. Isometric Contraction – Using Antagonist(s) (in an Acute Setting, Without Stretching)

Indications

- Relaxing acute muscular spasm or contraction
- Mobilising restricted joints
- Preparing joint for manipulation.

Contraction starting point: For acute muscle, or any joint problem, commence at 'easy' restriction barrier (first sign of resistance towards end of range).

Modus operandi: The patient is attempting to push towards the barrier of restriction against the practitioner's/therapist's precisely matched counterforce, therefore antagonist(s) to affected muscle(s) are being employed in an isometric contraction, so obliging shortened muscles to relax via reciprocal inhibition/'increased stretch tolerance'.

Forces: Practitioner's/therapist's and patient's forces are matched involving approximately 20% of patient's strength (or less).

Duration of contraction: 5–7 s; no pain should be induced by the effort.

Action following contraction: The tissues (muscle/joint) are taken to their new restriction barrier without stretch after ensuring complete relaxation. Movement to the new barrier should be performed on an exhalation.

Repetitions: Repeat one or two times.

Reminder: When using MET in an acute setting no stretching is involved, merely attempts to reduce excessive tone.

2. Isometric Contraction – Using Agonist(s) (in an Acute Setting, Without Stretching)

Indications

- Relaxing acute muscular spasm or contraction
- Mobilising restricted joints
- Preparing joint for manipulation.

Contraction starting point: At resistance barrier.

Modus operandi: The affected muscles (the agonists) are used in the isometric contraction, therefore the shortened muscles subsequently relax. If there is pain on contraction this method is contraindicated and the previous method (use of antagonist) is employed. The practitioner/therapist is attempting to push towards the barrier of restriction against the patient's precisely matched counter-effort.

Forces: Practitioner's/therapist's and patient's forces are matched involving approximately 20% of patient's strength.

Duration of contraction: 5–7 s.

Action following contraction: The tissues (muscle/joint) are taken to their new restriction barrier without stretch after ensuring patient has completely relaxed. Movement to new barrier should be performed on an exhalation.

Repetitions: Repeat one or two times.

Reminder: When using MET in an acute setting no stretching is involved, merely attempts to reduce excessive tone.

3. Isometric Contraction – Using Agonist OR Antagonist Contractions (in a Chronic Setting, With Stretching)

Indications

- Stretching chronic or subacute restricted, fibrotic, contracted soft tissues (fascia, muscle) or tissues housing active myofascial trigger points.

Contraction starting point: Short of the resistance barrier.

Modus operandi: The affected muscles (agonists) OR their antagonists are used in the isometric contraction, enhancing 'stretch tolerance' (see discussion in Chapter 4). The patient is attempting to push away from OR towards the barrier of restriction (or in a different direction altogether), against the practitioner's precisely matched counter-effort.

Forces: The practitioner's/therapist's and patient's forces are matched, involving no more than 30% of patient's strength.

Duration of contraction: 5–7 s.

> **! CAUTION**
>
> Longer, stronger contractions may predispose towards onset of cramping and so should be used with care.

Action following contraction: There should be a rest period of a few seconds to ensure complete relaxation before commencing the stretch. On an exhalation the area (muscle) is taken to its new restriction barrier, and a small degree beyond, painlessly, and held in this position for between 5 and 30 s. The patient should, if possible, participate in assisting in the move to, and through, the barrier, effectively further inhibiting the structure being stretched, and retarding the likelihood of a myotatic stretch reflex.

Repetitions: One or two times, or until no further gain in range of motion is possible, with each isometric contraction commencing from a position just short of the restriction barrier.

4. Isotonic Concentric Contraction (for Toning or Rehabilitation)

Indications

- Toning weakened musculature.

Contraction starting point: In a mid-range easy position.

BOX 5.4   MET Summary of Variations—cont'd

Modus operandi: The affected muscle is allowed to contract, with some (constant) resistance from the practitioner/therapist.

Forces: The patient's effort overcomes that of the practitioner/therapist since the patient's force is greater than the practitioner's/therapist's resistance. The patient uses maximal effort available, but force is built slowly, not via sudden effort. The practitioner/therapist maintains a constant degree of resistance.

Duration: 3–4 s.

Repetitions: Repeat five to seven times, or more if appropriate.

5. Isotonic Eccentric Contraction (Isolytic, for Reduction of Fibrotic Change, to Introduce Controlled Microtrauma)

Indications
- Stretching tight fibrotic musculature.

Contraction starting point: At the restriction barrier.

Modus operandi: The muscle to be stretched is contracted by the patient and is prevented from doing so by the practitioner/therapist, by means of superior practitioner/therapist effort, so that the contraction is rapidly overcome and reversed, introducing stretch into the contracting muscle.

The process should take no more than 4 s. Origin and insertion do not approximate. The muscle should be stretched to, or as close as possible to, full physiological resting length.

Forces: The practitioner's/therapist's force is greater than that of the patient. Less than maximal patient force should be employed at first. Subsequent contractions build towards this if discomfort is not excessive.

Duration of contraction: 2–4 s.

Repetitions: Repeat three to five times if discomfort is not excessive.

 CAUTION

Avoid using isolytic contractions on head/neck muscles or at all if patient is frail, very pain-sensitive or osteoporotic. The patient should anticipate soreness for several days in the affected muscles.

6. Slow Eccentric Isotonic Contraction – Slow Eccentric Isotonic Stretch for Strengthening Weak Postural Muscles and Preparing Their Antagonists for Stretching

Indications
- Strengthening weakened postural muscles
- Preparing tight antagonists to inhibited muscles for stretching.

Contraction starting point: At the restriction barrier.

Modus operandi: The muscle is contracted and is prevented from doing so by the practitioner/therapist, via superior practitioner/therapist effort, so that the contraction is *slowly* overcome and reversed, as the contracting muscle is stretched. The origin and insertion do not approximate but diverge. The muscle should be stretched to its full physiological resting length. This process tones the muscle and inhibits its antagonist(s), and these can subsequently be stretched as in other MET procedures.

Forces: The practitioner's/therapist's force is greater than the patient's. Less than maximal patient's force should be employed at first. Subsequent contractions build towards this if discomfort is not excessive.

Duration of contraction: 5–7 s.

Repetitions: Repeat three times if discomfort is not excessive.

> **! CAUTION**
>
> Avoid using isotonic eccentric contractions on head/neck muscles involved in rotation, or at all if the patient is frail, very pain-sensitive or osteoporotic.

7. Isokinetic (Combined Isotonic and Isometric Contractions)

Indications
- Toning weakened musculature
- Building strength in all muscles involved in particular joint function
- Training and balancing effect on muscle fibres.

Starting point of contraction: Easy mid-range position.

Modus operandi: The patient resists with moderate and variable effort at first, progressing to maximal effort subsequently, as the practitioner/therapist rapidly puts a joint (ankle or wrist for example) through as full a range of movements as possible. This approach differs from a simple isotonic exercise by virtue of the inclusion of whole ranges of motion, rather than single motions, and because the applied resistance varies, progressively increasing as the procedure progresses.

Forces: The practitioner's/therapist's force overcomes the patient's effort to prevent movement. First movements (taking an ankle, say, into all its directions of motion) may involve moderate force, progressing to full force subsequently. An alternative is to have the practitioner/therapist (or machine) resist the patient's effort to make all the movements.

Duration of contraction: Up to 4 s.

Repetitions: Repeat two to four times.

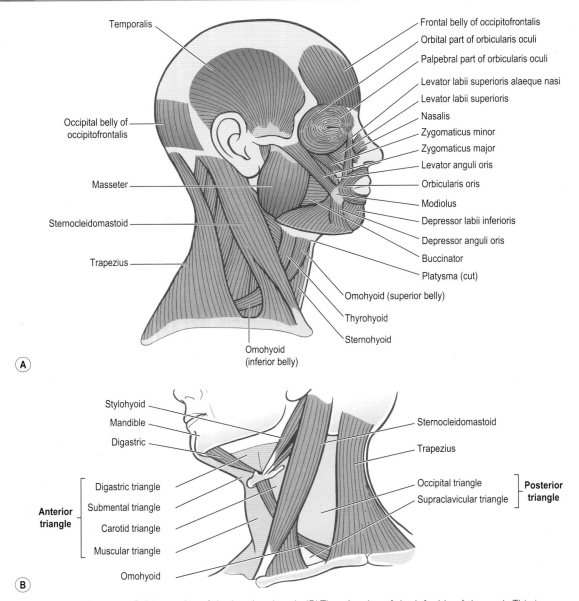

Fig. 5.6 (A) The superficial muscles of the head and neck. (B) The triangles of the left side of the neck. This is a highly schematic two-dimensional representation of what in reality are non-planar trigones distributed over a waisted column.

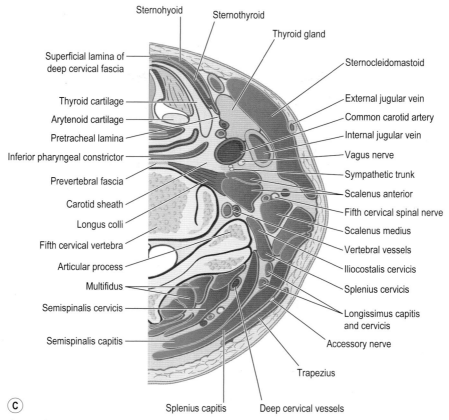

Sternohyoid

Sternothyroid

Thyroid gland

Superficial lamina of deep cervical fascia

Sternocleidomastoid

Thyroid cartilage

External jugular vein

Arytenoid cartilage

Common carotid artery

Pretracheal lamina

Internal jugular vein

Inferior pharyngeal constrictor

Vagus nerve

Prevertebral fascia

Sympathetic trunk

Carotid sheath

Scalenus anterior

Longus colli

Fifth cervical spinal nerve

Fifth cervical vertebra

Scalenus medius

Articular process

Vertebral vessels

Multifidus

Iliocostalis cervicis

Semispinalis cervicis

Splenius cervicis

Semispinalis capitis

Longissimus capitis and cervicis

Accessory nerve

Trapezius

(C)

Splenius capitis

Deep cervical vessels

Fig. 5.6 (cont'd) (C) Transverse section through the right half of the neck to show the arrangement of the deep cervical fascia. (Redrawn with permission from William, P.L., 1995. Gray's Anatomy, 38th ed. Churchill Livingstone.)

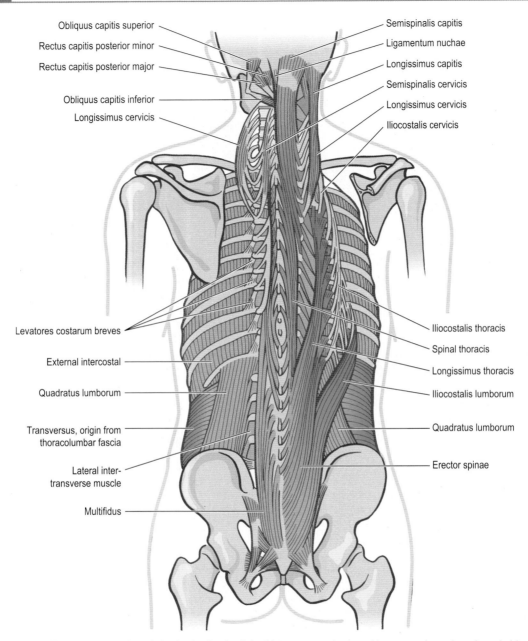

Fig. 5.7 The deep muscles of the back. On the left side erector spinae and its upward continuations (with the exception of longissimus cervicis, which has been displaced laterally) and semispinalis capitis have been removed. (Redrawn with permission from William, P.L., 1995. Gray's Anatomy, 38th ed. Churchill Livingstone.)

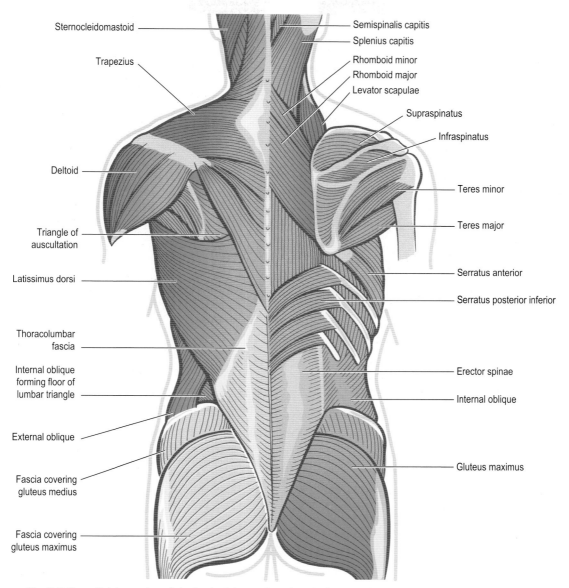

Fig. 5.8 Superficial muscles of the back of the neck and trunk. On the left only the skin, superficial and deep fasciae (other than gluteofemoral) have been removed; on the right, sternocleidomastoid, trapezius, latissimus dorsi, deltoid and external oblique have been dissected away. (Redrawn with permission from William, P.L., 1995. Gray's Anatomy, 38th ed. Churchill Livingstone.)

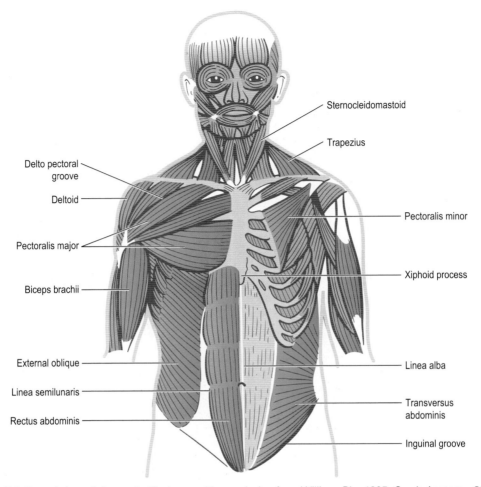

Fig. 5.9 Frontal view of the trunk. (Redrawn with permission from William, P.L., 1995. Gray's Anatomy, 38th ed. Churchill Livingstone.)

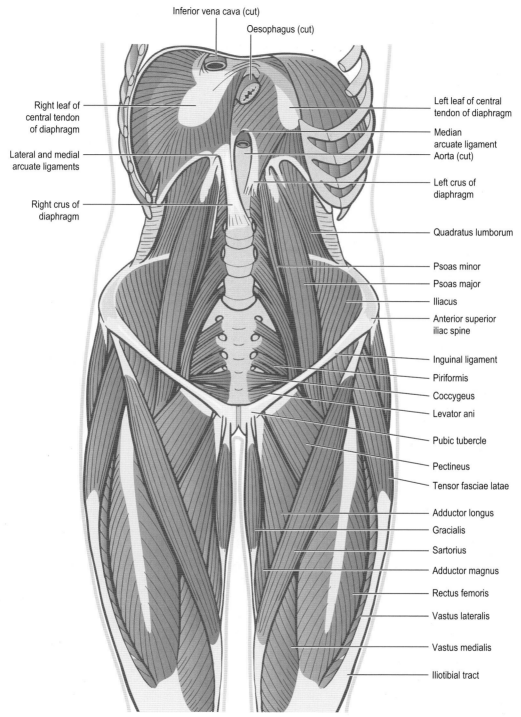

Fig. 5.10 View of the abdomen, pelvis and thighs, showing abdominal aspect of the diaphragm, hip flexors and superficial muscles of the thigh. (Redrawn with permission from William, P.L., 1995. Gray's Anatomy, 38th ed. Churchill Livingstone.)

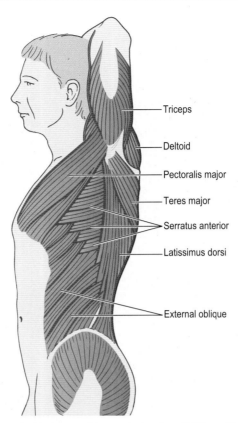

Fig. 5.11 Lateral view of the trunk. (Redrawn with permission from William, P.L., 1995. Gray's Anatomy, 38th ed. Churchill Livingstone.)

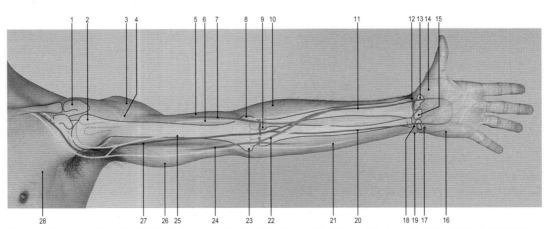

1. Acromion. 2. Greater tubercle (tuberosity). 3. Deltoid. 4. Axillary nerve. 5. Biceps brachii. 6. Radial nerve. 7. Cephalic vein. 8. Lateral epicondyle. 9. Head of radius. 10. Brachioradialis. 11. Radial artery. 12. Styloid process of radius. 13. Scaphoid. 14. Thenar eminence. 15. Lunate. 16. Hypothenar eminence. 17. Triquetrum. 18. Styloid process of ulna. 19. Proximal wrist crease. 20. Ulnar artery. 21. Ulnar nerve. 22. Median cubital vein. 23. Median epicondyle. 24. Basilic vein. 25. Median nerve. 26. Triceps. 27. Brachial artery. 28. Pectoralis major.

Fig. 5.12 Anterior view of the arm abducted at the shoulder. (Redrawn with permission from William, P.L., 1995. Gray's Anatomy, 38th ed. Churchill Livingstone.)

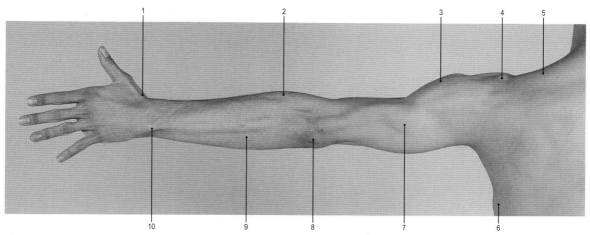

1. Anatomical snuffbox. 2. Brachioradialis. 3. Deltoid. 4. Acromion. 5. Trapezius. 6. Latissimus dorsi. 7. Triceps. 8. Olecranon process. 9. Common extensor muscle group. 10. Extensor carpi ulnaris.

Fig. 5.13 Posterior view of the arm abducted at the shoulder. (Redrawn with permission from William, P.L., 1995. Gray's Anatomy, 38th ed. Churchill Livingstone.)

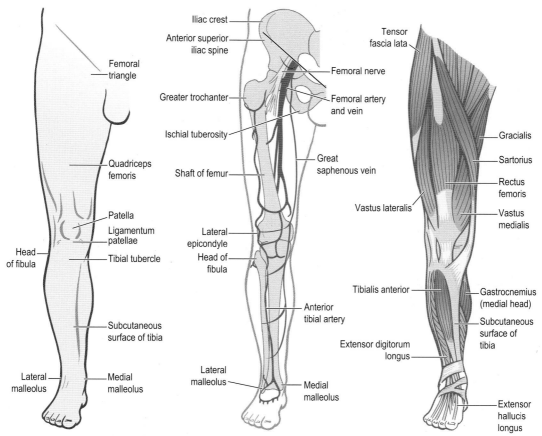

Fig. 5.14 Anterior aspect of lower limb to show surface anatomy, bony and soft tissue structures. (Redrawn with permission from William, P.L., 1995. Gray's Anatomy, 38th ed. Churchill Livingstone.)

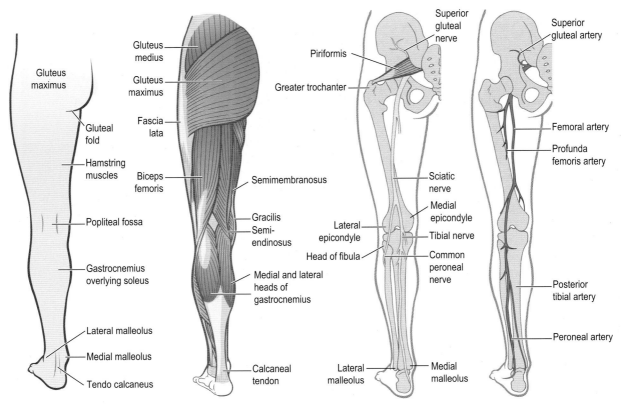

Fig. 5.15 Posterior view of the lower limb to show surface anatomy, bony and soft tissue structures and main nerves and arteries. (Redrawn with permission from William, P.L., 1995. Gray's Anatomy, 38th ed. Churchill Livingstone.)

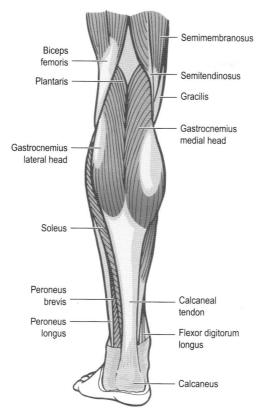

Semimembranosus

Semitendinosus

Gracilis

Gastrocnemius
medial head

Biceps
femoris

Plantaris

Gastrocnemius
lateral head

Soleus

Peroneus
brevis

Peroneus
longus

Calcaneal
tendon

Flexor digitorum
longus

Calcaneus

Fig. 5.16 Muscles of the left calf: superficial group. (Redrawn with permission from William, P.L., 1995. Gray's Anatomy, 38th ed. Churchill Livingstone.)

REFERENCES

Abizanda, P., Navarro, J.L., García-Tomás, M.I., López-Jiménez, E., Martínez-Sánchez, E., Paterna, G., 2012. Validity and usefulness of hand-held dynamometry for measuring muscle strength in community-dwelling older persons. Arch. Gerontol. Geriatr. 54, 21–27.

Affaitati, G., Constantini, R., Fabrizio, A., et al., 2011. Effects of treatment of peripheral pain generators in fibromyalgia patients. Eur. J. Pain 15 (1), 61–69.

Ali, A., Andrzejowski, P., Kanakaris, N.K., Giannoudis, P.V., 2020. Pelvic girdle pain, hypermobility spectrum disorder and hypermobility-type Ehlers–Danlos syndrome: a narrative literature review. J. Clin. Med. 9 (12), 3992. doi:10.3390/jcm9123992.

Batavia, M., 2006. Contraindications in Physical Rehabilitation: Doing No Harm. Saunders Elsevier, St Louis, MO.

Bhimani, R., Gaugler, J.E., Felts, J., 2020. Consensus definition of muscle tightness from multidisciplinary perspectives. Nurs. Res. 69 (2), 109–115.

Blood, S., 1980. Treatment of the sprained ankle. J. Am. Osteopath. Assoc. 79 (11), 689.

Carnes, D., Mars, T.S., Mullinger, B., Froud, R., Underwood, M., 2010. Adverse events and manual therapy: A systematic review. Man. Ther. 15, 355–363.

Clark, R.A., Franklyn-Miller, A., Falvey, E., Bryant, A.L., Bartold, S., McCrory, P., 2009. Assessment of mechanical strain in the intact plantar fascia. Foot 19, 161–164.

Cummings, J., Howell, J., 1990. The role of respiration in the tension production of myofascial tissues. J. Am Osteopath. Assoc. 90 (9), 842.

DiGiovanna, E., 1991. Treatment of the spine. In: DiGiovanna, E. (Ed.), An Osteopathic Approach to Diagnosis and Treatment. Lippincott, Philadelphia.

Falvey, E.C., Clark, R.A., Franklyn-Miller, A., Bryant, A.L., Briggs, C., McCrory, P.R., 2010. Iliotibial band syndrome: An examination of the evidence behind a number of treatment options. Scand. J. Med. Sci. Sports 20 (4), 580–587.

Franklyn-Miller, A., Falvey, E., Clark, R., 2009. The strain patterns of the deep fascia of the lower limb. Fascial Research II:

Basic Science and Implications for Conventional and Complementary Health Care. Elsevier GmbH, Munich.

Gajdosik, 1991. Effects of static stretching on short hamstring muscles. J. Sports Phys. Ther. 14 (6), 250–255.

Goodridge, J., 1981. MET—Definition, explanation, methods of procedure. J. Am. Osteopath. Assoc. 81 (4), 249.

Greenman, P., 1996. Principles of Manual Medicine, second ed. Williams and Wilkins, Baltimore.

Greenman, P.E., 2003. Principles of Manual Medicine, third ed. Lippincott, Williams & Wilkins, Baltimore.

Guissard, N., Duchateau, J., Hainaut, K., 1988. Muscle stretching and motoneuron excitability. Eur. J. Appl. Physiol. 58, 47–52.

Gunnari, H., Evjenth, O., 1983. Sequence Exercise. Dreyers Verlag, Oslo [Norwegian.].

Hammer, W., 1999. Functional Soft Tissue Examination and Treatment by Manual Methods. Aspen Publications, Gaithersburg, Md., pp. 535–540.

Hoover, H.V., 1969. Collected papers. Academy of Applied Osteopathy Year Book, pp. 16–68.

Hoppeler, H., 2016. Moderate load eccentric exercise; a distinct novel training modality. Front. Physiol. 7, 483. doi:10.3389/fphys.2016.00483.

Janda, V., 1978. Muscles, central nervous motor regulation, and back problems. In: Korr, I.M. (Ed.), Neurobiologic Mechanisms in Manipulative Therapy. Plenum, New York.

Janda, V., 1983. Muscle Function Testing. Butterworths, London.

Janda, V., 1986. Some aspects of extracranial causes of facial pain. J. Prosthet. Dent. 56 (4), 484–487.

Janda, V., 1990. Differential diagnosis of muscle tone in respect of inhibitory techniques. In: Paterson, J.K., Burn, L. (Eds.), Back Pain, an International Review. Springer, Dordrecht, 196–199.

Janda, V., 1993. Assessment and Treatment of Impaired Movement Patterns and Motor Recruitment. Presentation to Physical Medicine Research Foundation. Montreal.

Johns, R.J., Wright, Y., 1962. Relative importance of various tissues in joint stiffness. J. Appl. Physiol. 17, 824–828.

Jones, L.H., 1981. Strain and Counterstrain. Academy of Applied Osteopathy, Colorado Springs.

Jull, G., Janda, V., 1987. Muscles and motor control in low back pain: assessment and management. In: Twomey, L., Grieve, G. (Eds.), Physical Therapy of the Low Back. Churchill Livingstone, Edinburgh, pp. 253–278.

Kappler, R.E., Jones, J.M., 2003. Thrust (high-velocity/low-amplitude) techniques. In: Ward, R.C. (Ed.), Foundations for Osteopathic Medicine, second ed. Lippincott, Williams & Wilkins, Philadelphia, pp. 852–880.

Key, J., 2008. A model of movement dysfunction. J. Bodyw. Mov. Ther. 12 (2), 105–120.

King, H.H., 2010. Research related to clinical applications of manual therapy for musculoskeletal and systemic disorders from the osteopathic experience. In: King, H.H., Jänig, W., Patterson, M. (Eds.), The Science and Clinical Application of Manual Therapy. Elsevier, Amsterdam.

Kisselkova, H., Georgiev, J., 1976. Effects of training on postexercise limb muscle EMG synchronous to respiration. J. Appl. Physiol. 46, 1093–1095.

Kottke, F., 1982. Therapeutic exercise to maintain mobility. In: Krusen's Handbook of Physical Medicine and Rehabilitation, third ed. W B Saunders, Philadelphia.

Kraus, H., 1970. Clinical Treatment of Back and Neck Pain. McGraw Hill, New York.

Kuchera, W.A., Kuchera, M.L., 1992. Osteopathic Principles in Practice. Kirksville College of Osteopathic Medicine Press, Missouri.

LaStayo, P., Marcus, R., Dibble, L., Frajacomo, F., Lindstedt, S., 2014. Eccentric exercise in rehabilitation: Safety, feasibility, and application. J. Appl. Physiol. 116, 1426–1434. doi:10.1152/japplphysiol.00008.2013.

Lewit, K., 1991. Manipulative Therapy in Rehabilitation of the Motor System. Butterworths, London, p. 23.

Lewit, K., 1999. Manipulative Therapy in Rehabilitation of the Motor System, third ed. Butterworths, London.

Lewit, K., 2009. Manipulative Therapy: Musculoskeletal Medicine. Churchill Livingstone, Edinburgh.

Lewit, K., Janda, V., Veverkova, M., 1998. Respiratory synkinesis – polyelectromyographic investigation. J. Orthopaedic Med. 20, 2–6.

Li, R.C., Jasiewicz, J.M., Middleton, J., Condie, P., Barriskill, A., Hebnes, H., Purcell, B., 2006. The development, validity, and reliability of a manual muscle testing device with integrated limb position sensors. Arch. Phys. Med. Rehabil. 87, 411–417.

Liebenson, C., 1989. Active muscular relaxation techniques. Part I. Basic principles and methods. J. Manipulative Physiol. Ther. 12 (6), 446–454.

Liebenson, C., 1996. Rehabilitation of the Spine. Williams and Wilkins, Baltimore.

Liebenson, C., 2006. Rehabilitation of the Spine, second ed. Williams and Wilkins, Baltimore.

Liem, T., 2004. Cranial Osteopathy Principles and Practice. Churchill Livingstone, Edinburgh, pp. 340–342.

Lovering, R.M., Brooks, S.V., 2014. Eccentric exercise in aging and diseased skeletal muscle: Good or bad? J. Appl. Physiol. 116 (11), 1439–1445. doi:10.1152/japplphysiol.00174.2013.

Lucas, K., Polus, B.I., Rich, P.A., 2004. Latent myofascial trigger points: their effects on muscle activation and movement efficiency. J. Bodyw. Mov. Ther. 8 (3), 160–166.

Mattes, A., 1990. Active and Assisted Stretching. Mattes, Sarasota.

Mitchell, F., Moran, P., Pruzzo, N., 1979. An Evaluation and Treatment Manual of Osteopathic Muscle Energy Technique. Valley Park, Missouri.

Moore, M.A., Kukulka, C.G., 1991. Depression of Hoffmann reflexes following voluntary contraction and implications for proprioceptive neuromuscular facilitation therapy. Phys. Ther. 71 (4), 321–329.

Muller, K., A. Kreutzfeldt, R. Schwesig, J. Muller-Pfeil, U. Bandemer-Greulich, B. Schreiber, U. Bahrke, E. Fikentscher. 2003. Hypermobility syndrome and chronic back pain study. Man. Med. 41, no. 2 105–109.

Niddam, D.M., Chan, R.C., Lee, S.H., Yeh, T.C., Hsieh, J.C., 2008. Central representation of hyperalgesia from myofascial trigger point. Neuroimage 39, 1299–1306.

Nijls, J., Van Houdenhove, B., 2009. From acute musculoskeletal pain to chronic widespread pain and fibromyalgia: application of pain neurophysiology in manual therapy practice. Man. Ther. 14, 3–12.

Norris, C., 1999. Functional load abdominal training: part 1. J. Bodyw. Mov. Ther. 3 (3), 150–158.

Parmar, S., Shyam, A., Sabnis, S., Sancheti, P., 2011. The effect of isolytic contraction and passive manual stretching on pain and knee range of motion after hip surgery: a prospective, double-blinded, randomised study. Hong Kong Physiother. J. 29, 25–30.

Pruyn, E.C., Watsford, M.L., Murphy, A.J., 2016. Validity and reliability of three methods of stiffness assessment. J. Sport Health Sci. 5 (4), 476–483.

Reuter, P.R., Kaylee, R.F., 2019. Prevalence of generalized joint hypermobility, musculoskeletal injuries, and chronic musculoskeletal pain among American university students. PeerJ. 7, e7625.

Ruddy, T.J., 1962. Osteopathic rhythmic resistive technic. Academy of Applied Osteopathy Yearbook 1962, 23–31.

Russek, L.N., Patricia, S., Jane, S., 2019. Recognizing and effectively managing hypermobility-related conditions. Phys. Ther. 99 (9), 1189–1200.

Scariati, P., 1991. Neurophysiology relevant to osteopathic manipulation. In: DiGiovanna, E. (Ed.), An Osteopathic Approach to Diagnosis and Treatment. Lippincott, Philadelphia.

Sharan, D., 2018. Outcome of treatment of myofascial pain syndrome using a sequenced multidisciplinary rehabilitation protocol. Ann. Phys. Rehabil. Med. 61, e2.

Shellock, F.G., Prentice, W.E., 1985. Warming-up and stretching for improved physical performance and prevention of sports-related injuries. Sports Med 2 (4), 267–278.

Simons, D., Travell, J., Simmons, L., 1999. Myofascial Pain and Dysfunction: The Trigger Point Manual, vol 1, second ed. Williams and Wilkins, Baltimore.

Smith, M., Fryer, G., 2008. A comparison of two muscle energy techniques for increasing flexibility of the hamstring muscle group. J. Bodyw. Mov. Ther. 12 (4), 312–317.

Sucher, B.M., 1990. Thoracic outlet syndrome—a myofascial variant: part 2. Treatment. J. Am. Osteopath. Assoc. 90 (9), 810–823.

Sucher, B.M., 1994. Palpatory diagnosis and manipulative management of carpal tunnel syndrome. J. Am. Osteopath. Assoc. 94, 647–663.

Tunnell, P., 1997. Protocol for visual assessments. J. Bodyw. Mov. Ther. 1 (1), 21–27.

Ward, R., 1997. Foundations of Osteopathic Medicine. Williams and Wilkins, Baltimore.

Zaidi, F., Ishaq, A., 2020. Effectiveness of muscle energy technique as compared to Maitland mobilisation for the treatment of chronic sacroiliac joint dysfunction. J. Pak. Med. Assoc. 70 (10), 1693–1697.

Zhong, G., Zeng, X., Xie, Y., Lai, J., Wu, J., Xu, H., et al., 2021. Prevalence and dynamic characteristics of generalized joint hypermobility in college students. Gait Posture 84, 254–259.

6

Sequential Assessment and MET Treatment of Main Postural Muscles

Leon Chaitow, Sandy Fritz

CHAPTER CONTENTS

CLINICAL RESEARCH EVIDENCE

The approaches used for muscle energy technique (MET) application remain relatively consistent since first described in 1948 by Fred Mitchell Sr, DO As described in previous chapters, the progress of research has resulted in refinements of assessment and intervention and ongoing validation of efficacy. The most current research continues to validate benefits. The present chapter focuses on MET application in clinical practice.

As outlined in Chapter 4, research into the mechanisms associated with, and efficacy of MET use, is growing, but remains – as with many aspects of manual therapy – partial (Cayco et al., 2019; Shaha & Sharath, 2021).

Numerous studies show the benefits for enhanced muscle flexibility and increased range of motion (ROM) of joints following use of MET (Thomas et al., 2019; Osama, 2021). The variables discussed in previous chapters, including the length of contraction, number of repetitions, etc. remain open to debate (Bandy et al., 1997;

Shrier & Gossal, 2000; Feland et al., 2001; López-Bedoya et al., 2020), but as explained in Chapters 1 and 4, these matters have attracted the attention of researchers, and protocols, supported by evidence, are emerging.

A selection of examples of the value of MET in common clinical settings are described below.

MET and Myofascial Pain

- Lewit and Simons (1984) demonstrated the efficacy of MET in treatment of myofascial pain. A total of 244 patients with myofascial pain were shown among them to have muscle groups in which there were either (1) trigger points in a muscle and/or its insertion (2) excessive muscular tension during stretch or (3) muscular tension and shortening which was not secondary to joint dysfunction. The method used to treat these muscles involved Lewit's postisometric relaxation (PIR) approach in which mild isometric contractions against resistance were carried out for up to 10 seconds before releasing. Following complete 'letting go' by the patient, and on a subsequent exhalation, any additional slack was taken up and the muscle moved to its new barrier (*'stretch was stopped at the slightest resistance'*). From the new position, the process was repeated, although if no release was apparent, contractions, which remained mild, were extended for up to 30 seconds. The authors noted that it was only after the second or third contraction that a release was obtained, and three to five repetitions were usually able to provide as much progress as was likely at one session. When release was achieved the operator was careful not to move too quickly:

At this time the operator was careful not to interfere with the process and waited until the muscle relaxed completely. When the muscle reached a full range of motion, the tension and the tender (trigger) points in the muscle were gone.

Immediate relief of pain and/or tenderness was noted in 330 (94%) of the 351 muscles or muscle groups treated. The technique was required to be precise concerning the direction of forces, which needed to be aligned to stretch the fibres demonstrating greatest tension. The patient's effort therefore needed to involve contraction in the direction which precisely affected these fibres. This was most important in triangular muscles such as pectoralis major and trapezius. At a 3-month follow-up, lasting relief of pain was found to have been achieved in 63% of cases (referring to the pain originally complained of) and lasting relief of tenderness (relating to relief of tenderness in the treated muscles) in a further 23% of muscles. Among the muscles treated in this study, those

TABLE 6.1 Results of Use of MET in Myofascial Pain Study

Muscle	Number Treated	Pain Relief	Tenderness Relief	No Relief
Upper trapezius	7	7		
Wrist and finger flexors	5	5		
Lateral epicondyle of arm involving spinator, wrist and finger extensors and/or biceps brachii	20	19	1	
Suboccipital	23	21	2	
Soleus (Achilles tendon)	6	5	1	
Sternomastoid	9	7	2	
Hamstrings	8	5	2	1
Pelvic muscles/ligaments	29	22	4	3
Gluteus maximus (coccyx attachment)	27	15	9	3
Levator scapulae	19	10	7	2
Piriformis	21	11	6	4
Erector spinae	28	13	12	3
Deep paraspinal	15	7	5	3
Upper pectorals	22	10	5	7
Biceps femoris (fibula head)	18	8	6	4
Biceps femoris (long head)	7	2	0	5

MET, Muscle energy technique.

which were found to respond most successfully are given in Table 6.1. Lewit and Simons point out that:

The technique not only abolished trigger points in muscles, but also relieved painful ligaments and periosteum in the region of attachment. The fact that increasing the length of shortened muscles relieved tenderness and pain, supports a muscular origin of the pain.

The authors further pointed out that those patients achieving the greatest degree of long-term relief were those who carried out home treatment using MET stretches under instruction.

- Dhargalkar et al. (2017) concluded that MET has added beneficial effects for decreasing disability and improving function in patients with chronic nonspecific low back pain along with supervised exercises, hot pack and TENS. The subjects who were exposed to MET along with exercise therapy recovered to a greater extent than those treated with exercises alone. The MET and the exercises were operationally defined to allow the intervention to be easily reproduced in the clinical setting.
- Wendt and Waszak (2020) studied the effect of the combination therapy of MET and trigger point therapy (TPT) on ROM of the cervical spine and on the pressure pain threshold (PPT) of the trapezius muscle in asymptomatic individuals. The study involved 60 right-handed, asymptomatic students with a latent trigger point in the upper trapezius muscle. The MET + TPT method proved to be the most effective, as it caused changes in all examined goniometric and subjective parameters.
- Dearing and Hamilton (2008) compared the effects of ischaemic compression, with MET, or relaxing music, in 50 individuals with myofascial trigger points, identified in the upper trapezius muscle. MET and compression both resulted in significant reductions in pain sensitivity in the trigger point areas. See Chapter 14 for a full description of integrated neuromuscular inhibition technique (INIT) which combines ischaemic compression and MET (as well as positional release).
- Blanco et al. (2006) compared the efficacy of MET and strain/counterstrain (SCS) in treatment of trigger points in the masseter muscles of 90 individuals. A significant improvement in active mouth opening was observed and measured, following application

of MET (described as PIR technique) ($P = .001$), but not following application of SCS ($P = .8$).

- Jhaveri and Gahlot (2018) investigated treatment of trapezius pain, comparing the effectiveness of myofascial release technique (MFR) and MET. Forty subjects with chronic trapezius pain were randomised into two groups. Group A received five to seven repetitions of MFR, while Group B received three repetitions of MET for seven sessions. This study provided evidence to support the use of MFR and MET in management of chronic trapezius pain. The researchers also found that MET is more effective than MFR in improving pain, cervical disability and cervical ROM in patients with upper trapezitis because of the stretching effect on muscle and stimulation of nociceptive endings connected to A-delta fibres.

Shoulder Range of Motion, Impingement and Dysfunction

- Moore et al. (2011) compared MET applications to the glenohumeral joint (GHJ) horizontal abductors, with MET applied to the GHJ external rotators, to improve GHJ ROM in baseball players. They found that a single application of MET to the GHJ horizontal abductors provided immediate improvements in both GHJ horizontal adduction and internal rotation ROM, in asymptomatic collegiate baseball players.
- Portugal (2011) described a case study in which there was evidence of immediate benefit following MET application to a 76-year-old individual with left shoulder impingement syndrome, supraspinatus and subscapularis tendinopathy and cervical degenerative spine disease with multilevel foraminal stenosis. The patient had previously received occupational therapy with minimal benefit, as well as short-term relief following steroid injections. A modified osteopathic MET was performed. Pain immediately reduced from 10/10 to 1/10 with abduction and 7/10 to 0/10 at rest. Abduction ROM increased from 90 to 170 degrees.
- Knebl et al. (2002) treated chronic shoulder dysfunction in 29 elderly individuals, comparing the use of passive articulation/mobilisation of the shoulder, with the same protocol with MET added. A total of eight treatments over 14 weeks produced similar benefits in both groups (mobilisation alone, or mobilisation plus MET); however at follow-up it was noted that the MET group continued to demonstrate

improved ROM, in contrast to decreasing ROM in the group who received passive articulation only.

- Iqbal et al. (2020) compared the effects of Spencer MET and passive stretching in adhesive capsulitis (AC). The approach is a well-known multistep technique that combines Spencer's positioning, sequencing and slow stretching of the shoulder complex within pain-free limits while incorporating muscular energy with post-isometric contraction and relaxation. Spencer's joint mobility and MET were found to be more effective than passive stretching exercises to reduce pain, and to improve joint ROM and functionality in AC.

- In a case report, Veera et al. (2020) describe using Spencer technique to treat shoulder inflammation related to vaccine administration (SIRVA). SIRVA is an underdiagnosed phenomenon that involves inflammation of surrounding structures after a vaccine administration. Conventional therapies for SIRVA, such as non-steroidal anti-inflammatory drugs (NSAIDs), corticosteroid injections and physical therapy, may not be enough to manage symptoms in chronic settings. In these cases, commonly used osteopathic manipulative treatments, such as the Spencer technique augmented with MET, can be beneficial, and if assessed and performed correctly, patients with chronic SIRVA may respond well to this noninvasive alternative to surgical intervention.

Low-Back and Sacroiliac Pain

- Salvador et al. (2005) used MET to successfully treat lower back pain (LBP) in garbage workers by focusing attention on increasing extensibility of the hamstrings and quadratus lumborum (QL) muscles.

- Prachi et al. (2010) compared MET applied to QL, combined with transcutaneous electrical nerve stimulation (TENS), with TENS alone, in treatment of LBP. Pain was relieved in both, but the MET group demonstrated greater improvement in function, as well as spinal ROM.

- Selkow et al. (2009) focused attention, using MET, to treat the iliopsoas and hamstring muscles in the successful treatment of innominate dysfunction, in patients who tested positive following sacroiliac provocation tests.

- García-Peñalver et al. (2020) compared MET to osteopathic manipulation (thrust method) in the treatment of sacroiliac joint dysfunction. The study results found statistically significant differences between the MET and muscle energy groups compared with the placebo group. While it was observed that results of the thrust technique were significantly higher than the MET technique, MET did achieve benefits.

- Sachdeva et al. (2018) compared the effectiveness of MET and mobilisation on pain and disability in post-partum females with sacroiliac joint dysfunction. The study results concluded that MET was effective for this particular condition and population group.

MET – With Other Modalities – for Example in Treatment of Fibromyalgia

- Stotz and Kappler (1992) of the Chicago College of Osteopathic Medicine report having successfully treated patients with fibromyalgia (FM) using a variety of osteopathic approaches including MET. The results given below were achieved by incorporating MET alongside positional release methods, together with a limited degree of more active manipulation (personal communication 1994). FM is notoriously unresponsive to standard methods of treatment and continues to be treated, in the main, by resorting to mild anti-depressant medication, despite many of the primary researchers' insistence that in most instances depression is a result, rather than a cause of the condition (Block, 1993; Duna & Wilke, 1993). Stotz and Kappler measured the effects of treatment (including MET) on the intensity of pain reported from tender points in 18 patients, who met all the criteria for fibromyalgia syndrome (FMS) (Goldenberg, 1993). Each patient received six treatments over a 1-year period. Twelve of the patients responded well with a 14% pain reduction, as against a 34% increase in the six patients who did not respond well. Activities of daily living were significantly improved and general pain symptoms decreased.

- In another study, 19 FM patients were treated once weekly, for 4 weeks at Kirksville, Missouri, College of Osteopathic Medicine, using OMT which included MET as a major component: 84.2% showed improved sleep patterns, 94.7% reported less pain and most patients had fewer tender points on palpation (Rubin et al., 1990).

- Gamber et al. (2002) combined standard medical care with osteopathic treatment of 24 patients with confirmed FM diagnoses, in a randomised, observer-masked, placebo-controlled clinical trial of osteopathic treatment. Patients were randomly assigned to one of four treatment groups: (1) soft tissue manipulation group (including MET), (2) manipulation and teaching group, (3) moist heat group and (4) control group, which received no additional treatment other than current medication. The osteopathic attention involved a combination of MET, myofascial release and strain/counterstrain – individualised to the needs of each patient, that is, there was no formal protocol of manual treatment. This study found that OMT, combined with standard medical care, was more efficacious in the treatment of FM than standard care alone.

- Uysal et al. (2019) studied 37 women diagnosed with FM. MET was applied to cervical accessory respiratory muscles in patients with FM who had complaints in the neck and back region. They were assessed for their respiratory muscle strength, respiratory muscle endurance, pain and fatigue severity, flexibility and disability. The MET was applied to the scalene, upper trapezius and sternocleidomastoid (SCM) muscles after a superficial heat application. The treatment was continued for 3 weeks with three sessions per week, resulting in increased respiratory muscle strength and endurance, cervical flexibility and decreased pain intensity, fatigue and disability.

In these FM examples, MET is seen to have been used as part of a wider range of soft tissue modalities.

Before describing protocols for the use of MET in treating specific muscular dysfunction (such as shortness, tightness, weakness) the broader objectives of manual therapy deserve brief attention.

OBJECTIVES OF MANUAL TREATMENT

What are the focuses and objectives of manual treatment in general, and manipulation in particular?

- O'Sullivan (2005) and others have spearheaded a trend in manual therapy, away from focus on the treatment of pain and associated symptoms, towards methods that enhance function, performance and, almost as a by-product, reduce focus on, and experience of, pain.
- In that model of care, assessment of function takes precedence over assessment of pain sources, and single interventions – whether these involve particular exercise models (van Middelkoop et al., 2010) or forms of manual therapy such as MET (Salvador et al., 2005) – that are dismissed as outmoded. As discussed more extensively in Chapter 1, pain and dysfunction – it is suggested – should be managed from a biopsychosocial perspective, with physical, lifestyle,

neuro-physiological, psychosocial and genetic factors all taken into consideration as the unique features of each individual's problems are classified so that appropriate treatment can be offered.

- Such comprehensive perspectives are clearly likely to be of greater value in dealing with pain and dysfunction than 'magic bullet' thinking and practice. However, within comprehensive patient-centred frameworks of care, in which new, more functional patterns of use are being encouraged, there remains an essential need for facilitating strategies (including both active and passive treatment approaches) that promote function by removing obstacles to free motion.
- Apart from symptom control/modification, useful therapeutic interventions are characterised as having primary objectives that either encourage enhanced function or reduced adaptive load, or both. When appropriately utilised, MET can be shown to support such outcomes.
- Lewit (1985a) summarises what he believes manual therapy should be concerned with the phrase 'restricted mobility', with or without pain.
- Evjenth (1984) is equally succinct, and states that what is needed to become proficient in treating patients with symptoms of pain or 'constrained movement' is *experience gained by thoroughly examining every patient*. The only real measure of successful treatment is, he states, *restoration of muscle's normal pattern of movement with freedom from pain*.
- Janda (1988) seemed mainly to be concerned with 'imbalances' and the implications of dysfunctional patterns, in which some muscles become weaker (inhibited) and others progressively tighter. Such imbalances, if unchanged, clearly impede the learning of better functional use patterns, improved posture, more functional breathing, etc. (See crossed syndrome discussion Box 5.2, Chapter 5).
- Greenman (2003) reports on the conclusion of a 1983 workshop in which manual experts considered the question of the 'goal of manipulation'. The conclusion was: *To restore maximal pain-free movement of the musculoskeletal system in postural balance*.

Previous chapters have discussed concepts relating to 'tight–loose', 'ease–bind' and particular muscle groups – however they are categorised – are subject, as part of their adaptation to the stresses of life, to shortening, while other muscle groups are subject to weakening and/or lengthening. It is in the context of such adaptation, compensation and decompensation that soft tissue and articular changes can be identified by means of diligent palpation and assessment. It is hoped that attention will also be paid to any habits of use that have contributed to the dysfunctional pattern being treated.

Restoration of more normal function demands the availability of therapeutic tools by means of which change can be engineered. Biomechanical (manipulation, exercise, etc.) solutions and strategies that reduce the chances of recurrence may focus on key muscles that require strengthening, or on enhancing postural or breathing function.

Re-education strategies depend for success, at least partly, on correction or improvement of the structural and functional imbalances present at the outset. As these imbalances (hypo-or hypermobility, etc.) are modified, improved posture, better breathing, etc. become easier to achieve.

- No one with restricted and shortened accessory breathing/upper fixator muscles can learn to breathe correctly until these have, to an extent, been normalised (Perri & Halford, 2004).
- No one with short lumbar erector spinae and weak abdominal muscles can learn to use their spine correctly, until these muscular imbalances have, to an extent, been normalised (Key et al., 2008).
- No one with short-tight psoas muscles can either stand fully erect or breathe normally (Haugstad et al., 2006).

The structure–function continuum demands that therapeutic attention be paid to both aspects. Function cannot fully change until structure allows it to do so, and structure will continue to modify and adapt at the expense of optimal function until dysfunctional patterns of use are altered for the better.

Part of a solution is offered by the methods used in MET, in which the short and tight structures are identified and lengthened, while the weak and inhibited muscles are encouraged towards enhanced tone, strength and stamina. Rehabilitation and re-education methods can then work in a relatively unhindered environment as new habits of use are learned.

Greenman (1996) offers a summary of this clinical approach:

After short tight muscles are stretched, muscles that are inhibited can undergo retraining… as in all manual medicine procedures, after assessment, stretching, and strengthening, reevaluation of faulty movement patterns… is done.

Dommerholt (2000), discussing enhancement of posture and function in musicians, has summarised an important concept:

In general, assessment and treatment of individual muscles must precede restoration of normal posture and normal patterns of movement. Claims that muscle imbalances would dissolve following lessons in Alexander technique are not substantiated in the scientific literature (Rosenthal 1987). Instead, muscle imbalances must be corrected through very specific strengthening and flexibility exercises… myofascial trigger points must be inactivated… [and] … associated joint dysfunction… must be corrected with joint mobilisation. Once the musculoskeletal conditions of 'good posture' have been met, postural retraining can proceed.

EVALUATING MUSCLE SHORTNESS AND STRENGTH

Many of the problems of the musculoskeletal system seem to involve pain or restriction related to aspects of muscle shortening (Lewit, 1999). For example, simple dysfunctional patterns such as restricted hip extension can be shown to directly relate to shortness of hip flexors (Tyler et al., 1996). Where weakness (or lack of tone) is found to be a major element, it will often be noted that antagonists to these muscles are hypertonic and/or shortened, reciprocally inhibiting their tone. As discussed in Chapter 5 in relation to Figs. 5.3 and 5.4, some experts – such as Janda (1996) and Liebenson (2006) – hold that prior to any effort to strengthen weak muscles, shortened ones should be dealt with by appropriate means, after which spontaneous toning usually occurs in the previously 'weakened' muscles. If muscle tone remains inadequate, then, and only then, should exercise and/or isotonic procedures be initiated.

This is, however, not a universally accepted model, with many clinicians preferring to work on weak structures first, so reducing tone in their (usually) hypertonic antagonists. Attention to weak structures as a primary therapeutic effort may usefully reduce hypertonicity in antagonists; however, such treatment methods cannot reverse fibrotic states present in many chronically shortened structures, and until this is achieved the lead author contends that enhancing the strength of previously weak phasic (stabiliser, see Chapter 2) muscles is unlikely in itself to restore functional balance.

Janda (1983) tells us that short, tight muscles usually maintain their strength; however, in extreme cases of tightness some strength decrease occurs. In such cases stretching (as in MET use) of the tight muscle usually leads to a rapid recovery of strength (as well as toning of the antagonists via removal of reciprocal inhibition (RI)). As noted in Chapter 5, weakened postural muscles also benefit from slowly applied isotonic eccentric methods (Norris, 1999).

It is therefore important that short, tight muscles are assessed in a systematic, standardised manner. Janda (1983) suggests that in order to obtain a reliable evaluation of muscle shortness:

- The starting position, method of fixation and direction of movement must be observed carefully.
- The prime mover must not be exposed to external pressure.
- If possible, the force exerted on the tested muscle must not work over two joints.
- The examiner should perform, at an even speed, a slow movement that brakes slowly at the end of the range.
- Keep the stretch and the muscle irritability about equal, and the movement must not be jerky.
- Pressure or pull must always act in the required direction of movement.
- Muscle shortening can only be correctly evaluated if the joint range is not decreased, as might be the case should an osseous limitation or joint blockage exist.

It is also in shortened muscles that local reflex dysfunction is most commonly noted (Scudds et al., 1995; Gerwin & Dommerholt, 2002; Lewit, 2009) – variously called trigger points (Simons et al., 1999), tender points, zones of irritability, hyperalgesic zones (Lewit, 2009), neurovascular and neurolymphatic reflexes, etc. (Chaitow, 1991). Localising these areas of altered function is usually possible via normal palpatory methods. Identification and treatment of tight muscles may also be systematically carried out using the methods described later in this chapter.[1]

IMPORTANT NOTES ON ASSESSMENTS AND USE OF MET

1. When the term 'restriction barrier' is used in relation to soft tissue structures, it is meant to indicate the place where the first signs of resistance are noted (as palpated by sense of 'bind,' or sense of effort required to move the area, or by visual or other palpable evidence), and not the greatest possible range of pain-free movement obtainable. (Refer to the ease–bind palpation exercise involving the adductors in Chapter 5 and Fig. 5.1A and B.)

2. In all treatment descriptions involving MET (apart from the first set of assessment tests involving gastrocnemius and soleus later in this chapter) it will be assumed that the 'shorthand' reference to 'acute' and 'chronic' will be adequate to alert the reader to the variations in methodology which these variants call for, as discussed in Chapter 2, where appropriate barriers for use in acute and chronic situations were summarised (see also Box 6.1).

3. Assistance from the patient is valuable as movement is made to, or through, a barrier, provided that the patient can be educated to gentle cooperation and can learn not to use excessive effort.

4. In most MET treatment guidelines in this chapter, the method described will involve isometric contraction of the agonist(s) – that is, the muscle(s) that require stretching. It is assumed that the reader is now familiar

---

> ### BOX 6.1   *'Acute' and 'Chronic'*
>
> The words 'acute' and 'chronic' should alert the reader to the differences in methodology which these variants call for in applying MET, especially in terms of the starting position for contractions and whether or not stretching should take place after the contraction.
>
> In acute conditions the isometric contraction starts at the barrier, whereas in chronic conditions the contraction starts short of the barrier (Janda, 1983; Liebenson, 1996; Lewit, 1999). After the contraction the practitioner takes the area to the new barrier in acute conditions, or through the previous resistance barrier into slight sustained stretch in chronic conditions.
>
> The term 'acute' may be applied to strain or injury that has occurred within the past 3 weeks, or where the symptoms such as pain are acute, or where active inflammation is present.
>
> Use of the antagonists to the affected muscle(s) offers an alternative to activation of an isometric contraction in such muscles if this proves painful or difficult for the patient to perform.
>
> A further alternative is to use Ruddy's repetitive pulsing contractions, rather than a sustained contraction, if the latter is painful or difficult for the patient to perform (see Chapter 5).

---

[1]Note that the assessment methods presented are not themselves diagnostic but provide strong indications of probable shortness of the muscles being tested.

with the possibility of using the antagonists to achieve increased stretch tolerance before initiating stretch or movement to a new barrier, and will use this alternative when appropriate (e.g. if there is pain on use of agonist, or if there has been prior trauma to the agonist, or in an attempt to see if more release can be made available after the initial use of the agonist isometrically). See Chapter 4 for discussion of the current degree of research evidence relative to the choice of the terms *reciprocal inhibition* (RI) or *postisometric relaxation* (PIR) in MET usage. Recall also that, as discussed in Chapter 4, there exists some controversy relating to the use of the words 'antagonist' and 'agonist' in some MET-like methods.

5. Isolytic methods (rapidly stretched eccentric isotonic contractions) will be suggested in a few instances, for example in treating tensor fascia lata (TFL), but these are not generally recommended for application in sensitive patients or in potentially 'fragile' areas such as the muscles associated with the cervical spine.

6. Careful reading of earlier chapters is urged before commencing practice of the methods listed below.

7. There should be no pain experienced during application of MET, although mild discomfort (stretching) is acceptable.

8. The methods of assessment and treatment of postural muscles given here are far from comprehensive or definitive. There are many other assessment approaches, and numerous treatment/stretch approaches, using variations on the theme of MET, as evidenced by the excellent texts by Janda, Basmajian, Lewit, Liebenson, Greenman, Grieve, Mattes, Hartman, Evjenth and Dvorak, among others, found in the reference lists. The methods recommended below provide a sound basis for the application of MET to specific muscles and areas, as do the methods suggested for spinal, pelvic, neck and shoulder regions in Chapters 8, 9, 10 and 11. By developing the skills with which to apply the methods, as described, a repertoire of techniques can be acquired, offering a wide base of choices that will be appropriate in numerous clinical settings.

9. Some of the discussion of particular muscles will include notes containing information unrelated to the main objective, which is to outline assessment and MET treatment possibilities. These notes are included where the particular information they carry is likely to be useful clinically.

10. Breathing cooperation can, and should, be used as part of the methodology of MET. This, however, will not be repeated as an instruction in each example of MET use below. Basically, if appropriate (i.e if the patient is cooperative and capable of following instructions), the patient should be given the instructions outlined in Box 6.2. A note that gives the instruction to 'use appropriate breathing', or some variation on it, will be found in the text describing various MET applications, and this refers to the guidelines outlined in Box 6.2.

11. Various eye movements are sometimes advocated during contractions and stretches, particularly by Lewit (1999, 2009) who uses these methods to great effect. The only specific recommendations for use of visual synkinesis in this chapter will be found in regard to muscles such as the scalenes where this may be useful due to the gentleness of the contractions they induce.

12. 'Pulsed muscle energy technique' is based on Ruddy's work (see Chapters 2, 5 and 7). This approach can be substituted for any of the methods described in the text below for treating shortened soft tissue structures, or for increasing the ROM in joints (Ruddy, 1962).

13. There are times when 'co-contraction' seems to be clinically useful, involving contraction of both the

---

BOX 6.2   Notes on Respiratory Synkinesis During Muscle Energy Technique

Patients who are cooperative and capable of following instructions should be asked to:

- Inhale as they slowly build up an isometric contraction.
- Hold the breath during the 5–7-s contraction, and
- Release the breath as the contraction is slowly released.
- Inhale and exhale fully once more, following cessation of all effort, as the patient is requested to 'let go completely'.
- During this second exhalation the tissues are taken to their new barrier in an acute condition, or the barrier is passed as the muscle is stretched in a chronic condition (with patient assistance if possible).
- An exception to this sequence occurs for quadratus lumborum where stretch is introduced during an inhalation since the muscle is activated on exhalation.

Lewit (1999).

agonist and the antagonist. Studies have shown that this approach is particularly useful in treatment of the hamstrings, when both these and the quadriceps are isometrically contracted prior to stretch (Moore & Hutton, 1980).

14. It is seldom necessary to treat all the shortened muscles that are identified via the methods described below.

For example, Lewit and Simons (1984) mention that:

- PIR of the suboccipital muscles will also relax the SCM muscles.
- Treatment of the thoracolumbar muscles induces relaxation of iliopsoas, and vice versa.
- Treatment (MET) of the SCM and scalene muscles relaxes the pectorals.

These interactions are worthy of greater study.

What's Short? What's Tight? Postural Muscle Assessment Sequence Checklist

Note: Each muscle listed for assessment is named and has been given a code that refers to the listing in Box 6.3. This checklist can be used to follow (and record results of) the simple sequence of postural muscle assessments, as described below.

SEQUENTIAL ASSESSMENT AND MET TREATMENT OF POSTURAL MUSCLES

The assessment and treatment recommendations that follow represent a synthesis of information derived from personal clinical experience, as well as from the numerous sources cited, or are based on the work of named researchers, clinicians and therapists (Fryette, 1954; Ruddy, 1961, 1962; Cailliet, 1962; Mennell, 1964; Williams, 1965; Basmajian, 1974; Rolf, 1977; Mitchell et al., 1979; Janda, 1983, 2006; Dvorak & Dvorak, 1984; Greenman, 1989, 1996, 2003; Lewit, 1992, 1999, 2009; Mitchell Jr., 2009; Stiles, 2009).

▶ 1. Assessment of Gastrocnemius (01) and Soleus (02) (Fig. 6.1A and B)

- The patient lies supine with feet extended over the edge of the table.
- The practitioner stands at the foot of the table, facing the patient.
- For *right leg* examination the practitioner's left hand cradles the Achilles tendon just above the heel, avoiding pressure on the tendon.

BOX 6.3   Postural Muscle Assessment Sequence

NAME _____

E = Equal (circle both if both are short)

L or R are circled if left or right are short

Spinal abbreviations indicate low-lumbar, lumbodorsal junction, low-thoracic, mid-thoracic and upper thoracic areas (of flatness and therefore reduced ability to flex – short erector spinae)

1. Gastrocnemius E L R
2. Soleus E L R
3. Medial hamstrings E L R
4. Short adductors E L R
5. Rectus femoris E L R
6. Psoas E L R
7. Hamstrings
   a. upper fibres E L R
   b. lower fibres E L R
8. Tensor fascia lata E L R
9. Piriformis E L R
10. Quadratus lumborum E L R
11. Pectoralis major E L R
12. Latissimus dorsi E L R
13. Upper trapezius E L R
14. Scalenes E L R
15. Sternocleidomastoid E L R
16. Levator scapulae E L R
17. Infraspinatus E L R
18. Subscapularis E L R
19. Supraspinatus E L R
20. Flexors of the arm E L R
21. Spinal flattening:
    a. seated legs straight LL LDJ LT MT UT
    b. seated legs flexed LL LDJ LT MT UT
22. Cervical spine extensors short? Yes No

- The heel lies in the palm of the hand, fingers curving round it.
- The practitioner's right hand is placed so that the fingers rest on the dorsum of the foot (**Note:** the finger contact *does not* apply pulling force), with the thumb on the sole, lying along the medial margin. (This position is important for adequate control – it is a mistake to place the thumb too near the centre of the sole of the foot.)
- Stretch is introduced by means of a *pull on the heel with the left hand*, taking out the slack of the muscle, while at the same time the right hand maintains light cephalad pressure on the sole of the foot, via the

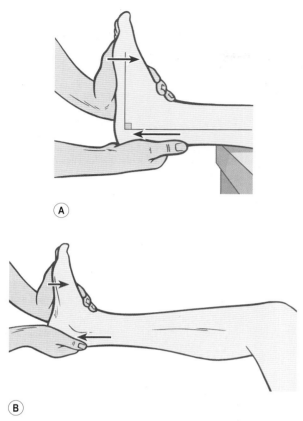

(A)

(B)

Fig. 6.1 (A) Assessment or treatment of gastrocnemius and soleus. During assessment the sole of the foot should achieve a vertical position without effort once slack is taken out via traction on the heel. Treatment would involve taking the tissues to or through (acute/chronic) the identified barrier following an isometric contraction. (B) With the knee flexed, the same assessment is evaluating the status of soleus alone. Treatment would involve taking the tissues to or through (acute/chronic) the identified barrier following an isometric contraction.

thumb (along its entire length). This directs the foot towards an upright position without force (Fig. 6.1A).
- The leg should remain resting on the table throughout the assessment. The arm and hand controlling the removal of slack via the contact on the heel should be placed so that it is an extension of the leg, not allowing an anteriorly directed (towards the ceiling) pull when slack is taken out.
- If the muscles being assessed are in a normal state, a range of movement should be achieved that takes the sole of the foot to a 90-degree angle with the leg, without any force being required.

- If this is not possible (i.e. if force is required to achieve the 90-degree angle between the sole of the foot and the leg), there is shortness in gastrocnemius and/or soleus. Further screening is then required to identify precisely which of these is involved (see soleus assessment below).

Assessment of Tight Soleus (O2)

The method described above assesses both gastrocnemius and soleus. To assess soleus alone, precisely the same procedure is adopted, with the knee passively flexed (over a cushion, for example) (Fig. 6.1B).
- If the sole of the foot fails to easily come to a 90-degree angle with the leg without force, once slack has been taken out of the tissues via traction through the long axis of the calf from the heel, soleus is considered short.
- If the previous test (in which the knee was not flexed) indicated shortness of gastrocnemius *or* soleus, and the soleus test (in which the knee is flexed) is normal, then gastrocnemius alone is short.

Squat Screening Test

A further screening test for soleus involves the patient being asked to squat, with the trunk in slight flexion, feet placed shoulder width apart, so that the buttocks rest between the legs (which face forwards, rather than outwards). If the soleus muscles are normal, then it should be possible to go fully into this position with the heels remaining flat on the floor. If not, and the heels rise from the floor as the squat is performed, the soleus muscles are considered to have shortened.

MET Treatment of Shortened Gastrocnemius and Soleus (See Fig. 6.1A and B)

Precisely the same position is adopted for treatment as for testing, with the knee flexed over a rolled towel or cushion if soleus is being treated, and with the knee straight if gastrocnemius is being treated.
- If the condition is acute (defined as a dysfunction/injury of less than 3 weeks' duration, or acutely painful) the area is treated with the foot dorsiflexed to the very first sign of a restriction barrier.
- If it is a chronic problem (longer duration than 3 weeks) the barrier is assessed and the muscle treated in a position of ease, slightly towards the mid-range, away from the restriction barrier.
- Starting from the appropriate position (at the restriction barrier or just short of it – based on the degree

of acuteness or chronicity), the patient is asked to exert a small effort (no more than 20% of available strength) towards plantarflexion, against unyielding resistance, with appropriate breathing (see Box 6.2).

- This effort isometrically contracts either gastrocnemius or soleus, or both (depending on whether the knee is unflexed or flexed).
- This contraction is held for 5 to 7 seconds.
- On slow release, on an exhalation, the foot/ankle is dorsiflexed (be sure to flex the whole foot and not just the toes) to its new restriction barrier if acute, or slightly and painlessly beyond the new barrier if chronic, *with the patient's assistance.*
- If chronic, the tissues should be held in slight stretch for between 5 and 30 seconds, to allow a slow lengthening of tissues (see notes on 'creep' and viscoelasticity in Chapter 2).
- This pattern is repeated until no further gain is achieved (backing off towards mid-range for the next contraction, if chronic, and commencing the next contraction from the new resistance barrier, if acute).
- Alternatively, if there is undue discomfort when contracting the agonists (the muscles being treated), the antagonists to the shortened muscles can be used, by introducing resisted dorsiflexion with the muscle at its barrier or just short of it, followed by a painless move to the new barrier (if acute) or beyond it (if chronic), ideally during an exhalation following the isometric contraction.
- Use of antagonists in this way is less effective than use of the agonist, but may be a useful strategy if trauma has taken place.

NOTE: Fig. 6.2 illustrates an alternative treatment position for gastrocnemius which can also be used for assessment. Flexion of the knee would allow this position to be used for treating soleus.

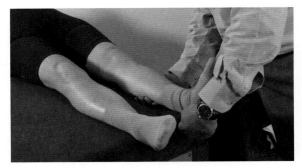

Fig. 6.2 Muscle energy technique treatment position for gastrocnemius. If knee were flexed the same position would focus on treatment of soleus only.

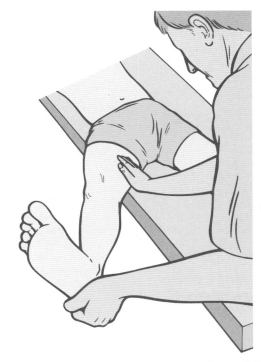

Fig. 6.3 Assessment and treatment position for medial hamstrings. Shortness of single joint adductors (e.g. adductor brevis, pectinius) may be evaluated and treated in the same relative position but with the knee of the leg to be treated in flexion.

▶ 2. Assessing for Shortness in Medial Hamstrings (03) (Semi-Membranosus, Semi-Tendinosus as Well as Gracilis) and Short Adductors (04) (Pectineus, Adductors Brevis, Magnus and Longus) (Figs. 6.3 and 6.4)

- The patient lies so that the non-tested leg is abducted slightly, heel over the end of the table.
- The leg to be tested should be close to the edge of the table, and the practitioner ensures that the tested leg is in its anatomically correct position, knee in full

extension and with no external rotation of the leg, which would negate the test.
- The practitioner should effectively stand between patient's leg and the table so that all control of the tested leg is achieved with their lateral (non-table-side) arm/hand, while the table-side hand can rest on,

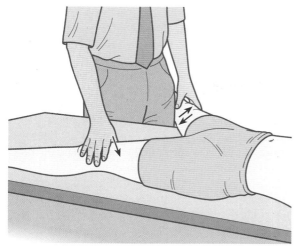

Fig. 6.4 Alternative position for treatment of shortness in adductors of the thigh.

and palpate, the inner thigh muscles for sensations of bind as the leg is eased into abduction.

- Abduction of the tested leg is introduced passively until the first sign of resistance is noted (see Fig. 6.3). There are effectively three indicators of this resistance, that is, that the barrier has been reached or passed:
  1. A sense of increased effort should be noted by the hand carrying the leg at the moment that the first resistance barrier is reached/passed.
  2. The sense of bind should be noted by the palpating hand on the muscle, at this same moment.
  3. A visual sign involving movement of the pelvis as a whole, laterally towards the tested side, should be observed as this barrier is passed.
- If abduction produces an angle with the midline of 45 degrees, or more, before a resistance barrier is reached, then no further test is needed, as that degree of abduction is normal, and there is probably no shortness in the short or long adductors (medial hamstrings or, more correctly, gracilis and biceps femoris).
- If, however, abduction ceases before a 45-degree angle is easily achieved (without effort, or a sense of bind in the tissues), then restriction exists in either the medial hamstrings or the short adductors of the thigh.

Screening Short Adductors (04) From Medial Hamstrings (03)

As in the tests for gastrocnemius and soleus, it is necessary to differentiate between shortness of the one joint

and two joint muscles (in this case the short adductors and the medial hamstrings).

- This is achieved by abducting the leg to its easy barrier, and then introducing flexion of the knee, allowing the lower leg to hang freely.
- If (after knee flexion has been introduced) further abduction is now easily achieved to 45 degrees when previously it was restricted, this indicates that any previous limitation into abduction was the result of medial hamstring shortness.
- If, however, restriction remains, as evidenced by continued 'bind', or obvious restriction in movement towards a 45-degree excursion, after knee flexion has been introduced, then the short adductors are continuing to prevent movement, and are short (see Fig. 6.4).

MET Treatment of Shortness in Short and Long Adductors of the Thigh

Precisely the same positions may be adopted for treatment as for testing.

- If the short adductors (pectineus, adductors brevis, magnus and longus) are being treated, then the leg, *with the knee flexed,* is held at the barrier (for an acute condition) or a little short of the barrier (if chronic).
- An isometric contraction is introduced by the patient using less than 20% of available strength, employing the agonists (the patient pushes away from the barrier of resistance) or the antagonists (the patient pushes towards the barrier of resistance) for 5 to 7 seconds.
- Appropriate breathing instructions should be given (see notes on breathing in Box 6.2).
- After the contraction ceases and the patient has relaxed, the leg is eased to its new barrier (if acute) or painlessly (assisted by the patient) beyond the new barrier and into stretch (if chronic), where it is held for between 5 and 30 seconds in order to stretch shortened tissue.
- The process is repeated at least once more.

If the medial hamstrings (semi-membranosus, semi-tendinosus, as well as gracilis) are being treated, all elements are the same, except that the *knee should be held in extension* (see Fig. 6.4). Whichever position is used, the subsequent movement, on an exhalation, is to the barrier (if acute), or through the barrier (if chronic), to commence normalisation of the shortened muscles.

NOTE: Either approach (knee straight or flexed) can be performed with the patient side-lying as in Fig. 6.5 – see description below.

Caution and Alternative Treatment Position (See Fig. 6.5)

A major error made in treating these particular muscles, using MET, relates to allowing a pivoting of the pelvis and a spinal side flexion to occur. Maintenance of the pelvis in a stable position is important, and this can most easily be achieved via suitable straps when supine or, during treatment, by having the patient side-lying with the affected side uppermost.

- Patient is side-lying.
- Practitioner stands behind and uses the caudad arm and hand to control the leg and to palpate for bind, with the treated leg flexed or straight as appropriate.
- The cephalad hand maintains a firm downwards pressure on the lateral pelvis to ensure stability during stretching.
- All other elements of treatment are identical to those described for supine treatment above.

▶ 3. Assessment and Treatment of Hip Flexors – Rectus Femoris (05), Iliopsoas (06) (See Also Box 6.4 and Fig. 6.6A)

- The patient lies supine with buttocks (coccyx) as close to the end of the table as possible, the non-tested leg held towards the chest to produce stability

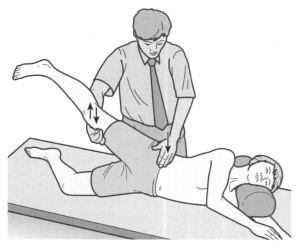

Fig. 6.5 Side-lying position for treatment of two-joint adductors of the thigh.

in the pelvis while the tested-side leg hangs freely off the end of the table, with the knee flexed.

- Full flexion of the non-tested-side hip helps to maintain the pelvis in full rotation with the lumbar spine flat. This is essential if the test (Thomas test) is to be meaningful, and stress on the spine avoided.
- If the thigh of the tested leg lies in a horizontal position, parallel to the floor/table (see Fig. 6.6A), as well as there being a degree of 'spring' as the thigh is moved passively towards the floor, then the indication is that iliopsoas is not short.
- If, however, the thigh rises above the horizontal (Fig. 6.6B) – or is parallel with the floor but has a rigid feel – then iliopsoas is probably short.
- Even if the thigh is able to lie parallel to the floor in this test position, a slight degree (±10 degrees) of hip extension should be possible in response to a gentle push downwards on the thigh by the practitioner, with no knee extension occurring as this is done.
- If effort is required to achieve 10 degrees of hip extension, this suggests iliopsoas shortening on that side.
- **Rectus femoris test in Thomas position:** Assessment of rectus femoris muscle length is an important part of the clinical examination because of its influence on both the hip and the knee. If the knee straightens when the thigh is eased towards the floor, this suggests rectus femoris (or possibly TFL) shortening, on that side. Corkery et al. (2007) found the Thomas test (as described here) is a reliable procedure. Magee (2002) has reported that 90 degrees is a normal angle between thigh and lower leg, for this test (i.e. the angle between the lower limb that is hanging free, and the angle of the femur which is more or less parallel with the floor). Gabbe et al. (2005) suggest that measuring rectus femoris flexibility by means of the modified Thomas test can be a predictor of future hamstring injury, with those with less than 51 degrees of knee flexion (suggesting shortened rectus femoris) being more likely to sustain a hamstring injury.
- Rectus femoris shortness can be further confirmed by seeing whether or not the heel on the tested side can easily flex to touch the buttock when the patient is prone. If rectus femoris is short, the heel will not easily (i.e. without force) reach the buttock (see Fig. 6.8).
- In the supine testing position, if the lower leg of the tested side fails to hang down to an almost 90-degree angle with the thigh, vertical to the floor, then shortness of rectus femoris is suggested (see Fig. 6.6B).

BOX 6.4 Notes on Psoas

- Lewit (1985b) mentions that in many ways the psoas behaves as if it were an internal organ. Tension in the psoas may be secondary to kidney disease, and one of its frequent clinical manifestations, when in spasm, is that it reproduces the pain of gall-bladder disease (often after the organ has been removed).
- The definitive signs of psoas problems are not difficult to note, according to Fryette (1954). He maintains that the distortions produced in inflammation and/or spasm in the psoas are characteristic and cannot be produced by other dysfunction. The origin of the psoas is from 12th thoracic to (and including) the fourth lumbar, but not the fifth lumbar. The insertion is into the lesser trochanter of the femur, and thus, when psoas spasm exists unilaterally, the patient is drawn forwards and side-bent to the involved side. The ilium on the side will rotate backwards on the sacrum, and the thigh will be everted. When both muscles are involved, the patient is drawn forward, with the lumbar curve locked in flexion. This is the characteristic reversed lumbar spine. Chronic bilateral psoas contraction creates either a reversed lumbar curve if the erector spinae of the low back are weak, or an increased lordosis if they are hypertonic.
- Lewit (1999) says, 'Psoas spasm causes abdominal pain, flexion of the hip and typical antalgesic (stooped) posture. Problems in psoas can profoundly influence thoracolumbar stability'.
- The fifth lumbar is not involved directly with psoas, but great mechanical stress is placed upon it when the other lumbar vertebrae are fixed in either a kyphotic or an increased lordotic state. In unilateral psoas spasms, a rotary stress is noted at the level of fifth lumbar. The main mechanical involvement is, however, usually at the lumbodorsal junction. Attempts to treat the resulting pain (frequently located in the region of the fifth lumbar and sacroiliac) by attention to these areas will be of little use. Attention to the muscular component should be a primary focus, ideally using muscle energy technique.
- Bogduk (Bogduk et al., 1992; Bogduk, 1997) provides evidence that psoas plays only a small role in the action of the spine, and states that it 'uses the lumbar spine as a base from which to act on the hip'. He goes on to discuss just how much pressure derives from psoas compression on discs: 'Psoas potentially exerts massive compression loads on the lower lumbar discs... upon maximum contraction, in an activity such as sit-ups, the two psoas muscles can be expected to exert a compression on the L5–S1 disc equal to about 100 kg of weight'.
- There exists in all muscles a vital reciprocal agonist-antagonist relationship that is of primary importance in determining their tone and healthy function.

Psoas-rectus abdominis have such a relationship and this has important postural implications (see notes on lower crossed syndrome in Chapter 5).
- Observation of the abdomen 'falling back' rather than mounding when the patient flexes indicates normal psoas function. Similarly, if the patient, when lying supine, flexes knees and 'drags' the heels towards the buttocks (keeping them together), the abdomen should remain flat or fall back. If the abdomen mounds or the small of the back arches, psoas is incompetent (Liebenson, 1996).
- If the supine patient raises both legs into the air and the belly mounds, it shows that the recti and psoas are out of balance. Psoas should be able to raise the legs to at least 30 degrees without any help from the abdominal muscles.
- Psoas fibres merge with (become 'consolidated' with) the diaphragm and it therefore influences respiratory function directly (as does quadratus lumborum). Haugstad et al. (2006) reported that women with chronic pelvic pain '"typically" displayed upper chest breathing patterns, with almost no movement of the thorax or the abdominal area'. They were also able to confirm 'a characteristic pattern of standing, sitting and walking, as well as lack of coordination and irregular high costal respiration'. Of interest in relation to diaphragmatic function was their finding that: 'the highest density, and the highest degree of elastic stiffness, [was] found in the iliopsoas muscles'.
- Basmajian (1974) informs us that the psoas is the most important of all postural muscles. If it is hypertonic and the abdominals are weak and exercise is prescribed to tone these weak abdominals (such as curl-ups with the dorsum of the foot stabilised), then a disastrous negative effect will ensue in which, far from toning the abdominals, increase of tone in psoas will result, due to the sequence created by the dorsum of the foot being used as a point of support. When this occurs (dorsiflexion), the gait cycle is mimicked and there is a sequence of activation of tibialis anticus, rectus femoris and psoas. If, on the other hand, the feet could be plantarflexed during curl-up exercises, then the opposite chain is activated (triceps surae, hamstrings and gluteals) inhibiting psoas and allowing toning of the abdominals.
- When treating, it is sometimes useful to assess changes in psoas length by periodic comparison of apparent arm length. Patient lies supine, arms extended above head, palms together so that length can be compared. A shortness will commonly be observed in the arm on the side of the shortened psoas, and this should normalise after successful treatment (there may of course be other reasons for apparent difference in arm length, and this method provides an indication only of possible changes in psoas length).

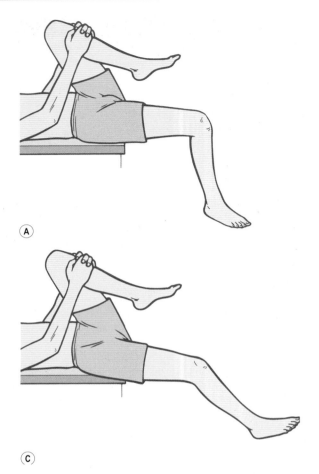

(A)

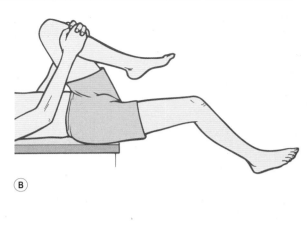

(B)

(C)

Fig. 6.6 (A) Test position for shortness of hip flexors. Note that the hip on the non-tested side must be fully flexed to produce full pelvic rotation. The position shown suggests that psoas is normal. (B) In the test position, if the thigh is elevated (i.e. not parallel to the table) probable psoas shortness is indicated. The inability of the lower leg to hang more or less vertically towards the floor indicates probable rectus femoris shortness (tensor fascia lata shortness can produce a similar effect). (C) The fall of the thigh below the horizontal indicates hypotonic psoas status. Rectus femoris is once again seen to be short, while the relative external rotation of the lower leg (see angle of foot) hints at probable shortened tensor fascia lata and/or piriformis involvement.

- If this is not clearly observed, application of light pressure towards the floor on the lower third of the thigh will produce a compensatory extension of the lower leg only, confirming that rectus femoris is short.
- If both iliopsoas and rectus femoris are short, passive flexion of the knee will result in compensatory lumbar lordosis and increased hip flexion. (See also functional assessment method for psoas in Chapter 9 and notes on psoas in Box 6.4.)
- If both psoas and rectus femoris are short, clinical experience suggests that rectus should be treated first.
- In the test position, if the suspended thigh hangs downwards, below a parallel (with the floor) position, this indicates a degree of laxity in iliopsoas (Fig. 6.6C).
- If TFL structure is short (a further test indicates this, see Test 5, later in this chapter), then there should be

an obvious groove apparent on the lateral thigh, and sometimes the whole lower leg will deviate laterally.

Mitchell's Strength Test

Before using MET methods to normalise a short psoas, Mitchell et al. (1979) recommended that the patient should lie at the end of the table, both legs hanging down, with feet turned in so that they can rest on the practitioner's lateral calf areas, as they stand facing the patient. To judge which psoas is weaker or stronger than the other, the patient should press firmly against the practitioner's calves with their feet, while the practitioner rests their hands on the patient's thighs. The patient should then attempt to lift the practitioner from the floor. In this way, the relative strength of one leg's effort should be able to be assessed compared with the other.

> **⚠ CAUTION**
>
> Readers are cautioned against excessive reliance on perceived muscle strength/weakness assessments, unless objective methods are being used – as discussed briefly in Chapter 5, for example using a dynamometer (Li et al., 2006).

If a psoas has tested short (as in the test described above) and also tests strong in this test, then it is suitable for MET treatment, according to Mitchell's guidelines (Mitchell et al., 1979). However, if it tests both *short and weak*, then other factors such as tight erector spinae muscles, or the presence of trigger points in the low-back muscles (multifidus, iliocostalis), or in psoas itself, should be treated first, until psoas tests *strong and short*, at which time MET should be applied to start the lengthening process (Simons et al., 1999).

As mentioned above, it has been found to be clinically useful, before treating a shortened psoas, to first address any ipsilateral shortness in rectus femoris.

What if One Psoas Is Inhibited, and the Other Tight?

Schamberger (2002) discusses an imbalance ('*malalignment syndrome*') in which the psoas on one side is inhibited, while the other is tight. A pelvic tilt may occur, with elevation on the short, tight, side. However, Schamberger reports that the work of Maffetone (1999) suggests that the reverse might also be true, with psoas inhibition being located on the side of pelvic elevation (Fig. 6.7A).

Testing for length and for weakness (as above – see Fig. 6.6A–C) would lead to disclosure of the true picture, whatever the underlying cause(s).

Alternative Psoas Strength Test and Toning Exercise (Norris, 1999) (Fig. 6.7B)

An alternative test for psoas weakness/inhibition can become a toning exercise when repeated regularly:

- The patient sits upright on a chair, with spine in neutral and with the knee flexed at 90 degrees.
- The leg on the side to be tested, or the side on which psoas requires toning (right in this example), should be raised about 5 cm from the floor.
- If psoas is strong, it should be possible to maintain this raised leg for 10 seconds, before lowering and repeating the raise and hold nine more times.

During this test, if psoas is strong, there should be:
1. No loss of the upright, neutral, spinal position, or
2. No quiver or twitch of the anterior thigh muscles and
3. It should be possible to perform the 10 repetitions of 10-second holds, without distress.
   - Precisely the same procedure as the test should be performed once or twice daily, until 10 repetitions of 10 seconds are possible without strain.

If shortness is still evident, once tone and strength are restored, MET stretching should be applied.

NOTE: It is worth recalling Norris's (1999) advice that a slowly performed isotonic eccentric exercise will normally strengthen a weak postural muscle. As discussed in Chapters 2 and 5, psoas is classified as a postural muscle, and a mobiliser, depending on the descriptive model being used – therefore prone to shortening when chronically stressed.

There is therefore virtually universal agreement that psoas will shorten in response to stress.

MET Treatment for Shortness of Rectus Femoris ⏵

- The patient lies prone, ideally with a cushion under the abdomen to help avoid hyperlordosis.
- The practitioner stands on the side of the table of the affected leg so that they can stabilise the patient's pelvis (hand covering the sacral area or ischial tuberosity) during the treatment, using the cephalad hand.
- The affected leg is flexed at hip and knee.
- The practitioner can either hold the lower leg at the ankle (as in Fig. 6.8) or the upper leg can be cradled so that the hand curls under the lower thigh and is able to palpate for bind, just above the knee, with the practitioner's upper arm offering resistance to the lower leg.
- Either of these holds allows flexion of the knee to the barrier, perceived either as increasing effort being required or as palpated bind in rectus femoris, or both.
- If rectus femoris is short, then the patient's heel will not easily be able to touch the buttock (see Fig. 6.8).
- Once the restriction barrier has been established (how close can the heel get to the buttock before the barrier is noted?), the decision will have been made as to whether to treat this as an acute problem (commencing the contraction from the barrier) or as a chronic problem (commencing the contraction from short of the barrier).
- Appropriate degrees of resisted isometric effort are then introduced. For an acute problem, a mild 15%

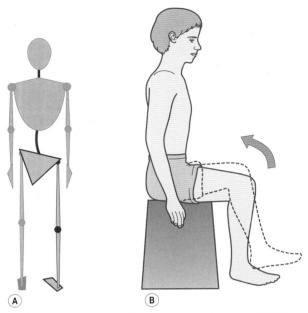

Fig. 6.7 (A) Static postural assessment of malalignment caused by psoas inhibition on the right, leading to medial rotation of the ipsilateral foot, with excessive pronation. The lumbar spine is shown to be convex on the left, involving a tight psoas. As noted by Maffetone (1999), the pelvis may be higher or lower on the side of the inhibited psoas. (Redrawn from Schamberger, 2002, p. 90, Fig. 3.2A.) (B) Psoas strength test.

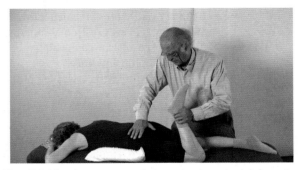

Fig. 6.8 Muscle energy technique treatment of left rectus femoris muscle. Note that the practitioner's right hand stabilises the sacrum and pelvis to prevent undue stress during the stretching phase of the treatment.

to 20% of MVC (maximum voluntary contraction) is used. For a chronic problem, a longer, stronger (up to 25% of MVC) effort may be used, as the patient tries to both straighten the leg and take the thigh towards the table (this activates both ends of rectus femoris).

- Appropriate breathing instructions should be given (see notes on breathing in Box 6.2).

- The contraction is followed, on an exhalation, by taking the muscle to (acute), or stretching through (chronic), the new barrier, by taking the heel towards the buttock with the patient's help.
- The stretch (in chronic conditions) should be held for up to 30 seconds.
- It may be helpful to increase slight hip extension before the next isometric contraction (using a cushion to support the thigh) as this removes slack from the cephalad end of rectus femoris.
- Repeat once or twice using agonists or antagonists.

Alternative Rectus Femoris MET Treatment, Using Slow Eccentric Isotonic Stretching of the Hamstrings (in Chronic, Not Acute, Settings)

- The patient lies prone, as in the previous description.
- The heel is eased towards the buttock to establish the *first sign of resistance* (bind).
- The heel should be held towards the buttock by the patient's own effort.
- The practitioner then *slowly* eases (forces) the leg towards a straightened position, the patient having been given the instruction that, '*I am going to try to*

straighten your leg. You should resist this but not totally, so that you allow me to slowly overcome your effort'.

- This slow eccentric stretch of the hamstrings tones these, and inhibits quadriceps/rectus femoris – or increases tolerance to the stretch that follows.
- After the slow eccentric isotonic stretching (SEIS) procedure the knee is flexed again, and the heel eased towards the buttock to stretch rectus femoris – as in the previous exercise.

Once a reasonable degree of increased range has been gained in rectus femoris, it is appropriate to treat psoas, if this has tested as short.

MET Treatment of Psoas

Method A prone (Fig. 6.9A and B). Psoas can be treated in the prone position, described for rectus femoris above. The stretch follows the patient's isometric effort to bring the thigh to the table against resistance (see Fig. 6.9A).

- The patient is prone with a pillow under the abdomen to reduce the lumbar curve (or the contralateral leg can be placed so that the foot touches the floor, neutralising the lumbar curve) and offering a stable pelvis from which to apply the subsequent stretch (see Fig. 6.9B).
- The practitioner stands contralateral to the side of psoas to be treated, with the table-side hand supporting the thigh.
- The non-table-side hand is placed so that the heel of that hand is on the sacrum, applying pressure towards the floor, to maintain pelvic stability.
- The fingers of that hand may be placed so that the middle, ring and small fingers are on one side of L2/3 segment and the index finger on the other. This allows these fingers to sense a forward (anteriorly directed) 'tug' of the vertebrae, when psoas is stretched past its barrier, as the thigh is elevated from the table.
- An alternative hand position is offered by Greenman (1996) who suggests that the stabilising contact on the pelvis should apply pressure towards the table, on the ischial tuberosity – not the sacrum, as thigh extension is introduced (see Fig. 6.9A and B). The author agrees that this is a more comfortable contact than the sacrum. However, it fails to allow access to palpation of the lumbar spine during the procedure.
- The practitioner eases the thigh (knee is flexed) off the table surface, and senses for ease of movement of extension of the hip. If there is a strong sense of

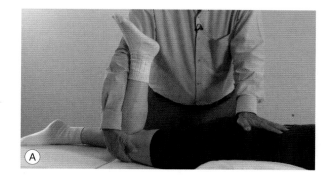

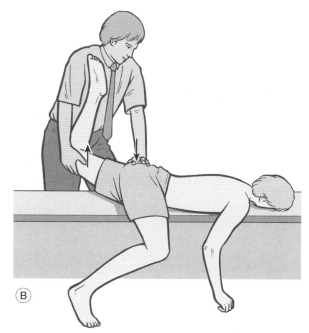

Fig. 6.9 Muscle energy technique treatment of psoas with stabilising contact on ischial tuberosity as described by Greenman (1996). (A) Position 1 and (B) Position 2.

resistance to this movement, there should be an almost simultaneous awareness of the palpated vertebral segment moving anteriorly.

- It should be possible – if psoas is normal – to achieve approximately 10 degrees of hip extension before that barrier is reached, without force. Greenman (1996) suggests that *'Normally the knee can be lifted 6 inches [15 cm] off the table. If less, tightness and shortness of psoas is present'*.
- Having identified the barrier, the practitioner either works from this (in an acute setting) or short of it

(in a chronic setting) as the patient is asked to bring the thigh towards the table against resistance, using 15% to 25% of their maximal voluntary contraction potential, for 5 to 7 seconds.

- Following release of the effort the thigh is eased to its new barrier if acute, or past that barrier, into stretch, with the patient's assistance ('gently "float" your foot towards the ceiling').
- If stretch is introduced, this is held for up to 30 seconds.
- It is important that as a stretch is introduced no lumbar hyperextension should occur. Pressure from the heel of the practitioner's hand on the sacrum or ischial tuberosity usually ensures that spinal stability is maintained.
- The process is then repeated.

Method B (Fig. 6.10A). Grieve's (1986) method involves using the supine test position, in which the patient lies with the buttocks at the very end of the table, with the non-treated leg fully flexed at the hip and knee, and either held in that state by the patient, or by placement of the patient's foot against the practitioner's lateral chest wall (see Fig. 6.10A).

- The leg on the affected side is allowed to hang freely, with the medio-plantar aspect of the foot resting on the practitioner's knee or shin.
- The practitioner stands sideways on to the patient, at the foot of the table, with both hands holding the thigh of the extended leg. The practitioner's far leg should be flexed slightly at the knee so that the patient's foot can rest, as described.
- This is used as a contact which, with the hands, resists the attempt of the patient to *externally rotate the leg* and, at the same time, *flex the hip* for 5 to 7 seconds. This combination of forces focuses the contraction effort into psoas, very precisely.
- The practitioner resists both efforts, and an isometric contraction of the psoas and associated muscles therefore takes place.
- Appropriate breathing instructions should be given (see notes on breathing, Box 6.2).
- If the condition is acute, the treatment commences from the restriction barrier, whereas if the condition is chronic, the leg is elevated into a slightly more flexed-hip position.
- After the isometric contraction, using an appropriate degree of effort, the thigh should, on an exhalation, either be taken to the new restriction barrier, without force (if acute), or through that barrier with slight, painless pressure towards the floor on the anterior

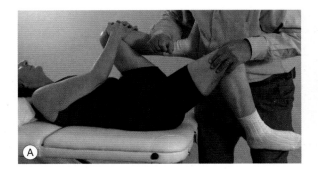

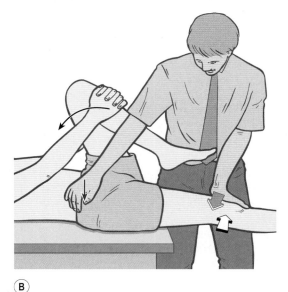

Fig. 6.10 (A) Muscle energy technique treatment of psoas using Grieve's method, in which there is placement of the patient's inverted foot, against the practitioner's thigh. This allows a more precise focus of contraction into psoas when the patient attempts to lightly flex the hip against resistance. (B) Psoas treatment variation, with the leg held straight and the pelvis stabilised.

aspect of the thigh (if chronic), and held there for up to 30 seconds (see Fig. 6.10A and also a variation, Fig. 6.10B).

- Repeat until no further gain is achieved.[2]

---

[2]Direct inhibitory pressure techniques applied to the vertebral attachments of psoas through the midline is an effective alternative approach, especially in acute psoas conditions. This is not usually applicable in overweight individuals.

MET Treatment of Psoas

Method C (Fig. 6.11A and B). This method is appropriate for chronic psoas problems only.

- The supine test position is used in which the patient lies with the buttocks at the very end of the table, the non-treated leg fully flexed at the hip and knee, and either held in that state by the patient (Fig. 6.11A), or by the practitioner's hand (Fig. 6.11B), or by placement

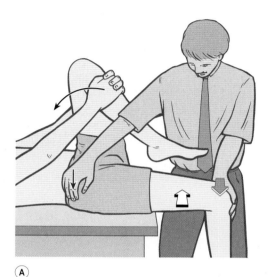

(A)

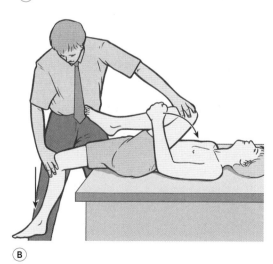

(B)

Fig. 6.11 (A) Muscle energy technique treatment involves the patient's effort to flex the hip against resistance. (B) Stretch of psoas, which follows the isometric contraction (see Fig. 6.10A) and is achieved by means of gravity plus additional practitioner effort.

of the patient's foot against the practitioner's lateral chest wall.

- The leg on the affected side is allowed to hang freely.
- The practitioner resists a light attempt by the patient to flex the hip for 5 to 7 seconds.
- Appropriate breathing instructions should be given (see notes on breathing, Box 6.2).
- After the isometric contraction, using an appropriate degree of effort, on an exhalation the thigh should be taken slightly beyond the restriction barrier, with a light degree of painless pressure towards the floor, and held there for up to 30 seconds (see Fig. 6.11B).
- Repeat until no further gain is achieved (see footnote 3).

Self-Treatment of Psoas

Method A.

- Lewit suggests self-treatment in a position as above in which the patient lies close to the end of a table as shown in Fig. 6.6B, with one leg fully flexed at the hip and knee and held in this position throughout, while the other leg is allowed to reach the limit of its stretch, as gravity pulls it towards the floor.
- The patient then lifts this leg slightly (say a further 2 cm) to contract psoas, holding this for 5 to 7 seconds, before slowly allowing the leg to ease towards the floor.
- This stretch position is held for a further 30 seconds, and the process is repeated once or twice more.
- The counterpressure in this effort is achieved by gravity.

Method B (Fig. 6.12).

- The patient stands facing a chair or stool onto which is placed the non-treated-side foot.
- The flexed knee should be above hip height.
- The treated-side leg is placed behind the trunk so that all hip flexion is eliminated, until a sense of light stretching is noted on the anterior thigh, but not in the low back.
- The patient places both hands on hips and ensures that no hyperextension of the lumbar spine is occurring.
- The patient is instructed to ease the trunk anteriorly, without any spinal flexion or extension, until a sense of additional stretch is noted on the anterior thigh.
- This is held for 30 seconds before a further movement anteriorly, of the patient's trunk, reproduces the sense of stretching in the anterior thigh.
- This again is held for 30 seconds.

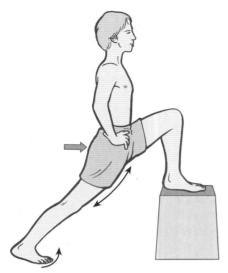

Fig. 6.12 Psoas self-stretch.

▶ 4. Assessment and Treatment of Hamstrings (07) (Fig. 6.13A and B)

Should tight hamstrings always be treated? Van Wingerden (1997), reporting on the earlier work of Vleeming (Vleeming et al., 1989), states that both intrinsic and extrinsic support for the sacroiliac joint derives – in part – from hamstring (biceps femoris) status. Intrinsically the influence is via the close anatomical and physiological relationship between biceps femoris and the sacrotuberous ligament (they frequently attach via a strong tendinous link):

Force from the biceps femoris muscle can lead to increased tension of the sacrotuberous ligament in various ways. Since increased tension of the sacrotuberous ligament diminishes the range of sacroiliac joint motion, the biceps femoris can play a role in stabilisation of the SIJ.

Van Wingerden also notes that in low-back pain patients, forward flexion is often painful as the load on the spine increases. This happens whether flexion occurs in the spine or via the hip joints (tilting of the pelvis). If the hamstrings are tight and short, they effectively prevent pelvic tilting:

In this respect, an increase in hamstring tension might well be part of a defensive arthrokinematic reflex mechanism of the body to diminish spinal load.

If such a situation is longstanding, the hamstrings (biceps femoris) will shorten, almost certainly influencing sacroiliac and lumbar spine dysfunction (Arab & Nourbakhsh, 2011). The decision to treat tight ('tethered') hamstrings should therefore take account of why they are tight, and consider that, in some circumstances, they might be offering beneficial support to the SIJ, or be reducing low-back stress.

Methodology

If the hip flexors (psoas, etc.) have previously tested as short, then the test position for the hamstrings needs to commence with the non-tested leg flexed at both knee and hip, foot resting flat on the treatment surface to ensure full pelvic rotation into neutral (as in Fig. 6.13B). If no hip flexor shortness was observed, then the non-tested leg should lie flat on the surface of the table.

Hamstring test A.

- The patient lies supine with non-tested leg either flexed or straight, depending on previous test results for hip flexors.
- The tested leg is taken into a straight-leg-raised (SLR) position, no flexion of the knee being allowed, with minimal force employed. Piva et al. (2006) found in studies that this method of hamstring assessment was the most reliable.
- The first sign of resistance (or palpated bind) is assessed as the barrier of restriction.
- If straight leg raising to 80 degrees is not easily possible, then there exists some shortening of the hamstrings and the muscles can be treated in the straight leg position (see below).

Hamstring test B (Fig. 6.13C). Whether or not an 80-degree elevation is easily achieved, a variation in testing is also needed to evaluate the lower hamstring fibres.

- To achieve this assessment, the tested leg is taken into *full* hip flexion (helped by patient holding the upper thigh with both hands (see Fig. 6.13C)). The knee is then straightened until resistance is felt, or bind is noted by palpation of the lower hamstrings.
- If the knee cannot straighten with the hip flexed, this indicates shortness in the lower hamstring fibres, and the patient will report a degree of pull behind the knee and lower thigh. MET treatment of this is carried out in the test position (Fig. 6.13A).
- If, however, the knee is capable of being straightened with the hip flexed, having previously not been capable of achieving an 80-degree straight leg raise, then

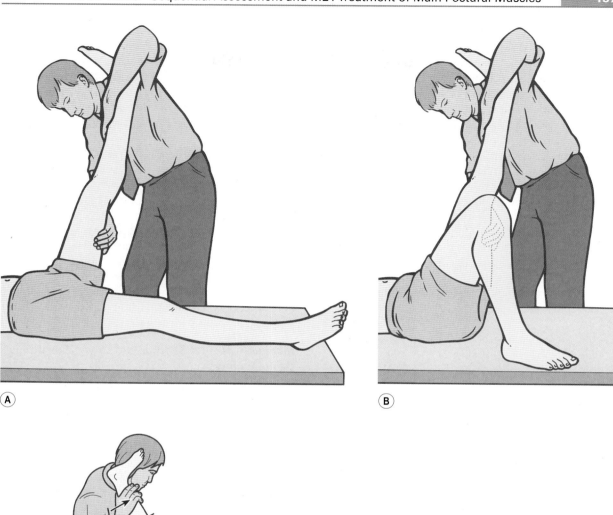

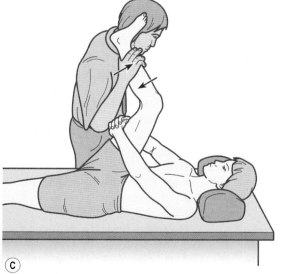

Fig. 6.13 (A) Assessment for shortness in hamstring muscles. The practitioner's right hand palpates for bind/the first sign of resistance, while the practitioner maintains the patient's knee in extension. (B) MET treatment of shortened hamstrings. Following an isometric contraction, the leg is taken to or through the resistance barrier (depending on whether the problem is acute or chronic). (C) Assessment and treatment position for lower hamstring fibres.

the lower fibres are not responsible for the restriction, and it is the upper fibres of hamstrings that require attention using MET, working from the SLR test position (Fig. 6.13A).

Janda's hip extension test (see Fig. 6.14). This functional assessment offers additional information to that gained from the hamstring tests described above:

- The patient lies prone and the practitioner stands to the side at waist level with the cephalad hand spanning the lower lumbar musculature and assessing erector spinae activity.
- The caudal hand is placed so that the heel lies on the gluteal muscle mass with the fingertips on the hamstrings.
- The patient is asked to raise their leg into extension as the practitioner assesses the firing sequence.

Janda (1996) suggests that the ideal activation sequence is (1) gluteus maximus, (2) hamstrings, followed by (3) erector spinae contralateral then (4) ipsilateral.

The poorest pattern occurs when the erector spinae on the ipsilateral side, or even the shoulder girdle muscles, initiate the movement and activation of gluteus maximus is weak and substantially delayed... the leg lift is achieved by pelvic forward tilt and hyperlordosis of the lumbar spine, which undoubtedly stresses this region.

If the hamstrings and/or erectors take on the role of gluteus maximus as prime mover, they will shorten and further inhibit gluteus maximus.

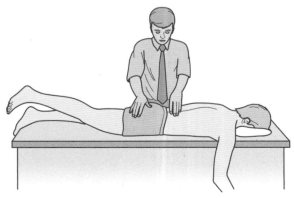

Fig. 6.14 Prone hip extension test. (Reproduced with permission from Chaitow and Fritz, 2007.)

Commentary on hip extension test. This firing sequence – as outlined above – is not always as described. Bruno and Bagust (2007) reported on the firing patterns of muscles (erector spinae, gluteus maximus and hamstrings) during a prone hip extension test, and demonstrated that, while there is no fixed pattern that could differentiate LBP and non-LBP subjects, LBP patients have greater consistency of the pattern compared to non-LBP subjects. Arab et al. (2011) have confirmed the findings of Bruno and Bagust, concluding that there exists: 'an altered activity pattern of the lumbo-pelvic muscles during hip extension in patients with chronic LBP'.

Alternative observational test. When the hip extension movement is performed the lower limb should be observed to be 'hinging' at the hip joint. If, instead, the hinge seems to take place in the lumbar spine, the indication is that the lumbar spinal extensors have adopted much of the role of gluteus maximus and that these extensors (and probably hamstrings) will have shortened.

Method A. MET for Shortness of Lower Hamstrings Using Agonists

If the lower hamstring fibres are implicated as being short (see hamstring test B above), then the treatment position is identical to the test position (see Fig. 6.13C).

- The non-treated leg needs to be either flexed (if hip flexors are short, as described above) or straight on the table.
- The treated leg should be flexed at both the hip and knee, and then straightened by the practitioner until the restriction barrier is identified (one hand should palpate the tissues behind the knee for sensations of bind as the lower leg is straightened).
- Depending upon whether it is an acute or a chronic problem, the isometric contraction against resistance is introduced at this 'bind' barrier (if acute) or a little short of it (if chronic).
- The instruction might be something such as 'try to gently bend your knee, against my resistance, starting slowly and using only a quarter of your strength'.
- It is particularly important with the hamstrings to take care regarding cramp, and so it is suggested that no more than 25% of patients' strength should ever be used during isometric contractions in this region.
- Following the 5 to 7 seconds of contraction (for notes on respiratory synkinesis see Box 6.2) followed by complete relaxation, the leg should, on an exhalation,

be straightened at the knee towards its new barrier (in acute problems) and through that barrier, with a degree of stretch (if chronic), with the patient's assistance.

- This slight stretch should be held for up to 30 seconds.
- Repeat the process until no further gain is possible (usually one or two repetitions achieve the maximum degree of lengthening available at any one session).

Method B. MET Treatment of Lower Hamstrings Using Antagonists (see Fig. 6.13C)

- The supine patient fully flexes the hip on the affected side.
- The flexed knee is extended by the practitioner to the point of initial resistance (identifying the barrier).
- The calf of the treated leg is placed on the shoulder of the practitioner, who stands facing the head of the table on the side of the treated leg.
- If the right leg of the patient is being treated, the calf will rest on the practitioner's right shoulder, and the practitioner's right hand stabilises the patient's extended unaffected leg against the table.
- The practitioner's left hand holds the treated leg at the thigh to both maintain stability and to palpate for bind when the barrier is being assessed.
- The patient is asked to attempt to *straighten* the lower leg (i.e. extend the knee) utilising the antagonists to the hamstrings, employing ~20% of the strength in the quadriceps.
- This is resisted by the practitioner for 5 to 7 seconds.
- Appropriate breathing instructions should be given (see notes in Box 6.2).
- The leg is then extended at the knee to its new hamstring limit if the problem is acute (or stretched slightly if chronic) – after relaxation, and the procedure is then repeated.

Method C. Co-Contraction MET Method of Hamstring Treatment

- Starting from the same position as Method B, above, a combined contraction may be introduced (Moore & Hutton, 1980).
- The instruction to the patient would be to pull the thigh towards their face (i.e. to flex the hip) and to push the lower leg downward onto the practitioner's shoulder (i.e. flexing the knee).
- This effectively contracts both the quadriceps and the hamstrings, facilitating subsequent easing to, or stretching through, the restriction barrier of the tight muscle, as described above.

Method D. Simultaneous Toning of Hamstring Antagonists (Quadriceps) and Preparation for Stretch of Shortened Hamstrings Using SEIS

Slow eccentric isotonic stretching (SEIS) of a muscle has a toning effect, while simultaneously preparing the antagonist for subsequent stretching.

- The patient is supine with hip and knee of the leg to be treated, flexed.
- The practitioner extends the flexed knee to its first barrier of resistance, palpating the tissues proximal to the knee crease for first sign of 'bind'.
- The patient is asked to resist, using a little more than half available strength, an attempt by the practitioner to slowly flex the knee fully (stretching the contracting quadriceps, and so toning these).
- An instruction should be given which makes clear the objective, 'I am going to slowly bend your knee, and I want you to partially resist this, but to let it slowly happen'.
- After performing the slow isotonic stretch of the quadriceps, the hamstrings should be retested for length, and ease of straight-leg raising, and if necessary, the hamstrings should be taken into a stretched position and held for up to 30 seconds before repeating the procedure.

MET for Shortness of the Upper Hamstrings

- If the upper fibres are involved (i.e. hamstring test A, above), then treatment is performed in the SLR position, with the knee maintained in extension at all times.
- The non-treated leg should be flexed at hip and knee or straight, depending on the hip flexor findings as explained above.
- In all other details, the procedures are the same as for treatment of lower hamstring fibres except that the leg is kept straight (see Fig. 6.13A and B).

   NOTE: In addition to the hamstring treatment methods described above, there may be clinical advantages in introducing positional variations, including internal and external rotation at the hip, as well as adduction and abduction of the limb, as barriers are identified. This strategy frequently unmasks areas of localised restriction that might not be evident when only straight-leg raising is performed.

5. Assessment and Treatment of Tensor Fascia Lata (08) (See Also Box 6.5)

The test recommended is a modified form of Ober's test (Fig. 6.15) which has been assessed by Baker et al. (2011) and found in clinical trials to be accurate and

BOX 6.5   Notes on Tensor Fascia Lata

- Mennell (1964) and Liebenson (1996) say that TFL shortness can produce all the symptoms of acute and chronic sacroiliac problems.
- Pain from TFL shortness can be localised to the posterior superior iliac spine (PSIS), radiating to the groin or down any aspect of the thigh to the knee.
- Although the pain may arise in the sacroiliac (SI) joint, dysfunction in the joint may be caused and maintained by taut TFL structures.
- Pain from the iliotibial band (ITB) itself can be felt in the lateral thigh, with referral to hip or knee.
- TFL and the ITB can be 'riddled' with sensitive fibrotic deposits and trigger point activity.
- There is commonly a posteriority of the ilium associated with short TFL.
- TFL's prime phasic activity (all postural structures also have some phasic function) is to assist the gluteals in abduction of the thigh.
- If TFL and psoas are short they may, according to Janda, 'dominate' the gluteals on abduction of the thigh, so that a degree of lateral rotation and flexion of the hip will be produced, rotating the pelvis backwards.
- Rolf (1977) points out that persistent exercise such as cycling will shorten and toughen the fascial ITB 'until it becomes reminiscent of a steel cable'. This band crosses both hip and knee, and spatial compression allows it to squeeze and compress cartilaginous elements such as the menisci. Ultimately, it will no longer be able to compress, and rotational displacement at knee and hip will take place.

TFL, Tensor fascia lata.

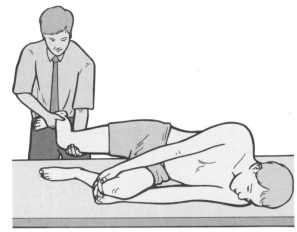

Fig. 6.15 Assessment for shortness of tensor fascia lata (TFL) – modified Ober's test. When the hand supporting the flexed knee is removed the thigh should fall to the table if TFL is not short.

reproducible. Piva et al. (2006) observed that: 'inter-tester reliability coefficients were substantial for measures of… ITB/TFL complex length… which ensures valid interpretation in clinical practice'.

- The patient is side-lying with back close to the edge of the table.
- The practitioner stands behind the patient, whose lower leg is flexed at hip and knee and held by the practitioner for stability.
- The tested leg is supported by the practitioner, who must ensure that there is *no hip flexion,* which would nullify the test.
- The leg is extended to the position where the iliotibial band (ITB) lies over the greater trochanter.

- The tested leg is held by the practitioner at ankle and knee, with the whole leg in its anatomical position, neither abducted nor adducted, and not forward or backward of the trunk. (Note: some clinicians (Baker et al., 2011) describe the leg being held in slight abduction for this test, and not in neutral. The method described in this text suggests no abduction, for patient comfort.)
- The practitioner carefully introduces flexion at the knee to 90 degrees, *without allowing the hip to flex,* and then, while supporting the limb at the ankle, allows the knee to fall towards the table.
- *If the TFL is normal,* the thigh and knee will fall easily, with the knee usually contacting the table surface (unless there is unusual hip width, or a short thigh length, that prevents this).
- If the upper leg remains aloft, with little sign of 'falling' towards the table, then either the patient is not letting go, or the TFL is short and does not allow it to fall.
- As a rule, the band will palpate as tender under such conditions.
- TFL may also test as weak, or not.
- Studies show that excessive TFL/ITB (iliotibial band) tightness – as evidenced by a positive Ober's test – does not necessarily equate with weakness (Arab & Nourbakhsh, 2010). Their clinical studies revealed that all patients with low-back pain had significant weakness of the hip abductors, *whether or not there*

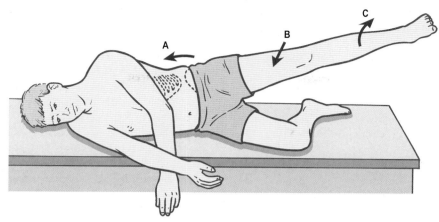

Fig. 6.16 Hip abduction observation test. (Reproduced with permission from Chaitow and Delany, 2011.)

was evidence of ITB/TFL shortness. ITB/TFL tightness might therefore not be due to a compensatory mechanism related to hip abductor weakness in subjects with LBP.

Lewit's (1999) TFL Palpation

See also the functional assessment method in Chapter 9.

- The patient is side-lying and the practitioner stands facing the patient's front, at hip level.
- The patient's non-tested leg is slightly flexed to provide stability, and there should be a vertical line to the table between one anterior superior iliac spine (ASIS) and the other (i.e. no forwards or backwards 'roll' of the pelvis).
- The practitioner's cephalad hand rests over the ASIS so that it can also palpate over the trochanter, with the fingers resting on the TFL and the thumb on gluteus medius.
- The caudad hand rests on the mid-thigh to apply slight resistance to the patient's effort to abduct the leg.
- The patient abducts the upper leg (which should be extended at the knee and slightly hyperextended at the hip) and the practitioner should feel the trochanter 'slip away' as this is done.
- If, however, the whole pelvis is felt to move rather than just the trochanter, there is inappropriate muscular imbalance.
- In balanced abduction, gluteus is activated at the beginning of the movement, with TFL operating later in the pure abduction of the leg.
- If there is an overactivity (and therefore shortness) of TFL, then there will be pelvic movement on the abduction, and TFL will be felt to come into play before gluteus medius.
- The abduction of the thigh movement will have been modified to include external rotation and flexion of the thigh (Janda, 1996).
- This indicates a stressed postural muscle (TFL), which implies shortness.
- It may be possible (depending on the practitioner's hand size and patient anatomical size) to increase the number of palpation elements involved by having the cephalad hand also palpate (with an extended small finger) QL during leg abduction.
- In a balanced muscular effort to lift the leg sideways, QL should not become active until the leg has been abducted to around 25 to 30 degrees.
- When quadratus is overactive it will often initiate the abduction along with TFL, thus producing a pelvic tilt (see also Fig. 6.11A and B).[3]

Janda's (1996) Observation Assessment – Hip Abduction Test (Fig. 6.16)

- The patient is side-lying, ideally with head on a cushion, with the upper leg straight and the lower leg flexed at hip and knee, for balance.

---

[3]Remember that a lateral 'corset' of muscles exists to stabilise the pelvic and low-back structures and that if TFL and quadratus (and/or psoas) shorten and tighten, the gluteal muscles will weaken. This test gives the proof of such imbalance existing. (See notes on lower crossed syndrome in Chapter 5, and Box 5.2 in particular.)

- The practitioner, who is observing, not palpating, stands in front of the patient and towards the head end of the table.
- The patient is asked to slowly raise the leg into abduction.
- Normal is represented by pure hip abduction to 45 degrees.
- Abnormal is represented by:
  - hip flexion during abduction, indicating TFL shortness
  - the leg externally rotating during abduction, indicating piriformis shortness
  - 'hip hiking', indicating QL shortness (and gluteus medius weakness)
  - posterior pelvic rotation, suggesting short antagonistic hip adductors.

Method A. Supine MET Treatment of Shortened TFL (Fig. 6.17)

- The patient lies supine with the unaffected leg flexed at hip and knee.
- The practitioner stands facing the contralateral leg at approximately knee level.

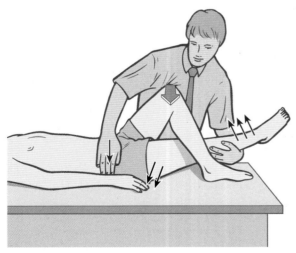

Fig. 6.17 Muscle energy technique (MET) treatment of tensor fascia lata. If a standard MET method is being used, the stretch will follow the isometric contraction in which the patient will attempt to move the right leg to the right against sustained resistance. It is important for the practitioner to maintain stability of the pelvis during the procedure.

- The affected-side leg is adducted to its barrier, requiring it to be brought under the contralateral leg/foot which is flexed at knee and hip.
- Observing the guidelines previously discussed for acute and chronic problems, TFL will be treated at, or short of, the barrier of resistance, using light to moderate degrees of effort involving isometric contractions of 5 to 7 seconds.
- The practitioner uses their trunk to stabilise the patient's pelvis by leaning against the flexed contralateral knee.
- The practitioner's caudad arm supports the affected leg so that the knee is stabilised by the hand. The other hand maintains a firm contact on the affected side ASIS stabilising the pelvis.
- The patient is asked to abduct the leg against resistance using minimal force ('using less than a quarter of your strength, slowly take your leg back towards the midline, against my resistance').
- After the contraction ceases, and the patient has relaxed, and on an exhalation, the leg should be taken to or through the new restriction barrier (into adduction past the barrier) to stretch the muscular fibres of TFL (the upper third of the structure).
- Care should be taken to ensure that the pelvis is not tilted during the stretch.
- Stability is achieved by the practitioner maintaining pressure against the flexed knee/thigh.
- The entire process should be repeated several times, or until no further gain is possible.

Method B. Greenman Alternative Supine MET Treatment of Shortened TFL (Fig. 6.18)

- The patient adopts the same position as for psoas assessment (Thomas position), lying at the end of the table with the non-treated-side leg in full hip flexion and held by the patient, with the tested leg hanging freely, knee flexed.
- For a right-sided TFL treatment the practitioner stands at the end of the table facing the patient so that their left lower leg can contact the patient's foot.
- The practitioner's left hand is placed on the patient's distal femur, and with this they introduce internal rotation of the thigh, while simultaneously introducing external rotation of the tibia, by means of light pressure on the distal foot from their lower leg.
- During this process, the practitioner senses for resistance (the movements should be easy and 'springy' without any hard end-feel).

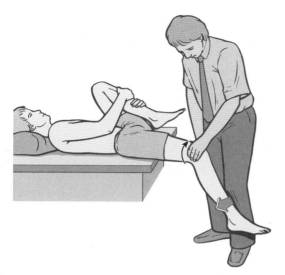

Fig. 6.18 Greenman tensor fascia lata treatment: the patient's right thigh is held at resistance barrier of internal rotation, together with external rotation of the tibia, as the patient introduces adduction of the femur and external rotation of the tibia against resistance. This is followed by the barriers being re-engaged and the stretch held for 30 seconds.

- If while maintaining these rotational holds a characteristic depression or groove can be observed on the lateral thigh, this strongly suggests shortness and tension involving TFL (Greenman, 1996, p. 464).
- Once the resistance barrier has been identified, the leg should be held just short of this for a chronic problem, as the patient is asked to *externally rotate the tibia,* and to *adduct the femur,* against resistance, for 5 to 7 seconds.
- Following this the practitioner eases the leg into a greater degree of internal hip rotation and external tibial rotation, and holds this stretch for up to 30 seconds.

Method C. Isolytic Variation

If an isolytic contraction is introduced to actively stretch the interface between elastic and non-elastic tissues, there is a need to stabilise the pelvis more efficiently, either by use of wide straps or by another pair of hands holding the ASIS to the table during the stretch.

- The procedure consists of the patient attempting to abduct the leg as the practitioner overcomes the muscular effort, forcing the leg into adduction.

- With the patient positioned as in Fig. 6.17, the contraction/stretch should be rapid (2 to 3 seconds at most to complete).
- Repeat several times.
- Caution the patient to anticipate local discomfort for a day or two.

Method D. Side-Lying MET Treatment of TFL

- The patient lies on the affected TFL side with the upper leg flexed at hip and knee and resting on the table, anterior to the affected leg.
- The practitioner stands behind the patient and uses their caudad hand and arm to (1) bring the hip into slight extension, (2) raise the affected leg (which is on the table) while stabilising the pelvis with the cephalad hand until an easy barrier is noted; or uses both hands to raise the affected leg into slight adduction towards the barrier (only appropriate if strapping is used to hold the pelvis to the table).
- The patient contracts the muscle against resistance by trying to take the leg into abduction (towards the table) using breathing assistance as appropriate (see notes on breathing, Box 6.2).
- After the effort, on an exhalation, the practitioner lifts the leg into further adduction, beyond the barrier to stretch the interface between elastic and non-elastic tissues (in chronic conditions).
- Repeat as appropriate or modify to use as an isolytic contraction (method C above) by rapidly stretching the structure past the barrier, during the contraction.

Additional Methods

Mennell (1964) has described efficient soft tissue stretching techniques for releasing the ITB. These involve a series of snapping actions applied by thumbs to the anterior fibres with patient side-lying, followed by a series of heel-of-hand thrusts across the long axis of the posterior ITB fibres.

Additional release may be possible by use of elbow or heel-of-hand 'stripping' of the structure, neuromuscular deep tissue approaches (using thumb or a rubber-tipped T-bar) applied to the upper fibres and those around the knee, and specific deep tissue release methods.

Most of these methods are distinctly uncomfortable and all require expert tuition.[4]

---

[4]These methods are fully described in Chaitow (2010).

Self-Treatment and Maintenance

- The patient lies on their side, on a bed or table, with the affected leg uppermost and hanging over the edge (lower leg comfortably flexed).
- The patient may then introduce an isometric contraction by slightly lifting the hanging leg a few centimetres, and holding this position for 10 seconds, before slowly releasing and allowing gravity to take the leg towards the floor, so introducing a greater degree of stretch.
- This is held for up to 30 seconds and the process is then repeated several times to achieve the maximum available stretch in the tight soft tissues.
- The counterforce in this isometric exercise is gravity.

6. Assessment and Treatment of Piriformis (09) (See Also Boxes 6.6 and 6.7)

Test A1. Piriformis Stretch Test

- When it is shortened, piriformis will usually cause the affected side leg of the supine patient to appear to be short, and externally rotated.
- The supine patient's tested leg should be placed into flexion at the hip and knee so that the foot rests on the table lateral to the contralateral knee (the tested leg is crossed over the straight non-tested leg, as shown in Fig. 6.19A).

- The angle of hip flexion should not exceed 60 degrees (see notes on piriformis in Box 6.6).
- The non-tested side ASIS is stabilised to prevent pelvic motion during the test and the knee of the tested side is pushed into adduction, to place a stretch on piriformis.

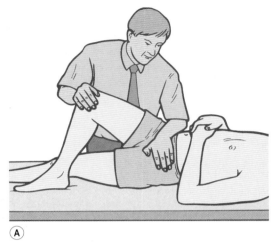

(A)

Fig. 6.19 (A) Muscle energy technique treatment of piriformis muscle with patient supine. The pelvis must be maintained in a stable position as the knee (right in this example) is adducted to stretch piriformis following an isometric contraction.

BOX 6.6   Notes on Piriformis

- Piriformis paradox. The performance of external rotation of the hip by piriformis occurs when the angle of hip flexion is 60 degrees or less. Once the angle of hip flexion is greater than 60 degrees piriformis function changes so that it becomes an internal rotator of the hip (Lehmkuhl & Smith, 1983; Gluck & Liebenson, 1997). The implications of this are illustrated in Figs. 6.19A and 6.21.
- This postural muscle, like all others which have a predominance of type I fibres, will shorten if stressed. In the case of piriformis, the effect of shortening is to increase its diameter and because of its location this allows for direct pressure to be exerted on the sciatic nerve, which passes under it in 80% of people. In the other 20% the nerve passes through the muscle so that contraction will produce veritable strangulation of the sciatic nerve.
- In addition, the pudendal nerve and the blood vessels of the internal iliac artery, as well as common perineal

nerves, posterior femoral cutaneous nerve and nerves of the hip rotators, can all be affected.
- If there is sciatic pain associated with piriformis shortness, then on straight leg raising, which reproduces the pain, external rotation of the hip should relieve it, since this slackens piriformis. (This clue may, however, only apply to any degree if the individual is one of those in whom the nerve actually passes through the muscle.)
- The effects can be circulatory, neurological and functional, inducing pain and paraesthesia of the affected limb as well as alterations to pelvic and lumbar function.
- Diagnosis usually hinges on the absence of spinal causative factors and the distributions of symptoms from the sacrum to the hip joint, over the gluteal region and down to the popliteal space. Palpation of the affected piriformis tendon, near the head of the trochanter, will elicit pain and the affected leg will probably be externally rotated.

BOX 6.6   Notes on Piriformis—cont'd

- The piriformis muscle syndrome is frequently characterised by such bizarre symptoms that they may seem unrelated. One characteristic complaint is a persistent, severe, radiating low-back pain extending from the sacrum to the hip joint, over the gluteal region and the posterior portion of the upper leg, to the popliteal space. In the most severe cases the patient will be unable to lie or stand comfortably, and changes in position will not relieve the pain. Intense pain will occur when the patient sits or squats since this type of movement requires external rotation of the upper leg and flexion at the knee.
- Compression of the pudendal nerve and blood vessels which pass through the greater sciatic foramen and re-enter the pelvis via the lesser sciatic foramen is possible because of piriformis contracture. Any compression would result in impaired circulation to the genitalia in both sexes. Since external rotation of the hips is required for coitus by women, pain noted during this act could relate to impaired circulation induced by piriformis dysfunction. This could also be a basis for impotency in men. (See also Box 6.7.)
- Piriformis involvement often relates to a pattern of pain which includes:
  - pain near the trochanter
  - pain in the inguinal area
  - local tenderness over the insertion behind trochanter
  - sacroiliac (SI) joint pain on the opposite side
  - externally rotated foot on the same side

- pain unrelieved by most positions with standing and walking being the easiest
- limitation of internal rotation of the leg which produces pain near the hip
- short leg on the affected side.
- The pain itself will be persistent and radiating, covering anywhere from the sacrum to the buttock, hip and leg including inguinal and perineal areas.
- Bourdillon (1982) suggests that piriformis syndrome and SI joint dysfunction are intimately connected and that recurrent SI problems will not stabilise until hypertonic piriformis is corrected.
- Janda (1996) points to the vast amount of pelvic organ dysfunction to which piriformis can contribute due to its relationship with circulation to the area.
- Mitchell et al. (1979) suggest that (as in the psoas example above) piriformis shortness should only be treated if it is tested to be short and stronger than its pair. If it is short and weak then whatever is hypertonic and influencing it should be released and stretched first (Mitchell et al., 1979). When it tests strong and short, piriformis should receive muscle energy technique treatment.
- Since piriformis is an external rotator of the hip it can be inhibited (made to test weak) if an internal rotator such as tensor fascia lata is hypertonic or if its pair is hypertonic, since one piriformis will inhibit the other.

BOX 6.7   Working and Resting Muscles

Richard (1978) reminds us that a working muscle will mobilise up to 10 times the quantity of blood mobilised by a resting muscle. He points out the link between pelvic circulation and lumbar, ischiatic and gluteal arteries and the chance this allows to engineer the involvement of 2400 square metres of capillaries by using repetitive pumping of these muscles (including piriformis).

The therapeutic use of this knowledge involves the patient being asked to repetitively contract both piriformis muscles against resistance. The patient is supine, knees bent, feet on the table; the practitioner resists an effort to abduct the flexed knees, using a pulsed muscle energy approach (Ruddy's method) in which two isometrically resisted pulsation/contractions per second are introduced for as long as possible (a minute seems a long time doing this).

- If piriformis is shortened the degree of adduction will be limited and the patient will report discomfort posterior to the trochanter.

Test A2. Alternative: FAIR Test = Flexion, Adduction, Internal Rotation

- The FAIR test is applied with the patient side-lying, on the unaffected side with the affected side up, the hip flexed to an angle of 60 degrees, and the knee flexed to an angle of 60 to 90 degrees. (See Fig. 6.19B).
- While stabilising the hip, the examiner internally rotates and adducts the hip by applying downward pressure to the knee.
- The test is both sensitive and specific to a high degree (Fishman et al., 2002) and is considered positive if sciatic pain is reproduced (see also Box 6.6).

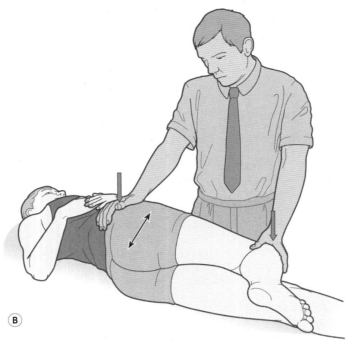

Fig. 6.19 (B) FAIR test. With patient side-lying, with flexed hip internally rotated and adducted, if downward pressure applied to the knee reproduces sciatic pain, the test is positive for piriformis involvement.

Test B. Piriformis Palpation Test (Fig. 6.20)

- The patient is side-lying, tested side uppermost.
- The practitioner stands at the level of the pelvis in front of and facing the patient, and, in order to contact the insertion of piriformis, draws imaginary lines between:
  - ASIS and the ischial tuberosity
  - PSIS and the most prominent point of trochanter.
- Where these reference lines cross, just posterior to the trochanter, is the insertion of the muscle, and digital pressure here will produce marked discomfort if the structure is short or irritated.
- To locate the most common trigger point site in the belly of the muscle, a line from the ASIS should be taken to the tip of the coccyx, rather than to the ischial tuberosity.
- The mid-point of the belly of piriformis, where triggers are common, is found where this line crosses the line from the PSIS to the trochanter. Light compression here that produces a painful response is indicative of a stressed muscle, and possibly an active myofascial trigger point.

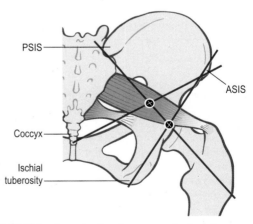

Fig. 6.20 Using bony landmarks as coordinates, the commonest tender areas are located in piriformis, in the belly and at the attachment of the muscle.

Piriformis Strength Test

- The patient lies prone, knees flexed to 90 degrees and touching, feet widely separated and flat on the table, with the practitioner at the foot of the table grasping the lower legs.

- This internally rotates the hips and therefore allows comparison of the range of movement permitted by shortened external rotators.
- The patient attempts to bring the ankles together as the practitioner assesses the relative strength of the two legs.

Mitchell et al. (1979) suggest that if there is relative shortness (as evidenced by the lower leg not being able to travel as far from the midline as its pair in this position), and if that same side also tests strong, then MET is called for. However, if there is shortness as well as relative weakness, then the reasons for the weakness (trigger points for example) need to be dealt with prior to stretching using MET.

MET Treatment of Piriformis

Method A: Supine. This method is based on the test position (see Fig. 6.19) and is described by Lewit (1999).

- With the patient supine, the treated leg is placed into flexion at the hip and knee, so that the foot rests on the table lateral to the contralateral knee (the leg on the side to be treated is crossed over the other, straight, leg).
- The angle of hip flexion should not exceed 60 degrees (see notes on piriformis, Box 6.6, for explanation).
- The practitioner places one hand on the contralateral ASIS to prevent pelvic motion, while the other hand is placed against the lateral flexed knee as this is pushed into resisted abduction to contract piriformis for 5 to 7 seconds.
- Following the contraction, the practitioner eases the treated-side leg into adduction until a sense of resistance is noted; this is held for 10 to 30 seconds.

Method B: Supine, with full hip flexion and external rotation.

- The position illustrated in Fig. 6.21A is adopted (see explanatory notes in Box 6.6, first bullet point).
- The hip is flexed beyond 60 degrees and the hip fully externally rotated to its barrier.
- The patient attempts – using minimal effort – to internally rotate the hip against resistance.
- Following this, and full relaxation, the hip is flexed further and externally rotated further and held for 30 seconds, before repeating the sequence.

Method C: Prone (see Fig. 6.21B)

- The patient is prone with the practitioner on the side to be treated, facing the table at thigh level.

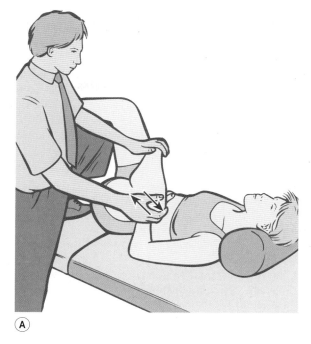

(A)

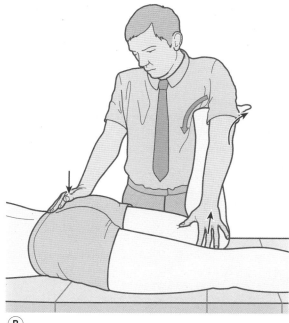

(B)

Fig. 6.21 (A) Muscle energy technique treatment of piriformis, patient supine, with hip fully flexed and externally rotated (see Box 6.6, first bullet point). (B) Muscle energy technique treatment of piriformis, patient prone, with hip fully flexed and externally rotated.

- The patient's knee is flexed to 90 degrees with the practitioner holding the leg in internal rotation to the barrier, while stabilising the pelvis with a hand on the pelvic crest above the hip.
- The patient attempts an external rotation against firm resistance, using no more than 25% of available strength, for 5 to 7 seconds.
- After complete relaxation, the practitioner introduces increased internal rotation at the hip to place piriformis at slight stretch.
- This is held for between 5 and 30 seconds before being repeated.

Hunt and Legal (2010) found this method to be effective in producing an immediate increase in piriformis extensibility as well as pain relief.

Method D: Side-lying – ischaemic compression together with MET.

- The patient should be side-lying, close to the edge of the table, affected side uppermost, both legs flexed at hip and knee.
- The practitioner stands facing the patient at hip level.
- The practitioner places their cephalad elbow tip gently over the point behind trochanter, where piriformis inserts.
- The patient should be close enough to the edge of the table for the practitioner to stabilise the pelvis against their trunk (Fig. 6.22).
- At the same time, the practitioner's caudad hand grasps the patient's ankle and uses this to bring the upper leg/hip into internal rotation, taking out all the slack in piriformis.

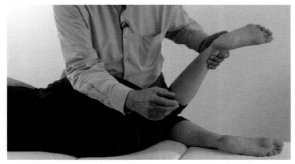

Fig. 6.22 A combined ischaemic compression (elbow pressure) and muscle energy technique side-lying treatment of piriformis. The pressure is alternated with isometric contractions/stretching of the muscle until no further gain is achieved.

- A degree of inhibitory pressure (sufficient to cause discomfort but not pain) is applied via the elbow for approximately 5 seconds while the muscle is kept at a reasonable but not excessive degree of stretch.
- The practitioner maintains contact on the point, but eases pressure, and asks the patient to introduce an isometric contraction (25% of strength for approximately 5 seconds) to piriformis, by bringing the lower leg towards the table, against resistance.
- The same acute and chronic rules as discussed previously are employed, together with cooperative breathing if appropriate (see Box 6.2).
- After the isometric contraction ceases, and the patient relaxes, the lower limb is taken to its new resistance barrier and elbow pressure is reapplied.
- This process is repeated until no further gain is achieved, commonly after 4 to 5 repetitions.

7. Assessment and Treatment of Quadratus Lumborum (10) (See Also Box 6.8)

QL is a very important muscle in relation to spinal and pelvic mechanics, directly linking the pelvis with the spine and diaphragm (Bergmark, 1989). Fryer (2000) observes:

Asymmetries in lumbo-pelvic rhythm, leg length, scoliosis, hip flexion, sacroiliac joint anatomy, hamstring, piriformis and quadratus lumborum muscle length [all] have a profound effect on pelvic symmetry during forward flexion.

QL is a postural muscle with a tendency to 'tightness, hypertonia and shortening' when overused or stressed (Janda, 1968). It is suggested that the reader reviews Janda's (1996) Observation assessment – hip abduction test, described earlier in this chapter (see Fig. 6.16).

Quadratus Lumborum Test A (Fig. 6.23, See Also Fig. 6.16)

- The patient is side-lying and is asked to take the upper arm over the head to grasp the top edge of the table, 'opening out' the lumbar area.
- The practitioner stands facing the back of the patient and has easy access for palpation of QLs lateral border – a major trigger point site (Travell & Simons, 1992) – with the cephalad hand.
- Activity of quadratus is tested (palpated for) with the cephalad hand as the leg is abducted, while also

BOX 6.8   Notes on Quadratus Lumborum

Norris (2000) describes the divided roles in which quadratus is involved:

- The quadratus lumborum has been shown to be significant as a stabiliser in lumbar spine movements (McGill et al., 1996), while tightening has also been described (Janda, 1983). It seems likely that the muscle may act functionally differently in its medial and lateral portions, with the medial portion being more active as a stabiliser of the lumbar spine, and the lateral more active as a mobiliser (see stabiliser/mobiliser discussion, Chapter 2). Such sub-division is seen in a number of other muscles, for example the gluteus medius, where the posterior fibres are more posturally involved (Jull, 1994); the internal oblique, where the posterior fibres attaching to the lateral raphe are considered stabilisers (Bergmark, 1989); and the external oblique, where the lateral fibres work during flexion in parallel to the rectus abdominis (Kendall et al., 1993).
- Janda (1983) observes that, when the patient is side-bending (as in method B) 'when the lumbar spine appears straight, with compensatory motion occurring only from the thoracolumbar region upwards, tightness of quadratus lumborum may be suspected'. This 'whole lumbar spine' involvement differs from a segmental restriction which would probably involve only a part of the lumbar spine.
- Quadratus fibres merge with the diaphragm (as do those of psoas), which makes involvement in respiratory dysfunction a possibility since it plays a role in exhalation, both via this merging and by its attachment to the 12th rib.
- Shortness of quadratus, or the presence of trigger points, can result in pain in the lower ribs and along the iliac crest if the lateral fibres are affected.
- Shortness of the medial fibres, or the presence of trigger points, can produce pain in the sacroiliac joint and the buttock.

- Bilateral contraction produces extension and unilateral contraction produces extension and side-bending to the same side.
- The important transition region, the lumbodorsal junction (LDJ), is the only one in the spine in which two mobile structures meet, and dysfunction results in alteration of the quality of motion between these structures (upper and lower trunk/dorsal and lumbar spines). In dysfunction there is often a degree of spasm or tightness in the muscles which stabilise the region, notably: psoas and erector spinae of the thoracolumbar region, as well as quadratus lumborum and rectus abdominis.
- Symptomatic differential diagnosis of muscle involvement at the LDJ is possible as follows:
  - psoas involvement usually triggers abdominal pain if severe and produces flexion of the hip and the typical antalgesic posture of lumbago
  - erector spinae involvement produces low-back pain at its caudad end of attachment and interscapular pain at its thoracic attachment (as far up as the mid-thoracic level)
  - quadratus lumborum involvement causes lumbar pain and pain at the attachment of the iliac crest and lower ribs
  - rectus abdominis contraction may mimic abdominal pain and result in pain at the attachments at the pubic symphysis and the xiphoid process, as well as forward-bending of the trunk and restricted ability to extend the spine.
- There is seldom pain at the site of the lesion in LDJ dysfunction. Lewit (1992) points out that even if a number of these muscles are implicated, it is seldom necessary, using postisometric relaxation methods, to treat them all since, as the muscles most involved (discovered by tests for shortness, overactivity, sensitivity and direct palpation) are stretched and normalised, so will others begin automatically to normalise.

palpating gluteus medius (and TFL) with the caudad hand.

- If the muscles act simultaneously, or if quadratus fires first, then it is stressed, probably short, and will benefit from stretching.
- When the leg of the side-lying patient is abducted, and the practitioner's palpating hand senses that quadratus becomes actively involved in this process before the leg has reached at least 25 degrees of elevation, then quadratus is probably overactive.

- If quadratus has been overactive for any length of time, then it is almost certainly hypertonic and short, and a need for MET can be assumed.

Quadratus Lumborum Test B

- The patient stands, back towards crouching practitioner.
- Any leg length disparity (based on pelvic crest height) is equalised by using a book or pad under the short-leg-side heel.

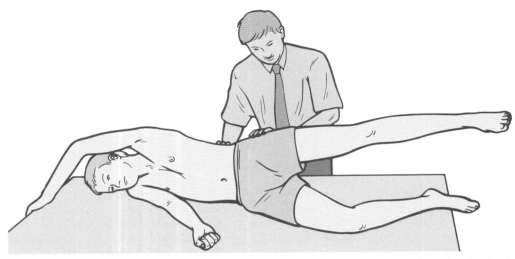

Fig. 6.23 Palpation assessment for quadratus lumborum overactivity. The muscle is palpated, as is gluteus medius, during abduction of the leg. The correct firing sequence should be gluteus, followed at around 25 degrees elevation by quadratus. If there is an immediate 'grabbing' action by quadratus it indicates overactivity, and therefore stress, so shortness can be assumed (see details of similar functional assessments in this chapter).

- With the patient's feet shoulder-width apart, a pure side-bending is requested so that the patient runs a hand down the lateral thigh/calf. (Normal level of side-bending excursion allows the fingertips to reach to just below the knee.)
- The side to which the fingertips travel furthest is assessed.
- If side-bending to one side is limited, then quadratus on the opposite side is probably short.
- Combined evidence from palpation (test A) and this side-bending test indicate whether or not it is necessary to treat quadratus.

▶ Treatment of Shortened QL

Method A. MET for shortness in quadratus lumborum ('banana') (Fig. 6.24).
- The patient lies supine with the feet crossed (the side to be treated crossed under the non-treated-side leg) at the ankle.
- The patient is arranged in a light side-bend, away from the side to be treated so that the pelvis is towards that side and the feet and head away from that side ('banana-shaped').
- As this side-bend is being achieved, the lateral border of the affected quadratus can be palpated for bind so that the barrier is correctly identified.

- The patient's heels are placed just off the side of the table, anchoring the lower extremities and pelvis.
- The patient places the arm of the side to be treated behind their neck as the practitioner, standing on the side opposite that being treated, slides their cephalad hand under the patient's shoulders to reach the treated-side axilla.
- The patient grasps the practitioner's cephalad arm at the elbow, with the treated-side hand, making the contact more secure.
- The patient's non-treated-side hand should be interlocked with the practitioner's cephalad hand.
- The patient's treated-side elbow should, at this stage, be pointing superiorly.
- The practitioner's caudad hand is placed on the ASIS, on the side to be treated.
- The patient is instructed to very lightly side-bend towards the treated side.
- This produces an isometric contraction in QL on the side being treated.
- After 5 seconds the patient is asked to relax completely, *to inhale* (QL fires on exhalation) and to simultaneously side-bend towards the non-treated side, as the practitioner transfers their body weight from the cephalad leg to the caudad leg and leans backwards slightly, to assist in side-bending the patient.

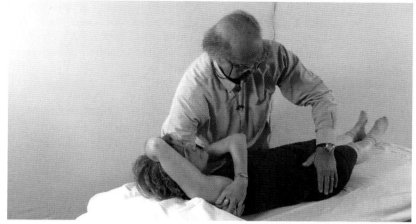

Fig. 6.24 Muscle energy technique treatment of quadratus lumborum utilising 'banana' position.

- This effectively stretches QL. The stretch is held for up to 30 seconds, allowing a lengthening of shortened musculature in the region, including QL.
- Repeat as necessary.

Method B. Quadratus lumborum side-lying MET (Fig. 6.25).

- The practitioner stands behind the side-lying patient, at waist level.

- The patient has the uppermost arm extended over the head to firmly grasp the top end of the table and, on an inhalation, abducts the uppermost leg until the practitioner palpates quadratus activity (elevation of around 30 degrees usually).
- The patient holds the leg (and, if appropriate, the breath, see Box 6.2) isometrically in this manner, allowing gravity to provide resistance.

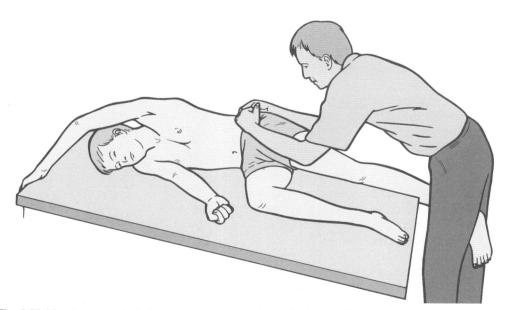

Fig. 6.25 Muscle energy technique treatment of quadratus lumborum. Note that it is important after the isometric contraction (sustained raised/abducted leg) that the muscle be eased into stretch, avoiding any defensive or protective resistance which sudden movement might produce. For this reason, body weight rather than arm strength should be used to apply traction.

- After the 10-second (or so) contraction, the patient allows the leg to fall towards the floor, slightly behind them over the back of the table.
- The practitioner straddles this leg (to stabilise its position) and, cradling the pelvis with both hands (fingers interlocked over the crest of the pelvis), leans back to take out all slack of the soft tissues, including quadratus, easing the pelvis away from the lower ribs, *during an inhalation.*
- This stretch should be held for between 10 and 30 seconds.
- The method will be more successful if the patient is grasping the top edge of the table, thus providing a fixed point from which the practitioner can induce stretch (see Fig. 6.25).
- Contraction followed by stretch is repeated once or twice more with the leg raised in front of the trunk, and once or twice with raised leg behind the trunk in order to activate, and subsequently stretch different quadratus fibres. This calls for the practitioner changing from the back to the front of the table for the best results.
- When the leg hangs to the back of the trunk the long fibres of the muscle are mainly affected; and when the leg hangs forward of the body the diagonal fibres are mainly involved.
- The direction of stretch should be varied so that it is always in the same direction as the long axis of the abducted leg.

Method C. Quadratus lumborum gravity-induced MET – self-treatment.

- The patient stands, legs apart, bending sideways.
- The patient inhales and slightly raises the trunk (a few centimetres) at the same time as looking (moving the eyes only) away from the side to which side flexion is taking place.
- *On an inhalation,* the side-bend is allowed to slowly go further to its elastic limit, while the patient looks towards the floor, in the direction of the side flexion. (Care is needed that very little, if any, forward or backward bending is taking place at this time.)
- This sequence is repeated a number of times.

Eye positions (visual synkinesis) influence the tendency to flex and side-bend (eyes look down) and extend (eyes look up) (Lewit, 1999).

Gravity-induced stretches of this sort require holding the stretch position for at least as long as the contraction, and ideally longer. More repetitions may be needed with

a large muscle such as quadratus, and home stretches should be advised several times daily.

Method D. Quadratus lumborum MET. The side-lying treatment of latissimus dorsi described later in this chapter also provides an effective quadratus stretch when the stabilising hand rests on the pelvic crest (Fig. 6.32).

8. Assessment and Treatment of Pectoralis Major (11) and Latissimus Dorsi (12)

Latissimus and Pectoral Test A

Observation can be as accurate as palpation for evidence of pectoralis major shortening. The patient will have a rounded shoulder posture – especially if the clavicular aspect is involved. Or:

- The patient lies supine with upper arms on the table, hands resting palm down on the lower abdomen.
- The practitioner observes from the head and notes whether either shoulder is held in an anterior position (protraction) in relation to the thoracic cage.
- If one or both shoulders are forward of the thorax, pectoralis muscles are short (Fig. 6.26).

Latissimus and Pectoral Test B

- The patient lies supine with the head several feet from the top edge of the table and is asked to rest the arms, extended above the head, on the treatment surface, palms upwards (Fig. 6.27).

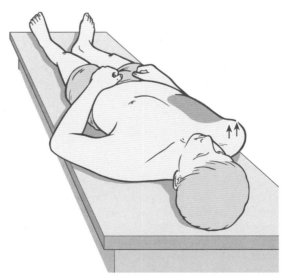

Fig. 6.26 Observation assessment in which pectoral shortness on the right is suggested by the inability of the shoulder to rest on the table.

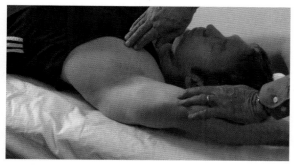

Fig. 6.27 Assessment of shortness in pectoralis major and latissimus dorsi. Visual assessment is used: if the arm on the tested side is unable to rest along its full length, shortness of pectoralis major is probable; if there is obvious deviation of the elbow laterally, probable latissimus shortening is indicated.

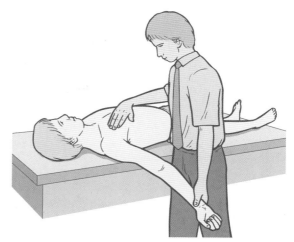

Fig. 6.28 Palpation assessment for shortness of subclavicular portion of pectoralis major.

- If these muscles are normal, the arms should be able to easily reach the horizontal when directly above the shoulders, and also to be in contact with the surface for almost all of the length of the upper arms, with no arching of the back or twisting of the thorax.
- If either arm cannot reach the vertical above the shoulder, but is held laterally, elbow pulled outwards, then latissimus dorsi is probably short on that side. If an arm cannot rest with the dorsum of the upper arm in contact with the table surface without effort, then pectoral fibres are almost certainly short.

Assessment of Shortness in Pectoralis Major (Fig. 6.28)

- Assessment of the subclavicular portion of pectoralis major involves abduction of the arm to 90 degrees (Lewit, 1985b).
- In this position, the tendon of pectoralis major at the sternum should not be found to be unduly tense, even with maximum abduction of the arm, unless the muscle is shortened.
- For assessment of sternal attachment, the arm is brought into elevation and abduction, as the muscle, as well as the tendon on the greater tubercle of the humerus, is palpated.
- If the sternal fibres have shortened, tautness will be visible and tenderness of the tissues under palpation will be reported.

Assessment for Strength of Pectoralis Major

- The patient is supine with arm in abduction at the shoulder joint, and medially rotated (palm is facing down) with the elbow extended.

- The practitioner stands at the head and secures the opposite shoulder with one hand to prevent any trunk torsion and contacts the dorsum of the distal humerus, on the tested side, with the other hand.
- The patient attempts to lift the arm and to adduct it across the chest, against resistance, as strength is assessed in the sternal fibres.
- Different arm positions can be used to assess clavicular and costal fibres. For example:
  - with an angle of abduction/elevation of 135 degrees costal and abdominal fibres will be involved
  - with abduction/elevation of 45 degrees the clavicular fibres will be assessed.
- The practitioner should palpate to ensure that the 'correct' fibres contract when assessments are being made.
- If this postural muscle tests as weak, it may be useful to use Norris's (1999) approach of strengthening it by application of a slow eccentric isotonic contraction, before proceeding to an MET stretching procedure – see Method D below.

Method A. MET Treatment of Short Pectoralis Major (Fig. 6.29A and B)

- The patient lies supine with the arm abducted in a direction which produces the most marked evidence of pectoral shortness (assessed by palpation and visual evidence of the particular fibres involved, as described in tests above).

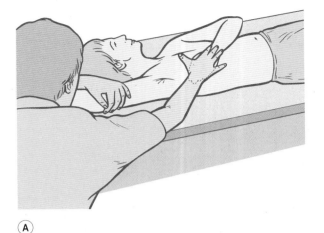

(A)

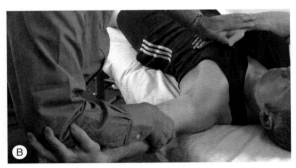

(B)

Fig. 6.29 (A) Muscle energy technique treatment of pectoral muscle – abdominal attachment. Note that the fibres being treated are those which lie in line with the long axis of the humerus. (B) An alternative hold for application of muscle energy technique to pectoral muscle – sternal attachment. Note that the patient needs to be close to the edge of the table to allow the arm to be taken towards the floor once the slack has been removed, during the stretching phase after the isometric contraction.

- The more elevated the arm (i.e. the closer to the head), the more focus there will be on costal and abdominal fibres.
- With a lesser degree of abduction (to around 45 degrees), the focus is more on the clavicular fibres.
- Between these two extremes lies the position which influences the sternal fibres most directly.
- The patient lies as close to the side of the table as possible so that the abducted arm can be brought below the horizontal level to apply gravitational pull and passive stretch to the fibres, as appropriate.
- The practitioner stands on the side to be treated and grasps the humerus.

- A useful arm hold, which depends upon the relative size of the patient and the practitioner, involves the practitioner grasping the anterior aspect of the patient's flexed upper arm just above the elbow, while the patient cups the practitioner's elbow and holds this contact throughout the procedure (see Fig. 6.29B).
- *The patient's hand is placed on the contact (attachments of shortened fibres) area* on the thorax so that their hand acts as a 'cushion'. This is more physically comfortable and also prevents physical contact with emotionally sensitive areas such as breast tissue.
- The practitioner's thenar or hyperthenar eminence is placed over the patient's 'cushion' hand to stabilise the area during the contraction and stretch, preventing movement of it.
- Commencing with the patient's arm in a position which takes the affected fibres to just short of their restriction barrier (for a chronic problem), the patient introduces a light contraction (20% of strength) involving adduction against resistance from the practitioner, for 5 to 7 seconds.
- As a rule, the long axis of the patient's upper arm should be in a straight line with the fibres being treated.
- If a trigger point has previously been identified in pectoralis, the practitioner should ensure – by means of palpation if necessary, or by observation – that the fibres housing the trigger point(s) are involved in the contraction.
- As the patient exhales following complete relaxation of the area, a stretch through the new barrier is activated by the patient and maintained by the practitioner.
- Stretch is achieved via the positioning and leverage of the arm, while the contact hand on the thorax acts as a stabilising point only.
- *There are two distinct phases to the stretch and these need to be carefully achieved to avoid irritation of the shoulder.*
- The stretch needs to be one in which the arm is first pulled away (distracted) from the thorax, with the patient's assistance ('ease your arm away from your shoulder'), before the stretch is introduced. If the patient grasps the practitioner's elbow effectively, this distraction (to 'take out the slack') is achieved by a simple lean backwards by the practitioner.
- The stretch itself is then introduced, and this involves the humerus being taken carefully and slowly below

the horizontal, achieved by means of the practitioner lowering their centre of gravity (bending the knees).

- During the stretching phase it is essential for the entire thorax to be stabilised and the practitioner needs to be very sensitive to the point at which the muscle's end-of-range (length) barrier is engaged. No rolling or twisting of the thorax in the direction of the stretch should be permitted.

- **To recapitulate**: *There are two phases of the stretching procedure, the first in which slack is removed by distracting the arm away from the contact/stabilising hand on the thorax, and the second involving movement of the arm towards the floor, initiated by the practitioner bending their knees.*

- Stretching (after an isometric contraction) should be repeated once or twice in each position, so involving different pectoral fibres.

- All attachments should be treated, which calls for the use of different arm positions, as discussed above, each with different stabilising ('cushion') contacts as the various fibre directions and attachments are isolated.

Method B. Pectoralis Major MET (Fig. 6.30)

- The patient lies supine close to the edge of the table on the side to be treated.

- The treated-side arm is taken into 90 degrees of abduction at the shoulder and the elbow is flexed to 90 degrees.

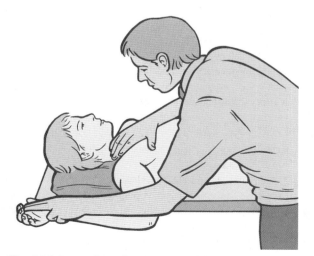

Fig. 6.30 Pectoralis major muscle energy technique stretch. (Redrawn with permission from Kostopoulos & Rizopoulos, 2001.)

- The practitioner stands at waist level facing the head of the table.

- The practitioner's table-side hand is placed on the anterior shoulder area, holding this to the table throughout the procedure.

- The practitioner's non-table-side hand holds the ventral surface of the patient's wrist, with their forearm in contact along the length of the patient's forearm to provide a firm contact.

- The patient is asked to use no more than 20% of available strength to attempt adducting the arm, pressing it against the resistance offered by the practitioner's arm, for 5 to 7 seconds.

- On an exhalation the practitioner eases the arm into greater horizontal abduction, stretching pectoralis major.

- This is held for 30 seconds, before relaxing the stretch, repeating the contraction and stretching again.

Method C. Slow Eccentric Isometric Contraction MET Treatment of Pectoralis Major

- The patient lies supine with the arm abducted in a direction which produces the most marked evidence of pectoral shortness (assessed by palpation and visual evidence of the particular fibres involved, as described in the assessment tests above).

- The patient is asked to maintain the arm in extension and adduction, at the resistance barrier, as the practitioner slowly eases (forces) it into flexion and abduction (taking the arm across the chest), so slowly isotonically stretching the antagonists to pectoralis major (such as – depending on the arm position – latissimus dorsi).

- After this, the arm is replaced at the barrier and the stretching procedure described in method A is used to lengthen pectoralis major.

  MET treatment of short pectoralis minor (Fig. 6.31).

- If there is evidence of shoulder protraction, pectoralis minor is probably short, and this should be addressed.

- The patient is side-lying, arms are lightly folded across the lower thorax, with the side to be treated uppermost, and the practitioner standing behind the patient, close to the edge of the table.

- The practitioner threads their caudad arm anterior to the patient's elbow so that their caudad hand rests on pectoralis minor, with their other hand on the scapula.

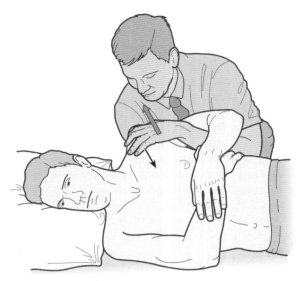

Fig. 6.31 The practitioner uses retraction of the scapula together with contact hand on pectoralis minor to introduce stretch following an isometric contraction.

- Posteriorly directed pressure is gradually applied to the shoulder to induce retraction, coupled with a guiding effort from the hand on the scapula.
- If the shoulder cannot be easily placed in its correct anatomical position, suggesting tension/shortness of pectoralis minor, the patient is asked to lightly push the shoulder anteriorly, against the restraining hand of the practitioner, for 7 to 10 seconds.
- After this, slack is taken out of the muscle and a small degree of stretch is induced for between 5 and 30 seconds. Repeat once or twice more.

Latissimus Dorsi (12) Test For Shortness

- To screen latissimus dorsi, the standing patient is asked to bend forward and allow the arms to hang freely from the shoulders they hold a half-bend position, trunk parallel to the floor.
- If the arms are hanging other than perpendicular to the floor, there is probably some muscular restriction involved, and if this involves latissimus the arms will be held closer to the legs than perpendicular (if they hang markedly forward of such a position then trapezius shortening is probable, see below).
- To further screen latissimus in this position, one side at a time, the practitioner stands in front of the patient (who remains in this half-bend position) and,

stabilising the scapula area with one hand, grasps the arm at elbow level and gently draws the tested side (straight) arm forwards.
- It should, without undue effort or excessive bind in the tissues being held, allow itself to be taken to a position where the elbow is higher than the level of the back of the head.
- If this is not possible, then latissimus is short on that side.

Method A. MET Treatment of Shortened Latissimus Dorsi

NOTE: The positioning for this method is virtually identical to that described for treatment of QL earlier and illustrated in Fig. 6.24.

- The patient lies supine with the feet crossed (the side to be treated crossed under the non-treated-side leg at the ankle).
- The patient is arranged in a light side-bend away from the side to be treated so that the pelvis is towards that side, and the feet and head away from that side.
- The heels are placed just off the edge of the table, so anchoring the lower extremities.
- The patient places their arm on the side to be treated behind their neck, as the practitioner, standing on the side opposite that to be treated, slides their cephalad hand under the patient's shoulders to grasp the treated-side axilla.
- The patient grasps the practitioner's cephalad arm at the elbow, making this contact more secure. The patient's treated-side elbow should point superiorly.
- The patient's non-treated-side hand should be interlocked with the practitioner's cephalad hand.
- The practitioner's caudad hand is placed on the ASIS on the side being treated, and the patient is instructed to very lightly take the pointed elbow towards the sacrum and also to lightly try to bend backwards and towards the treated side. This should produce a light isometric contraction in latissimus dorsi on the side to be treated.
- After 5 to 7 seconds the patient is asked to relax completely as the practitioner transfers their body weight from the cephalad leg to the caudad leg, to side-bend the patient further while simultaneously standing more erect and leaning in a caudad direction.
- This effectively lifts the patient's thorax from the table surface and introduces a stretch into latissimus (especially if the patient has maintained a grasp on

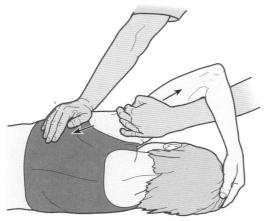

Fig. 6.32 Treatment of latissimus dorsi. A variety of different positions are required for the stabilising hand (on the chest wall, or even as far as the crest of the pelvis) to allow for precise application of stretches of fibres with different attachments, following the sequence of isometric contractions.

the practitioner's elbow and the practitioner has a firm hold on the patient's axilla).

- This stretch is held for 5 to 30 seconds allowing a lengthening of shortened musculature in the region.
- Repeat at least once more.

Method B. MET of Shortened Latissimus Dorsi (see Fig. 6.32)

- The patient is side-lying, affected side up.
- The arm is taken into abduction to the point of resistance, with the elbow flexed and patient's hand resting on their head.
- It should be possible to visualise, or palpate, the attachment of the shortened fibres on the lateral and posterior thorax.
- The muscle is treated in either the acute or chronic mode of MET, close to – or short of – the restriction barrier, as appropriate.
- As shown in Fig. 6.32, the practitioner stands near the head of the patient, and depending on the fibres to be stretched, slightly behind, at the head of, or slightly in front of, the patient.
- The practitioner holds the patient's upper arm as shown in Fig. 6.32, while using the other hand to stabilise the posterior thorax area, or the pelvic crest.[5]

---

[5]When the contact/stabilising hand is on the crest of the pelvis, the stretch using the arm as a lever will effectively also stretch quadratus lumborum.

- A build-up of tension should be palpated under the stabilising hand as the patient introduces an isometric contraction by attempting to bring their arm back towards the side against firm resistance, using only a modest amount of effort (20%).
- After 5 to 7 seconds, the effort should be released as the patient relaxes completely, at which time the practitioner takes out available slack and – if a chronic condition – introduces stretch through, the restriction barrier, bringing the humerus into greater adduction, while applying a stabilising contact on the trunk, anywhere between the lateral chest wall and the crest of the pelvis.
- A downward movement of the humerus, towards the floor, assists the stretch following a separation of the practitioner's two contact hands to remove all slack.
- As in the stretch of pectoralis major described above (method A), there should be two phases – a distraction, taking out the slack, and a movement towards the floor by the practitioner, flexing the knees, to induce a safe stretch.
- Repeat as necessary.

Latissimus should be retested following stretching to evaluate the degree of improvement.

9. Assessment and Treatment of Upper Trapezius (13)

Lewit (1999) simplifies the need to assess for shortness of this muscle, by stating, 'The upper trapezius should be treated if tender and taut'. Since this is an almost universal state in modern life, it seems that everyone requires MET application to this muscle. Lewit also notes that a characteristic mounding of the muscle can often be observed when it is very short, producing the effect of 'Gothic shoulders', similar to the architectural supports of a Gothic church tower.

Upper Trapezius Shortness Test A (Fig. 6.33)

Greenman (1996) describes a functional 'firing sequence' assessment that identifies general imbalance and dysfunction involving the upper and lower fixators of the shoulder (see Fig. 6.33).

- The patient is seated and the practitioner stands behind.
- The practitioner rests their right hand over the right shoulder area to assess the firing sequence of muscles during shoulder abduction.

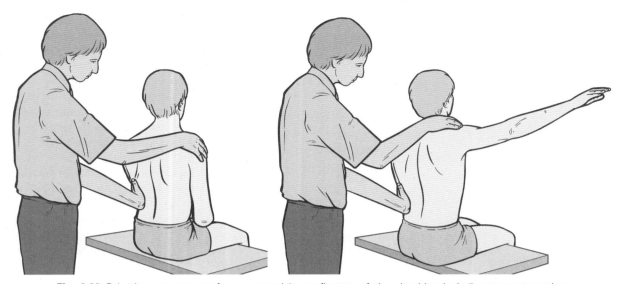

Fig. 6.33 Palpation assessment for upper and lower fixators of the shoulder, including upper trapezius. (Greenman, 1996).

- The other hand can be placed either on the mid-thoracic region, mainly on the side being assessed, or spanning the lower back to palpate quadratus firing.
- The assessment should be performed several times so that various hand contacts are used to evaluate the behaviour of different muscles during abduction.

Greenman (1996) bases his findings on the work of Janda (1983), who described the 'correct' sequence for shoulder abduction, when seated, as involving:

1. Supraspinatus
2. Deltoid
3. Infraspinatus
4. Middle and lower trapezius
5. Contralateral quadratus.

In dysfunctional states the most common substitutions are said to involve shoulder elevation by *levator scapulae and upper trapezius,* as well as early firing by *quadratus lumborum, ipsilateral and contralateral.*

As explained by Janda, abduction of the arm, in this position, should not employ upper trapezius as a prime mover, although it does increase in tone during the procedure.

Inappropriate activity of any of the upper fixators results in a tendency to shorten. When overactivity involves the lower fixators of the shoulder/scapula, weakness and possible lengthening results (Norris, 1999).

See Chapter 2 for discussion of postural/phasic, etc. muscle characteristics.

Upper Trapezius Shortness Test B

- The patient is seated and the practitioner stands behind with one hand resting on the shoulder of the side to be tested, stabilising it.
- The other hand is placed on the ipsilateral side of the head as the head/neck is taken into contralateral side-bending without force, while the shoulder is stabilised (Fig. 6.34).
- The same procedure is performed on the other side with the opposite shoulder stabilised.
- A comparison is made as to which side-bending manoeuvre produced the greater range, and whether the neck can easily reach 40 degrees of side flexion in each direction, which it should.
- If neither side can achieve this degree of side-bending, then both trapezius muscles are probably short.
- The relative shortness of one, compared with the other, is evaluated.

NOTE 1: When the shoulder *towards which* the head is being side-bent is being stabilised, the assessment is of the mobility of the cervical structures. By stabilising the side *from which* the bend is occurring, the muscular component is being evaluated (see Fig. 6.34).

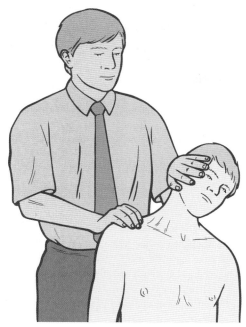

Fig. 6.34 Assessment of the relative shortness of the right-side upper trapezius. One side is compared with the other (for both the range of unforced motion and the nature of the end-feel of motion) to ascertain the side most in need of muscle energy technique attention.

NOTE 2: The range of side flexion motion has been studied in both symptomatic and asymptomatic individuals (Bush et al., 2010).

The average composite ranges of motion were asymptomatic 40.0 degrees and asymptomatic 33.2 degrees. The aging factor predisposed the symptomatic group [average age 32 years, asymptomatic 22.2 years] to various compromising conditions, including tissue changes (e.g. loss of series elastic component, that result in decreased range of motion).

NOTE 3: Gemmell and Dunford (2007) have evaluated cervical ranges of motion, as well as pain symptoms, in amateur rugby players – comparing forwards with backs. They found that:

there was an 83% prevalence of neck pain in forwards, compared to 41% prevalence for backs [and] a decreased cervical range in motion was present for all of the backs and forwards.

The information deriving from these studies (Bush et al., 2010; Gemmell & Dunford, 2007) should be kept in mind during assessment of cervical ranges of motion, as described in upper trapezius shortness tests B and C.

Upper Trapezius Shortness Test C

- The patient is supine with the neck fully side-bent contralaterally (away from the side being assessed) *to its easy end-of-range* which should be in the region of 30 to 40 degrees depending on whether the individual has cervical symptoms or not, with age as another potential factor in reduced range (see Notes 2 and 3 above).
- The practitioner is standing at the head of the table and uses a cupped hand contact on the ipsilateral shoulder (i.e. on the side being tested) to assess the ease with which it can be depressed (moved caudally) (Fig. 6.35A–C for head and neck positions).
- There should be an easy 'springing' sensation as the practitioner eases the shoulder towards the feet, with a *soft* end-feel to the movement.
- If depression of the shoulder is difficult or if there is a *hard,* sudden end-point, upper trapezius shortness is confirmed, particularly if the side-flexion range is limited.
- This same assessment (always with full lateral flexion) should be performed with the head fully rotated away from the side being tested, half turned away from the side being tested, and slightly turned *towards* the side being tested, to assess the relative shortness and functional efficiency respectively of posterior, middle and anterior subdivisions of the upper portion of upper trapezius.

Method A. MET Treatment of Chronically Shortened Upper Trapezius (See Fig. 6.35A–C)

In order to treat all the fibres of upper trapezius, it is the clinical experience of the author that MET should be applied sequentially. In this clinical approach, upper trapezius is arbitrarily subdivided into anterior, middle and posterior fibres. The flexed neck should be placed into three different positions of rotation (full rotation away from side being treated, half rotation away from side being treated, and slight rotation towards side being treated), *always* coupled with full (easy end of range) *side flexion away* from the side being assessed, for treatment of the posterior, middle and anterior fibres, respectively.

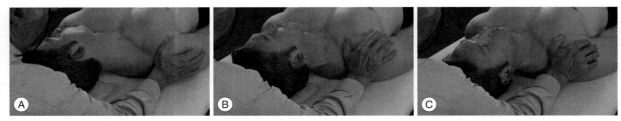

Fig. 6.35 Muscle energy technique treatment of right-side upper trapezius muscle. (A) Posterior fibres, (B) middle fibres, (C) anterior fibres. Note that stretching in this (or any of the alternative positions which access the middle and posterior fibres) is achieved following the isometric contraction by means of an easing of the shoulder away from the stabilised head, with no force being applied to the neck and head itself.

- The patient lies supine, arm on the side to be treated lying alongside the trunk, head/neck side-bent away from the side being treated to just short of the restriction barrier (the *'feather-edge'* of the barrier, see Chapter 2 for explanation), while the practitioner stabilises the shoulder with one hand and supports the cervical spine and the ipsilateral atlanto-occipital area, with the other.
- With the neck slightly flexed or in neutral, depending on patient comfort, and fully side-bent, and *fully rotated contralaterally*, the *posterior* fibres of upper trapezius are involved in the contraction (see below) (Fig. 6.35A).
- This will facilitate subsequent stretching of this aspect of the muscle.
- When the neck is fully side-bent, and *half contralaterally rotated*, the more central ('middle') fibres are involved in the contraction (Fig. 6.35B).
- When the neck is fully side-bent and *slightly rotated towards the side being treated*, the *anterior* fibres of upper trapezius are engaged (Fig. 6.35C).
- The various contractions and subsequent stretches can be performed with practitioner's arms crossed, with hands stabilising the cervical spine and sub-occipital area, as well as the shoulder (see Fig. 6.35).
- The patient introduces a light resisted effort (20% of available strength) to take the stabilised shoulder towards the ear (a semi-shrug movement) and the ear/cervical spine towards the shoulder.
- The double movements (or efforts towards movement) are important to introduce a contraction of the muscle from both ends, simultaneously.
- The degree of effort should be mild and no pain should be felt.

- The contraction should be sustained for 5 to 7 seconds and, upon complete relaxation of effort, the practitioner gently eases the head/neck into an increased degree of side-bending and rotation, where it is stabilised, as the shoulder is stretched caudally *with the patient's active participation*.
- This patient cooperation can easily be achieved by saying something such as: *'as you breathe out please slide your hand gently towards your feet'*. The practitioner then follows the patient's effort – rather than initiating the stretch, to just beyond the new barrier.
- Patient participation in the stretch reduces the chances of a stretch reflex being initiated.
- Once the muscle is in a stretched position, the patient relaxes and the stretch is held for up to 30 seconds.

> **! CAUTION**
>
> No stretch should be introduced from the cranial/cervical end of the muscle, as this could stress the neck. The head is stabilised at its side-flexion and rotation barrier.

Disagreement: There is some disagreement as to the head/neck rotation position as described in the treatment method above, which calls for side-bending and rotation away from the affected side to engage posterior and middle fibres:

- Liebenson (1996) suggests that the patient should 'lie supine with the head supported in anteflexion and laterally flexed away and rotated towards the side of involvement'.
- Lewit (1985b) suggests: 'The patient is supine... the therapist fixes the shoulder from above with one

hand, side-bending the head and neck with the other hand so as to take up the slack. They then ask the patient to look towards the side away from which the head is bent, resisting the patient's automatic tendency to move towards the side of the lesion'. (This method is described below.)

The author has used method A, described above, with good effect and urges readers to compare these approaches with those of Liebenson and Lewit, and to evaluate results for themselves.

Method B. MET Treatment of Acutely Shortened Upper Trapezius, With Visual Synkinesis

Lewit (1985b) suggests the use of eye movements to facilitate initiation of a contraction before stretching, is an ideal method for *acute problems* in this region.

- The patient is supine, while the practitioner fixes the shoulder and the side-bent (away from the treated side) head and neck at the restriction barrier, and asks the patient to look, *moving the eyes only* (not the head), towards the side away from which the neck is bent.
- This eye movement is maintained, while the practitioner resists the slight isometric contraction this will have created.
- On an exhalation, and complete relaxation, the head/neck is taken to a new barrier and the process repeated – *with no stretching, simply engagement of the new barrier.*
- If the shoulder is brought into the process, this should be firmly resisted as the patient attempts to lightly push it into a shrug, during the isometric contraction phase.
- After a 5- to 7-second contraction, slack should again be removed, as the head and neck are repositioned, before a repetition.

Cervical mobility and MET. Before discussion of MET for key cervical muscles it may be useful to reflect on the suggestion by Fred Mitchell Jr (1998) that:

Treating a joint restriction as if the cause were tight muscle(s) is one approach that makes possible restoration of normal joint motion. Regardless of the cause, MET treatment, based on a 'short muscle' paradigm, is usually effective in eliminating blockage, and restoring normal range of motion, even when the blockage is due to non-muscular factors.

More recently, Burns and Wells (2006) conducted a study to evaluate the usefulness of MET in treatment of cervical restriction (in asymptomatic individuals). They noted that:

the muscle energy procedure was used to lengthen potentially shortened cervical muscles and fascia, to normalize the gross cervical range of motion.

They postulated that:

segmental motion is limited by hypertonic short restrictor muscles and possibly arthroidal locking, and that regional cervical motion restrictions [may be] caused by shortened, hypertonic long restrictor muscles of the cervical spine.

They suggested that by lengthening these larger muscle groups, restoration of gross physiologic ROM in the neck might be achieved, via a combination of reduced hypertonicity, improved articular relationships and reduced joint compression. This hypothesis was confirmed by the outcome of the study that demonstrated: 'a significant increase in overall regional cervical ROM in the treatment group when compared with control subjects'.

Mitchell's hypothesis, that restricted joints would benefit if treatment is focused on the associated soft tissues, appears to be correct. The protocol used in this study is discussed in Chapter 6.

10. Assessment and Treatment of Scalenes (14) (See Also Box 6.9)

Observation of the individual's breathing pattern offers an immediate alert as to the likelihood of scalene dysfunction since the scalenes are *primarily* respiratory muscles, whatever other functions they perform.

- If the individual is prone to upper chest breathing, the scalenes will have shortened and will almost certainly house trigger points. Hudson et al. (2007) have observed that human scalenes are *obligatory* inspiratory muscles that have a greater mechanical advantage than the *accessory* breathing muscle, such as SCM.
- Schleifer et al. (2002) have noted that:

a thoracic breathing pattern… imposes biomechanical stress on the neck/shoulder region due to the

---

BOX 6.9   Notes on Scalenes

- The scalenes are controversial muscles since they seem to be both postural and phasic (Lin et al., 1994), their status being modified by the type(s) of stress to which they are exposed (see Chapter 2 for discussion of adaptation in the evolution of dysfunction).
- Janda (1988) reports that 'spasm and/or trigger points are commonly present in the scalenes as also are weakness and/or inhibition'.
- The attachment sites of the scalene muscles vary, as does their presence. The scalene posterior is sometimes absent, and sometimes blends with the fibres of scalenus medius.
- Scalenus medius is noted to frequently attach to the atlas (Gray, 1995) and sometimes extend to the second rib (Simons et al., 1999).
- Scalenus minimus (pleuralis), which attaches to the pleural dome, is present in one-third (Platzer, 1992) to three-quarters (Simons et al., 1999) of people, on at

least one side and, when absent, is replaced by a transverse cupular ligament (Platzer, 1992).
- The brachial plexus exits the cervical column between the scalenus anterior and medius. These, together with the first rib, form the scalene hiatus (also called the 'scalene opening' or 'posterior scalene aperture') (Platzer, 1992). It is through this opening that the brachial plexus and vascular structures for the upper extremity pass. When scalene fibres are taut, they may entrap the nerves (scalenus anticus syndrome) or crowd the 1st rib against the clavicle and indirectly impinge on the vascular, or neurologic, structures (compromising of both neural and vascular structures is rare) (Stedman, 1998). Any of these conditions may be diagnosed as 'thoracic outlet syndrome', 'a collective title for a number of conditions attributed to compromised blood vessels or nerve fibers (brachial plexus) at any point between the base of the neck and the axilla' (Stedman, 1998).

---

ancillary recruitment of sternocleidomastoid, scalene, and trapezius muscles in support of thoracic breathing.

- Masubuchi et al. (2001) used fine-wire electrodes inserted into muscles, and high-resolution ultrasound, to identify the activity of three muscle groups, in response to various respiratory and postural manoeuvres. They concluded that the scalenes are the most active, and trapezius the least active, cervical accessory inspiratory muscles, while SCM is intermediate.
- Scalene dysfunction and the presence of trigger points ('functional pathology') were identified in more than 50% of individuals, in a series of 46 hospitalised patients who demonstrated paradoxical (i.e. upper chest rather than diaphragmatic) patterns of respiration. A combination of MET ('postisometric relaxation') and self-stretching of the scalenes was used during rehabilitation (Pleidelová et al., 2002).

Assessment A: Scalene Observation – The Paradoxical Breathing Assessment

During the history-taking interview, the patient can be asked to place one hand on the abdomen just above the umbilicus, and the other flat against the upper chest (Fig. 6.36).

On inhalation, the hands are observed and if the upper hand moves first during inhalation, particularly if it rises

significantly towards the chin, rather than moving slightly anteriorly, a pattern of upper chest breathing can be assumed, and therefore stress, and therefore shortness of the scalenes, as well as other accessory breathing muscles, notably SCM. See notes below, regarding the influence of exhalation on SCM, during a functional test.

Assessment B: Scalene Functional Observation and Palpation

There is no easy test for shortness of the scalenes apart from observation, palpation and assessment of trigger point activity/tautness. However, a functional observation may prove useful.

- In most people who have marked scalene shortness there is commonly a tendency to overuse these (and other upper fixators of the shoulder and neck) as accessory breathing muscles (Peper & Tibbetts, 1992; Middaugh et al., 1994; Hudson et al., 2007; Schleifer et al., 2002).
- There may also be a tendency to hyperventilation (with a possible history of anxiety, phobic behaviour, panic attacks and/or fatigue symptoms) (Goldstein, 1996).
- These muscles seem to be excessively tense in many people with chronic fatigue and anxiety symptoms (George, 1964).

Observation assessment consists of the practitioner placing their relaxed hands over the patient's shoulders

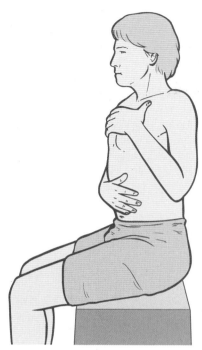

Fig. 6.36 Observation assessment of respiratory function. Any tendency for the upper hand to move cephalad, or earlier than the caudad hand, suggests scalene overactivity.

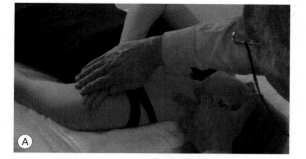

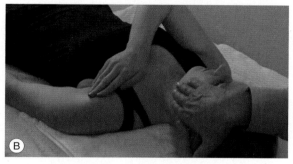

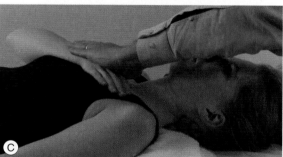

so that the fingertips rest on the clavicles, at which time the seated patient is asked to inhale moderately. If the practitioner's hands noticeably rise towards the patient's ears during such inhalation, then there exists inappropriate overuse of the scalenes, indicating that they are stressed, which also means that, by definition, they will probably have shortened and would benefit from some form of stretching (as well as breathing rehabilitation!).

MET Treatment of Short Scalenes (Fig. 6.37A–C)

- The patient lies supine with a cushion or folded towel under the upper thoracic area so that, unless supported by the practitioner's contralateral hand, the head would fall into extension.
- The head is rotated contralaterally (away from the side to be treated).
- There are three positions of rotation required, all with the head/neck in slight extension:
  1. Full contralateral rotation, and side flexion, of the head/neck produces involvement of the posterior scalene muscle.

Fig. 6.37 (A) Muscle energy technique for scalenus posticus. On stretching, following the isometric contraction, the neck is allowed to move into slight extension while a mild stretch is introduced by the contact hand which rests on the second rib, below the lateral aspect of the clavicle. (B) Muscle energy technique treatment for the middle fibres of scalenes; hand placement (thenar or hypothenar eminence of relaxed hand) is on the second rib below the centre of the clavicle. (C) Muscle energy technique treatment of the anterior fibres of the scalenes; hand placement is on the sternum.

  2. A contralateral 45-degree rotation, and side flexion, of the head/neck involves the middle scalene.
  3. A position of only slight contralateral rotation and side flexion involves the anterior scalene.
- The practitioner's free hand is placed on the side of the patient's face/forehead to restrain the isometric

contraction, which will be used to initiate the release of the scalenes.

- The patient's head/neck is in one of the degrees of rotation mentioned above, supported by the practitioner's contralateral hand.

- The patient is instructed to attempt to lift the forehead a fraction and to attempt to turn the head towards the affected side, resisted by the practitioner's hand to prevent both movements, together with appropriate breathing cooperation ('breathe in and hold your breath as you "lift and turn", and hold this for 5 to 7 seconds').

- Both the effort and the counterpressure should be modest and painless at all times.

- After a 5 to 7-second contraction, the head/neck is placed into extension, and one hand stabilises the neck to prevent movement during the scalene stretch. This hand should ideally be placed so that it restrains ('fixes') that part of the neck to which that aspect of the scalenes attach.

- Previous to the contraction, the thenar eminence of the patient's contralateral hand should have been placed (palm down) just inferior to the lateral end of the affected side clavicle (for full contralateral rotation of the head/neck, for attention to the posterior scalenes).

- The practitioner's hand which was acting to produce resistance to the isometric contraction is now placed onto the dorsum of the patient's 'cushion' hand.

- As the patient slowly exhales, the practitioner's contact hand, resting on the patient's hand, which is itself resting on the upper thorax, pushes obliquely away and towards the ipsilateral foot, following the rib movement into its exhalation position and locking it there, so stretching the attached musculature and fascia.

- This stretch is held for 20 to 30 seconds after each isometric contraction, while the patient breathes normally.

- The process is then repeated at least once more.

- Next, the head is rotated 45 degrees contralaterally and the thenar eminence of the 'cushion' hand contact is placed just inferior to the middle aspect of the clavicle.

- The sequence as described for the posterior scalenes is then repeated for the middle scalenes (and associated musculature and fascia).

- When the head is in the side-flexed and in an almost upright facing position, for treatment of the anterior scalenes, the 'cushion' hand contact rests on the upper sternum itself.

- In all other ways, the methodology is as described for the first position above (with a stretch induced by exhalation, after an isometric contraction, and with the neck being stabilised.)

NOTE: It is important to avoid heroic degrees of neck extension during any phase of this treatment. There should be some extension, but it should be appropriate to the age and condition of the individual.

A degree of eye movement can usefully assist scalene treatment and may be used as an alternative to the 'lift and turn' muscular effort described above, especially in acute conditions where pain and sensitivity demand a gentle approach – for example post-whiplash – where no actual stretching would be introduced, merely isometric contractions to encourage reduced hypertonicity.

If the patient makes the eyes look caudally (towards the feet), and towards the affected side, during the isometric contraction, they will increase the degree of contraction in the muscles. If during the resting phase, when stretch is being introduced, or relaxation of the muscle encouraged, they look away from the treated side, with eyes looking towards the top of the head, this will enhance the efficacy of the procedure (Lewit, 1999).

This whole sequence should be performed bilaterally several times in each of the three head positions.

Scalene stretches, with all their variable positions, clearly also influence many of the other anterior neck structures (such as platysma).

11. Assessment for Shortness of Sternocleidomastoid (15) (See Also Box 6.10)

Assessment for SCM is as for the scalenes – there is no absolute test for shortness but observation of posture (hyperlordotic neck, chin poked forward, upper crossed syndrome (Janda, 1983; Lewit, 1999)) and palpation of the degree of induration, fibrosis and trigger point activity can all alert to probable shortness of SCM. This is an accessory breathing muscle and, as with the scalenes, will be shortened by inappropriate breathing patterns which have become habitual. Observation is an accurate assessment tool.

Since SCM is barely observable when normal, if the clavicular attachment is easily visible, or any part of the muscle is prominent, this can be taken as a clear sign of excessive tightness of the muscle. If the patient's posture involves the head being held forward of the body, often accompanied by cervical lordosis and dorsal kyphosis

BOX 6.10   Notes on Sternocleidomastoid

- Sternocleidomastoid (SCM) is a prominent muscle of the anterior neck and is closely associated with the trapezius. SCM often acts as postural compensator for head tilt associated with postural distortions found elsewhere (e.g. spinal, pelvic or lower extremity functional or structural inadequacies) although they seldom cause restriction of neck movement.
- SCM is synergistic with anterior neck muscles for flexion of the head and flexion of the cervical column on the thoracic column, when the cervical column is already flattened by the prevertebral muscles. However, when the head is placed in extension and SCM contracts, it accentuates lordosis of the cervical column, flexes the cervical column on the thoracic column, and adds to extension of the head. In this way, SCM is both synergist and antagonist to the prevertebral muscles (Kapandji, 1974).
- SCM trigger points are activated by forward head positioning, 'whiplash' injury, positioning of the head to look upwardly for extended periods of time and structural compensations. The two heads of SCM each have their own patterns of trigger point referral which include (among others) into the ear, top of head, into the temporomandibular joint, over the brow, into the throat, and those which cause proprioceptive disturbances, disequilibrium, nausea and dizziness. Tenderness in SCM may be associated with trigger points in the digastric muscle and digastric trigger points may be satellites of SCM trigger points (Simons et al., 1999).
- Simons et al. (1999) report:

  When objects of equal weight are held in the hands, the patient with unilateral trigger point [TrP] involvement of the clavicular division [of SCM] may exhibit an abnormal Weight Test. When asked to judge which is heaviest of two objects of the same weight that look alike but may not be the same weight (two vapocoolant dispensers, one of which may have been used) the patient will [give] evidence [of] dysmetria by underestimating the weight of the object held in the hand on the same side as the affected sternocleidomastoid muscle. Inactivation of the responsible sternocleidomastoid TrPs promptly restores weight appreciation by this test. Apparently, the afferent discharges from these TrPs disturb central processing of proprioceptive information from the upper limb muscles as well as vestibular function related to neck muscles.*

- Lymph nodes lie superficially along the medial aspect of the SCM and may be palpated, especially when enlarged. These nodes may be indicative of chronic cranial infections stemming from a throat infection, dental abscess, sinusitis or tumour. Likewise, trigger points in SCM may be perpetuated by some of these conditions (Simons et al., 1999).
- Lewit (1999) points out that tenderness noted at the medial end of the clavicle and/or at the transverse process of the atlas is often an indication of SCM hypertonicity. This will commonly accompany a forward head position and/or tendency to upper chest breathing, and will almost inevitably be associated with hypertonicity, shortening and trigger point evolution in associated musculature, including scalenes, upper trapezius and levator scapula (see crossed syndrome notes in Chapter 5 box 5.2).

(see notes on upper crossed syndrome in Chapter 5, Box 5.2), weakness of the deep neck flexors and tightness of SCM can be suspected.

Functional SCM Test

- The craniocervical flexion test (CCF-T) evaluates deep cervical flexor status. The supine patient is asked to: 'very slowly raise your head and touch your chin to your chest'.
- The practitioner stands to the side with their eyes at the same level as the patient's head.
- At the beginning of the movement of the head, as the patient lifts this from the table, the practitioner would (if SCM were short) note that the chin was lifted first ('chin poke'), allowing it to jut forwards, rather than the forehead leading the arc-like progression of the movement.
- When shortness of SCM is very marked the chin moves forward in a jerky manner, as the head is lifted. If the reading of this sign is unclear then Janda (1988) suggests that a slight resistance pressure be applied to the forehead, as the patient makes the 'chin to chest' attempt. If SCM is short, this will ensure the jutting of the chin at the outset.

NOTE: The multiple influences on muscle function are highlighted by a study by Cagnie et al. (2008). In a research study the EMG of SCM activity was recorded during normal breathing, as well as during slow expiration. During normal inhalation significantly higher ($P < .05$) EMG activity of the SCM was observed in those individuals who had an upper costal breathing pattern, compared to those with diaphragmatic breathing. During the test, EMG activity of the SCM was lowered when slow exhalation was introduced – leading to a more optimal performance of the test. The request to the patient should therefore be stated in terms such as: 'Slowly breathe out, and as you do so please lift you head and touch your chin to your chest'.

▶ MET Treatment of Shortened SCM (Fig. 6.38)

- The patient is supine with the head supported in a neutral position by one of the practitioner's hands.
- The shoulders rest on a cushion or folded towel so that, when the head is placed on the table, the neck will be in slight extension at which time the degree of extension of the neck should be slight, 10 to 15 degrees at most.
- The patient's contralateral hand rests on the upper aspect of the sternum to act as a cushion when pressure is applied during the stretch phase of the operation (as in scalene and pectoral treatment described above).
- The patient's head is fully but comfortably rotated, contralaterally.
- The patient is asked to lift the fully rotated head a small degree towards the ceiling, and to hold the breath.
- When the head is raised there is no need for the practitioner to apply resistance as gravity effectively provides this.

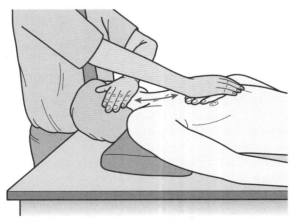

Fig. 6.38 Muscle energy technique of sternocleidomastoid on the right.

- After 5 to 7 seconds of isometric contraction, the patient is asked to slowly release the effort (and the breath) and to place the head (still in rotation) on the table, so that a small degree of extension occurs.
- The practitioner's hand should be placed over the patient's 'cushion' hand (which rests on the sternum) to apply oblique pressure/stretch to the sternum, to ease it away from the head and towards the feet.
- The hand not involved in applying pressure to the sternum caudally should be in contact with the mastoid process in order to gently restrain the tendency the head will have to follow this stretch but *should not under any circumstances apply pressure to stretch the head/neck while it is in this vulnerable position of rotation and slight extension.*
- This stretch of SCM, which is applied as the patient exhales, is maintained for not less than 30 seconds to begin the release/stretch of hypertonic and fibrotic structures.
- Repeat at least once.
- The other side should then be treated in the same manner.

> **! CAUTION**
>
> Care is required, especially with middle-aged and elderly patients, in applying this useful stretching procedure. Appropriate tests should be carried out to evaluate cerebral circulation problems. The presence of such problems indicates that this particular MET method should be avoided as described.

12. Assessment and Treatment of Levator Scapulae (16)
Test A (Spring Test) for Levator Scapula Shortness

- The patient lies supine with the arm of the side to be tested stretched out with the supinated hand and lower arm tucked under the buttocks, to help restrain movement of the shoulder/scapula.
- For the right-side levator scapula, the practitioner's left hand supports the patient's neck and eases it into full flexion, side flexion and rotation, away from the side to be treated.
- The practitioner's right hand is under the patient's shoulder so that the scapula lies against the palm of the hand, the heel of which engages the superior surface of the scapula.

- With the scapula held caudally and the neck/head in the position described (at the resistance barrier), all easily available slack will have been removed from the muscle.
- If dysfunction exists, and/or if levator scapula is short, there will be discomfort reported at the attachment on the upper medial border of the scapula, and/or pain reported near the levator attachment on the spinous process of C2.
- The hand on the scapula should then gently 'spring' it caudally.
- If levator is short there will be a *harsh*, 'blocked' feel to this action.
- If it is normal there will be a soft springing response.

Test B for Levator Scapula Shortness (Observation)

- A functional assessment involves applying the evidence of the imbalances that commonly occur between the upper and lower stabilisers of the scapula.
- In this process, shortness is often noted in pectoralis minor, levator scapulae and upper trapezius (as well as SCM), while weakness develops in serratus anterior, rhomboids, middle and lower trapezius – as well as the deep neck flexors.
- Observation of the patient from behind will often show a 'hollow' area between the shoulder blades, where interscapular weakness has occurred, as well as an increased (above normal) distance between the medial borders of the scapulae and the thoracic spine, if the scapulae have 'winged' away from it.

Test C for Levator Dysfunction

- To see the imbalance described in test B in action, Janda (1996) has the patient in the press-up position.
- On very slow lowering of the chest towards the floor from a maximum push-up position, the scapula(e) on the side(s) where stabilisation has been compromised will move laterally and superiorly – often into a winged position – rather than medially towards the spine.
- This is diagnostic of weak lower stabilisers, which implicates tight upper stabilisers, including levator scapulae, as probably inhibiting them.
- If there is such evidence, then levator scapula will have shortened.

MET Treatment of Levator Scapula (Fig. 6.39)

Treatment of levator scapula using MET enhances the lengthening of the extensor muscles attaching to the occiput and upper cervical spine. The position described below is used for treatment, either at the limit of easily reached ROM or a little short of this, depending upon the degree of acuteness or chronicity of the dysfunction.

- The patient lies supine with the arm of the side to be tested stretched out with the supinated hand and lower arm tucked under the buttocks, to help restrain movement of the shoulder/scapula.
- For the right-side levator scapula, the practitioner's left hand supports the patient's neck and eases it into full flexion, side flexion and rotation, away from the side to be treated.
- The practitioner's right hand is under the patient's shoulder so that the scapula is lying on the hand and

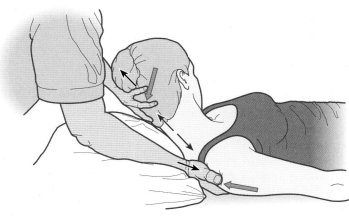

Fig. 6.39 Muscle energy technique test A and treatment position for levator scapula (right side).

its superior border being engaged by the thenar and hyperthenar eminences.

- With the scapula held caudally by the practitioner's hand, and the head/neck in full flexion, side flexion and rotation (each at its resistance barrier), all available slack will have been removed from levator, from both ends.
- The patient is asked to take the head backwards towards the table, and slightly to the side from which it was turned, against the practitioner's unmoving resistance, while at the same time a slight (20% of available strength) shoulder shrug (or superior movement of the scapula) is asked for, and resisted.
- Following the 5- to 7-second isometric contraction and complete relaxation of all elements of this combined contraction, the neck is taken to further flexion, side-bending and rotation, where it is maintained, as the scapula is depressed caudally with the patient's assistance, following the instruction, 'As you breathe out, take your shoulder blade towards your pelvis'.
- The stretch is held for 30 seconds, and the process is repeated at least once.

> **! CAUTION**
> Avoid overstretching this sensitive area.

Facilitation of Tone in Lower Shoulder Fixators Using Pulsed MET (Ruddy, 1962)

Method A. In order to commence rehabilitation and proprioceptive re-education of weakened rhomboids, middle and lower trapezii and serratus anterior:

- The practitioner places a single digit contact very lightly against the lower medial scapula border, on the side of the treated upper trapezius, of the seated or standing patient.
- The patient is asked to attempt to ease the scapula, at the point of digital contact, towards the spine.
- An instruction is given such as: 'Press against my finger with your shoulder blade, towards your spine, just as hard (i.e. very lightly) as I am pressing against your shoulder blade, for less than a second'.
- Once the patient has learned to establish control over the particular muscular action required to achieve this subtle movement (which can take a significant number of attempts), and can do so for 1 second at a time, repetitively, they are ready to begin the sequence based on Ruddy's 'pulsed MET' methodology.

- The patient is told something such as: 'Now that you know how to activate the muscles which push your shoulder blade lightly against my finger, I want you to try to do this 20 times in 10 seconds, starting and stopping, so that no actual movement takes place, just a contraction and a stopping, repetitively'.
- This repetitive contraction will activate the rhomboids, middle and lower trapezii and serratus anterior – all of which are likely to be inhibited if upper trapezius is hypertonic.
- The repetitive contractions also produce an automatic RI of potentially hypertonic upper trapezius, and levator scapula.
- The patient can be taught to make a light finger or thumb contact against the medial scapula (by placing the opposite arm behind the back) so that home application of this method can be performed several times daily.

Method B.

- A similar process of facilitation of the lower fixators of the scapula combined with inhibition of overactivity of the upper fixators (levator scapula, upper trapezius, etc.) can be achieved by introducing the same sequence with a finger contact on the lower angle of the scapula.
- An instruction can be offered, such as: 'Pulse your shoulder blade towards the floor in a rhythmic way, one pulse per second, for 20 repetitions, then rest and repeat the process'.
- It is important that the patient be taught to achieve these pulsations without undue movement occurring other than very locally. Ruddy (1962) used the term, 'No wobble, no bounce' to help to achieve this.

Pulsed MET Treatment for Eye Muscles (Ruddy, 1962)

Ruddy's treatment method for the muscles of the eye is outlined in Box 6.11.

13. Assessment and Treatment of Shortness in Infraspinatus (17)

Infraspinatus Shortness Test A

- The patient is asked to reach backwards, upwards and across to touch the upper border of the opposite scapula, so producing external rotation of the humeral head.
- If this effort is painful, infraspinatus shortness should be suspected.

BOX 6.11 Ruddy's Treatment for the Muscles of the Eye

Osteopathic eye specialist Dr. T. Ruddy described a practical treatment method for application of muscle energy technique principles to the muscles of the eye:

- The pads of the practitioner's index, middle and ring fingers and the thumb are placed together to form four contacts into which the eyeball (eye closed) can rest (middle finger is above the cornea and the thumb pad below it).
- These contacts resist the attempts the patient is asked to make to move the eyes downwards, laterally, medially and upwards – as well as obliquely between these compass points – up and half medial, down and half medial, up and half lateral, down and half lateral, etc.
- The fingers resist and obstruct the intended path of eye motion.
- Each movement should last for a count 'one' and then rest between efforts for a similar count, and in each position there should be 10–20 repetitions before moving on around the circuit.

Ruddy maintained the method released muscle tension, permitted better circulation, and enhanced drainage. He applied the method as part of treatment of many eye problems.

Ruddy's Self-Treatment Method

- The patient is asked to close the eyes and to move the gaze (eyes closed) around the clock face – 12 o'clock, 1 o'clock, etc., until a full circle has been covered. When a particular direction of gaze produces a sense of discomfort, even if mild, it is assumed that the muscles antagonist to those active in moving towards that direction, are short, hypertonic.
- The patient creates a 'circle' by placing the thumb, index, middle and ring fingers of either hand together and placing these to surround the closed eyeball. These digits provide a barrier against which the eye can be pulsed, towards the direction of mild discomfort previously noted; 10–20 very small, pulsed movements are made in that direction, after which the eyes are relaxed and the direction again tested for discomfort. It should be far easier and more relaxed.
- This procedure is carried out on each eye, wherever a direction of discomfort is noted.

Ruddy (1962).

Infraspinatus Shortness Test B (Fig. 6.40)

- Visual evidence of shortness is obtained by having the patient supine, the upper arm of the side to be

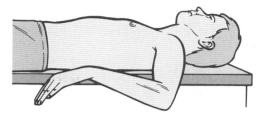

Fig. 6.40 Assessment and self-treatment position for infraspinatus. If the upper arm cannot rest parallel to the floor, possible shortness of infraspinatus is indicated.

tested at right angles to the trunk, elbow flexed so that the lower arm is parallel to the trunk, pointing caudally with the palm downwards.

- This brings the arm into internal rotation and places infraspinatus at stretch.
- The practitioner ensures that the shoulder remains in contact with the table during this assessment by means of light compression.
- If infraspinatus is short, the lower arm will not be capable of resting parallel to the floor, obliging it to point somewhat towards the ceiling.

Assessment for Infraspinatus Weakness

- The patient is seated.
- The practitioner stands behind.
- The patient's arms are flexed at the elbows and held to the side, and the practitioner provides isometric resistance to external rotation of the lower arms (externally rotating them and also the humerus at the shoulder).
- If this effort is painful, an indication of probable infraspinatus shortening exists.
- The relative strength is also judged.
- If weak, the method discussed by Norris (1999) should be used to increase strength (slow isotonic eccentric contraction performed slowly).

NOTE: In this, as in other tests for weakness, there may be a better degree of cooperation if the practitioner applies the force, and the patient is asked to resist as much as possible. Force should always be built slowly and not suddenly.

MET Treatment of Infraspinatus (Fig. 6.41)

- The patient is supine, upper arm at right angles to the trunk, elbow flexed so that the lower arm is parallel to the trunk, pointing caudally, with the palm downwards.
- This brings the arm into internal rotation and places infraspinatus at stretch.

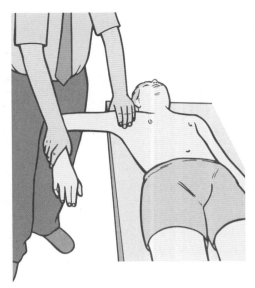

Fig. 6.41 Muscle energy technique treatment of infraspinatus. Note that the practitioner's left hand maintains a downward pressure to stabilise the shoulder to the table during this procedure.

- The practitioner ensures that the posterior shoulder remains in contact with the table by means of light compression.
- The patient slowly and gently lifts the dorsum of the wrist towards the ceiling, against resistance from the practitioner, for 5 to 7 seconds.
- After this isometric contraction, on relaxation, the forearm is taken towards the floor (combined patient and practitioner action), so increasing internal rotation at the shoulder and stretching infraspinatus (mainly at its shoulder attachment).
- Care needs to be taken to prevent the shoulder from rising from the table as rotation is introduced, so giving a false appearance of stretch in the muscle.
- The stretch is held for up to 30 seconds.
  And/or:
- In order to initiate stretch of infraspinatus at the scapular attachment, the patient is seated with the arm (flexed at the elbow) fully internally rotated and taken into full adduction across the chest.
- The practitioner holds the upper arm and applies sustained traction from the shoulder to prevent subacromial impingement.
- The patient is asked to use a light (20% of strength) effort to attempt to externally rotate and abduct the

arm, against resistance offered by the practitioner, for 5 to 7 seconds.
- After this isometric contraction, and with the traction from the shoulder maintained, the arm is taken into increased internal rotation and adduction (patient and practitioner acting together) with the stretch held for up to 30 seconds.

14. Assessment and Treatment of Subscapularis (18)
Subscapularis Shortness Test A
Direct palpation of subscapularis is often required to define problems in it, since pain patterns in the shoulder, arm, scapula and chest may all derive from subscapularis or from other sources.
- The patient is supine and the practitioner grasps the affected-side hand and applies traction while the fingers of the other hand palpate over the edge of latissimus dorsi in order to make contact with the ventral surface of the scapula, where subscapularis can be palpated.
- There may be a marked reaction from the patient when this is touched, indicating acute sensitivity.

Subscapularis Shortness Test B (Fig. 6.42A)
- The patient is supine with the arm abducted to 90 degrees, the elbow flexed to 90 degrees, and the forearm in external rotation, palm upwards.
- The whole arm is resting at the restriction barrier, with gravity as its counterweight.
- If subscapularis is short the forearm will be unable to easily rest parallel to the floor but will be somewhat elevated.
- Care is needed to prevent the anterior shoulder becoming elevated in this position (moving towards the ceiling) and so giving a false normal picture.

Assessment of Weakness in Subscapularis
- The patient is prone with humerus abducted to 90 degrees and elbow flexed to 90 degrees, hand directed caudally.
- The humerus should be in internal rotation so that the forearm is parallel to the trunk, palm towards the ceiling.
- The practitioner stabilises the scapula with one hand and with the other applies pressure to the patient's wrist and forearm as though taking the humerus towards external rotation, while the patient resists.

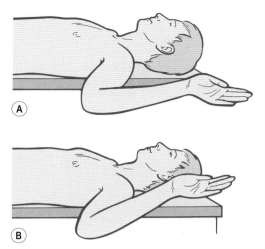

Fig. 6.42 (A and B) Assessment position for subscapularis. If the upper arm cannot rest parallel to the floor, possible shortness of subscapularis is indicated.

The relative strength is judged and the method discussed by Norris (1999) should be used to increase strength (slow isotonic eccentric contraction performed slowly).[6]

MET Treatment of Subscapularis

- The patient is supine with the arm abducted to 90 degrees, the elbow flexed to 90 degrees, and the forearm in external rotation, palm upwards.
- The whole arm is resting at the restriction barrier, with gravity as its counterweight (care is needed to prevent the anterior shoulder becoming elevated in this position, i.e. moving towards the ceiling, and so giving a false normal picture).
- The patient raises the forearm slightly, against minimal resistance from the practitioner, for 5 to 7 seconds and, following relaxation, gravity or slight assistance from the operator takes the arm into greater external rotation, through the barrier, where it is held for 30 seconds.

15. Assessment for Shortness of Supraspinatus (19)
Supraspinatus Shortness Test
- The practitioner stands behind the seated patient, with one hand stabilising the shoulder on the side to

be assessed while the other hand reaches in front of the patient to support the flexed elbow and forearm.
- The patient's upper arm is adducted to its easy barrier and the patient then attempts to abduct the arm.
- If pain is noted in the posterior shoulder region during this attempt, this is diagnostic of supraspinatus dysfunction and, by implication because it is a postural muscle, of probable shortness.

Assessment for Supraspinatus Weakness
- The patient sits or stands with arm abducted 15 degrees, elbow extended.
- The practitioner stabilises the shoulder with one hand, while the other hand offers a resistance contact, which, if forceful, would adduct the arm.
- The patient attempts to resist this, and the degree of effort required to overcome the patient's resistance is graded as weak or strong.

The relative strength is judged and the method discussed by Norris (1999) should be used to increase strength (slow isotonic eccentric contraction performed slowly).

MET Treatment of Supraspinatus (Fig. 6.43)
- The practitioner stands behind the seated patient, with one hand stabilising the shoulder on the side to be treated while the other hand reaches in front of the patient to support the flexed elbow and forearm.
- The patient's upper arm is adducted to its easy barrier and the patient then attempts to abduct the arm using 20% of strength against practitioner resistance.
- After a 7- to 10-second isometric contraction, the arm is taken gently towards its new resistance barrier into greater adduction, with the patient's assistance.
- Repeat several times, holding each painless stretch for not less than 30 seconds.

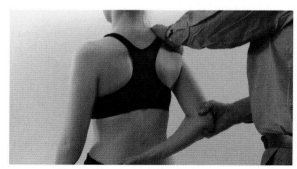

Fig. 6.43 Position for assessment and muscle energy technique treatment of supraspinatus.

---

[6]There could be other reasons for a restricted degree of external rotation, and accurate assessment calls for direct palpation as in test A above.

16. Assessment and Treatment of Flexors of the Arm (20)

Biceps Tendon Shortness Test A

The long biceps tendon can be considered to be stressed if pain arises when the semi-flexed arm is raised against resistance.

Biceps Tendon Shortness Test B

- The patient fully flexes the elbow and the practitioner holds it in one hand while holding the patient's hand in the other.
- The patient is asked to resist as the practitioner attempts to externally rotate the elbow and to straighten the arm.
- If unstable, the tendon may momentarily leave its groove and pain will result.

Biceps Tendon Shortness Test C

- The patient sits with extended arm (taking it backwards from the shoulder) and half flexes the elbow so that the dorsum of the hand approximates the contralateral buttock.
- The patient attempts to flex the elbow further against resistance.
- If pain is noted, there is stress on the tendon and the flexor muscles are probably shortened.

MET Treatment for Shortness in Biceps Tendon

Lewit (1992) describes the following method:
- The patient sits in front of the practitioner, with the affected arm behind the back, the dorsal aspect of that hand passing beyond the buttock on the opposite side.
- The practitioner grasps this hand, bringing it into pronation, to take up the slack (Fig. 6.44).
- The patient is instructed to attempt to take the hand back into supination.
- This is resisted for about 10 seconds by the practitioner, and the relaxation phase is used to take it further into pronation, with simultaneous extension of the elbow.
- Repeat several times more.
  Self-treatment is possible, with the patient applying counterpressure with the other hand.

Flexors of the Forearm – MET Treatment

A painful medial humeral epicondyle usually accompanies tension in the flexors of the forearm.
- The patient is seated facing the practitioner, with flexed elbow supported by the practitioner's fingers.

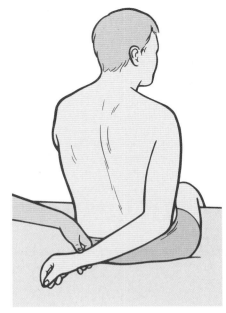

Fig. 6.44 Assessment and muscle energy technique treatment for dysfunction affecting biceps tendon.

- The patient's hand is dorsiflexed at the wrist so that the palm is upwards and fingers face the shoulder (Fig. 6.45).
- The practitioner guides the wrist into greater flexion to an easy barrier, with pronation exaggerated by pressure on the ulnar side of the palm.
- This is achieved by means of the practitioner's thumb being placed on the dorsum of the patient's hand, while the fingers stabilise the palmar aspect, fingertips pressing this towards the floor on the patient's ulnar side of the palm.
- The patient attempts to gently supinate the hand against resistance for 5 to 7 seconds following which, after relaxation (depending on whether it is an acute or chronic problem), dorsiflexion is increased to, or through, the new barrier.
- Repeat as needed.
  This method is easily capable of adaptation to self-treatment by means of the patient applying the counterpressure.

Biceps Brachii – Assessment and MET Treatment

If extension of the arm is limited, the flexors are probably short.

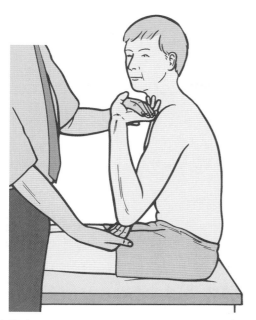

Fig. 6.45 Assessment and muscle energy technique treatment for shortness of the flexors of the forearm.

- Treatment of biceps brachii involves the affected arm being held in extension at the easy barrier.
- The practitioner holds the patient's wrist to restrain a light effort to flex the elbow for 5 to 7 seconds after which, following appropriate relaxation of the effort, the arm is extended to or through (depending on whether it is an acute or chronic problem), the new resistance barrier.
- Repeat several times.

17. Assessment and Treatment of Paravertebral Muscles (21)

Paravertebral Muscle Shortness Test A

- The patient is seated on a treatment table, legs extended, pelvis vertical.
- Flexion is introduced to approximate forehead to knees.
- An even 'C'-shaped curve should be observed and a distance of about 4 inches (10 cm) from the knees achieved by the forehead.
- No knee flexion should occur and the movement should be a spinal one, not involving pelvic tilting (Fig. 6.46).

Interpretation of what is observed is described below and also in the caption of Fig. 6.46.

Paravertebral Muscle Shortness Test B

- The assessment position is then modified to remove hamstring shortness from the picture by having the patient sit at the end of the table, knees flexed over it.
- Once again the patient is asked to perform full flexion, without strain, so that forward bending is introduced to bring the forehead towards the knees.
- The pelvis should be fixed by the placement of the patient's hands on the pelvic crest.
- If bending of the trunk is greater in this position than in test A above, then there is probably shortened hamstring involvement.

Interpretation of Paravertebral Muscle Shortness Tests A and B

- During these assessments, areas of shortening in the spinal muscles may be observed as 'flatness', or even, in the lumbar area, as a reversed curve.
- For example, on forward bending, a lordosis may be maintained in the lumbar spine, or flexion may be very limited even without such lordosis.
- There may be evidence of obvious overstretching of the upper back and relative tightness of the lower back.
- All areas of 'flatness' are charted since these represent an inability of those segments to flex, which involves the erector spinae muscles as a primary or a secondary feature.
- Even if the flexion restriction relates to articular factors, the erector group may benefit from MET.
- If the soft tissues are primary features of the flexion restriction, then MET attention is even more indicated.

NOTE: Lewit (1999) points out that patients with a long trunk and short thighs may perform the flexion movement without apparent difficulty, even if the erectors are short, whereas if the trunk is short and the thighs long, even if the erectors are supple, flexion will not allow the head to approximate the knees.

In the modified position, with patient's hands on the crest of the pelvis, and the patient 'hunching' their spine, Lewit suggests observation of the presence or otherwise of lumbar kyphosis for evidence of shortness in that region. If it fails to appear, erector spinae shortness in the lumbar region is likely. This, together with the presence of flat areas, provides significant evidence of shortness.

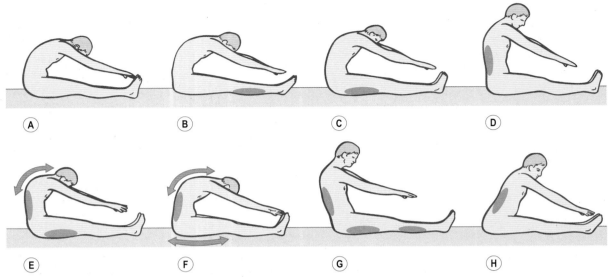

Fig. 6.46 Tests for shortness of the erector spinae and associated postural muscles. (A) Normal length of erector spinae muscles and posterior thigh muscles. (B) Tight gastrocnemius and soleus; the inability to dorsiflex the feet indicates tightness of the plantar-flexor group. (C) Tight hamstring muscles, which cause the pelvis to tilt posteriorly. (D) Tight low-back erector spinae muscles. (E) Tight hamstrings; slightly tight low-back muscles and overstretched upper back muscles. (F) Slightly shortened lower back muscles, stretched upper back muscles and slightly stretched hamstrings. (G) Tight low-back muscles, hamstrings and gastrocnemius/soleus. (H) Very tight low-back muscles, with lordosis maintained even in flexion.

▶ Paravertebral Muscle Shortness Test C – the 'Breathing Wave' (Fig. 6.47)

- Once all flat areas are noted and charted, the patient is placed in prone position.
- The practitioner squats at the side and observes the spinal 'wave' as deep breathing is performed.
- There should be a wave of movement starting at the sacrum and finishing at the base of the neck on inhalation.
- Areas of restriction ('flat areas'), lack of movement, or where motion is not in sequence should be noted and compared with findings from tests A and B above.
- Periodic review of the relative normality of this wave is a useful guide to progress (or lack of it) in normalisation of the functional status of the respiratory and spinal structures.

▶ MET Treatment of Erector Spinae Muscle – Seated

- The patient sits on the treatment table, back towards the practitioner, legs hanging over the side and hands clasped behind the neck.

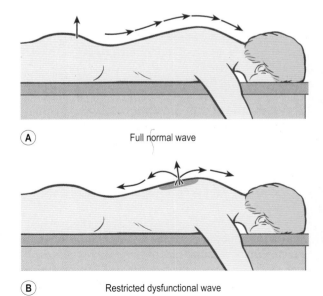

(A)   Full normal wave

(B)   Restricted dysfunctional wave

Fig. 6.47 Observation of the prone breathing wave indicates areas of paravertebral stiffness or vertebral fixation. Rigid areas tend to move as a block, rather than as a wave.

- The practitioner stands on the side towards which the patient will be positioned, or behind the patient, and passes a hand across the front of the patient's chest, to rest on the contralateral shoulder, or to grasp the patient's upper arm (for variations see Figs. 6.1A–F and 6.2A and B).
- The patient is drawn into flexion, side-bending and rotation to take out slack in the area being treated.
- The practitioner's free hand monitors the area of tightness (as evidenced by 'flatness' in the flexion test) and ensures that the various forces localise at the point of maximum contraction/tension.
- When the patient has been taken to the comfortable limit of flexion and/or side flexion, and/or rotation, they are asked either to look (moving the eyes only) towards the direction from which movement has been made or to do so while also introducing a very slight degree of effort towards returning to the upright position, against firm resistance from the practitioner.
- During the contraction it may be useful to have the patient 'breathe into' the tight spinal area which is being palpated and monitored by the practitioner. This will cause an additional increase in isometric contraction of the shortened muscles.
- The patient is then asked to release the breath, and completely relax.
- The practitioner waits for the patient's second full exhalation and then takes the patient further in all the directions of restriction, towards the new barrier, but not through it.
- This whole process is repeated several times, at each level of restriction/flatness.
- The patient may also be asked to gently attempt to move towards the restriction barrier. This involves contraction of the antagonists.
- After relaxation of the effort, the new barrier is again approached.

MET Transverse Stretching of Paraspinal Musculature

'C' bend and 'S' bend techniques (Figs. 6.48 and 6.49). In order to lengthen local areas of muscle and/or connective tissue, the tissues may be 'bent' (into a 'C' or an 'S' shape), to a first barrier of resistance so that the thumbs engage the barrier. At this stage, an isometric contraction should be introduced, achieved by having the patient slightly lift one leg or the other, for 3 to 5

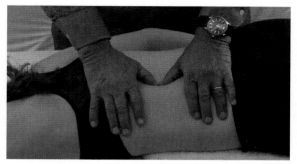

Fig. 6.48 Application of 'C' bend to paraspinal muscles.

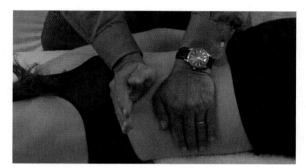

Fig. 6.49 Application of 'S' bend to paraspinal muscles.

seconds. After this, a new barrier is engaged for a period of 10 to 30 seconds.

As an alternative to thumb contacts, heel of hand (thenar/hyperthenar for example) can replace these, thus addressing a broader section of paraspinal muscle.

Patient assistance can be further employed by, for example, requesting: 'slowly and gently begin to lengthen your leg/extend your arm towards the far wall'.

By means of a maintained transverse pressure ('C' or 'S' bend) following an isometric contraction – together with a longitudinal lengthening effort from the patient – the paraspinal musculature should rapidly relax.

Lewit (1992) points out that shortness of the connective tissue is most characteristic for short (taut) muscles – usually overactive muscles. Producing a tissue fold and stretching it is the most effective way to obtain lengthening, because the stretch reflex can be avoided.

Figs. 6.48 and 6.49 show examples of 'C' and 'S' bends.
- Fig. 6.48 shows a 'C' bend being slowly applied to paraspinal muscles, allowing a gentle lengthening to occur (Lewit, 1992).
- Fig. 6.49 shows application of an 'S' bend to paraspinal muscles using the alternative 'heel of hand' contact.

- To achieve a relaxation of a specific area of muscle tension using an 'S' bend, the hands should be positioned in such a way as to allow thumb or hand pressure to be applied across the fibres of a contracted or indurated muscle so that the contacts are travelling in opposite directions to each other (Lewit, 1999).
- As pressure is applied simultaneously with each thumb or hand ('C' bend or 'S' bend), the tissues between the two contacts will progressively have the slack removed, and be placed in a lightly lengthened situation, in which they can be held until release occurs.
- As a rule, tissues are held in a lengthened state for upwards of 30 seconds, before different fibres are selected to receive the same attention.

Thoracolumbar Dysfunction

This important region was discussed briefly in the section dealing with QL (heading 7 above), and deserves special attention due to its particularly vulnerable 'transition' status involving the powerful effect that spasm and tightness of the major stabilising muscles of the region can have on it: notably psoas, the thoracolumbar erector spinae and QL, as well as the influence of rectus abdominis in which weakness is all too common (see lower crossed syndrome notes in Chapter 5, Box 5.2).

Screening for lumbodorsal dysfunction involves having the patient straddle the table (so locking the pelvis) in a slightly flexed posture (slight kyphosis). Rotation in either direction then enables segmental impairment to be observed at the same time that the spinous processes are monitored.

Restriction of rotation is the most common characteristic of this dysfunction.

MET Treatment of Thoracolumbar Dysfunction

Psoas and/or QL should be assessed and if found to be dysfunctional (most probably shortened), treated as described earlier in this chapter.[7]

NOTE: Thoracic spinal restriction treatment is covered in Chapter 6, which evaluates MET and joints.

---

[7]Not all the muscles involved in thoracolumbar dysfunction pattern described above may need treatment, since when one or other is treated appropriately the others commonly normalise. Underlying causes of dysfunction must also always receive attention.

Assessment for Shortness in Erector Spinae Muscles of the Neck (22)

- The patient is supine and the practitioner stands at the head of the table, or to the side, supporting the neck in one hand, and the occiput in the other, to afford complete support for both.
- When the head/neck is eased into flexion, the chin should easily be able to be brought into contact with the suprasternal area, *without force.*
- If there remains a noticeable gap between the tip of the chin (ignore double chin tissues!) and the upper chest wall, then the neck extensors are considered to be short.

Assessment of Weakness of Deep Neck Flexors

NOTE: In applying this test, it is helpful for the supine patient if the practitioner maintains a hand contact on the lower thorax to stabilise the trunk, especially if weak abdominal muscles are a feature.

- The patient is asked to flex the neck to approximately 45 degrees, and to maintain this position for 10 seconds.
- If this is not possible, or if visible tremor is noted as the patient attempts to maintain the position, weakness of the deep neck flexors can be assumed.
- It is also possible to test relative strength by offering resistance against the forehead as the patient attempts to flex the neck.

If weakness is shown, in conjunction with shortness of the extensor muscles of the neck, then weakness should be treated initially.

Toning the Deep Neck Flexors Using Slow Eccentric Isotonic Stretching (See Chapter 5)

- The neck of the supine patient is taken into flexion, as described for the weakness test above.
- The practitioner stands at the head of the table and supports the neck with one hand. This hand should be placed just below the occiput so that it supports the suboccipital and upper neck region.
- The other hand is on the patient's forehead.
- The patient is asked to 'tuck your chin in' (to activate the deep neck flexors) and this additional flexion is 'locked in' by the practitioner's hand on the forehead.
- The patient is asked to resist the effort the practitioner will make to extend the neck over their hand, slowly.
- This action is performed and then repeated.

The effect is to tone the deep neck flexors and to inhibit the shortened extensors, which can then be taken into stretch, as described in the MET method below.

MET Treatment of Short Neck Extensor Muscles

- The neck of the supine patient is flexed to its easy barrier of resistance (if acute), or short of this (if chronic), and the patient is asked to extend the neck ('take the back of your head back to the table, gently') using minimal effort on an inhalation, against resistance.
- If the hand positions as described in the test above are not comfortable, then try placing the hands, arms crossed, so that a hand rests on the anterior surface of each shoulder, while the head rests on the crossed forearms.
- After the contraction, the neck is flexed further to the new barrier of resistance, ensuring that the suboccipital muscles receive focused stretching attention.
- A further aid during the contraction phase may be achieved by having the practitioner contact the top of the patient's head with their abdomen, and to use this contact to prevent the patient tilting the head upwards.
- This allows for an additional isometric contraction which involves the short extensor muscles at the base of the skull ('Try to tip your chin upwards').
- The subsequent stretch, as above, will involve these muscles as well.
- Repetitions of the stretch to the new barrier should be performed until no further gain is possible, or until the chin easily touches the chest on flexion.

NOTE: No force should be used, or pain produced during this procedure.

MET Treatment Methods for Joint Problems

A variety of MET treatment methods for pelvic and spinal joint restrictions, as well as the shoulder, clavicular and cervical area, can be found in Chapter 7, and these can be used alongside the more general, muscle-orientated, approaches detailed in this chapter.

REFERENCES

Arab, A.M., Ghamkhar, L., Mahnaz, E., Nourbakhsh, M.R., 2011. Altered muscular activation during prone hip extension in women with and without low back pain. Chiropr. Man. Ther. 19, 18.

Arab, A.M., Nourbakhsh, M.R., 2010. The relationship between hip abductor muscle strength and iliotibial band tightness in individuals with low back pain. Chiropr. Osteopat. 18, 1–5.

Arab, A.M., Nourbakhsh, M., Mohammadifar, A., 2011. The relationship between hamstring length and gluteal muscle strength in individuals with sacroiliac joint dysfunction. J. Man. Manip. Ther. 19 (1), 5–10.

Baker, R.L., Souza, R.B., Fredericson, M., 2011. Iliotibial band syndrome: soft tissue and biomechanical factors in evaluation and treatment. Phys. Med. Rehabil. 3, 550–561.

Bandy, W.D., Irion, J.M., Briggler, M., 1997. The effect of time and frequency of static stretching on flexibility of the hamstring muscles. Phys. Ther. 77, 1090–1096.

Basmajian, J., 1974. Muscles Alive. Williams and Wilkins, Baltimore.

Bergmark, A., 1989. Stability of the lumbar spine. A study in mechanical engineering. Acta Orthop. Scand. Suppl. 230 (6), 2–54.

Blanco, C.R., de las Penas, C.F., Xumet, J.E.H., Algaba, C.P., Rabadán, M.F., de la Quintana, M.C.L., 2006. Changes in active mouth opening following a single treatment of latent myofascial trigger points in the masseter muscle involving post-isometric relaxation or strain/counterstrain. J. Bodyw. Mov. Ther. 10, 197–205.

Block, S., 1993. Fibromyalgia and the rheumatisms. Controversies Rheumatol. 119 (1), 61–78.

Bogduk, N., 1997. Clinical Anatomy of the Lumbar Spine and Sacrum, third ed. Churchill Livingstone, Edinburgh.

Bogduk, N., Pearcy, M., Hadfield, G., 1992. Anatomy and biomechanics of psoas major. Clin. Biomech. 7, 109–119.

Bourdillon, J., 1982. Spinal Manipulation, third ed. Heinemann, London.

Bruno, P.A., Bagust, J., 2007. An investigation into motor pattern differences used during prone hip extension between subjects with and without low back pain. Clin. Chiropr. 10, 68–80.

Burns, D.K., Wells, M.R., 2006. Gross range of motion in the cervical spine: the effects of osteopathic muscle energy technique in asymptomatic subjects. J. Am. Osteopath. Assoc. 106 (3), 137–142.

Bush, T.R., Vorro, J., Alderink, G., Gorbis, S., Li, M., Leitkam, S., 2010. Relating a manual medicine diagnostic test of cervical motion function to specific three-dimensional kinematic variables. Int. J. Osteopath. Med. 13, 48–55.

Cagnie, B., Danneels, L., Cools, A., Dickx, N., Cambier, D., 2008. The influence of breathing type, expiration and cervical posture on the performance of the cranio-cervical flexion test in healthy subjects. Man. Ther. 13 (3), 232–238.

Cailliet, R., 1962. Low Back Pain Syndrome. Blackwell, Oxford.

Cayco, C.S., Labro, A.V., Gorgon, E.J.R., 2019. Hold-relax and contract-relax stretching for hamstrings flexibility: a systematic review with meta-analysis. Phys. Ther. Sport 35, 42–55.

Chaitow, L., 1991. Soft Tissue Manipulation. Healing Arts Press, Rochester.

Chaitow, L., Fritz, S., 2007. A Massage Therapist's Guide to Lower Back & Pelvic Pain. Elsevier Health Sciences.

Chaitow, L., 2010. Modern Neuromuscular Techniques, third ed. Churchill Livingstone, Edinburgh.

Corkery, M., Briscoe, H., Ciccone, N., Foglia, G., Johnson, P., Kinsman, S., Legere, L., et al., 2007. Establishing normal values for lower extremity muscle length in college-age students. Phys. Ther. Sport 8, 66–74.

Dearing, J., Hamilton, F., 2008. An examination of pressure-pain thresholds (PPT's) at myofascial trigger points (MTrP's), following muscle energy technique or ischaemic compression treatment. Man. Ther. 13, 87–88.

Dhargalkar, P., Kulkarni, A., Ghodey, S., 2017. Added effect of muscle energy technique for improving functional ability in patients with chronic nonspecific low back pain. Int. J. Physiother. Res. 5 (3), 2082–2087.

Dommerholt, J., 2000. Posture. In: Tubiana, R., Amadio, P. (Eds.), Medical Problems of the Instrumentalist Musician. Martin Dunitz, London, pp. 405–406.

Duna, G.F., Wilke, W.S., 1993. Diagnosis, etiology, and therapy of fibromyalgia. Compr. Ther. 19 (2), 60–63.

Dvorak, J., Dvorak, V., 1984. Manual Medicine – Diagnostics. George Thieme Verlag, New York.

Evjenth, O., 1984. Muscle Stretching in Manual Therapy. Alfta RehabAlfta, Sweden.

Feland, J.B., Myrer, J.W., Schulthies, S.S., Fellingham, G.W., Measom, G.W., 2001. The effect of duration of stretching of the hamstring muscle group for increasing range of motion in people aged 65 years or older. Phys. Ther. 81, 1100–1117.

Fishman, L.M., Dombi, G.W., Michaelsen, C., Ringel, S., Rozbruch, J., Rosner, B., et al., 2002. Piriformis syndrome: diagnosis, treatment, and outcome – a 10-year study. Arch. Phys. Med. Rehabil. 83, 295–301.

Fryer, G., 2000. Muscle energy concepts-a need for change. J. Osteopath. Med. 3 (2), 54–59.

Fryette, H., 1954. Principles of osteopathic technic. Yearbook of the Academy of Applied Osteopathy 1954, Indianapolis.

Gabbe, B.J., Finch, C.F., Bennell, K.L., Wajswelner, H., 2005. Risk factors for hamstring injuries in community level Australian football. Br. J. Sports Med. 39, 106–110.

Gamber, R.G., Shores, J.H., Russo, D.P., Jimenez, C., Rubin, B.R., 2002. Osteopathic manipulative treatment in conjunction with medication relieves pain associated with fibromyalgia syndrome: results of a randomized clinical pilot project. J. Am. Osteopath. Assoc. 102 (6), 321–325.

Gemmell, H., Dunford, P.J., 2007. A cross-sectional study of the prevalence of neck pain, decreased cervical range of motion and head repositioning accuracy in forwards and backs in rugby union. Clin. Chiropr. 10, 187–194.

García-Peñalver, U.J., Palop-Montoro, M.V., Manzano-Sánchez, D., 2020. Effectiveness of the muscle energy technique versus osteopathic manipulation in the treatment of sacroiliac joint dysfunction in athletes. Int. J. Environ. Res. Public Health 17 (12), 4490.

George, W.K., George Jr., W.D., Smith, J.P., Gordon, F.T., Baird, E.E., Mills, G.C., 1964. Changes in serum calcium, serum phosphate and red-cell phosphate during hyperventilation. N. Engl. J. Med. 270, 726–728.

Gerwin, R., Dommerholt, J., 2002. Treatment of myofascial pain syndromes. In: Weiner, R. (Ed.), Pain Management: A Practical Guide for Clinicians. CRC Press, Boca Raton, pp. 235–249.

Gluck, N., Liebenson, C., 1997. Paradoxical muscle function. J. Bodyw. Mov. Ther. 1 (4), 219–222.

Goldenberg, D.L., 1993. Fibromyalgia, chronic fatigue syndrome and myofascial pain syndrome. Curr. Opin. Rheumatol. 5, 199–208.

Goldstein, J., 1996. Betrayal by the Brain. Haworth Press, New York.

Gray, 1995. Gray's Anatomy, thirty-eighth ed. Churchill Livingstone, Edinburgh.

Greenman, P., 1989. Principles of Manual Medicine, first ed. Williams and Wilkins, Baltimore.

Greenman, P., 1996. Principles of Manual Medicine, second ed. Williams and Wilkins, Baltimore.

Greenman, P., 2003. Principles of Manual Medicine, third ed. Williams and Wilkins, Baltimore.

Grieve, G.P., 1986. Modern Manual Therapy of the Vertebral Column. Churchill Livingstone, Edinburgh.

Haugstad, G.K., Haugstad, T.S., Kirste, U.M., Leganger, S., Wojniusz, S., Klemmetsen, I., et al., 2006. Posture, movement patterns, and body awareness in women with chronic pelvic pain. J. Psychosom. Res. 61 (5), 637–644.

Hudson, A.L., Gandevia, S.C., Butler, J.E., 2007. The effect of lung volume on the co-ordinated recruitment of scalene and sternomastoid muscles in humans. J. Physiol. 584 (1), 261–270.

Hunt, G.M., Legal, L., 2010. Comparative study on the efficacy of thrust and muscle energy techniques in the piriformis muscle. Osteopatía Científi. 5 (2), 47–55.

Iqbal, M., Riaz, H., Ghous, M., Masood, K., 2020. Comparison of Spencer muscle energy technique and passive stretching in adhesive capsulitis: a single blind randomized control trial. J. Pak. Med. Assoc. 70 (12), 2113–2118.

Janda, V., 1968. Postural and phasic muscles in the pathogenesis of low back pain, Proceedings of the XIth Congress ISRD. Dublin, 553–554.

Janda, V., 1983. Muscle Function Testing. Butterworths, London.

Janda, V., 1988. In: Grant, R. (Ed.), Physical Therapy of the Cervical and Thoracic Spine. Churchill Livingstone, New York.

Janda, V., 1996. Evaluation of muscular imbalance. In: Liebenson, C. (Ed.), Rehabilitation of the Spine. Williams and Wilkins, Baltimore.

Janda, V., Frank, C., Liebenson, C., 2006. Evaluation of muscular imbalance. In: Liebenson, C. (Ed.), Rehabilitation of the Spine, second ed. Lippincott Williams and Wilkins, Baltimore.

Jhaveri, A., Gahlot, P., 2018. Comparision of effectiveness of myo facial release technique versus muscle energy technique on chronic trapezitis-an experimental study. Int. J. Innov. Res. Adv. Stud. 5 (7), 89–94.

Jull, G., 1994. Active Stabilisation of the Trunk. Course Notes, Edinburgh.

Kapandji, I., 1974, second ed. The Physiology of the Joints, vol. 3. Churchill Livingstone, Edinburgh.

Kendall, F.P., McCreary, E.K., Provance, P.G., 1993. Muscles, Testing and Function, fourth ed. Williams and Wilkins, Baltimore.

Key, J., Clift, A., Condie, F., Harley, C., 2008. A model of movement dysfunction. J. Bodyw. Mov. Ther. 12 (1), 7–21.

Knebl, J.A., Shores, J.H., Gamber, R.G., Gray, W.T., Herron, K.M., 2002. Improving functional ability in the elderly via the Spencer technique, an osteopathic manipulative treatment: a randomized, controlled trial. JAOA 102 (7), 387–396.

Kostopoulos, D., Rizopoulos, K., 2001. The Manual of Trigger Point and Myofascial Therapy. Slack Inc., Thorofare, NJ.

Lehmkuhl, L., Smith, L., 1983. Brunnstrom's Clinical Kinesiology, fourth ed. F.A. Davis, Philadelphia.

Lewit, K., 1985a. Muscular and articular factors in movement restriction. Man. Med. 1, 83–85.

Lewit, K., 1985. Manipulative Therapy in Rehabilitation of the Motor System. Butterworths, London.

Lewit, K., 1992. Manipulative Therapy in Rehabilitation of the Locomotor System, second ed. Butterworths, London.

Lewit, K., 1999. Manipulative Therapy in Rehabilitation of the Locomotor System, third ed. Butterworths, London.

Lewit, K., 2009. Manipulative Therapy: Musculoskeletal Medicine. Churchill Livingstone, Edinburgh.

Lewit, K., Simons, D.G., 1984. Myofascial pain: relief by post-isometric relaxation. Arch. Phys. Med. Rehabil. 65, 452–456.

Li, R.C., Jasiewicz, J.M., Middleton, J., Condie, P., Barriskill, A., Hebnes, H., et al., 2006. The development, validity, and reliability of a manual muscle testing device with integrated limb position sensors. Arch. Phys. Med. Rehabil. 87, 411–417.

Liebenson, C., 1996. Rehabilitation of the Spine. Williams and Wilkins, Baltimore.

Liebenson, C., 2006. Rehabilitation of the Spine, second ed. Williams and Wilkins, Baltimore.

Lin, J.P., Brown, J.K., Walsh, E.G., 1994. Physiological maturation of muscles in childhood. Lancet 343, 1386–1389.

López-Bedoya, J., Vernetta-Santana, J., Lizaur-Girón, P., Martínez-Patiño, M.J., Ariza-Vargas, L., 2020. Effectiveness and pain perception with holdrelax stretching technique and electrostimulation. Revista Internacional de Medicina y Ciencias de la Actividad Física y del Deporte 20 (80), 623–640. DOI:10.15366/rimcafd2020.80.011.

Maffetone, P., 1999. Complementary Sports Medicine. Human Kinetics, Champaign, IL.

Magee, D.J., 2002. Orthopedic Physical Assessment, fourth ed. WB Saunders, New York.

Masubuchi, Y., Abe, T., Yokoba, M., Yamada, T., Katagiri, M., Tomita, T., 2001. Relation between neck accessory inspiratory muscle electromyographic activity and lung volume. J. Jpn. Respir. Soc. 39 (4), 244–249.

McGill, S., Juker, D., Kropf, P., 1996. Quantitative intramuscular myoelectric activity of quadratus lumborum during a wide variety of tasks. Clin. Biomech. 11, 170–172.

Mennell, J., 1964. Back Pain. T and A Churchill, Boston.

Middaugh, S., 1994. Muscle overuse and posture as factors in the development and maintenance of chronic musculoskeletal pain. In: Grzesiak, R., Ciccone, D. (Eds.), Psychological Vulnerability to Chronic Pain. Springer, New York, pp. 55–89.

Mitchell Jr., F., 1998. Muscle Energy Manual. MET Press, East Lansing, p. 1.

Mitchell Jr., F., 2009. Interview. In: Franke, H. (Ed.), The History of MET. Muscle Energy Technique History-Model-Research. Verband der Osteopathen Deutschland, Wiesbaden.

Mitchell, F., Moran, P., Pruzzo, N., 1979. An Evaluation and Treatment Manual of Osteopathic Muscle Energy Procedures. Mitchell Moran and Pruzzo Associations, Valley Park, Missouri.

Moore, M.A., Hutton, R.S., 1980. Electromyographic investigation manual of muscle stretching techniques. Med. Sci. Sports Exerc. 12, 322–329.

Moore, S.D., Laudner, K.G., McLoda, T.A., Shaffer, M.A., 2011. The immediate effects of muscle energy technique on posterior shoulder tightness: a randomized controlled trial. J. Orthop. Sports Phys. Ther. 41 (6), 400–407.

Norris, C.M., 1999. Functional load abdominal training: part 1. J. Bodyw. Mov. Ther. 3 (3), 150–158.

Norris, C.M., 2000. The muscle designation debate. J. Bodyw. Mov. Ther. 4 (4), 225–241.

Osama, M., 2021. Effects of autogenic and reciprocal inhibition muscle energy techniques on isometric muscle strength in neck pain: a randomized controlled trial. J. Back Musculoskelet. Rehabil. 34 (4), 555–564.

O'Sullivan, P., 2005. Diagnosis and classification of chronic low back pain disorders: maladaptive movement and motor control impairments as underlying mechanism. Man. Ther. 10 (4), 242–255.

Peper, E., Tibbetts, V., 1992. Fifteen-month follow-up with asthmatics utilizing EMG/incentive inspirometer feedback. Biofeedback Self Regul. 17 (2), 143–151.

Perri, M., Halford, E., 2004. Pain and faulty breathing: a pilot study. J. Bodyw. Mov. Ther. 8, 297–306.

Piva, S.R., Fitzgerald, K., Irrgang, J.J., Jones, S., Hando, B.R., Browder, D.A., et al., 2006. Reliability of measures of impairments associated with patellofemoral pain syndrome. BMC Musculoskelet. Disord. 7, 33.

Platzer, W., 1992. Color Atlas/Text of Human Anatomy, fourth ed. Locomotor System, vol. 1. Thieme, Stuttgart.

Pleidelová, J., Balážiová, M., Porubská, V., 2002. Frequency of scalenal muscle disorders. Rehabilitacia 35 (4), 203–207.

Portugal, S., 2011. Poster 165 osteopathic muscle energy technique in the management of shoulder impingement syndrome: a case report. PM&R 10 (3), S226–S227.

Prachi, P.N., Basavaraji, C., Santosh, M., Khatri, S., 2010. Effectiveness of muscle energy technique on quadratus lumborum in acute low back pain-randomized controlled trial. Ind. J. Physiother. Occup. Ther. 4 (1), 54–58.

Richard, R., 1978. Lésions Ostéopathiques du Sacrum. Maloine, Paris.

Rolf, I., 1977. Rolfing – Integration of Human Structures. Harper and Row, New York.

Rosenthal, E., 1987. Alexander technique and how it works. Med. Probl. Perform. Art. 2, 53–57.

Rubin, B.R., Gamber, R.G., Cortez, C.A., Wright, T.J., Shores, J., Davis, G., 1990. Treatment options in fibromyalgia syndrome. J. Am. Osteopath. Assoc. 90 (9), 844–845.

Ruddy, T., 1962. Osteopathic rapid rhythmic resistive technic. Academy of Applied Osteopathy Yearbook, 23–31 196258–68.

Ruddy, T.J., 1961. Resistive Rhythmic Duction. White Paper with black text. Lecture notes. Still National Osteopathic Museum call# 1992.1473.07.

Sachdeva, S., Sheetal, K., Sonia, P., 2018. Effects of muscle energy technique versus mobilization on pain and disability in post-partum females with sacroiliac joint dysfunction. Ind. J. Health Sci. Care 5 (1), 11–17.

Salvador, D., Neto, P.E.D., Ferrari, F.P., 2005. Application of muscle energy technique in garbage collectors with acute mechanical lumbar pain. Fisioterapia e Pesquisa 12 (2), 20–27.

Schamberger, W., 2002. The Malalignment Syndrome. Churchill Livingstone, Edinburgh, pp. 90.

Schleifer, L., Ley, R., Spalding, T.W., 2002. A hyperventilation theory of job stress and musculoskeletal disorders. Am. J. Ind. Med. 41 (5), 420–443.

Scudds, R.A., Landry, M., Birmingham, T., et al., 1995. The frequency of referred signs from muscle pressure in normal healthy subjects (abstract). J. Musculoskelet. Pain 3 (Suppl 1), 99.

Selkow, N.M., Grindstaff, T.L., Cross, K.M., Pugh, K., Hertel, J., Saliba, S., 2009. Short-term effect of muscle energy technique on pain in individuals with non-specific lumbopelvic pain: a pilot study. J. Man. Manip. Ther. 17 (1), E14–E18.

Shaha, S., Sharath, U.R., 2021. Comparing the effect of static, ballistic and contract-relax stretching on hamstring muscles flexibility in young individuals. Int. J. Phys. Educ. Sports Health. 8 (1), 9–15.

Shrier, I., Gossal, K., 2000. Myths and truths of stretching: individualized recommendations for healthy muscles. Phys. Sports Med. 28 (8), 1–7.

Simons, D., Travell, J., Simons, L., 1999, second ed. Myofascial Pain and Dysfunction: The Trigger Point Manual1. Williams and Wilkins, Baltimore.

Stedman, T.L., 1998. Stedman's Electronic Medical Dictionary. Version 4.0. Williams and Wilkins, Baltimore.

Stiles, E., 2009. Muscle energy techniques. In: Franke, H. (Ed.), The History of MET. Muscle Energy Technique History-Model-Research, Verband der Osteopathen Deutschland, Wiesbaden.

Stotz, A., Kappler, R., 1992. Effects of osteopathic manipulative treatment on tender points associated with fibromyalgia. J. Am. Osteopath. Assoc. 92 (9), 1183–1184.

Thomas, E., Cavallaro, A.R., Mani, D., Bianco, A., Palma, A., 2019. The efficacy of muscle energy techniques in symptomatic and asymptomatic subjects: a systematic review. Chiropr. Man. Therap. 27 (1), 1–18.

Travell, J., Simons, D., 1992. Myofascial Pain and Dysfunction: The Trigger Point Manual, vol. 2. Williams and Wilkins, Baltimore.

Tyler, T., Zook, L., Brittis, D., Gleim, G., 1996. A new pelvic tilt detection device: roentgenographic validation and application to assessment of hip motion in professional ice hockey players. J. Orthop. Sports Phys. Ther. 24 (5), 303–308.

Uysal, S.C., Tüzün, E.H., Eker, L., Angın, E., 2019. Effectiveness of the muscle energy technique on respiratory muscle strength and endurance in patients with fibromyalgia. J. Back Musculoskelet. Rehabil. 32 (3), 411–419.

van Middelkoop, M., Rubinstein, S.M., Verhagen, A.P., Ostelo, R.W., Koes, B.W., van Tulder, M.W., 2010. Exercise therapy for chronic nonspecific low-back pain. Best Pract. Res. Clin. Rheumatol. 24 (2), 193–204.

van Wingerden, J.-P., 1997. The role of the hamstrings in pelvic and spinal function. In: Vleeming, A. (Ed.), Movement, Stability and Low Back Pain. Churchill Livingstone, New York.

Veera, S., Chin, J., Kleyn, L., Spinelli, S., Tafler, L., 2020. Use of osteopathic manipulation for treatment of chronic shoulder injury related to vaccine administration. Cureus 12 (7), e9156.

Vleeming, A., Van Wingerden, J.P., Snijders, C.J., Stoeckart, R., Stijnen, T., 1989. Load application to the sacrotuberous ligament; influences on sacroiliac joint mechanics. Clin. Biomech. 4, 204–209.

Wendt, M., Waszak, M., 2020. Evaluation of the combination of muscle energy technique and trigger point therapy in asymptomatic individuals with a latent trigger point. Int. J. Environ. Res. Public Health 17 (22), 8430.

Williams, P., 1965. Lumbosacral Spine. McGraw Hill, New York.

7

MET and the Treatment of Joints

Leon Chaitow, Sandy Fritz

CHAPTER CONTENTS

JOINTS AND MET

This chapter targets muscle energy techniques (MET) focused on joint functions. Specific applications of MET are described for various (but not all) spinal, pelvic, cervical, shoulder, acromioclavicular and sternoclavicular joints, and the temporomandibular joint (TMJ). In these examples no stretching is ever called for, merely a movement following the isometric contraction (or employment of pulsed MET), to engage a new barrier, without force.

In order to apply the principles embodied in MET methodology to any joint dysfunction that is not specifically covered in this chapter (for example the knee or elbow), an appreciation of the normal physiological and anatomical barriers associated with the restricted joint, as well as sound palpation and assessment skills, are required. With awareness of normal ranges of motion, and a keen sense of end-feel (what the end of a movement *should* feel like, compared with what is actually presented – as discussed in Chapters 2 & 5.) should come an appreciation of what is needed in order to position a joint, for receipt of MET input, irrespective of which joint is involved.

If end-feel is sharp or sudden, it probably represents protective spasm of joint pathology, such as arthritis, and benefits of MET to such pathologically restricted joints will be limited to what the pathology will allow; however, even in arthritic settings, a modification of soft-tissue tone commonly produces benefits.

It is reasonable to question the suggestion above as to the reliability of palpation assessment, since end-feel and range-of-motion assessments are not universally regarded as reliable, with mixed reports of accuracy. As examples of the mixed evidence consider that:

- In a systematic review of 17 studies, van Trijffel et al. (2010) found that there was acceptable reliability when measuring range of motion of knee extension using a goniometer, while visual assessment of knee flexion was also reliable. However, most but not all studies of measurements of end-feel were unreliable for all hip and knee movements.
- In contrast the findings of a randomised controlled trial by Lakhani et al. (2009) demonstrated that motion palpation of end-feel appears to be a reliable assessment tool in the cervical spine, for determining whether perceived motion restriction found before treatment improves after manual treatment. This observation may however be limited to symptomatic participants.

There is further discussion of what methods are most reliable in assessment of end-feel in Chapters 2 and 5. Technological advancements may increase the reliability of palpation and visual assessment. There are applications for smartphone devices now available that are easy to incorporate into the assessment process (Awatani et al., 2018; Ramos et al., 2019; Stanek et al., 2020). A variety of clinicians are increasingly using smartphone apps for assessing joint range of motion, adding confidence and precision to what the practitioner observes and feels.

Opinion or Evidence?

As far as possible, the recommendations and statements in this chapter (as in other chapters) are based on such validated sources as are available. However, as with much manual therapy, a great deal of what therapists do is based on experience and clinical tradition – with research support only intermittently evident.

Research for the present edition showed little change in the methods developed in the past but instead focuses on clinical efficacy showing benefit for multiple conditions involving musculoskeletal function. The most current research also focuses on ongoing exploration of underlying mechanisms, but it should be noted that focusing on individual mechanisms in isolation will always fall short of providing meaningful insight, because manual therapy in all its forms is a complex intervention involving multiple interactions of complementary mechanisms (Bialosky et al., 2018). A scoping review of animal models described limits in mechanistic investigations regarding the effects of manual therapy. However, a recent shift towards the neurophysiological and psychological effects of manual therapy has also been observed in the literature (Lima et al., 2020). Application of methods such as MET remains consistent and unchallenged by current research or expert opinion. Clinical benefits continue to be supported by the literature, even though the precise mechanisms remain elusive (Anggiat et al., 2020; Pfluegler et al., 2020). How methods are applied based on expert opinion remains valid. The statements and advice in Box 7.1 can be seen to largely comprise opinion, and readers therefore need to exercise critical judgment as to the degree to which they choose to accept the opinions expressed – despite their derivation being from acknowledged experts.

Before examining what evidence there is to support the opinions and suggestions summarised in Box 7.1,

BOX 7.1 MET for Joints – Guidelines and Advice

NOTE: Some of the quotes in this box appear elsewhere in the book. They are deliberately repeated here because of their pertinence to this chapter's focus – MET in relation to joints.

What might be causing the joint restriction that is being treated?

Treating a joint motion restriction as if the cause were tight muscle(s) is one approach that makes possible restoration of normal joint motion. Regardless of the cause of restriction, MET treatment, based on a 'short muscle' paradigm, is usually completely effective in eliminating blockage, and restoring normal range of motion, even when the blockage is due to non-muscular factors.

Mitchell, Jr. (1998)

What forms the barrier of restriction?

As the [restriction] barrier is engaged, increasing amounts of force are necessary and the distance decreases. The term barrier may be misleading if it is interpreted as a wall or rigid obstacle to be overcome with a push. As the joint reaches the barrier, restraints in the form of tight muscles and fascia serve to inhibit further motion. We are pulling against restraints rather than pushing against some anatomic structure.

Kappler and Jones (2003)

Whose force should be employed in MET?

The therapist's force is always the counterforce. A common mistake is to ask the patient to 'resist my effort'. This ignores the factor of intentionality that ensures that core muscles are re-educated and rehabilitated. What works best is to tell the patient the exact direction of the action, the amount of force, and when to stop.

Mitchell Jr. (2009)

In what direction(s) should forces be directed during the post-contraction phase of MET, in treatment of joint restrictions?

Originally (1940s) MET was taught with joints being taken to their end of range (restriction) in three planes – for example flexion, side-flexion, rotation. MET applied in this way was often 'very difficult, if not impossible'. However, Lewit demonstrated that because segmental vertebral motions are coupled, if normal ROM can be restored in the coronal plane, normal motion will be restored in the other planes. Clinical experience suggests that MET procedures

applied, using side-flexion (or translation), will usually release restrictions in other planes'.

Mitchell Jr. (2009)

How long should an isometric contraction be maintained in MET treatment of joints?

The sensory (spinal) adaptive response in the ... proprioceptor mechanism ... probably takes no more than one tenth of second. Once that (sensory) adaptive response occurs, passive mobilization, during the post-isometric phase, can usually be accomplished without effort. ... For joints, more than two seconds of isometric contraction is a waste of energy.

Mitchell Jr. (2009)

How strong should isometric contractions be in MET treatment of joints?

Strong or moderate force contractions – as initially used in MET – recruited too many of the 'wrong' motor units, and results were less that were hoped for. It was Lewit who drastically reduced the force generated by muscle contractions.

Mitchell Jr. (2009)

The use of MET in paediatric settings is the same as that for adults:

There are six steps used in muscle energy treatment and they are repeated twice. 1) The area is positioned to engage the restrictive barrier. 2) The patient is instructed to contract the involved muscles with a specific intensity and in a specific direction (move the area in a specific direction). 3) The patient's contraction is met with the appropriate counterforce (isometric, isotonic, isolytic) for 3–5 seconds. 4) The patient is instructed to slowly relax, and the physician relaxes the counterforce. 5) There is a pause to allow for muscle relaxation. 6) The area is repositioned to the new restrictive barrier and the sequence is repeated.

Carreiro (2009a)

Ruddy's description of Rapid Resistive Duction (known in this text as 'pulsed MET'):

Resistive duction is a rapid succession of rhythmic muscle contractions against resistance by the [practitioner] for the purpose of establishing normal muscle tone, removing fascial tension and fixation, permitting freedom to tissue and body fluids.

Ruddy (1962)

Within that approach Ruddy famously cautioned that there should be 'No wobble; no bounce' so emphasising

(Continued)

BOX 7.1   MET for Joints – Guidelines and Advice—cont'd

the need for a rhythmic series of controlled contractions, as described later in this chapter.

Summary

1. When treating complex joints, where there are numerous muscle attachments (e.g. pelvis, neck) clinical experience – and logic – suggests that before specifically focusing on the restricted joint, all major attaching muscles should receive MET attention in order to reduce hypertonicity.

2. Treatment commences at the restriction barrier for all acute soft tissue conditions, and for all joint MET.

3. For a joint, following a light isometric contraction (of agonist, antagonist, or other muscle(s) – depending on chosen direction of effort) – or the use of pulsed MET, tissues are taken to the new barrier, without force or stretching. One or two repetitions, using alternative directions of force application if the initial one was unsuccessful, are commonly recommended.

4. Complex joint restrictions, for example involving a spinal segment, may be treated by attention to single directions of restriction, e.g. flexion or extension, or by taking the joint to its easy end-of-range in, for example, flexion, side flexion and rotation – and then using a quite different direction for the pulsed or sustained contraction, for example translation.

5. No stretch is *ever* used with joint mobilisation, when using MET.

6. When using pulsed MET, the initial rhythmic resisted pulsation is usually towards the barrier. After approximately 20 rhythmic contractions, the muscle or joint is positioned at the new barrier. This process is repeated until there is no more gain – frequently using different directions of isometric effort.

7. Visual and/or respiratory synkinesis may be useful, particularly in acute settings.

aspects of joint stiffness or laxity and behaviour deserve our attention.

What Makes Joints Stiff?

Landmark research in the 1960s by Johns and Wright identified those features of joints that contribute to their stiffness. Their research is still regularly cited in current research papers on this topic, and it has not been challenged (Wright & Johns, 1960a, 1960b; Johns & Wright, 1962).

They observed that contributions to joint restriction derived from the following influences in the proportions shown: joint capsule (47%), surrounding muscles and intermuscular fasciae (41%), tendons (10%), skin tissue (2%).

- Citing Johns and Wright (1962), Lebiedowska and Fisk (2009) confirm that:

The passive stiffness of a joint reflects properties of the muscle tissue, joint capsule, tendons, skin and geometry of the joint.

- Wu et al. (2009) note that with arthritic changes – in this case involving the thumb, which they were

studying – stiffness can increase by up to 100%. During that degenerative process the degree of muscular force required to use the joint is seen to increase proportionally, and that:

it is possible, theoretically, to improve the range of motion for OA patients in [the] early stages, by increasing muscle strength through exercise.

This study highlights the influence of pathology on joint stiffness.

- Hasson et al. (2011) highlight the influence of age on stiffness, in their research into ankle joint features:

Many clinical studies use maximal isometric strength as a marker of functional ability. However, the present study has shown additional age-related differences in the dynamic properties of the ankle muscles, with slower concentric force capabilities and stiffer series elasticity in the older adults.

This study highlights the influence of aging on joint stiffness.

What Is Hypermobility and Joint Laxity?

Hypermobility syndrome was first described in 1967 by Kirk and colleagues as a condition where joint laxity is associated with various musculoskeletal complaints (Kirk et al., 1967). The most common presenting complaint related to hypermobility is joint pain (Tinkle, 2020). Lewit (2009) also described the implications of hypermobility.

In recent years, 14 subtypes of hypermobility syndrome have been identified, with a range of genetic and environmental predisposing factors. Hypermobility can be acquired by an injury to a joint or progressively though ongoing flexibility activities (Sacks et al., 2019; Solecki et al., 2020), and joint hypermobility is commonly associated with younger age groups (Van Meulenbroek et al., 2021). Joint laxity is typically identified based on joint movement assessment and determination of hypermobility. Generalised joint laxity (GJL), also known as systemic joint laxity, is a condition in which the majority of synovial joints have range of motion beyond normal. Joint laxity can be caused by genetic disorders affecting collagen, such as Ehlers-Danlos or Marfan syndrome. Specific neurodevelopmental factors affecting hypermobility, motor coordination, and proprioception have been identified and are the subject of ongoing research (Ghibellini et al., 2015).

Myofascial pain and hypermobility are commonly found together and, as a result, assessment may identify stiffness which could be related to compensation promoting stability (Tewari et al., 2017; Qureshi et al., 2019; Hastings et al., 2019; Ahmed et al., 2020). Interestingly, neither body composition, muscle flexibility, muscle strength, nor muscle power in those with hypermobility were found to be significantly different to those with normal function, confounding the process of assessment and understanding of symptoms experienced (Ewertowska et al., 2020; Thijs et al., 2020).

Logically, treatment to address stiffness without understanding the source of underlying hypermobility can result in a reduction in stability.

There are multiple assessment tools related to the diagnosis of hypermobility. A simple screening using a patient reported questionnaire consisting of five questions is helpful (Hakim & Grahame 2003; Schlager et al., 2020):

- Can you now (or could you ever) place your hands flat on the floor without bending your knees?
- Can you now (or could you ever) bend your thumb to touch your forearms?
- As a child did you amuse your friends by contorting your body into strange shapes or could you do the splits?
- As a child or teenager, did your shoulder or kneecap dislocate on more than one occasion?
- Do you consider yourself double-jointed?

A positive answer to two or more questions suggests hypermobility, while additional investigation is needed to establish the presence of Ehlers-Danlos or related syndromes.

In suspected or confirmed cases of hypermobility, manual therapy should be used cautiously, but may afford benefits in managing pain and dysfunction in hypermobile patients (Boudreau et al., 2020; Song et al., 2020). Treatment adaptation and suggestions are provided in this chapter.

Age, Disease and MET

There is evidence for MET having beneficial effects on elderly patients with chronic shoulder restrictions, most of which involved arthritic changes (Knebl et al., 2002). That study compared use of an osteopathic shoulder mobilisation sequence (Spencer technique) with and without the addition of MET as part of the protocol. While both treatments produced increased mobility, it was noted that there was a continuing trend for the range of motion of the shoulder to improve in those who received the additional MET during mobilisation (see later in this chapter for description of the protocol, as well as the video clip for demonstrations of the Spencer methodology). In contrast, those who improved with mobilisation alone, gradually lost the benefit gained during the period when the MET group continued to improve. A more current study by Iqbal et al. (2020) found that in individuals with an average age of 45, the Spencer technique was more effective than passive stretching in treating patients with adhesive capsulitis.

MET's potential for influencing the features of joint stiffness, identified by Johns and Wright and the studies of others, would – unsurprisingly – therefore seem to relate to changes in muscular and fascial structures, the very tissues that MET so directly targets.

Viscoelasticity in relation to MET/PNF contractions and stretching) indicated that:

1. There are direct fascial influences during isometric contractions – specifically affecting the series, and

parallel elastic components of sarcomeres (Lederman, 2005).

2. There is a 'hydraulic' influence on connective tissue during contractions, reducing the stiffness, albeit temporarily, but potentially allowing a window of opportunity for enhanced mobilisation efforts (Klingler et al., 2004).

End-of-Range, End-Feel, Restrictions to Normal Motion

Kaltenborn et al. (2008) have summarised some of the major reasons for joint restrictions, and the tissues involved in these, as well as optimal treatment options:

- Periarticular restrictions may be due to adaptive shortening of neuromuscular and inert structures (including skin, retinacula and scar tissue), as well as extra-articular structures (capsule and ligaments) that, it is suggested, are best treated with sustained mobilisation techniques.
- Periarticular restrictions that are due to muscle hypertonicity are said to respond best to neurophysiological inhibitory techniques – including the use of isometric contractions (Exelby 1996; Hsieh et al., 2002).
- Intra-articular restrictions respond to (traction) manipulation initiated from the actual resting position and by restoration of joint roll/glide function. De las Penas et al. (2011), Kaltenborn et al. (2008) and Mulligan (2004) offer descriptions of methods to achieve mobilisation, that involve both active and passive interventions – however discussion of these methods lies outside the scope of this text.

Kaltenborn's (1985) Description of Normal End-Feel Variations

- Normal soft end-feel results from soft tissue approximation (as in flexing the knee) or soft tissue stretching (as in ankle dorsiflexion).
- Normal firm end-feel is the result of capsular or ligamentous stretching (internal rotation of the femur for example).
- Normal hard end-feel occurs when bone meets bone as in elbow extension.

Kaltenborn's Definition of Abnormal End-Feel Variations

- A firm, elastic feel is noted when scar tissue restricts movement or when shortened connective tissue is present.

- An elastic, less soft end-feel occurs when increased muscle tonus prevents free movement.
- An empty end-feel is noted when the patient stops the movement, or requests that it be stopped, before a true end-feel is reached, usually as a result of extreme pain such as might occur in active inflammation, or a fracture, or because of psychogenic factors.
- As noted above, a sudden, hard end-feel is commonly due to interosseous changes such as arthritis.
- By engaging the barrier (*always* the barrier, never short of the barrier for joint conditions) and using appropriate degrees of isometric effort, the barriers can commonly be modified.

The evidence supplied in this, and other chapters suggests that many joint restrictions – irrespective of aetiology – are amenable to appropriate MET methods involving variations on the theme of isometric, isotonic and rhythmic (pulsed) contractions.

Lewit's Anaesthetised Patients

The emphasis of MET on soft tissues should not be taken to indicate that intra-articular causes of dysfunction are not acknowledged. Indeed, Lewit (1985) addressed this controversy in an elegant study that demonstrated that some typical restriction patterns remain intact even when the patient is observed under narcosis with myorelaxants.

He attempts to direct attention towards a more balanced view when he states:

> The naive conception that movement restriction in passive mobility is necessarily due to articular lesion has to be abandoned. We know that taut muscles alone can limit passive movement, and that articular lesions are regularly associated with increased muscular tension.

He then goes on to point to the other alternatives, including the fact that many joint restrictions are not the result of soft tissue changes, using as examples those joints not under the direct control of muscular influences, such as tibiofibular, sacroiliac (SI) and acromioclavicular. He also points to the many instances where joint play is more restricted than normal joint movement. Since joint play is a feature of joint mobility that is not subject to muscular or voluntary control, the conclusion has to be made that there are indeed joint problems in which the soft tissues represent a secondary rather than primary factor in any general dysfunctional pattern of pain and/or restricted range of motion (blockage). He continues:

> This is not to belittle the role of the musculature in movement restriction, but it is important to re-establish the role of articulation, and even more to distinguish clinically between movement restriction caused by taut muscles, and that due to blocked joints, or very often, to both.

Fortunately MET seems capable of offering assistance towards normalisation of both forms of dysfunction.

Muscles or Joints?

Janda (1988) suggested that it is not known whether dysfunction of muscles causes joint dysfunction or vice versa; he points to the undoubted fact that each massively influences the other, and that it is possible that a major element in the benefits noted following joint manipulation derives from the effects such methods (high-velocity thrust, mobilisation, etc.) have on associated soft tissues.

When discussing the influence of muscles in disc and facet syndromes, Steiner (1994) described a possible sequence as follows:

- A strain involving body torsion, rapid stretch, loss of balance, etc., produces a myotatic stretch reflex response in, for example, a part of the erector spinae.
- The muscles contract to protect excessive joint movement, and spasm may result if (for any of a range of reasons) there is an exaggerated response and they fail to resume normal tone following the strain.
- This limits free movement of the attached vertebrae, approximates them and causes compression and bulging of the intervertebral discs, and/or a forcing together of the articular facets.
- Bulging discs might encroach on a nerve root, producing disc syndrome symptoms.
- Articular facets, when forced together, produce pressure on the intra-articular fluid, pushing it against the confining facet capsule that becomes stretched and irritated.
- The sinu-vertebral capsular nerves may therefore become irritated, provoking muscular guarding, initiating a self-perpetuating process of pain-spasm-pain. Steiner continued:

> From a physiological standpoint, correction or cure of the disc or facet syndromes should be the reversal of the process that produced them, eliminating muscle spasm and restoring normal motion.

He argues that before discectomy, or facet rhizotomy is attempted, with the all too frequent 'failed disc syndrome surgery' outcome, attention to the soft tissues and articular separation to reduce the spasm should be tried, in order to allow the bulging disc to recede, and/or the facets to resume normal motion.

Clearly, osseous manipulation (high-velocity thrust) often has a place in achieving this objective (Gibbons & Tehan, 1998), but clinical experience suggests that a soft tissue approach that either relies largely on MET, or at least incorporates MET as a major part of its methodology, is likely to produce excellent results in at least some such cases, and fortunately in this era of evidence-based medicine, research validation of this is available.

MET Mechanisms in Treatment of Joints

In the early years of MET's evolution the mechanisms that were assumed to be operating in MET were postisometric relaxation (PIR) and reciprocal inhibition (RI). The accuracy of these conceptualised mechanisms is now questioned, as explained in detail in Chapter 4, where more recent interpretations are described and discussed in relation to 'how MET works'.

Nevertheless, as recently as 2011, Walkowski and Baker continued to suggest that:

> The physiology of muscle energy treatment is suspected to be an activation of intramuscular proprioceptive fibers called Golgi tendon organs (Kuchera & Kuchera, 1994). These sensory units are found at the musculotendinous junctions and, when activated, will reflexively cause the motor units to temporarily shut down and relax the muscle tissue. They are thought to have a protective function against overstretching the muscle. By placing the muscle in a position of restriction and then having the patient isometrically contract, these fibers are thought to be activated and then reflexively allow for muscle relaxation.

As Gary Fryer details in Chapter 4, PIR and RI mechanisms cannot fully explain the effects of MET. Further studies listed in the relevant discussion in Chapter 10 also reach the same conclusion. As a result, different influences on MET outcomes need to be considered – such as:

- Increased tolerance to stretch – an as-yet unexplained phenomenon, possibly deriving from influences such as those described in this list, or from as-yet unknown mechanisms (Magnusson et al., 1996).
- Neurological (e.g. mechanoreceptor activation, stimulation-produced analgesia), fluid flow reducing concentrations of inflammatory cytokines, etc. (Fryer & Fossum, 2009; Espejo et al., 2018).
- Hydraulic changes (Klingler et al., 2004; Schleip, 2011).
- Viscoelastic/fascial changes (Lederman, 1997; Timanin et al., 2020).
- Release of analgesia-inducing endocannabinoids (McPartland, 2008; Onifer et al., 2019). Therefore, realistically, while none of the newer MET explanations can be shown to provide complete answers, the older concepts of PIR and RI are no longer appropriate, except as indications as to whether agonists are being employed in the contractions (PIR) or their antagonists (RI).

It would also be as well to remember Ruddy's pulsed MET variations, which are useful in treating joint problems (see Chapter 5). Clinical use, and anecdotal reports accumulated over approximately 60 years, support employment of these safe methods alongside or instead of sustained isometric or isotonic versions of MET.

It is hoped that the suitably trained reader will be able to employ the principles and methodology of MET, as explained in this and in other chapters, to those joints described in this chapter (using visual images on the DVD-ROM as aids if necessary). It should also be possible to adapt and extrapolate the use of MET methods to joint conditions that are not specifically discussed in this chapter.

EVIDENCE FOR MET

Examples of Joint Range of Motion (ROM) Increases Following MET

Factors such as duration of post-contraction stretch, and the number of isometric contraction repetitions, appear to be major variables that determine clinical outcomes. For example, a 30-second duration of stretch seems to be a key element in determining whether or not MET procedures are successful in changing muscle ROM, with some evidence that a single, long-held, 30-second stretch offers the same benefits as two 15-second or five 6-second stretches (Bandy et al., 1997).

The question of results enhancement using MET methods is ongoing. A recent study comparing MET and passive stretching showed a significant improvement in hamstring flexibility in both the groups and that both MET and passive stretching techniques have an immediate effect on reducing hamstring muscle tightness, with MET being slightly more effective than passive stretching (Sathe et al., 2020).

There are particular suggestions regarding length of stretch of soft tissues, where age is a factor. For example, Feland et al. (2001) demonstrated that in elderly subjects a 60-second stretch, repeated four times, was more effective in increasing knee extension ROM than a 15- or 30-second stretch (also repeated four times).

It is clear from the evidence in relation to stretching that, while the ROM of joints increases following appropriate stretching of particular muscles, the individual responses of different joints to soft tissue stretching varies.

- The *hip joint* was more responsive to flexion with a ROM improvement of ±9 degrees on average, than was the ankle joint, where only a modest increase (±3 degrees) in dorsiflexion was achieved (Shrier & Gossal, 2000).
- Lenehan et al. (2003) were able to show a greater than 10 degrees increase in rotation ROM of the *thoracic spine,* after a single MET isometric contraction – utilising a side flexion effort during the isometric contraction.
- Schenk et al. (1994) investigated the effect of MET over a 4-week period, on *cervical* ROM of 18 asymptomatic subjects with limitations (10 degrees or more) of active motion, in one or more planes. Those treated underwent seven treatment sessions in which the joint was positioned against the restrictive barrier, using three repetitions of light 5-second isometric contractions. Pre- and post-ROM was measured using a cervical ROM device, and the post-test range was measured 1 day after the last session. Those in the MET group achieved significant gains in rotation (approximately 8 degrees), and smaller non-significant gains in all other planes. The control group demonstrated little change.
- Moore et al. (2011) demonstrated an increase in ROM following a single application of an MET

for the *glenohumeral joint* horizontal abductors, in both horizontal adduction (mean ± SD, 6.8 ± 10.5 degrees) and internal rotation ROM (4.2 ± 5.3 degrees) in asymptomatic collegiate baseball players. Reed et al. (2018), identified similar results as Moore et al. using similar methods finding that the MET group had significantly more horizontal adduction ROM post-treatment compared to the control group

- Fryer and Ruskowski (2004) demonstrated a 6.65-degree increase in *cervical rotation* ROM using MET. However, the results differed depending on the length of the sustained isometric contraction (see below).

Ideal Length of Contraction for Increasing Joint ROM

Fryer and Ruskowski (2004) evaluated different lengths of contraction in a study involving 52 asymptomatic individuals.

- Results showed that a 5-second isometric contraction, using mild degrees of effort, was more effective in increasing cervical ROM than a 20-second contraction.
- ROM increased in those using 5-second contractions by 6.65 degrees (after three repetitions of the isometric contraction).
- ROM only increased in those using 20-second contractions by 4.34 degrees (after three repetitions of the isometric contraction).
- A sham group (bogus 'functional' technique) increased by 1.41 degrees.

There clearly remains much to learn as to ideal contraction times, with many different opinions, and very little actual evidence (Thomas et al., 2019).

Burns and Wells (2006): Cervical ROM Study

Burns and Wells (2006) conducted a study to evaluate the usefulness of MET in treatment of cervical restriction (in asymptomatic individuals). Their study demonstrated: 'a significant increase in overall regional cervical range of motion in the treatment group (MET) when compared with control subjects', supporting Mitchell's hypothesis that restricted joints would benefit if treatment focused on the associated soft tissues. The protocol used to deliver muscle energy treatment to subjects in the treatment group in this study was as follows:

1. The practitioner localised the joint or body tissues at a resistance barrier, i.e. initial range of motion

resistance to a specific movement (such as flexion/extension, side-bending and rotation).

2. The subject was instructed as to the amount (ounces to a few pounds) and duration (3 to 5 seconds) of contractile force to use – when requested.
3. The practitioner then asked the subject to push their head and neck in an appropriate direction,[1] while the practitioner provided isometric counterforce until an appropriate level of force was perceived.
4. This was maintained for 3 to 5 seconds, with the length of contraction varying with the size of the muscle being treated.
5. The subject was directed to gently cease the contraction.
6. After 3 to 5 seconds of relaxation the practitioner passively engaged a new barrier.
7. Steps 1 through 6 were repeated two to four times. The researchers noted that '*the quality of subject response often peaked at the third excursion with diminishing returns thereafter*'.

The recommendations of the author of this chapter are in accord with the protocols described – with a suggestion that there is probably not much to be gained by more than 2 further repetitions after the initial isometric contraction.

The reader is reminded of the study by Lenehan et al. (2003), in which gross trunk rotation was markedly increased by using side flexion as the contraction direction.

Burns and Wells (2006) offer a strong statement of support for the use of MET on a wide scale:

> MET may be useful in the treatment of numerous clinical syndromes, such as cervicogenic headache (Grimshaw, 2001), nerve compression syndromes (Luckenbill-Edds & Bechill, 1995), acute and chronic neck pain from motor vehicle accidents, or minor trauma to the neck (Cassidy et al., 1992a). There seems to be an inverse correlation between an increase in cervical range of motion and a decrease in neck pain (Cassidy et al., 1992b). Cervical

---

[1]Note: The 'appropriate' direction towards which the patient/subject should be asked to 'push' is unpredictable. Just because restriction is, say, towards rotation does not mean that a rotational force should be employed. Since it is almost impossible to predict precisely which soft tissues may be involved in any given joint restriction, a variety of directions of contraction should be explored.

manipulation was shown to be much safer, when compared with the use of nonsteroidal anti-inflammatory drugs in the treatment of neck pain by a factor of over 100% (Dabbs & Lauretti, 1995). Muscle energy technique may be applied in the treatment of somatic dysfunctions not only of the spine, but also of the ribs, extremities and pelvis (Goodridge, 1981).

Selkow et al. (2009): MET and Lumbopelvic Pain

Selkow et al. (2009) conducted a randomised controlled trial involving individuals with lumbopelvic pain (LPP). In those receiving treatment, MET was applied to the hamstrings and iliopsoas utilising 5-second isometric contractions, followed by engagement of a new barrier (repeated four times in all). The control group received sham treatment.

Significant pain reduction was noted immediately following the MET intervention, and 24 hours later. Selkow et al. observed that:

MET can be used to treat LPP, particularly low levels of pain. The touch of the clinician, along with stimulation of agonist and antagonist muscles, seems to alter perception of pain. This technique could be performed prior to other rehabilitation techniques, such as strengthening exercises, to decrease pain and allow more efficient exercises to then be executed. This technique may be better than others in decreasing pain for several reasons. The time it takes to administer MET is very short (less than 1 minute). It also allows the clinician to have physical contact with the patient, helping the patient to trust the clinician. Lastly, MET is a low-force isometric contraction in a pain-free position. This technique can be accomplished without causing further pain or harm to the patient.

The relative simplicity of application as well as the brief clinical time involved, offer compelling reasons for use of MET in such conditions.

Wilson et al. (2003): Acute Low-Back Pain and MET (See Chapter 8)

A detailed description of MET use in treatment of acute low-back pain is given by Wilson et al. (2003). They conclude:

Results from this pilot study suggest that MET, combined with supervised neuromuscular re-education and resistance training exercises, may be superior to supervised neuromuscular re-education and resistance training exercises alone, in improving function in patients with acute low back pain.

MET Versus HVLA Thrust

- High-velocity, low-amplitude (HVLA) thrust treatment has been compared with MET in treatment of cervical joint problems (Scott-Dawkins, 1997).
- Thirty patients with chronic cervical pain were randomised to receive either HVLA or MET manipulation.
- Each group was treated twice weekly for 3 weeks.

Patients treated with HVLA thrust experienced a greater immediate relief of pain but at the end of the treatment period there was no difference in pain levels, with pain decreasing in both groups to the same extent.

- A 2013 study of 60 healthy students compared a bilateral HVLA thrust to MET focused on the cervical C2 region and sub-occipital muscles respectively, measuring improvement in active cervical ROM. The study included a control group. Both techniques showed significant improvement to ROM, with MET demonstrating a greater significance in P value (Uong, 2013).
- In a 2020 study, 10 male workers with low back pain were randomised to HVLA and MET treatment groups and treated for a total of 7 weeks. Both methods were recorded as offering immediate relief which remained 2 weeks later. Trunk muscular activation patterns and postural balance were unaffected by either technique (Sturion et al., 2020).

Brodin (1987): MET Treatment of Chronic Low-Back Pain

Research at the Karolinska Hospital in Stockholm investigated the effects of MET application in a group of long-term, low-back pain (lumbar area only) sufferers, specifically excluding patients with signs of disc compression, spondylitis or SI lesions, but not those with radiographic evidence of common degenerative signs – such as spondylosis deformans (Brodin, 1987).

The group comprised 41 patients (24 female, 17 male) who had suffered pain in one or two lumbar segments, with reduced mobility that had lasted for at least 2 months. The patients were randomly assigned to two groups, one receiving no treatment and the other receiving MET treatment three times weekly for 3 weeks. The MET approach used is described by Brodin as 'a modification of the technique described by Lewit … a variation of Mitchell's MET'. Both groups of patients recorded their pain level at rest and during activity according to a 9-graded scale each week.

Results: After 3 weeks, the group receiving treatment showed significant pain reduction, statistically greater than in the non-treated group, as well as an increase in mobility of the lumbar spine:

- Of the 21 in the treated group, four remained the same or were worse, while 17 were improved, of whom seven became totally pain free.
- Only one in the non-treated group ($n = 20$) became totally pain free, while 16 remained the same or were worse. A total of four in this group, including the one who was totally improved, showed some improvement.

MET Approaches Used in the Brodin Study

- The patient was side-lying, with the lumbar spine rotated by moving the upper shoulder backwards, with the table-side shoulder drawn forwards until the restricted segment of the spine was engaged.
- The practitioner stabilised the patient's pelvis and the patient then pushed the shoulder forwards, using a very small amount of effort, against resistance from the practitioner, for 7 seconds.
- During relaxation, the practitioner increased the degree of lumbar rotation to the new barrier, and repeated the isometric resistance phase again, until no further gain was made, usually involving four or five repetitions.
- Additionally, active, rhythmic, small rotatory movements against the resistance barrier were carried out. See the description in Chapter 5 of 'pulsed MET' (Ruddy, 1962) that calls for this type of active engagement of the barrier.
- Aspects of respiratory and visual synkinesis were also employed (see Chapter 6).

- Patients were advised to use pain-free movements and positions during everyday life.

The author states:

From this study we can conclude that in pre-selected cases, muscle energy technique is an effective treatment for lower back pain (particularly when) mobility is decreased, or its end-feel abnormally distinct.

Brodin, 1982

MET Treatment of Joints Damaged by Haemophilia

Just how useful MET can be in treating joint problems in severely ill patients is illustrated by a Polish study of the effects of the use of MET in a group of haemophiliac patients, in whom bleeding had occurred into the joints. There had also been bleeding into muscles such as iliopsoas, quadriceps and gastrocnemius (Kwolek, 1989). The study notes that:

As a result of haemorrhage into the joints and muscles the typical signs and symptoms of inflammation develop; if they are untreated, or treated incorrectly, or rehabilitation is neglected, motion restriction, deformation, athrodesis, muscle atrophy, scarring and muscular contractures may occur.

Standard medical treatment used included electromagnetic field applications, heat, paraffin baths and massage, as well as (where appropriate) the use of casts for limbs and other medical and surgical procedures.

All patients received instruction as to self-application of breathing, relaxation and general fitness exercise, as well as rehabilitation methods for the affected joints using PIR methods (MET). These were performed twice daily, for a total of 60 minutes.

Range of movement was assessed, and it was found that those patients using PIR (MET) methods achieved an improvement in range of movement of between 5 and 50 degrees in 87% of the 49 joints treated – mainly involving ankles, knees and elbows (there was a reduction in motion range of 5 to 10 degrees in just six joints). These impressive results for MET, in a group of severely ill and vulnerable patients, highlight the safety of the method, since anything approaching aggressive intervention in treating such patients would be contraindicated.

The researchers, having pointed to frequent complications arising in the course of more traditional approaches, concluded:

The 87% improvement in movement range of 5 to 50°, and the lack of complications when rehabilitating articulations with haemophiliac arthropathy, speaks in favour of routine application of the post isometric relaxation methods for patients with haemophilia.

PREPARING JOINTS FOR HVLA MANIPULATION USING MET

What if high-velocity thrust or mobilisation methods of joint manipulation are the appropriate method of choice in treatment of a restricted joint? How can MET fit into the picture?

Muscle energy methods are versatile, and while they certainly have applications which are aimed at normalising soft tissue structures, such as shortened or tense muscles, with no direct implications as to the joints associated with these, they can also be used to help to improve joint mobility via their influence on dysfunctional soft tissues, which may be the major obstacle to the restoration of free movement.

MET may be employed to relax tight, tense musculature, or even spasm, and can also help in reduction of fibrotic changes in chronic soft tissue problems, as well as toning weakened structures which may be present in the antagonists of shortened soft tissues or in cases of hypermobility.

MET may therefore be employed in a *pre-manipulative* mode. In this instance, the conventional manipulative procedure is prepared for, as it would normally be, whether this involves leverage or a thrust technique. The practitioner – having adopted an appropriate position, made suitable manual contacts, prepared the tissues for the high-velocity or mobilisation adjustment, and engaged the restriction barrier by taking out available slack – could then ask the patient to 'push back' from this position against solid resistance. The practitioner will have engaged the barrier in this preparation for manipulation and will have taken out the slack that was available in the soft tissues of the joint(s), in order to achieve this position.

When the patient is asked to firmly but painlessly resist or 'push back', against the practitioner's contact hands, this produces a patient-indirect (practitioner pushing towards the resistance barrier while the patient pushes away from it) isometric contraction, which would have the effect of contracting the presumably shortened muscles associated with the restricted joint. After holding this effort for several seconds, both practitioner and patient would simultaneously release their efforts, in a slow, deliberate manner.

This could be repeated several times, with the additional slack being taken out after appropriate relaxation by the patient.

Having engaged and re-engaged the barrier a number of times, the practitioner would decide when adequate release of restraining tissues had taken place and would then make the high-velocity adjustment or mobilisation movement, as normal.

Hartman (1985) states that:

If the patient is in the absolute optimum position for a particular thrust technique during one of these repetitions [of MET], the joint in question will be felt to release. Even if this has not occurred, when retesting the movement range there is often a considerable increase in range and quality of play.

He suggests that the practitioner use the temporary rebound reflex relaxation in the muscles, which will have followed the isometric contraction, to perform the manipulative technique. This will allow successful completion of the adjustment with minimal force. This refractory period of relaxation lasts for quite a few seconds and is valuable in all cases, but especially where the patient is tense or resistant to a manipulative effort.

Avoid Wrestling

Walkowski and Baker (2011) note that difficulties with application of MET, particularly in relation to joints, commonly relate to poor localisation of force by the practitioner, lack of stabilisation against the isometric contraction, and the patient using excessive force, which needs to be great enough only to engage the tissues at the level of the localised, treated segment. Too much force becomes difficult to localise and may be too strong to control by the practitioner. 'Muscle Energy Technique, when properly applied, should not look like a wrestling match'.

BASIC CRITERIA FOR TREATING JOINT RESTRICTION WITH MET (FIG. 7.1A–F)

Because most MET treatment requires resistance against the patient's activating force to produce an isometric contraction, it is important to consider how best to stabilise the body of the patient, while still being able to monitor tissue changes in the dysfunctional structures. Good body mechanics, and an optimal choice of positioning, is called for.

In treating joint restriction with MET, Sandra Yates (1991) suggests the following simple criteria be maintained:

1. The joint should be positioned at its physiological barrier (specific in three planes if spinal segments are being treated: flexion or extension, side-bending and rotation).
2. The patient should be asked to statically contract muscles towards the direction of their freedom of motion (i.e. away from the barrier(s) of restriction) as the practitioner resists totally any movement of the part.
3. If the contraction is sustained, Yates suggests, it should be held for about 3 seconds (many MET experts suggest longer – up to 10 seconds).
4. The patient is asked to relax for 2 seconds or so, between the contraction efforts, at which time the practitioner re-engages the joint at its new motion barrier(s).

This process is repeated until free movement is achieved, or until no further gain is apparent following a contraction. The advice of the author of this chapter is that the isometric contraction could be in a different direction altogether – OR – that a pulsed, rhythmic, series of contractions should be introduced for 10 seconds or so.

Precise Focus of Forces – Example of Lumbar Dysfunction

Stiles (1984a), like most other practitioners using muscle energy methods, places emphasis on the importance of accurate and precise structural diagnosis, if MET is to be used effectively in treatment of joint dysfunction. By careful motion palpation, determination is made as to restricted joints or areas, and which of their motions is limited.

Precise, detailed localisation is required if there is to be accuracy in determining the direction in which the patient is to apply their forces, so that the specific restricted barrier can be engaged. If MET applications are poorly focused, it may be possible to actually create hypermobility in neighbouring segments, instead of normalising the restricted segment, by inappropriately introducing stretch into already adequately mobile tissues, above or below the restricted area.

For example, if a particular restriction is present between lumbar vertebrae – say limitation in gapping of the L4–L5 left-side facets on flexion – should a general MET mobilisation attempt be used that is not localised to this segment, and which involved the joints above and/or below the restricted segment, hypermobility of these joints could result, leading, on retesting for general mobility, to an incorrect assumption that the restriction had been reduced.

In order to localise the effort at the appropriate segment, the patient would require to be positioned so as to precisely engage the barrier in that joint. For example:

- One of the practitioner's hands would palpate the facets of L4–L5, while the seated patient is guided into a flexed and side-bent position which brings the affected segment to its barrier of motion (see Fig. 7.1B).
- At that point an instruction would be given for the patient to attempt to return to an upright position so involving the muscles (agonists) restraining the joint from movement to its normal barrier.
- At the same time the practitioner's force would restrain any movement.
- This isometric contraction should ideally be maintained for 3 to 5 seconds (Stiles's timing) with no more than perhaps 20% of the patient's strength being employed in the effort (ideally synchronised to breathing, see Chapter 6, Box 6.2).

After this, when all efforts have ceased, the barrier should have retreated, so that greater flexion and side-bending can be achieved, without effort, before re-engaging the barrier. Repetition would continue several times, until the maximum degree of motion had been obtained. Alternatively:

- Precisely the opposite method could also be employed, in which, having engaged the barrier, the patient would be asked to attempt to move through it, while being restrained. This would bring into play RI of any overly contracted muscles that might be restraining normal range of motion. In treating an acute condition, using RI reduces the likelihood of pain being produced during the procedure.

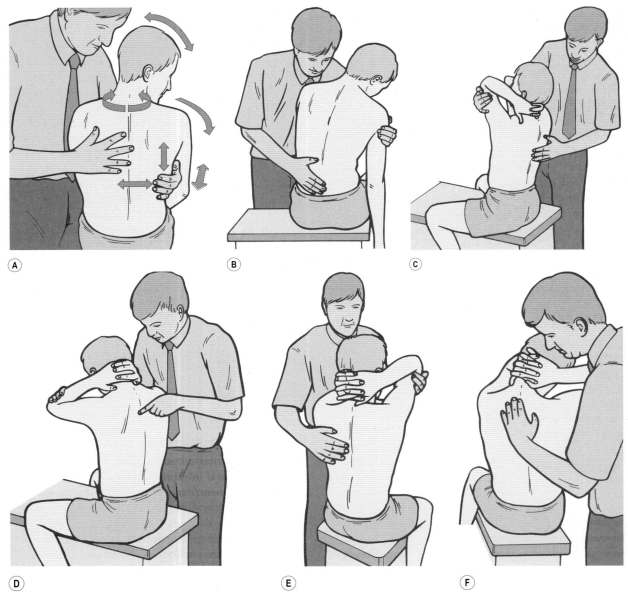

Fig. 7.1 (A) General assessment for restriction in thoracic spine, showing the possible directions of movement: flexion, extension, side-bending and rotation right and left, translation forwards, backwards, laterally in both directions, compression and distraction. MET treatment can be applied from any of the restriction barriers (or any combination of barriers) elicited in this way, with the area stabilised at the point of restriction. (B) Assessment and possible MET treatment position for restriction in side-bending and rotation to the right, involving the lumbar spine. (C) Assessment and possible MET treatment position for flexion restriction (inability to adequately extend) in the mid-thoracic area. MET treatment should commence from the perceived restriction barrier. (D) Assessment and possible MET treatment position for extension restriction (inability to adequately flex) in the upper thoracic area. MET treatment should commence from the perceived restriction barrier. (E) Assessment and possible MET treatment position for side-bending restriction (inability to adequately side-bend left) in the mid-thoracic area. MET treatment should commence from the perceived restriction barrier. (F) Assessment and possible MET treatment position for rotation restriction (inability to adequately rotate right) in the upper thoracic area. MET treatment should commence from the perceived restriction barrier.

Focus Rather than Force

Goodridge (1981) cautions that:

Monitoring of force is more important than intensity of force. Localisation depends on the practitioner's palpatory proprioceptive perception of movement (or resistance to movement) at or about the specific articulation. ... Monitoring and confining forces to the muscle group, or level of somatic dysfunction involved, are important in achieving desirable changes. Poor results are most often due to improperly localised forces, usually too strong.

Precise localisation of restrictions and identification of muscular contractions and fibrotic changes depend on careful palpation, a set of skills requiring constant refinement and maintenance by virtue of use. Identification of the particulars of each restriction can only be achieved via the development of the skills required to assess joint mechanics, combined with a sound anatomical knowledge.

Assessment, via motion palpation, is also called for. If forces are misdirected, then results will not only be poor but may also exacerbate the problem. In joint problems, localisation of the point of restriction seems to be the major determining factor of the success (or otherwise) of MET (as in all manipulation).

Harakal's Cooperative Isometric Technique (Harakal, 1975) (Fig. 7.2A–D)

Harakal's 1975 protocol is listed below, with comments regarding possible modifications based on subsequent studies.

When there is a specific or general restriction in a spinal articulation (for example):
- The area should be placed in neutral (usually with the patient seated).
- The permitted range of motion of a particular spinal segment should be determined by noting the patient's resistance to further motion.
- The patient should be rested for some seconds at a point just short of the resistance barrier, termed the 'point of balanced tension', to 'permit anatomic and physiologic response' to occur.
- The patient is asked to reverse the movement towards the barrier by 'turning back towards where we started', thus contracting any agonist muscles that may be influencing the restriction.

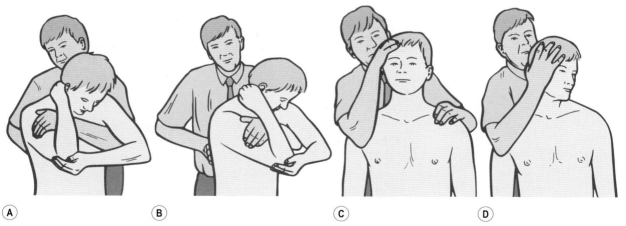

(A)　　　(B)　　　(C)　　　(D)

Fig. 7.2 (A) Harakal's approach requires the dysfunctional area (mid-thoracic in this example, in which segments cannot easily side-bend right and rotate left) to be taken to a position just short of the assessed restriction barrier. This is termed a point of 'balanced tension' where, after resting for a matter of seconds, an isometric contraction is introduced as the patient attempts to return towards neutral (sitting upright) against the practitioner's resistance. (B) Following this effort, the restriction barrier should have eased and the patient can be guided through it towards a new point of balanced tension, just short of the new barrier, and the procedure is repeated. (C) In this example the patient, who cannot easily side-bend and rotate the neck towards the left, is held just short of the present barrier in order to introduce an isometric contraction by turning the head to the right against resistance. (D) Following the contraction described in Fig. 7.2C, it is possible for the practitioner to ease the neck into a greater degree of side-bending and rotation towards the left.

NOTE: Ample evidence now suggests that 'reversing the motion' from the restriction barrier is not necessary – since use of alternative directions (side flexion, or translation, as examples) appear to be more efficient (Lenehan et al., 2003).

- The degree of patient participation at this stage can be at various levels, ranging from 'just think about turning' to 'turn as hard as you would like', or by giving more specific instructions.

NOTE: Lighter degrees of effort – as opposed to 'as hard as you like' are now considered more appropriate, as discussed in Chapter 5.

- Following a holding of this effort for a few seconds, and then relaxing completely, the patient is taken further in the direction of the previous barrier, to a new point of restriction determined by resistance to further motion, as well as tissue response (as a sense of 'bind' is palpated).
- The procedure is repeated until no further gain is being achieved.

NOTE: As explained in the descriptions of Ruddy's methodology (pulsed MET), the direction of effort is frequently commenced 'towards the barrier', with variations in direction subsequently being employed.

NOTE: An important issue in this description is that it does not involve any attempt whatsoever to move the tissues forcefully. Following the isometric contraction, and complete relaxation, the joint is carefully positioned at its new barrier, without force. This is in complete contrast to MET applied to a muscle, in which lengthening is the objective, and where stretching beyond the barrier would be both appropriate and essential for a positive outcome.

Grieve (1984) and MET for the Low Back

Grieve (1984) describes a low-back approach, using MET, that provides insights that can be adapted for use in other spinal regions. He discusses a spine, capable of full flexion, but in which palpable left side-bending and left rotation fixation exists (i.e. it is locked in left side-bending rotation, and therefore cannot freely side-bend and rotate to the right) in the lumbar spine.

Grieve's Low-Back Approach (Fig. 7.3)

NOTE: Using the current terminology, in use in 1984, it was appropriate for Grieve to mention RI and PIR. As

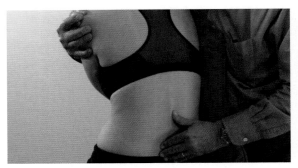

Fig. 7.3 Localisation of forces before using MET to release low-back restriction.

discussed earlier in this chapter, and elsewhere, these terms are now regarded as inaccurate in relation to the effects of MET.

In Grieve's example:

- The patient sits on a stool, feet apart and flat on the floor.
- The patient's left arm hangs between their knees, taking him into slight flexion and right rotation/side-bending.
- The practitioner stands at the patient's left side, with their left leg straddling the patient's left leg.
- The practitioner reaches across and holds the patient's right shoulder, while the right hand palpates the vertebral interspace between the spinous processes immediately below the restricted vertebra for its ability to rotate to the right.
- The patient is asked to slump forwards in this twisted posture until the segment under inspection is most prominent, posteriorly.
- At this point the practitioner presses their left pectoral area against the patient's left shoulder and, with the patient still flexed, the spine is side-bent by the practitioner, without resistance, so that the patient's right hand approximates the floor.
- The practitioner then rotates the patient to the right until maximum tension (bind) is felt to build at the segment being palpated. This is the restriction barrier.

At this time the first MET procedure is brought into play:

- The patient is asked to attempt to reach the floor with their right hand, and this effort is resisted by the practitioner – in order to produce RI.

- The isometric contraction may last for 5 to 10 seconds, after which the patient relaxes.
- As the patient exhales, the practitioner increases the side-bending and rotation to the right, before increasing the degree of flexion to the barrier of resistance. No force is used, simply removal of whatever additional degree of slack has been produced by the isometric effort.
- The procedure of attempting to increase these directions of spinal movement (side-bending and rotation to the right and flexion) is then repeated, against resistance, until no additional gain is achieved.
- After the repetitions, the patient (who is still flexed and rotated, and side-bent to the right) attempts to push against the practitioner's chest with the left shoulder (i.e. attempts to rotate left and side-bend left, as well as to extend).
- This effort is maintained for 5 to 10 seconds before relaxation, re-engagement of the barrier, and repetition.
- This contraction involves those structures which have shortened, and so the isometric contraction produces PIR in them.
- After each such contraction the slack is again taken out by taking the patient further into right side-bending, rotation and flexion.
- The practitioner's position alters after the isometric efforts to the left and right, so that they now stand behind the patient with a hand on each shoulder.
- Grieve then suggests that the patient be asked to perform a series of stretching movements to the floor, first with the left hand and then with the right hand, against resistance, before being brought into an upright position by the practitioner, against slight resistance of the patient.
- The condition is then reassessed.

Discussion of Grieve's Method

Notice that Grieve uses both RI and PIR in this manoeuvre. He states: 'Whether autogenic (PIR) or reciprocal inhibition is used is totally dependent on which technique effects the best neurophysiological change in the joint environment'.

In practice, however, it may not be clear which to choose; the author's experience is that use of the agonists – those structures thought to be most restricted and negatively influencing joint movement – produces the most beneficial results. Use of the antagonists in isometric contractions may also prove beneficial – for example, in situations in which agonist contractions are painful, or where agonist and antagonist both require therapeutic attention (e.g. following trauma such as whiplash in which all soft tissues will have been stressed).

In reality, since it is not usually possible to have certainty as to which soft tissues are involved in a particular joint restriction, it is suggested that almost any group of muscles related to a restricted joint, might be usefully isometrically contracted, as long as the guideline is adhered to that no pain should be produced, and if no attempt is made to force or 'stretch' joint structures.

Unlike the approach adopted in treatment of restricted muscles, joint applications of MET require that the barrier is engaged, with no attempt to push through it.

Additional Choices

Goodridge (1981) describes two additional MET procedures (the same pattern of dysfunction, described above, is assumed):

- *If the left transverse process of L5 is more posterior, when the patient is flexed, one postulates that the left caudad facet did not move anteriorly and superiorly along the left cephalad facet of S1, as did the right caudad facet.*
- *There would therefore seem to be restrictions in movements in the directions of flexion, lateral flexion (side-bending) to the right, and rotation to the right.*
- *It is conceptualised that the restricted motion involves hypertonicity (or shortening) of some muscle fibres.*
- *Therefore, the practitioner devises a muscle energy procedure to decrease the tone of (or to lengthen) the affected shortened or hypertonic fibres.*

Method (See Fig. 7.3)

- The position described by Grieve (see above) is adopted.

- The patient is seated, left hand hanging between thighs, with the practitioner at their left, the patient's right hand lateral to their right hip and pointing to the floor.
- The practitioner's right hand monitors either L5 spinous or transverse process.
- The patient's left shoulder is contacted against the practitioner's left axillary fold, and upper chest.
- The practitioner's left hand is holding the patient's right shoulder.
- The patient slouches in order to flex the lumbar spine, so that the apex of the posterior convexity is located at the L5–S1 articulation.
- The practitioner induces first a right side-bend, and then right rotation (patient's right hand approaches the floor) and localises movement at L5, when a sense of bind and restriction is noted there by the palpating hand.
- The patient is then asked to attempt to move in one or more directions, singly or in combination.
- These movements might involve left side-bending, translation, rotation left and/or extension, all against practitioner's counterforces.
- The patient is, in all of these efforts, contracting muscles on the left side of the spine, but is not changing the distance between the origin and insertion in muscles on either side of the spine.
- Subsequent contractions would be initiated after appropriate taking up of slack and engagement of the new barrier.
- *Additionally,* as in the Grieve example above, having attained the position of flexion, right side-bending and right rotation, localised at the joint in question, the patient might be asked to move both shoulders in a translation to the left, against resistance from the practitioner's chest and left anterior axillary fold.
- Neither of the shoulders should rise or fall as this is done, during the translation effort.
- While the patient is attempting to move in this manner, the practitioner palpates the degree of increased right side-bending which it induces, at L5–S1.
- As the patient eases off from this contraction, as described, the practitioner should be able to increase right rotation and side-bending until once again resistance is noted.
- The objective of Goodridge's alternative method is the same as in Grieve's example, but the movement

involves a concentric-isotonic procedure, because it allows right lateral flexion of the thoracolumbar spine during the effort.

As this method demonstrates, some MET methods are very simple, while others involve conceptualisation of multiple movements and the localisation of forces to achieve their ends.

The principles remain the same, however, and can be applied to any muscle or joint dysfunction, since the degree of effort, duration of effort and muscles utilised provide so many variables that can be tailored to meet most needs.

What if it Hurts?

What if pain is produced when using MET in joint mobilisation?

- Evjenth and Hamberg (1984) have a practical solution to the problem of pain being produced when an isometric contraction is employed. They suggest that the degree of effort be markedly reduced and the duration of the contraction increased from 10 seconds to 30 seconds. If this fails to allow a painless contraction, then use of the antagonist muscle(s) for the isometric contraction is another alternative.

Following the contraction, when the joint is being moved to a new resistance barrier, what variations are possible if this produces pain?

- If, following an isometric contraction, and movement towards the direction of restriction, there is pain, or if the patient fears pain, Evjenth suggests, 'then the therapist may be more passive and let the patient actively move the joint'.
- Pain experienced may often be lessened considerably if the therapist applies gentle traction while the patient actively moves the joint.
- Sometimes pain may be further reduced if, in addition to applying gentle traction, the therapist simultaneously either aids the patient's movement at the joint, or provides gentle resistance while the patient moves the joint.

Adaptation When Hypermobility Is a Factor

Adaptation will be determined based on the cause and extent of hypermobility. For example:

- an ankle or knee is hypermobile due to multiple sprains and strains

- hypermobility is acquired in an area related to performance in a sport such as shoulder hypermobility in baseball or basketball
- generalised increase in flexibility creating hypermobility found in individuals such as dancers, gymnasts or those who practice yoga
- hypermobility related to connective tissue disorders.

Hypermobility conditions can overlap resulting in commonly reported symptoms (Essles and Davies, 2021). Generally, the most commonly reported pain locations are the lower back, neck, shoulders, and knees (Feldman et al., 2020).

There are three distinct phases of generalised hypermobility syndrome (Tinkle et al., 2017; Song et al., 2020; Ali et al., 2020).

- The first 'hypermobility phase' occurs from childhood into adolescence. During this period symptoms include joint instability, recurrent dislocations, coordination/fine motor instability, fatigue, incontinence, developmental dyspraxia, and hypotonia.
- The second 'pain' phase most commonly occurs between the age ranges of 20 to 40 years old. The symptomatology of this phase includes generalised pain, and fatigue which is sometimes confused with fibromyalgia or chronic fatigue syndrome. Also common is pelvic pain, headaches, paresthesias, gastrointestinal (GI) disorders, and orthostatic imbalance.
- The final 'stiffness' stage, which is seen those older than 40, results from deconditioning and can cause muscle loss, proprioception deficits, and joint damage.

These same three phases occur with injury and performance-related hypermobility but may not follow the same time sequence. Repeated ankle sprain, for instance, will act like phase one instability, followed by the pain phase, and eventually the stiffness phase.

Multiple studies indicate the application of a multimodal treatment approach including manual therapy, therapeutic exercise, controlled stretching, postural and body mechanics education to treat hypermobility (Engelbert et al., 2017; Chopra et al., 2017; Song et al., 2020; Sirajudeen 2020). In general, exercise programs should focus on improving joint stability, preventing spasms, and optimising muscle tone and proprioception. Overstretching or hyperextension activities need to be avoided. Interventions should be limited to gentle, controlled, and focused methods. The various MET methods described in this text would meet these recommendations.

MET FOR THORACIC SPINAL DYSFUNCTION

NOTE: The example described below, of a specific thoracic vertebral restriction, should be seen as an example. It should be possible for anyone trained in assessment and treatment of spinal dysfunction (physiotherapist, osteopath, chiropractor, physiatrist, etc.) to take this example and relate it to *any spinal restriction.*

ADDITIONAL NOTE: This example describes a particular way of using MET in relation to a complex restriction. The reader is asked to recall the words of Mitchell Jr. (2009), Kappler and Jones (2003) and in Box 7.1, that emphasise the possibility of using a direction that is apparently unrelated to the restriction pattern, for an isometric contraction – with translation and side flexion being recommended based on clinical experience as well as research evidence (Lenehan et al., 2003).

Stiles (1984b) has described a similar protocol for use in the cervical spine (see below).

T3 Restriction: MET Protocol Summary

NOTE: In treatment of all joint restrictions, whether or not this is mentioned in the individual descriptions, before a joint is treated using any form of MET, associated muscles should be assessed and if necessary treated. In many instances, focused joint MET may then not be necessary.

NOTE: While this technique specifically mentions T3 being in an extended side-bent and rotated restriction, it may be used in treatment of any of the upper thoracic segments, either flexed or extended, and may be adapted for use anywhere in the spine.

- In this example the 3rd thoracic vertebra (T3) is extended, side-bent left, and rotated left.
- The objective is to use MET to increase the ability of T3 to flex, side-bend to the right and rotate to the right T4.
- The patient should be seated with the practitioner standing behind the patient.
- The practitioner places the middle finger of their left hand between the spinous processes of T3–T4; the index finger between T2 and T3, and the third finger between T4 and T5.
- The right hand is placed on top of the patient's head to passively produce flexion, right side-bending, and right rotation of T3, in order to engage the barrier.

- The palpating hand, using the three-finger palpation outlined above, should be able to precisely identify the moment that motion, directed by the hand on the head, reaches the involved segment as flexion, side flexion and rotation are introduced.
- Once the soft-end-of-range barrier is achieved ('feather edge of resistance') the patient is asked to gently extend the lower cervical and upper thoracic areas to include T3, against the practitioner's counterforce that is equal to the patient's force.
- This isometric contraction should be maintained for no more than 3 to 4 seconds, after which the patient should gently cease the effort, matched by reduction of counterforce.
- After a few seconds, during which the patient is asked to relax completely and to breathe normally, the practitioner takes up the slack and engages the new barriers (i.e. by introducing increased flexion, side-flexion right, rotation right).
- The process should be repeated once or twice more or until the greatest possible increase of motion is achieved.

Reminders

- The direction of contraction should vary, as it is impossible to predict which soft tissues are most involved in restrictions of this sort.
- Pulsed MET may also be usefully attempted instead of sustained contractions (see Box 7.1 and discussion of Pulsed MET in Chapters 5 and 6).

CERVICAL APPLICATION OF MET

Stiles (1984b) has described some of the most interesting applications of MET in treatment of joint restrictions. Some of his thoughts on cervical assessment and treatment are outlined below.

General Procedure Using MET for Cervical Restriction

Prior to any testing, Stiles suggests a general manoeuvre in which the patient is sitting upright. The practitioner stands behind and holds the head in the midline, with both hands stabilising it, and possibly employing their chest to prevent neck extension.

The patient is told to try (gently) to flex, extend, rotate and side-bend the neck, in all directions, alternately. (No particular sequence is necessary as long as all directions are engaged a number of times.) Each muscle group should undergo slight contraction against unyielding force. This relaxes the tissues in a general manner. Traumatised muscles will commonly relax without much pain via this method.

Localised Cervical Restriction Assessment and MET Treatment

There are predictable motion patterns in the cervical spine, below C1. Side flexion of any segment from C3 to C7 will induce automatic rotation in the same direction.

This is a clinically useful feature of the spinal mechanics of the cervical area, enabling precise use of various MET procedures in response to segmental restrictions. Cook et al. (2006) confirm that:

> *Coupled spinal motion is the rotation or translation of a vertebral body about or along one axis, that is consistently associated with the main rotation or translation about another axis. There is complete agreement among investigations regarding the directional coupling pattern of the lower cervical spine [C2–3 and lower] – i.e. side flexion and rotation to the same side.*

There is, however, less predictability in relation to movements of the occiput–C1, and C1–2 segments.

- If C3–C4 facets close appropriately as the neck of the supine patient is side-bent to the left, a characteristic physiological 'springing' will be noted as the barrier is reached.
- However, if on side-bending to the right, there is restriction, the facets will not be felt to close, and a pathological barrier will be noted, characterised by a lack of 'give', or increased resistance.
- Further assessment would reveal that not only is side flexion to the right restricted, but those same segments would be limited in their rotational potential to the right (Fryette, 1954; Mimura et al., 1989; Greenman, 1996; Cook et al., 2006). See Box 7.2 for further discussion on coupling.

This restriction may be expressed in two ways:

1. The positional diagnosis would be that the segment is flexed, rotated and side-bent to the left.
2. The functional diagnosis would be that the joint cannot freely extend, side-bend, or rotate to the right.
   - The patient should be in the same position used in assessment (supine, neck slightly flexed).

BOX 7.2 Spinal Coupling Notes

Fryette (1954) described an early model of spinal biomechanics when he defined basic 'laws' as follows:

Law 1 – side-bending with the spine in neutral results in rotation: the vertebra rotates towards the contralateral side (i.e. rotation into the convexity). This is known as type 1 coupling. Rotation is in the opposite direction to the side flexion.

Law 2 – side-bending with the spine in hyperextension or hyperflexion results in rotation to the ipsilateral side (i.e. into the concavity). This is known as type 2 coupling. Rotation is in the same direction as the side flexion.

Law 3 – when motion is introduced to a joint in one plane its mobility in other planes is reduced.

In the past MET has been taught with this model utilised to predict probable directions of motion.

Gibbons and Tehan (1998, 2006) have extensively examined current research and maintain that:

1. Coupled motion does indeed occur in all regions of the spine.
2. Coupled motion occurs independently of muscular activity but muscular activity might influence the direction and the magnitude of coupled movement.
3. Coupling of side-bending and rotation in the lumbar spine is variable in degree and direction.
4. There are many variables that can influence the degree and direction of coupled movement including pain, vertebral level, posture and facet tropism.
5. There does not appear to be any simple and consistent relationship between conjunct rotation and intervertebral motion segment level in the lumbar spine.

However, they state that the evidence of research and the literature is that *'in the cervical spine, below C2, Fryette's laws do seem to be applicable'*. This has been confirmed by Cook et al. (2006).

Systematic reviews of the literature conclude that consensus appears to have been reached regarding coupling direction and pattern variation in the cervical spine (Cook et al., 2006); whereas questions remain regarding thoracic coupling patterns due to inconsistencies in study designs and a lack of in vivo studies (Sizer et al., 2007). More recent cadaveric studies were used to produce a three-dimensional reconstruction of cervical spinal coupling, noting marked differences between lateral flexion and axial rotation (Liao, 2015).

The use of these biomechanical laws therefore allows application of Greenman's cervical spine method, as described in this chapter, to be used with confidence.

- The practitioner's right middle fingers would be placed over the right pillars of C3–C4 and the neck taken into *side-bending rotation to the right*, engaging the first sign of resistance of the barrier – not the extreme limit of motion.
- As this barrier is lightly engaged, the ability of that segment to rotate to the right should be tested, and the easy barrier identified.
- The left hand is placed over the patient's left parietal and temporal areas, and with this hand offering counterforce, the patient is invited to *side-bend and rotate to the left*, using minimal effort, for a few seconds, employing the muscles that may be contributing to the restriction.
- OR alternatively – avoiding either the side flexion, or the rotational element of restriction – the patient could be requested to introduce a side-shunt/translation effort, for a few seconds, mobilisation to the segment in question: *'Use translation whenever positioning against the "feather-edge" of the restrictive barrier'* (E. Stiles – personal communication 2011).
- A degree of relaxation should follow, after which the segment can be taken to its new barrier, and the same procedure repeated once or twice more – possibly employing different directions of translation, or side flexion, for example involving the patient initiating the isometric effort towards the barrier.
- A further alternative would be to have the patient use Ruddy's pulsating contractions, either into translation, or towards or away from the barrier. (See more detailed descriptions of Pulsed MET in Chapters 5 and 6, as well as Box 7.1.)

Greenman's Exercise in Cervical Palpation and Use of MET

The following exercise sequence is based on the work of Philip Greenman (1996), DeStefano (2010), and is suggested as a useful way of becoming familiar with both the mechanics of the neck joints, and safe and effective MET applications to whatever is found to be restricted.

In performing this exercise it is important to be aware that normal physiology dictates that side-bending and rotation in the cervical area (C3–C7) is usually Type 2 (see Box 7.2), which means that segments that are side-bending will automatically rotate towards the same side (i.e. a side-bend to the right means that rotation will take place to the right). Most cervical restrictions are compensations and will involve several segments, all of which will adopt this Type 2 pattern.

Exceptions occur if a segment is traumatically induced into a different format of dysfunction, in which case there could be side-bending to one side and rotation to the other – termed Type 1. The concept of general spinal coupling taking place in a predictable manner (apart from in the cervical region) has been challenged (Gibbons & Tehan, 1998; Cook et al., 2006) as discussed in Box 7.2.

Exercise in Cervical Palpation (Fig. 7.4A and B)

To easily palpate for side-bending and rotation, a side-to-side *translation* ('shunt') movement is used, with the neck in moderate flexion or extension. When the neck is in absolute neutral (no flexion or extension – an unusual state in the neck), true translation side-to-side is possible.

As any segment of the cervical spine below C2 is translated to one side, it automatically creates a side-bending effect and, because of the anatomical and physiological rules governing it, rotation to the same side occurs (Fryette, 1954; Mimura et al., 1989; Gibbons & Tehan, 1998; Cook et al., 2006).

In order to evaluate cervical function using this knowledge, Greenman suggests that the practitioner places the fingers as follows, on each side of the spine (see Fig. 7.4A):

- The index finger pads rest on the articular pillars of C6, just above the transverse processes of C7, which can be palpated just anterior to the upper trapezius.
- The middle finger pads will be on C6, and the ring fingers on C5, with the little finger pads on C3. Then:

1. With these contacts (the practitioner should be seated at the head of the supine patient) it is possible to examine for sensitivity, fibrosis, hypertonicity, as well as being able to apply lateral translation to cervical segments with the head in neutral, flexion or extension. In order to do this effectively, it is necessary to mobilise the superior segment to the one being examined. The heel of the hand helps to control movement of the head.

2. With the head/neck in relative neutral (no flexion and no extension), translation to the right and then left is introduced (any segment) to assess freedom

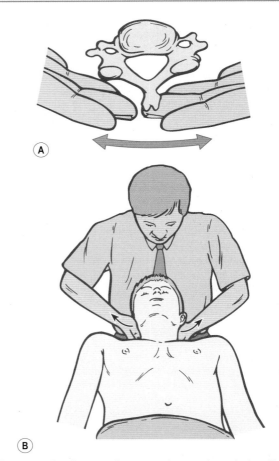

Fig. 7.4 (A) The finger pads rest as close to the articular pillars as possible, to be able to palpate and guide vertebral motion in a translatory manner. (B) With the neck/head in a neutral position, the practitioner sequentially guides individual segments into translation in both directions in order to sense indications of restriction and tissue modification. If a restriction is sensed, its increase or decrease is evaluated by retesting with the segment held in slight flexion and then extension. MET would be applied from the position of greatest unforced bind/restriction, using muscles which would either take the area through (i.e. antagonists to shortened muscles) or away from (i.e. shortened muscles themselves – the agonists) the barrier.

of movement (and by implication, side-bending and rotation) in each direction. Say C5 is being stabilised with the finger pads, as translation to the left is introduced, the ability of C5 to freely side-bend and rotate on C6 is being evaluated when the neck is in neutral. If the joint (and/or associated soft tissues) is normal, this translation will cause a gapping of the left facet and a 'closing' of the right facet as left translation is performed, and vice versa. There will be a soft end-feel to the movement, without harsh or sudden braking. If, however, translation of the segment towards the right from the left produces a sense of resistance/bind, then the segment is restricted in its ability to side-bend left and (by implication) to rotate left.

3. If such a restriction is noted, the translation should be repeated, but this time with the head in slight extension instead of neutral. This is achieved by lifting the contact fingers on C5 (in this example) slightly towards the ceiling before reassessing the side-to-side translation.

4. The head and neck are then taken into slight flexion, and left-to-right translation is again assessed.

The objective is to ascertain which position (neutral, flexion, extension) creates *the greatest degree of bind as the translation barrier is engaged*. Is movement more restricted in neutral, extension or flexion?

If this restriction is greater with the head extended, the diagnosis is of a joint restricted or locked in flexion, side-bent right and rotated right (meaning that there is difficulty in the joint extending and of side-bending and rotating to the left).

If this (C5 on C6 translation left to right) restriction is greater with the head flexed, then the joint is said to be restricted or locked in extension, and side-bent right and rotated right (meaning there is difficulty in the joint flexing, side-bending and rotating to the left).

▶ MET Treatment of the Cervical Area to Treat Translation Restriction

Using MET, and using the same example (C5 on C6 as above, translation right is restricted with the greatest degree of restriction noted in extension) the procedure would be as follows:

- One hand palpates both of the articular pillars of the inferior segment of the pair that testing (above) has shown to be dysfunctional.
- In this instance, this hand (index finger and thumb contacts) will stabilise the C6 articular pillars, holding the inferior vertebra so that the superior segment can be moved on it.
- The other hand will introduce movement to, and control the head and neck, above the restricted vertebra.
- The articular pillars of C6 are held and are guided anteriorly, introducing slight extension at that level,

while the other hand introduces side-bending and rotation to the left, involving the head and cervical spine down to C5, until the restriction barrier is engaged.

- A slight isometric contraction is asked for, with the patient incorporating side-bending, rotation to the right, and/or flexion – or pure translation.
- For example, the patient could be asked to try to lightly turn their head to the right, and to side-bend it right, while straightening the neck (or any one of these movements individually, if the combination is painful) OR the patient could be asked to translate towards, or away from, the restricted side.
- Whichever isometric effort is used should be firmly restrained.
- After 5 to 7 seconds the patient relaxes, and extension, side-bending and rotation to the left are increased to the new resistance barrier, with no force at all.
- Repeat several times – using different directions of isometric effort.
  OR:
- Have the patient introduce rhythmically pulsing mini-contractions in a chosen (by the practitioner) direction – aiming for around 20 rapid pulsations, without actual perceptible motion being observed ('no wobble, no bounce'). On cessation, the new barrier should be engaged and the process repeated.

NOTE: Eye movement can be used instead of muscular effort in cases where effort results in pain. Looking upwards will encourage isometric contraction of the extensors and vice versa, and looking towards a direction encourages contraction of the muscles on that side (see Chapters 5 and 6).

MET IN JOINT TREATMENT

It is not the aim of this chapter, or indeed the text as a whole, to provide a comprehensive body-wide, joint-by-joint description of MET application in joint restriction. Nevertheless, sufficient information is provided in this chapter (and elsewhere) to allow the interested practitioner to pursue this approach further, providing insights into possible technique applications involving spinal joints quite specifically, as well as generally, and also, more surprisingly perhaps, for dealing with joints that have no obvious muscular control, the iliosacral (IS) and acromioclavicular joints, both of which commonly respond well to MET use.

As a learning exercise in practical clinical application of MET to a dysfunctional joint, the well-known osteopathic Spencer shoulder sequence has been modified (see below). This sequence is based on a clinically useful and practical approach, first described nearly a century ago and still taught in most osteopathic schools in its updated form utilising MET or positional release methods (Spencer, 1976; Patriquin, 1992).

▶ Spencer Shoulder Sequence Incorporating MET

The Spencer shoulder treatment is a traditional osteopathic procedure (Spencer, 1976; Patriquin, 1992) that has in recent years been modified by the addition to its mobilisation procedures (described below) of MET. Clinical research has validated application of the Spencer sequence in a study involving elderly patients (Knebl et al., 2002).

- In a study 29 elderly patients with pre-existing shoulder problems were randomly assigned to a treatment (Spencer sequence osteopathic treatment) or a control group.
- The histories of those in the two groups were virtually identical: approximately 76% had a history of arthritis, 21% bursitis, 21% neurological disorders, 10% healed fractures.
- Sixty-three percent had reduced shoulder ROM as their chief complaint, and 33% pain (4% had both reduced ROM and pain).
- Treatment of the control (placebo) group involved the patients being placed in the same seven positions (see descriptions and Fig. 7.5A–F) as those receiving the active treatment; however, the one element that was not used in the control group was MET (described as the 'corrective force') as part of the protocol. Home exercises were also prescribed.
- Over the course of 14 weeks there were a total of eight 30-minute treatment sessions. Functional, pain and ROM assessments were conducted during alternate weeks, as well as 5 weeks after the end of treatment.
- Over the course of the study both groups demonstrated significantly increased ROM and a decrease in perceived pain. However, after treatment: 'Those subjects who had received osteopathic manipulative treatment [i.e. muscle-energy-enhanced Spencer sequence] demonstrated continued improvement in ROM, while the ROM of the placebo group decreased'.

The researchers concluded: 'Clinicians may wish to consider OMT [i.e. Muscle Energy Technique combined with Spencer sequence] as a modality for elderly patients with restricted ROM in the shoulder'.

Treating Muscles for Shoulder Restrictions

Carreiro (2009b) has described the Spencer sequence in relation to paediatric usage. She observes that the sequencing of the various stages of the protocol (involving between 7 and 9 stages, depending on the source): 'addresses all of the muscles of the shoulder girdle, using the arm as a long lever'.

For that reason, she argues:

The sequence should be carried out in the order described … because of the increasing complexity of movements required of the patient with each stage. Patients should be progressed through the sequence as tolerated. Pain is an indication that progression should be stopped until the next visit.

The sequence of eight stages, recommended by Carreira, is as follows: Extension, Flexion, Circumduction without traction, Circumduction with traction, Abduction, Adduction, Internal rotation, Abduction with resisted traction.

The descriptions below follow that recommended sequence apart from two elements:

1. Circumduction without traction is described below as circumduction with mild compression.
2. Abduction with resisted traction is not described.
3. Other major variations in the descriptions of the sequences in this text involve:
4. The introduction of pulsed MET into the protocol.
5. The use of variations in the directions of effort requested of the patient.

These suggested variations are based on clinical experience, and the reader is encouraged to experiment with further variations as clinical challenges demand.

A. Assessment and MET Treatment of Shoulder Extension Restriction (See Fig. 7.5A)

In this phase of the sequence the objective is to increase extension range of motion, and to help to normalise tone and length of pectoralis major, pectoralis minor as well as anterior deltoid muscles.

NOTE: For this phase of the sequence the practitioner can usefully stand in front of, or behind, the side-lying patient.

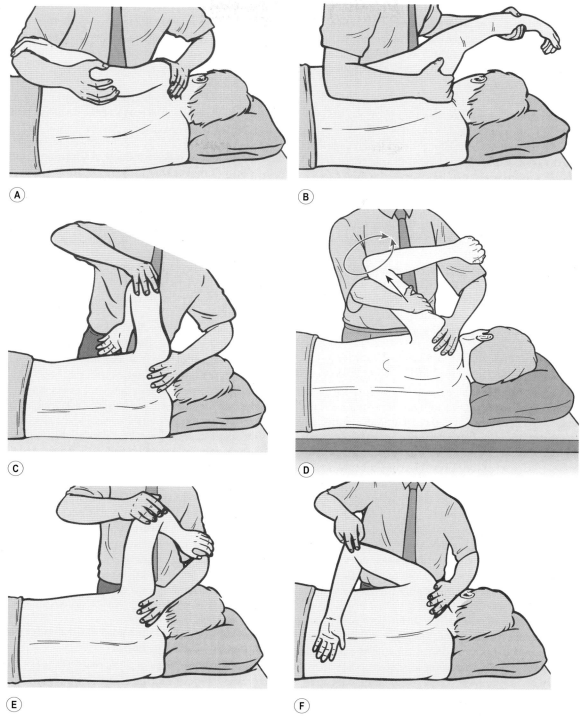

Fig. 7.5 (A) Shoulder extension. (B) Shoulder flexion. (C) Circumduction with compression. (D) Circumduction and traction. (E) Start position for both abduction and adduction of shoulder. (F) Internal rotation of the shoulder.

- The practitioner's cephalad hand cups the shoulder of the side-lying patient, firmly compressing the scapula and clavicle to the thorax, while the patient's flexed elbow is held in the practitioner's caudad hand, as the arm is taken into extension towards the optimal 90 degrees of extension.
- The first indication of resistance to movement should be sensed, indicating the beginning of the end of range of that movement.
- At that 'first sign of resistance' barrier the patient is instructed to push the elbow towards the feet, or anteriorly, or to push further towards the direction of extension – utilising no more than 20% of available strength, building up force slowly.
- This effort is firmly resisted by the practitioner, and after 5 to 7 seconds the patient is instructed to slowly cease the effort.
- After complete relaxation, and on an exhalation, the practitioner moves the shoulder further into extension, to the next restriction barrier, and the MET procedure is repeated, possibly using a different direction of effort. No stretching is involved.

B. Assessment and MET Treatment of Shoulder Flexion Restriction (See Fig. 7.5B)

In this phase of the sequence the objective is to increase flexion range of motion, and to help to normalise tone and length of latissimus dorsi, teres major and minor, as well as posterior deltoid muscles.

- The patient has the same starting position as in A, above, and the practitioner can usefully stand in front of, or behind, the side-lying patient.
- The practitioner stands at chest level, half-facing cephalad. The practitioner's non-table-side hand grasps the patient's forearm while the table-side hand holds the clavicle and scapula firmly to the chest wall.
- The practitioner slowly introduces shoulder flexion in the horizontal plane, as range of motion to 180 degrees is assessed, by which time the elbow will be in extension.
- At the position of very first indication of restriction in movement (palpated by the hand stabilising the shoulder, and by the hand/arm moving the patient's arm towards the direction being assessed), the patient is instructed to pull the elbow towards the feet, or to direct it posteriorly, or to push further towards the direction of flexion – utilising no more than 20% of available strength, building up force slowly.

- This effort is firmly resisted, and after 5 to 7 seconds the patient is instructed to slowly cease the effort.
- After complete relaxation, and on an exhalation, the practitioner moves the shoulder further into flexion, to the next restriction barrier, where the MET procedure is repeated.
- A degree of active patient participation in the movement towards the new barrier may be helpful, but no stretching is involved.

C. Articulation and Assessment of Circumduction With Mild Compression (See Fig. 7.5C)

In this phase of the sequence the objective is to increase the passive range of motion of the glenohumeral joint.

NOTE: For this phase of the sequence the practitioner can usefully stand in front of, or behind, the side-lying patient.

- The patient is side-lying with flexed elbow.
- The practitioner's cephalad hand cups the patient's shoulder, firmly compressing scapula and clavicle to the thorax.
- The practitioner's caudad hand grasps the patient's elbow and takes the shoulder through a slow clockwise circumduction, while adding compression through the long axis of the humerus.
- This is repeated several times to assess range, freedom and comfort of the circumduction motion, as the humeral head moves on the surface of the glenoid fossa.
- The same procedure is then performed anticlockwise.
- If any restriction is noted, Ruddy's pulsed MET may be usefully introduced, in which the patient attempts to execute a series of minute contractions, towards the restriction barrier, 20 times in a period of 10 seconds, before articulation is continued.
- Or a simple effort towards or away from the direction of restriction may be introduced against resistance, as described in previous Spencer positions.
- This would be followed by resumption of the circumduction movement until another barrier was identified.

D. Articulation and Assessment of Circumduction With Traction (See Fig. 7.5D)

In this phase of the sequence the objective is to increase the passive range of motion of the glenohumeral joint.

- The patient is side-lying with arm flexed at the elbow, and the practitioner can usefully stand in front of, or behind, the side-lying patient.

- The practitioner's cephalad hand cups the patient's shoulder, compressing scapula and clavicle to the thorax, while the caudad hand grasps the patient's upper arm close to the elbow and introduces slight traction, before taking the arm through slow clockwise circumduction.
- This articulates the joint while assessing range of motion in circumduction, as well as the status of the joint capsule.
- The same process is repeated anticlockwise.
- If any restriction is noted, Ruddy's pulsed MET (as described above), or a regular MET contraction against resistance, can usefully be introduced before articulation is continued.

E. Assessment and MET Treatment of Shoulder Abduction Restriction (See Fig. 7.5E)

In this phase of the sequence the objective is to assist in increasing abduction potential, while reducing motion limitations potentially resulting from impingement syndrome and/or subacromial bursa inflammation. The main muscular involvement is likely to relate to pectoralis minor, teres minor and infraspinatus.

NOTE: For this phase of the sequence the practitioner can usefully stand in front of, or behind, the side-lying patient.
- The patient is side-lying.
- The practitioner cups the patient's shoulder and compresses the scapula and clavicle to the thorax with the cephalad hand, while cupping flexed elbow with the caudad hand.
- The patient's hand is supported on the practitioner's cephalad forearm/wrist to stabilise the arm.
- The elbow is moved towards the patient's head, to abduct the shoulder, and range of motion is assessed.
- A degree of internal rotation is involved in this abduction.
- Pain-free easy abduction should be close to 180 degrees.
- Any restriction in range of motion is noted.
- At the position of the very first indication of resistance to movement, the patient is instructed to pull the elbow towards the waist, or to push further towards the direction of abduction, utilising no more than 20% of available strength, building up force slowly.
- This effort is firmly resisted, and after 7 to 10 seconds the patient is instructed to slowly cease the effort simultaneously with the practitioner.

- After complete relaxation, and on an exhalation, the practitioner, using their contact on the elbow, moves the shoulder further into abduction, to the next restriction barrier, where the MET procedure is repeated if necessary (i.e. if there is still restriction).
- A degree of active patient participation in the movement towards the new barrier may be helpful.

F. Assessment and MET Treatment of Shoulder Adduction Restriction (See Fig. 7.5E)

In this phase of the sequence the objective is to increase adduction range of motion. Muscular involvement in such a restriction is likely to include subscapularis and teres major.

NOTE: For this phase of the sequence the practitioner can usefully stand in front of, or behind, the side-lying patient.
- The patient is side-lying.
- The practitioner cups the patient's shoulder and compresses the scapula and clavicle to the thorax with the cephalad hand, while cupping the elbow with the caudad hand.
- The patient's hand is supported on the practitioner's cephalad forearm/wrist to stabilise the arm.
- The elbow is taken in an arc forward of the chest so that it moves both cephalad and medially, as the shoulder adducts and externally rotates.
- The action is performed slowly, and any signs of resistance are noted.
- At the position of the very first indication of resistance to movement, the patient is instructed to pull the elbow towards the ceiling, or to push further towards the direction of adduction – utilising no more than 20% of available strength, building up force slowly.
- This effort is firmly resisted, and after 5 to 7 seconds the patient is instructed to slowly cease the effort.
- After complete relaxation, and on an exhalation, the elbow is moved to take the shoulder further into adduction, to the next restriction barrier, where the MET procedure is repeated if restriction remains.
- A degree of active patient participation in the movement towards the new barrier may be helpful.

G. Assessment and MET Treatment of Internal Rotation Restriction (See Fig. 7.5F)

In this phase of the sequence the objective is to increase internal rotation range of motion most probably involving supraspinatus and infraspinatus shortness.

- The patient is side-lying.
- The patient's flexed arm is placed behind their back to evaluate whether the dorsum of the hand can be painlessly placed against the dorsal surface of the ipsilateral lumbar area (see Fig. 7.5F).
- This arm position is maintained throughout the procedure.
- The practitioner stands facing the side-lying patient and cups the patient's shoulder and compresses the scapula and clavicle to the thorax with their cephalad hand while cupping the flexed elbow with the caudad hand.
- The practitioner slowly brings the patient's elbow (ventrally) towards their body, and notes any sign of restriction as this movement, which increases internal rotation, is performed.
- At the position of first indication of resistance to this movement, the patient is instructed to pull their elbow away from the practitioner, either posteriorly, or medially, or both simultaneously – utilising no more than 20% of available strength, building up force slowly.
- This effort is firmly resisted, and after 5 to 7 seconds the patient is instructed to slowly cease the effort simultaneously with the practitioner.
- After complete relaxation, and on an exhalation, the elbow is moved to take the shoulder further into abduction and internal rotation, to the next restriction barrier, where the MET procedure is repeated.

Variable Directions of Effort

In any of the Spencer assessments, treatment of identified restrictions may involve isometric contractions towards, or away from, the barrier, or in any other directions that result in an increased range of movement. Alternatively, pulsed MET may be employed.

Modified PNF 'Spiral Stretch' Techniques

Proprioceptive neuromuscular facilitation (PNF) methods have been incorporated into useful assessment and treatment sequences (McAtee & Charland, 1999). These methods have been modified to take account of MET principles (Chaitow, 2001).

Spiral MET Method 1. Shoulder 'Spiral' Stretch Into Extension to Increase the Range of Motion in Flexion, Adduction and External Rotation (Fig. 7.6A)

- The patient lies supine and ensures that their shoulders remain in contact with the table throughout the procedure.

- The head is turned left.
- The patient flexes, adducts and externally rotates the (right) arm fully, maintaining the elbow in extension (palm facing the ceiling).
- The practitioner stands at the head of the table and supports the patient's arm at proximal forearm and elbow.
- The patient is asked to begin the process of returning the arm to their side, in stages, against resistance.
- The amount of force used by the patient should not exceed 25% of available strength.
- The first instruction is to pronate and internally rotate the arm ('turn your arm so that your palm faces the other way'), followed by abduction and then extension ('bring your arm back outwards and to your side').
- All these efforts are combined by the patient into a sustained effort which is resisted by the practitioner so that a 'compound' isometric contraction occurs, involving infraspinatus, middle trapezius, rhomboids, teres minor, posterior deltoid and pronator teres.
- On complete relaxation the practitioner, with the patient's assistance, takes the arm further into flexion, adduction and external rotation, stretching these muscles to a new barrier.
- The same procedure is repeated two or three times.

Spiral MET Method 2. Shoulder 'Spiral' Stretch into Flexion to Increase the Range of Motion in Extension, Abduction and Internal Rotation (See Fig. 7.6B)

- The patient lies supine and ensures that their shoulders remain in contact with the table throughout the procedure.
- They extend, abduct, and internally rotate the (right) arm fully, maintaining the elbow in extension (wrist pronated).
- The practitioner stands at the head of the table and supports the patient's arm at proximal forearm and elbow.
- The patient is asked to begin the process of returning the arm to their side, in stages, against resistance. The amount of force used by the patient should not exceed 25% of available strength.
- The first instruction is to supinate and externally rotate the arm ('turn your arm outwards so that your palm faces the other way'), followed by adduction and then flexion ('bring your arm back towards the table, and then up to your side').

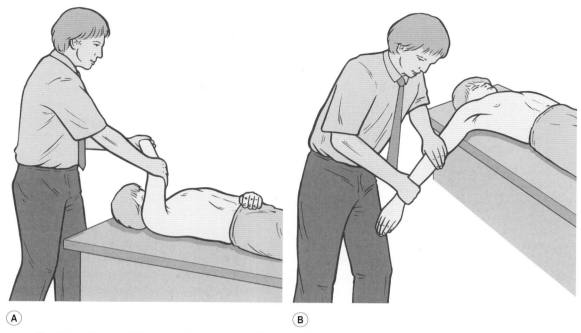

Fig. 7.6 (A) Spiral MET starts with shoulder in flexion, adduction and external rotation. Following compound isometric contraction all these directions are taken to new barriers. (B) Spiral MET2 starts with shoulder in extension, abduction and internal rotation. Following compound isometric contraction all these directions are taken to new barriers.

- All these efforts are combined by the patient into a sustained effort that is resisted by the practitioner, so that a 'compound' isometric contraction occurs, involving the clavicular head of pectoralis major, anterior deltoid, coracobrachialis, biceps brachii, infraspinatus and supinator.
- On complete relaxation the practitioner, with the patient's assistance, takes the arm further into extension, abduction and internal rotation, stretching these muscles to a new barrier.
- The same procedure should be repeated two or three times.

MET Treatment of Acromioclavicular and Sternoclavicular Dysfunction

Whereas spinal and most other joints are seen to be moved by, and to be under, the postural influence of muscles, and therefore to an extent to be capable of having their function modified by MET, articulations such as those of the sternoclavicular, acromioclavicular and IS joints seem far less amenable to such influences. It is hoped that, some of the methods detailed below will modify this impression, since MET is widely used in the osteopathic profession to help normalise the functional integrity of these joints.

In regard to the SI joint, the work of Vleeming et al. (1995) and Lee (2000), in particular, has shown that force closure of the joint provides stability. Simple logic suggests that if laxity of soft tissues removes stability, excessive tone and/or tightness, shortness of the soft tissues in question (which includes latissimus dorsi and the hamstrings) could produce restrictions to normal SI joint motion. It can be hypothesised that similar influences doubtless apply to other joints that lie outside voluntary control, such as the acromioclavicular (AC) joint (possibly involving structures such as upper trapezius, pectoralis minor, subclavius and/or the scalenes).

Acromioclavicular Dysfunction (Fig. 7.7A and B)

Stiles (1984b) suggests beginning evaluation of AC dysfunction at the scapulae, the mechanics of which closely relate to AC function.

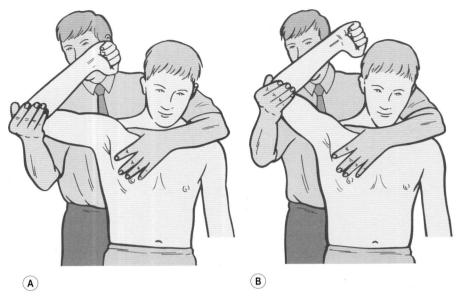

Fig. 7.7 (A) MET treatment of right-side acromioclavicular restriction. Patient attempts to return the elbow to the side against resistance. (B) Following the isometric contraction, the arm is elevated further while firm downward pressure is maintained on the lateral aspect of the clavicle.

- The patient sits erect and the spines of both scapulae are palpated by the practitioner, standing behind. The hands are moved medially, until the medial borders of the scapulae are identified, at the level of the spine of the scapula.
- Using the palpating fingers as landmarks, the levels are checked to see whether they are the same. Inequality suggests AC dysfunction.
- The side of dysfunction remains to be assessed, and each side is then tested separately (see Fig. 7.7A).
- To test the right-side AC joint, the practitioner is behind the patient, with the left hand palpating over the joint. The right hand holds the patient's right elbow. The arm is lifted in a direction, 45 degrees from the sagittal and frontal planes.
- As the arm approaches 90-degree elevation, the AC joint should be carefully palpated for hinge movement, between the acromion and the clavicle.
- In normal movement, with no restriction, the palpating hand should move slightly caudad, as the arm is abducted beyond 90 degrees. If the AC is restricted, the palpating hand/digit will move cephalad and little or no action will be noted at the joint itself as the arm goes beyond 90-degree elevation.

- MET is employed with the arm held at the restriction barrier, as for testing above.
- If the scapula on the side of dysfunction had been shown to be more proximal than that on the normal side, then the humerus is placed in external rotation, which takes the scapula caudad against the barrier, before the isometric contraction commences.
- If, however, the scapula on the side of the AC dysfunction was more distal than the scapula on the normal side, then the arm is internally rotated, taking the scapula cephalad against the barrier before the isometric contraction commences.
- The left hand (we assume this to be a right-sided problem in this example) stabilises the distal end of the clavicle, with caudad pressure being applied by the left thumb which rests on the proximal surface of the scapula. The first finger of the left hand lies on the distal aspect of the clavicle.
- The combination of the rotation of the arm as appropriate (externally if the scapula on that side was high and internally if it was low) as well as the caudad pressure exerted by the left hand on the clavicle and the scapula, provides an unyielding counterforce.
- The arm will have been raised until the first sign of inappropriate movement at the AC joint was noted

(as a sense of 'bind'). This is the barrier, and at this point the various stabilising holds (internal or external arm rotation, etc.) are introduced.

- An unyielding counterpressure is applied at the point of the patient's elbow by the right hand, and the patient is asked to try to take that elbow towards the floor with less than full strength.
- After 5 to 7 seconds the patient and practitioner relax, and the arm is once more taken towards the barrier.
- Again, greater internal or external rotation is introduced to take the scapula higher or lower, as appropriate, as firm but not forceful pressure is sustained on the clavicle and scapula in a caudad direction.
- The mild isometric contraction is again called for, and the procedure repeated several times. (It is worth recalling that respiratory accompaniment to the efforts described is helpful, with inhalation accompanying effort, and exhalation accompanying relaxation and the engagement of the new barrier.)
- The procedure is repeated until no further improvement is noted in range of motion or until it is sensed that the clavicle has resumed normal function.

Assessment and MET Treatment of Restricted Abduction in the Sternoclavicular Joint ('Shrug' Test)

- As the clavicle abducts, it rotates posteriorly.
- To test for this motion, the patient lies supine, or is seated, with arms at side (Fig. 7.8A).
- The practitioner places their index fingers on the superior surface of the medial end of the clavicle.
- The patient is asked to shrug the shoulders as the practitioner palpates for the expected caudal movement of the medial clavicle. If it fails to do so, there is a restriction retarding vertical motion.

MET Treatment of Restricted Abduction in the Sternoclavicular Joint (See Fig. 7.8B)

- The practitioner stands behind the seated patient with their thenar eminence on the superior margin of the medial end of the clavicle to be treated.
- The other hand grasps the patient's flexed elbow and holds this at 90 degrees, with the upper arm externally rotated and abducted.
- The patient is asked to adduct the upper arm for 5 to 7 seconds against resistance, using about 20% of available strength.

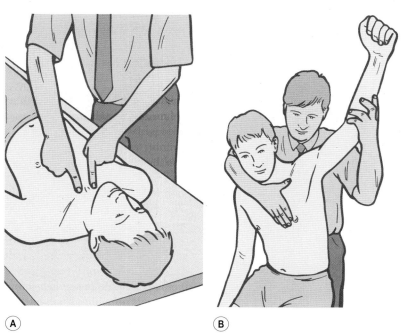

(A)   (B)

Fig. 7.8 (A) Assessment ('shrug test') for restriction in clavicular mobility. (B) MET treatment of restricted sternoclavicular joint. Following an isometric contraction, the arm is elevated and extended while firm downward pressure is maintained on the medial aspect of the clavicle with the thenar eminence.

- Following the effort and complete relaxation, the arm is abducted further, and externally rotated further, until a new barrier is sensed, with the practitioner all the while maintaining firm caudad pressure on the medial end of the clavicle.
- The process is repeated until free vertical movement of the medial clavicle is achieved.

Assessment ('Prayer' Test) and MET Treatment of Restricted Horizontal Flexion of the Upper Arm (Sternoclavicular Restriction)

- The patient lies supine and the practitioner stands to one side with the index fingers resting on the antero-medial aspect of each clavicle.
- The patient is asked to extend their arms forwards in front of their face in a 'prayer' position, palms together, pointing to the ceiling (Fig. 7.9A).
- On the patient pushing the hands forwards towards the ceiling, the clavicular heads should drop towards the floor and not rise up to follow the hands. If one or both fail to drop, there is a horizontal restriction.

MET Treatment of Restricted Horizontal Flexion of the Upper Arm (Sternoclavicular Restriction)

- The patient is supine and the practitioner stands on the contralateral side facing the patient at shoulder level. The practitioner places the thenar eminence of their cephalad hand over the medial end of the dysfunctional clavicle, holding it towards the floor. Their caudad hand lies under the shoulder on that side to embrace the dorsal aspect of the lateral scapula (Fig. 7.9B).
- The patient is asked to stretch out the arm on the side to be treated so that the hand can rest behind the practitioner's neck or shoulder.
- The practitioner leans back to take out all the slack from the extended arm and shoulder while at the same time lifting the scapula on that side slightly

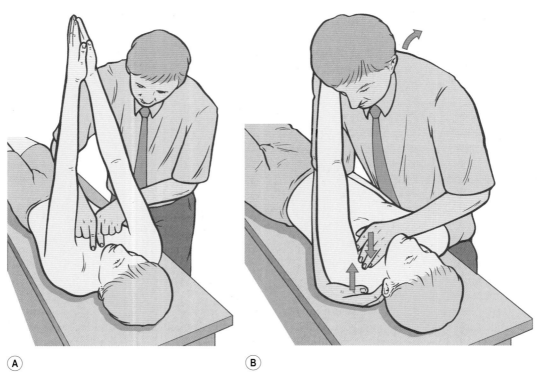

(A)   (B)

Fig. 7.9 (A) Assessment ('prayer test') for restricted horizontal flexion of the sternoclavicular joint. (B) MET treatment of horizontal flexion restriction. After isometric contraction (patient attempts to pull practitioner towards himself) the practitioner simultaneously lifts the shoulder while maintaining firm downwards pressure (to the floor) with the hypothenar eminence on the medial aspect of the clavicle.

from the table. At this time the patient is asked to pull the practitioner towards himself, against firm resistance, for 5 to 7 seconds.

- Following complete release of all the patient's efforts, the downwards (to the floor) thenar eminence pressure is maintained (painlessly) and more slack is taken out (practitioner keeps in place all elements of the procedure throughout, only the patient releases effort between contractions).
- The process is repeated once or twice more or until horizontal motion is restored.

NOTE: No pain should be noted during this procedure.

MET for Rib Dysfunction (Greenman, 1996, Goodridge & Kuchera, 1997)

In order to use MET successfully to normalise rib dysfunction the nature of the problem requires identification. In this section of the chapter only a limited number of rib problems are considered, in order to illustrate MET usefulness.

A search of the current literature offers a variety of opinions as to assessment of rib function, but very little appears to be based on evidence (Gray & Grimsby, 2004; Olsén & Romberg, 2010; Egan et al., 2011), and with reliability questioned regarding the accuracy of thoracic and rib evaluation/assessment (Heiderscheit & Boissonnault, 2008).

For example, many of the currently employed assessment approaches for rib dysfunction appear to be confined to testing for hypomobility, rather than attempting to identify specific rib dysfunction patterns (see below). Egan et al. (2011) note that when screening the ribs for mobility and pain, a crossed handed technique may be used, in which the clinician stabilises the opposite side of the thoracic spine with their hypothenar eminence lateral to the spinous process, and then applies a springing pressure over each rib angle, using the hypothenar eminence of the opposite hand. This approach is then acknowledged as having poor reliability, for both pain and mobility assessment, in patients with neck pain. The poor reliability element is noted as being successfully circumvented by changing the definition of what constitutes accurate assessment – so that a fairly close identification of location (within one spinal segment), is regarded as sufficient (described as an *expanded definition*), rather than precise identification (Christensen et al., 2002; Heiderscheit & Boissonnault, 2008).

Even if this approach was shown to be accurate, while pain provocation, and/or a judgement of hypomobility might confirm dysfunction, it would not be able to identify the actual nature of underlying dysfunction.

Preferred Approach

Rib dysfunction may be described both in relation to quality ('restricted', 'hypomobile', 'painful on springing') *as well as* function – i.e. whether an individual rib (or group of ribs) moves normally on both inhalation and exhalation. When a rib (group of ribs) fails to fully expand on inhalation, compared with the contralateral rib(s) (or with norms), the descriptor used is that it is/they are 'depressed'. Alternatively, if a rib/group of ribs fails to move normally on exhalation, compared with the contralateral rib(s) (or with norms), the descriptor used is 'elevated'. In this context, therefore, pain provocation tests have no particular value, as depressed and elevated ribs may or may not be painful on compression/provocation.

Terminology

There are various ways of describing the manner in which a rib, or group of ribs, might be restricted. For example:

- A rib that fails to move fully into its inhalation position can be variously described as being 'locked in exhalation', 'an exhalation restriction', 'limited in inhalation', or 'depressed'.
- A rib that fails to move fully into its exhalation position can variously be described as being 'locked in inhalation', 'an inhalation restriction', 'limited in exhalation', or 'elevated'.

In this text the shorthand terms 'elevated' and 'depressed' will be used.

Study is recommended of Greenman (1996), DeStefano (2010) and Ward (1997) for more on this topic, and for a wider range of MET choices for treating such restrictions than are described below.

Rib Treatment Guidelines

As a rule, clinical experience suggests that unless there has been direct trauma, rib restrictions are compensatory, and involve groups of ribs.

When treating a group of depressed ribs, it is suggested that the 'key' rib to receive primary attention should be the most superior of these. If this is successfully released it will tend to 'unlock' the remaining ribs in that group. Similarly, if a group of elevated ribs is being treated, the key rib is likely to be the most inferior of these, which if successfully released will unlock the remaining ribs in that group.

If palpation commences at the most cephalad aspect of the supine patient's thorax, the 2nd rib is the most easily palpated.

The ribs should be sequentially palpated and assessed as the patient inhales and exhales slowly and deliberately. If a depressed rib is noted (fails to rise symmetrically on inhalation) this is clearly the most cephalad and is the one to be treated (see below). Similarly, if an elevated rib is identified (fails to fall symmetrically on exhalation), the ribs continue to be evaluated until a normal pair is located, and the dysfunctional rib cephalad to these is treated.

MET methods described below are one way of releasing such restrictions. However, there are also extremely useful positional release methods for treating such problems, based on Jones's strain/counterstrain methods (Jones, 1981; Chaitow, 2010).

As in all forms of somatic dysfunction, causes should be sought and addressed in addition to mobilisation of restrictions, using MET or other methods as described in this text.

▶ Rib Palpation Test: Rib 1 (Fig. 7.10)

- The patient is seated and the practitioner stands behind.
- The practitioner places their hands so that the fingers can draw posteriorly the fibres of upper trapezius that lie superior to the 1st rib.
- The tips of the practitioner's middle and index (or middle and ring) fingers can then most easily be placed on the superior surface of the posterior shaft of the 1st rib.

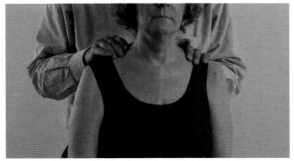

Fig. 7.10 Palpation of 1st rib anterior to upper trapezius fibres.

- Symmetry is evaluated as the patient breathes lightly.
- The commonest dysfunction is for one of the pair of 1st ribs to be 'locked' in an elevated position ('inhalation restriction').
- The superior aspect of this rib may palpate as tender, and attached scalene structures are likely to be short and tight (Greenman, 1996; DeStefano, 2010).

Or:

- The patient is seated and the practitioner stands behind.
- The practitioner places their hands so that the fingers can draw posteriorly the fibres of upper trapezius that lie superior to the 1st rib.
- The tips of the practitioner's middle and index (or middle and ring) fingers can then most easily be placed on the superior surface of the posterior shaft of the 1st rib.
- The patient exhales and shrugs their shoulders and the palpated 1st ribs behave asymmetrically (one moves superiorly more than the other), or the patient inhales fully and the palpated 1st ribs behave asymmetrically (one moves more than the other).
- The commonest restriction of the 1st rib is into elevation and the likeliest soft tissue involvement is of anterior and medial scalenes (Goodridge & Kuchera, 1997; DeStefano, 2010).

Rib Palpation Test: Ribs 2 to 10: Patient Seated (Fig. 7.11)

- The patient is supine or seated.
- If supine, the practitioner stands at waist level facing the patient's head, with an index finger contact on the superior aspect of one pair of ribs.
- The practitioner's dominant eye determines the side of the table from which they are approaching the observation of rib function (right-eye dominant calls for standing on the patient's right side).
- The fingers are observed as the patient inhales and exhales fully (eye focus is on an area between the palpating fingers so that peripheral vision assesses symmetry of movement).
- If, on inhalation, one of a pair of ribs fails to rise as far as its pair, it is described as a depressed rib, unable to move fully to its end of range on inhalation (an 'exhalation restriction').
- If, on exhalation, one of a pair of ribs fails to fall as far as its pair, it is described as an *elevated rib*, unable

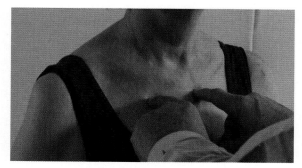

Fig. 7.11 Palpation of ribs 2–10.

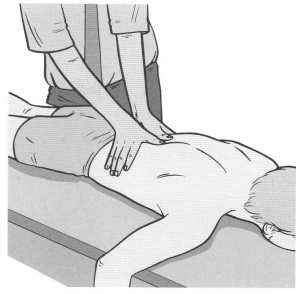

Fig. 7.12 Palpation of ribs 11 and 12.

to move fully to its end of range on exhalation (an 'inhalation restriction').

Rib Palpation Test: Ribs 11 and 12 (Fig. 7.12)

- Assessment of 11th and 12th ribs is usually performed with the patient prone and palpation performed with a hand contact on the posterior shafts to evaluate full inhalation and exhalation motions.
- The 11th and 12th ribs usually operate as a pair so that if any sense of reduction in posterior motion is noted on one side or the other, on inhalation, the pair is regarded as depressed, unable to fully inhale ('exhalation restriction').
- If any sense of reduction in anterior motion is noted on one side or the other, on exhalation, the pair (or individual rib) is regarded as elevated, unable to fully exhale ('inhalation restriction').

General Principles of MET for Rib Dysfunction

Before using MET on rib restrictions identified in tests such as those outlined above, appropriate attention should be given to the attaching musculature, for example the scalenes for the upper ribs, and pectorals, latissimus, quadratus lumborum and others for the lower ribs.

Additionally, before specific attention is given to rib restrictions, evaluation and appropriate treatment should be given to any thoracic spine dysfunction that may be influencing the function of associated ribs. Attention should also be given to postural and breathing habits that may be contributing to thoracic spine and/or rib dysfunction, and appropriate re-education and exercise protocols prescribed (Chaitow et al., 2002).

MET Treatment for Elevated 1st Rib, Patient Seated (Fig. 7.13A)

- The patient is seated on the treatment table, and the practitioner stands behind.
- To treat a right elevated 1st rib, the practitioner's left foot is placed on the table and the patient's left arm is 'draped' over the practitioner's flexed knee.
- The practitioner's left arm is flexed, with the elbow placed anterior to the patient's shoulder and with the left hand supporting the patient's (side of) head.
- The practitioner makes contact with the tubercle of the 1st rib with the fingers or thumb of their right hand, taking out available soft tissue slack as steady force is applied in an inferior direction.
- The practitioner eases their flexed leg to the left and simultaneously uses their left hand to encourage the patient's neck into a side flexion and rotation to the right, so unloading scalene tension on that side and encouraging the 1st rib shaft to move anteriorly and inferiorly.
- The contact thumb or fingers on the rib tubercle/ shaft take out available slack, and the patient is asked to 'inhale and hold your breath for a few seconds and at the same time gently press your head

MET Treatment for Elevated 1st Rib, Patient Supine (Fig. 7.13B)

- The patient lies supine and the practitioner sits at the head of the table.
- For an elevated left 1st rib the practitioner cradles the patient's neck with their right hand and applies *firm*, inferiorly directed, thumb contact to the superior surface of the posterior shaft of left 1st rib.
- The patient is requested to inhale fully and to hold the breath for 5 seconds, while simultaneously attempting to extend (or side flex) the neck against resistance offered by the practitioner's right hand.
- The practitioner maintains constant firm pressure on the 1st rib throughout, and as the patient exhales, and releases the extension effort, the firm pressure on the rib continues, accentuating its intended direction of movement, and subsequently resisting its tendency to move superiorly on the next inhalation.
- This cycle is repeated through three to four inhalation-exhalation cycles (see Fig. 7.13B).

MET Treatment for Elevated 2nd to 10th Ribs (Fig. 7.14)

- The most inferior of a group of elevated ribs should be identified.
- The patient lies supine and the practitioner stands at the head of the table, slightly to the left of the patient's head, with the right hand (for left-side rib dysfunction) supporting the patient's upper thoracic region, forearm supporting the neck and head.
- The left hand is placed so that the thenar eminence rests on the superior aspect of the costochondral junction of the designated rib, close to the mid-clavicular line (for upper ribs; for ribs 7 to 10 the contact would be more lateral, closer to the mid-axillary line), directing the rib caudally.

NOTE: If the rib to be contacted is in a gender-sensitive area, the patient's contralateral hand can be used as a 'cushion' to contact the rib, with the practitioner's hand covering it – as used in treatment of pectoralis major and scalene application of MET, as described in Chapter 6.

- The upper thoracic and cervical spine is then eased into flexion, as well as side flexion towards the treated side, until motion is sensed at the site of the rib stabilisation.

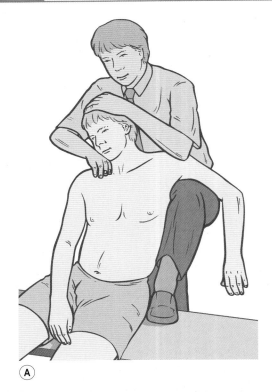

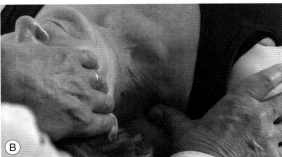

Fig. 7.13 (A) Position for MET treatment of restricted (elevated) 1st rib on the right with patient seated. (B) Position for MET treatment of restricted (elevated) 1st rib on the left with patient supine.

towards the left against my hand'. This 5- to 7-second effort will activate and isometrically contract the scalenes.

- On releasing the breath, slack is taken out of the soft tissues as all the movements which preceded the contraction are repeated.
- Two or three repetitions usually results in greater rib symmetry and functional balance.

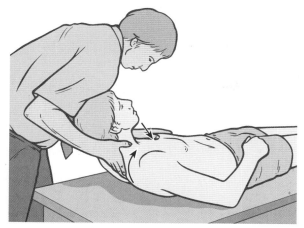

Fig. 7.14 MET treatment of elevated 2nd to 10th rib.

- If introduction of side flexion is difficult, the patient should be asked to ease the left hand (in this example) towards the feet until motion is noted at the palpated rib.
- The patient should then be asked to 'inhale fully and hold your breath' (producing an isometric contraction of the intercostal muscles, as well as the scalenes) and to attempt to return the trunk and head to the table, against the practitioner's firm resistance (producing an isometric contraction of multiple extensor muscles of the thorax).
- On release and full exhalation, slack is removed from the local tissues (with the thenar eminence holding the rib towards its caudad position) as increased flexion and side flexion is introduced.
- This sequence is repeated once or twice only, and usually results in release of the group of 'elevated' ribs.

▶ MET Treatment for Depressed 1st to 5th Ribs, Patient Supine (Fig. 7.15)

- The patient lies supine with the practitioner standing contralateral to the side of the rib being treated (1st to 5th).
- The practitioner leans across the patient's trunk, insinuating their table-side arm under the patient's scapula region and, with their table-side hand, grasps (hooks fingertips onto) the superior surface of the rib angle.

- The patient should have turned their head slightly away from the side to be treated and have their treatment-side arm fully abducted and flexed, with the back of their hand resting on their forehead.
- The practitioner places their non-table-side hand onto the patient's hand that is resting on their forehead.
- The patient is requested to simultaneously do one of the following – depending on which muscular forces are thought appropriate relative to the rib being treated:
  1. Inhale and hold the breath.
  2. Attempt to lift and turn the head towards the treatment side.
  3. Attempt to bring their (treatment side) arm to their side.

All these efforts would be light, and would be resisted by the practitioner (so contracting the neck flexors, scalenes, SCM, pectoralis major and/or latissimus as well as the diaphragm).

- The contraction and held breath should be held for 5 seconds.
- Following exhalation (and release of all muscular effort) and on the subsequent deep inhalation, the practitioner applies inferolateral traction to the posterior aspect of the shaft of the rib being treated, thereby guiding the anterior aspect towards its normal excursion.

MET Treatment for Elevated 11th to 12th Ribs (Fig. 7.16)

- The patient is prone, arms at their side, and the practitioner stands on the contralateral side to the dysfunctional ribs.

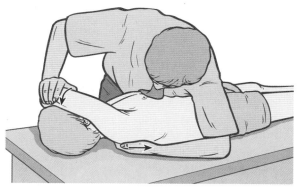

Fig. 7.15 MET treatment of depressed 1st–5th ribs.

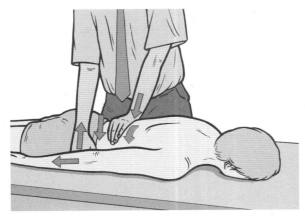

Fig. 7.16 MET treatment of elevated 11th and/or 12th ribs.

- For right-side 11th and 12th elevated ribs, the practitioner places the thenar and hypothenar eminences of their cephalad hand on the medial aspects of the shafts of both the 11th and 12th ribs (these two ribs usually act in concert in the way they become dysfunctional).
- The practitioner's caudad hand grasps the patient's right anterior superior iliac spine (ASIS).
- The patient is asked to exhale fully, and hold this out, and to reach towards the right foot with the right hand, so introducing side-bending to the right, taking the elevated ribs towards their normal position.
- At the end of the exhalation the patient is asked to bring the ASIS firmly into the practitioner's hand ('push your pelvis towards the table').
- After 5 to 7 seconds and complete relaxation, the practitioner takes out all slack with their contact hand and the process is repeated, before retesting.

MET Treatment for Depressed 11 to 12th Ribs (Fig. 7.17)

- The patient is prone, and the practitioner stands on the ipsilateral side, facing the patient.
- For left-side depressed 11th rib, the patient places their left arm above their head and the practitioner holds that elbow with their cephalad hand.
- The practitioner locates the depressed 11th rib and draws it superiorly to its barrier, with their finger pads.
- The patient is asked to breathe in and hold the breath, while simultaneously attempting to bring the elevated and abducted left elbow sideways, back towards the side, against resistance.

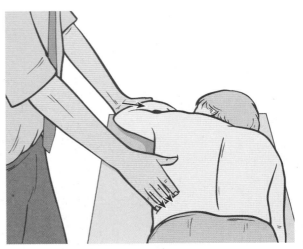

Fig. 7.17 MET treatment for depressed 11th–12th ribs.

- After 5 to 7 seconds, and complete relaxation by the patient, the rib is drawn superiorly towards its new barrier via the finger contact.
- A repetition of the procedure should then be carried out and the rib reassessed for motion.

General Mobilisation

Two methods are described below, in which no specific joint is addressed, but by means of which general mobilisation may be achieved – in one method involving the lower thoracic cage to which the diaphragm is attached, and in the other a general thoracic rotational mobilisation.

Lower Thorax and Diaphragm Attachment Release Using MET (Fig. 7.18)

- The patient is supine and the practitioner stands at waist level facing cephalad, and places their hands over the middle and lower thoracic structures, fingers along the rib shafts, curling towards the spine.
- Treating the structure being palpated as a cylinder, the hands test the preference this cylinder has to rotate around its central axis, one way and then the other:

'Does the lower thorax rotate with more difficulty to the right or to the left?'

- Once the direction of greatest rotational restriction has been established, the potential for side flexion one way or the other is evaluated:

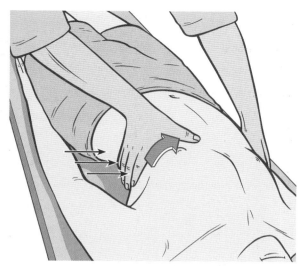

Fig. 7.18 General MET for release of lower thorax and diaphragm.

'Does the lower thorax side-flex with more difficulty to the right or to the left?'

- Once these two pieces of information have been established, the combined positions of restriction are introduced.
- By side-bending and rotating the lower thoracic cage *towards the tighter* directions, the combined directions of restriction are engaged, at which time the patient is asked to inhale deeply and to hold the breath.
- After a few seconds the patient is asked to pinch (block) the nose while forcibly attempting to exhale through the nose (Valsalva manoeuvre) for 2 to 3 seconds. This produces isometric contraction of the diaphragm and intercostal muscles.
- On complete exhalation and relaxation, the diaphragm should be found to function more normally, accompanied by a relaxation of associated soft tissues and by a more symmetrical rotation and side-flexion potential of the previously restricted tissues.

> ❗ **CAUTION**
>
> Avoid the Valsalva manoeuvre if the patient is hypertensive or has glaucoma.

General Thoracic Release Using MET (Lenehan et al., 2003) (See Fig. 2.3)

- The patient is seated at the end of a treatment table, arms folded, hands on opposite shoulders, with the practitioner alongside.
- Employing their non-table-side hand as a contact, the practitioner uses the patient's arms as levers to introduce rotation towards himself, to an easy, end-of-range, position (see Fig. 2.3).
- The practitioner's table-side arm is behind the patient's upper back, with a hand on the contralateral shoulder.
- After the restriction barriers have been engaged, the patient is requested to introduce an isometric contraction, by side-bending away from the direction of rotation against the unyielding resistance of the practitioner's hand.
- In the example in Fig. 2.3 the patient is rotated right and is attempting to side-flex left – or translate the shoulders left.
- After 3 to 5 seconds of mild isometric effort, and on an exhalation, the practitioner engages the new barrier, with no attempt to stretch or force the movement.
- An alternative would be for the patient to utilise pulsed isometric contractions against one or other of the practitioner's resistant hand contacts.

Assessment and MET Treatment of Sacroiliac and Iliosacral Restrictions

In order to usefully apply MET to SI and/or IS (or other pelvic) dysfunction, it is necessary to assess the implicated joint accurately. This seems to be easier said than done.

A survey of Australian osteopaths by Peace and Fryer (2004) evaluated which tests were most commonly used, and whether correlation existed between the tests and clinical experience. The results revealed that, amongst the 168 responders (representing approximately 30% of those surveyed), the commonest assessment tools for the sacroiliac joint (SIJ) involved:

- Asymmetry of bony landmarks (most commonly PSIS, ASIS and iliac crests).
- Motion tests (most commonly prone sacral springing, standing flexion and ASIS compression).
- Pain provocation tests (prone sacral spring, ASIS compression and SIJ spring/'thigh thrust'). Additionally, piriformis assessment was reported as being

commonly tested for tenderness and tissue texture change.

Few, if any, of the tests mentioned have been shown to consistently offer accurate clinical information, and some have been shown to produce positive results in asymptomatic individuals (Dreyfuss et al., 1994; Meijne & van Neerbos, 1999; Kokmeyer & van der Wurff, 2002).

Additionally, factors such as differences in leg length, body type and dimension, and asymmetrical bone structure, as well as the limited experience and skill of the examiner, create questions as to the clinical useful-ness of static assessment findings (Cibulka & Koldehoff, 1999; Levangie, 1999; Lewit & Rosina, 1999).

It is further suggested that the distinction, initially made by Mitchell et al. (1979) regarding the need to dif-ferentiate between IS and SI dysfunction, remains clin-ically useful.

> **! CAUTION**
>
> Evidence derived from, for example, the standing flex-ion test (as described below) might be compromised by concurrent shortness in the hamstrings, since this will effectively give either:
> - A false positive sign at the contralateral SIJ when there is unilateral hamstring shortness. For exam-ple, left hamstring shortness could prevent left iliac movement during flexion, helping to encourage a compensating right iliac movement during flexion, or
> - False negative signs if there is bilateral hamstring shortness. That is, there may be IS motion which is being masked by the restriction placed on the ilia via bilateral hamstring shortness.
>
> The hamstring shortness tests, as described in Chapter 6, should therefore be carried out before a stand-ing flexion test, and if shortness is found these structures should be normalised, as far as is possible, prior to the IS (standing) flexion tests, described below, being used.
>
> **NOTE**: See also notes on possible postural muscle involvement in apparent iliosacral restrictions, later in this chapter.

Which Spinal and SIJ Tests Do American Practitioners Use?

Fryer et al. (2009) carried out a similar survey of osteopathic physicians in the USA in relation to their assessment and treatment approaches to SI and spinal dysfunction. A total of 171 respondents provided data, from over 750 osteopathic physician members of the American Academy of Osteopathy who were contacted.

The most commonly reported findings for assess-ment of spinal somatic dysfunction were:
- Paraspinal tissue texture (98%)
- Transverse process asymmetry (89%)
- Tenderness (85%)

See discussion of STAR (or TART) assessment in Chapter 2.

The most commonly used spinal treatment methods were:
- Myofascial release (78%)
- Soft tissue technique (77%)
- Patient self-stretches (71%)
- MET (63%)

Assessment of pelvic landmark asymmetry employed during palpation were the following:
- ASIS (87%)
- Sacral base (82%)
- Posterior superior iliac spine (81%)
- Sacral sulci (78%)
- Iliac crests (77%)
- Inferior lateral angle of the sacrum (74%)

For assessment of sacroiliac joint motion the fol-lowing methods were most frequently employed:
- ASIS compression (68%)
- SI pain provocation tests were also used, although their use was less common than asymmetry or motion tests.
- Standing flexion test, and active straight leg raising were both used by approximately 55% of responders.

In treatment of pelvic and sacroiliac dysfunction, the following methods were most frequently employed:
- Muscle energy (70%)
- Myofascial release (67%)
- Patient self-stretches (66%)
- Osteopathy in the cranial field (59%)
- Muscle strengthening exercises (58%)
- Soft tissue technique (58%)
- Articulatory technique (53%)

The effect of the practitioners' gender was signifi-cant for many of the treatment procedures, with females using more soft tissue and muscle energy, and males more high-velocity technique.

Validity of such tests? Fryer et al. (2009) observe that: 'Assessment of pelvic and SI dysfunction, landmark asymmetry and tests that assess SI motion have been criticized for poor reliability and lack of validity' (Vleeming et al., 2008; Wurff et al., 2000). Fryer et al. (2009) conclude their survey by suggesting that:

Using the results from this study, which provides information about tests that are in common use, future studies could be designed to improve the reliability of these procedures.

The lead author suggests that 'form and force closure' assessments (as described below) should be carried out before moving on to use of other test procedures, in order to establish that the SIJ is indeed involved in the individual's symptoms. Other tests used should be those with which the clinician is comfortable, well trained, has personal confidence in using, and which have not been shown, categorically, to have no validity.

To understand the concept of form and force closure, the functional stability of the SIJ, particularly during the gait cycle, is briefly summarised in Box 7.3.

Form and Force Assessment

Active straight leg raise (ASLR) test

- Both ASLR and the Trendelenburg test measure the efficiency of load transfer between the lumbopelvic region and the lower limbs – one weightbearing, and one non-weightbearing. Roussel et al. (2007) have reported strong degrees of reliability when both tests are used for assessment of individuals with low-back pain.
- Liebenson et al. (2009) confirm that the ASLR test is reliable as a screen of lumbar spinal stability. The recommendation is for use of light abdominal bracing (AB) during performance of the test, an action which significantly improves stabilisation. This is achieved via the giving of verbal cues such as '*tighten your stomach*' or '*stiffen your abdominals and back*'.
- O'Sullivan et al. (2002) have tested and confirmed the usefulness and validity of ASLR test in patients with SI pain.

ASLR test supine: functional SI assessments (form/force closure) (Vleeming et al., 1995, 1996, 1997; Barker et al., 2004; Lee, 1997, 2000, 2010) (Fig. 7.20A and B)

- The patient is supine and is instructed to raise one leg.

- If there is evidence of compensatory rotation of the pelvis towards the side of the raised leg, during performance of the movement, or if pain is reported in the SIJ during the effort, dysfunction is suggested. Form closure assessment:
- The same leg should then be raised after the practitioner has applied compressive, medially directed force across the pelvis, with a hand on the lateral aspect of each innominate at the level of the ASIS (this augments form closure of the SIJ) (see Fig. 7.20A).
- If this *form* closure strategy, applied by the practitioner, enhances the ability to easily raise the leg, this suggests that structural factors within the joint may require externally enhanced support, such as a trochanter belt.
  Force closure assessment:
- To test for the influence of *force* closure, the same leg is raised with the patient simultaneously attempting to slightly flex and rotate the trunk towards the side being tested, against the practitioner's resistant counter-pressure, applied to the contralateral shoulder (see Fig. 7.20B).
- This increases oblique muscular activity and force-closes the SIJ being assessed (i.e. on the side of the raised leg).
- If the initial leg raising suggests SI dysfunction, and this is markedly reduced or absent with force closure, the prognosis is good provided that appropriate balancing of the musculo-ligamentous status can be achieved after the patient engages in appropriate rehabilitation exercise.

A variation on the ASLR test. Roussel et al. (2007) describe a variation of the ASLR as outlined above:

- The patient is positioned supine and instructed to raise a straight leg 20 cm above the table.
- The patient is then asked to score the perceived effort to perform the test on a 6-point scale: (a) not difficult at all, (b) minimally difficult, (c) somewhat difficult, (d) fairly difficult, (e) very difficult, or (f) unable to perform.
- In addition, during the performance of the ASLR, movement of the rib cage and abdomen during inspiration was observed and palpated.
- Patients were asked to hold the extended straight leg for 20 seconds during this breathing pattern assessment.
- While the patient's evaluation of the degree of difficulty correlated well with observed dysfunction – as

BOX 7.3   The Sacroiliac Joint During Gait

As the right leg swings forward the right ilium rotates backward in relation to the sacrum (Greenman, 1996). Simultaneously, sacrotuberous and interosseous ligamentous tension increases to brace the sacroiliac joint (SIJ) in preparation for heel strike.

Just before heel strike, the ipsilateral hamstrings are activated, thereby tightening the sacrotuberous ligament (into which they merge) to further stabilise the SIJ.

Vleeming et al. (1997) have demonstrated that, as the foot approaches heel strike there is a downward movement of the fibula, increasing (via biceps femoris) the tension on the sacrotuberous ligament, while simultaneously tibialis anticus fires, in order to dorsiflex the foot in preparation for heel strike.

Tibialis anticus links, via fascia, to peroneus longus under the foot, thus completing this elegant sling mechanism (the 'anatomical stirrup') which both braces the SIJ and engages the entire lower limb in that process.

Biceps femoris, peroneus longus and tibialis anticus together form this longitudinal muscle-tendon-fascial sling, which is loaded to create an energy store to be used during the next part of the gait cycle.

As Lee (1997) points out: 'Together, gluteus maximus and latissimus dorsi tense the thoracolumbar fascia and facilitate the force closure mechanism through the SIJ' (see functional form and force assessment, above).

During the latter stage of the single support period of the gait cycle, biceps femoris activity eases, as compression

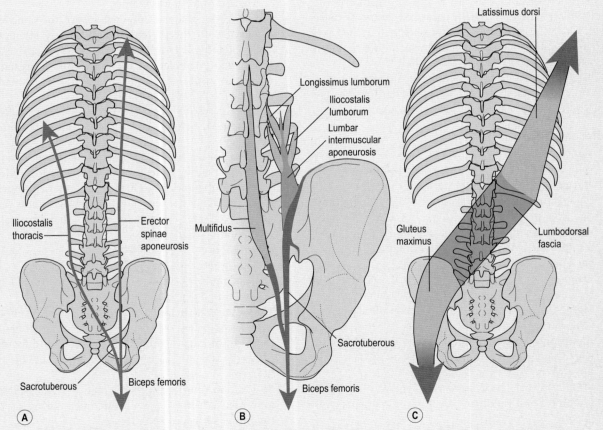

Fig. 7.19 (A) The biceps femoris is directly connected to the upper trunk via the sacrotuberous ligament, the erector spinae aponeurosis and iliocostalis thoracis. (B) Enlarged view of the lumbar spine area showing the link between biceps femoris, the lumbar intermuscular aponeurosis, longissimus lumborum, iliocostalis lumborum and multifidus. (C) Relations between gluteus maximus, lumbodorsal fascia and latissimus dorsi. (Reproduced with permission from Vleeming et al., 1997.)

BOX 7.3   The Sacroiliac Joint During Gait–cont'd

of the SIJ reduces and the ipsilateral iliac bone rotates anteriorly.

As the right heel strikes, the left arm swings forward – and the right gluteus maximus activates to compress and stabilise the SIJ.

There is a simultaneous coupling of this gluteal force with the contralateral latissimus dorsi by means of thoracolumbar fascia in order to assist in counter-rotation of the trunk on the pelvis (Fig. 7.19).

In this way, an oblique muscle-tendon-fascial sling is created across the torso, providing a mechanism for further energy storage to be utilised in the next phase of the gait cycle.

As the single support phase ends, and the double support phase initiates, there is a lessened loading of the SIJs and gluteus maximus reduces its activity, and as the next step starts, the leg swings forward and nutation at the SIJ starts again.

---

described in the form and force tests above – the observed breathing pattern changes were less reliably correlated.

ASLR test prone: functional SIJ assessment (form/force closure) (Vleeming et al., 1995, 1996, 1997; Barker et al., 2004; Lee, 1997, 2000, 2010) (Fig. 7.21A and B)

- The prone patient is asked to extend the leg at the hip by approximately 10 degrees.
- Hinging should occur at the hip joint, not the low back, and the pelvis should remain in contact with the table throughout.
- If there is an excessive degree of pelvic rotation in the transverse plane (anterior pelvic rotation), or if pain is reported in the SIJ during the effort, possible SIJ dysfunction is suggested.

Form closure assessment:

- If *form* features (i.e. structural) of the SIJ are at fault, the prone straight leg raise will be more normal (and painless) when medial compression of the joint is introduced by the practitioner applying firm bilateral medial pressure towards the SIJs, with hands on the innominates (see Fig. 7.21A).

Force closure assessment:

- *Force* closure may be enhanced during the assessment if latissimus dorsi can be recruited to increase tension on the thoracolumbar fascia.
- Lee (1997) states:

This is done by [the practitioner] resisting extension of the medially rotated [contralateral] arm prior to lifting the leg (see Fig. 7.21B).

- As in the supine straight leg raising (SLR) test, if force closure enhances more normal (and less painful) SIJ function, the prognosis for improvement is good; to

be achieved by means of appropriate balancing of soft tissue status, rehabilitation exercises and reformed use patterns.

It is suggested that normalisation of the status of dysfunctional postural muscles, attaching to the pelvis (from above and below), by means of stretching, toning and trigger point deactivation, as well as via postural re-education, will contribute greatly to removal of many instances of SIJ pain. In addition, methods such as IS joint and general pelvic normalisation, as described below, can prove extremely useful clinically, but this is only likely to be of lasting benefit if soft tissue balance has been achieved.

Modified Trendelenburg test. Various versions have been described of the Trendelenburg test that was originally developed as a means of assessing hip stability and function. The method outlined below is based on that developed by Hardcastle and Nade (1985).

- The patient is asked to flex one hip to 30 degrees and to lift the pelvis of the non-stance side above the transiliac line, and to maintain this position for 30 seconds.
- The pelvis should not tilt or rotate as weight is shifted to the supporting leg.
- To maintain balance the patient is permitted to touch a table or the wall, with one finger, but not for actual support.
- If the patient is unable to hold the test position for 30 seconds, or if the pelvis of the non-weightbearing side does not elevate above the transiliac line, the test is regarded as positive.
- Additionally, following the test, the patient is asked to score the perceived effort required to perform the test using a 6-point scale: (a) not difficult at all, (b) minimally difficult, (c) somewhat difficult, (d) fairly

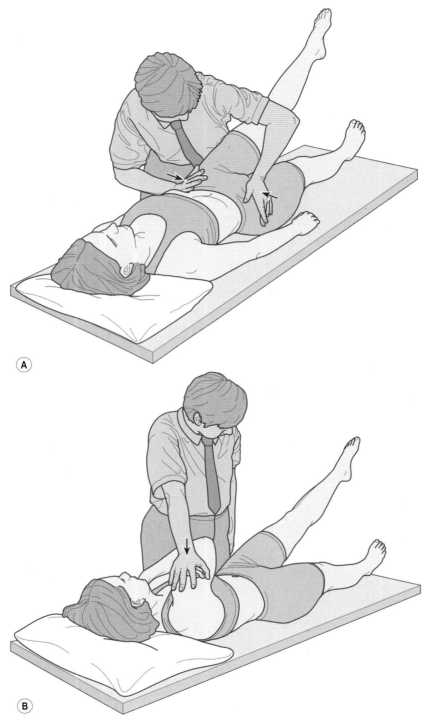

Fig. 7.20 Functional test of supine active straight leg raise: (A) with form closure augmented; (B) with force closure augmented.

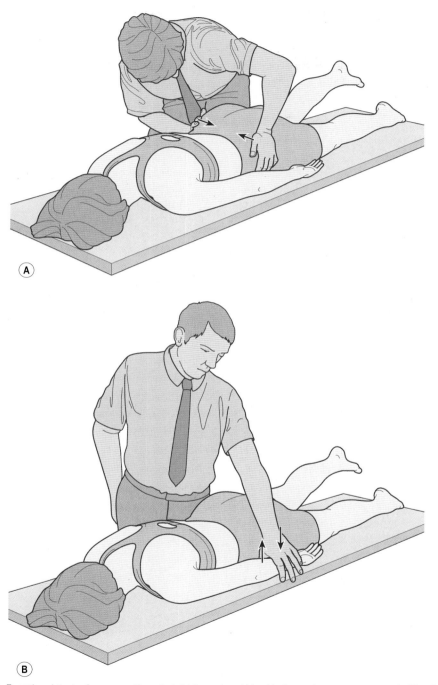

Fig. 7.21 Functional test of prone active straight leg raise: (A) with form closure augmented; (B) with force closure augmented.

difficult, (e) very difficult, or (f) unable to perform (Roussel et al., 2007).

- If the test proves positive, the precise nature of the dysfunction needs to be evaluated and treated/rehabilitated, whether this involves muscular imbalances, SI, lumbosacral or hip dysfunction.
- The advantage of using both ASLR and Trendelenburg tests is that these offer reasonably assured evidence of dysfunction when positive.
- Subsequent retesting, following appropriate treatment and rehabilitation, provides evidence of progress, or lack of progress.

NOTE: The various pelvic assessments described in this chapter, apart from the ASLR and Trendelenburg tests, remain unvalidated, despite being in widespread use. They are described here as representing methods used by the lead author, and should be employed with caution rather than certainty as to their reliability. As noted by Fryer et al. (2009), assessment of pelvic and SI dysfunction, landmark asymmetry and tests that assess SI motion have been criticised for poor reliability and lack of validity.

Tests and MET Treatment for Pelvic and Sacroiliac Joint Dysfunction

Standing flexion (iliosacral) test

- The patient is standing, with any inequality of leg length having been compensated for by insertion of a pad under the foot on the short side so that iliac crest height is equal on both sides.
- The practitioner's thumbs are placed firmly (a light contact is useless) on the inferior slope of the PSIS with fingers spread antero-laterally to offer a 'bracing' influence for the thumb contacts.
- The patient is asked to move into full flexion while the thumb contact is maintained (Fig. 7.22A).
- The patient's knees should remain extended during lumbar flexion.
- The practitioner observes, *especially near the end of the excursion of the bend,* whether one or other thumb seems to start to travel with the PSIS on which it rests.

Interpretation. If one thumb moves superiorly during flexion it indicates that the ilium is 'fixed' to the sacrum on that side (or that the contralateral hamstrings are

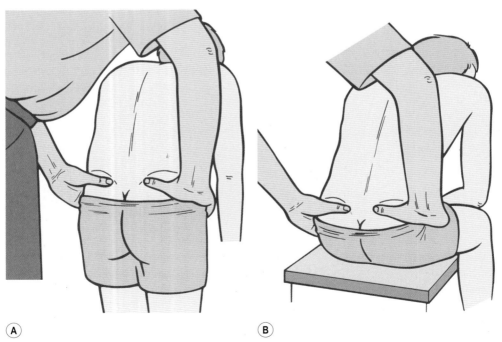

(A)   (B)

Fig. 7.22 (A) Standing flexion test for iliosacral restriction. The dysfunctional side is that on which the thumb moves during flexion. (B) Seated flexion test for sacroiliac restriction. The dysfunctional side is that on which the thumb moves during flexion.

short, or that the ipsilateral quadratus lumborum is short – therefore these muscles should have been assessed, and if necessary treated, prior to the standing flexion test).

- If muscle status is normal, a positive standing flexion test suggests IS dysfunction on the side on which the thumb moved superiorly.

Seated flexion (sacroiliac) test

- The seated flexion test involves exactly the same hand placement as in the standing flexion test (above) and observation of the thumb movement, if any, during full flexion, while the patient is seated on the table, legs over the side, knees in flexion (Fig. 7.22B).
- The patient's feet should be flat on floor, knees spread slightly, so that hands can pass freely between them, during flexion.

Interpretation. In this test, since the ischial tuberosities are being 'sat upon', the ilia cannot easily move, and if one thumb travels superiorly during spinal flexion, it suggests that the sacrum is relatively 'fixed' to the ilium on that side, dragging the ilium with it into flexion, indicating possible SI dysfunction on the side on which the thumb moved.

A positive standing flexion test result indicates a somatic dysfunction, in the sacral region or in the lower lumbar vertebrae, on the side of the positive test result.

Seffinger and Hruby (2007)

Paravertebral 'fullness' assessment

- The patient should be evaluated when standing and with the spine fully flexed, as well as when seated and fully flexed.
- In both settings the practitioner stands in front and looks down the spine in order to compare relative fullness, prominence of the paravertebral muscles in the lumbar area.
- If greater fullness exists in one paraspinal area of the lumbar spine with the patient standing, as opposed to when seated and flexed, this suggests a compensatory process, involving the lower limbs and/or pelvic area, as a prime influence.
- If, however, fullness in the lumbar paraspinal region is the same or greater when seated, compared with standing, this suggests a primary spinal dysfunction and not a compensation for pelvic or lower limb imbalance/dysfunction.

Confirmation of iliosacral dysfunction: standing hip flexion test

- The patient stands and the practitioner is behind, kneeling, with thumbs placed so that on the side being assessed the contact is on the PSIS, while the other hand palpates the median sacral crest directly parallel to the PSIS.
- The patient is asked to slowly and fully flex the ipsilateral hip to waist level.
- A normal response is for the thumb on the ipsilateral PSIS to move caudally in relation to the thumb on the sacral base, as the hip and knee are flexed.
- If on the flexing of the hip there is a movement of the PSIS and the median sacral crest 'as a unit', together with a compensating adaptation in the lumbar spine, this indicates *iliosacral* restriction on the side being palpated.
- If this combined (PSIS and sacral thumb contact) movement occurred when the contralateral hip is flexed, it suggests a *sacroiliac* restriction on the side being palpated.

What Type of Iliosacral Dysfunction Exists?

Once an IS restriction has been identified (by means of the seated flexion test, or the confirmation test described immediately above), it is necessary to define as far as possible what type of restriction exists. In this text only anterior rotation, posterior rotation, inflare and outflare will be considered. This part of the evaluation process depends upon observation of landmarks.

Landmark test. The patient lies supine and straight, while the practitioner locates the inferior slopes of the two ASISs, with thumbs, and views these contacts from directly above the pelvis with the dominant eye over the centre line (bird's eye view – see Fig. 7.23A):

- Which thumb is nearer the head and which nearer the feet?
- Is one side superior or is the other inferior?

In other words, has one ilium rotated posteriorly or the other anteriorly? This is determined by referring back to the standing flexion test that defines the side of dysfunction.

The side of dysfunction – as determined by the standing flexion test ('travelling thumb') and/or the standing hip flexion test – defines which observed anterior landmark is taken into consideration (Fig. 7.23Bi–Biv).

The practitioner's eyes should be directly over the pelvis with the thumbs resting on the ASISs.

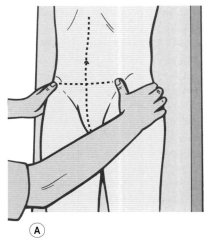

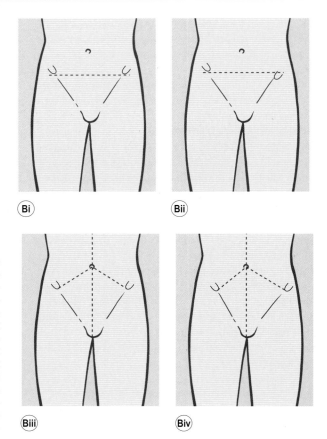

Fig. 7.23 A Practitioner adopts a position providing a bird's-eye view of ASIS prominences on which rest the thumbs. **Bi** The ASISs are level and there is no rotational dysfunction involving the iliosacral joints. **Bii** The right ASIS is higher than the left ASIS. If a thumb 'travelled' on the right side during the standing fl exion test this would represent a posterior right iliosacral rotation dysfunction. If a thumb 'travelled' on the left side during the test this would represent an anterior left iliosacral rotation dysfunction. **Biii** The ASISs are equidistant from the umbilicus and the midline, and there is no iliosacral fl are dysfunction. **Biv** The ASIS on the right is closer to the umbilicus/midline, which indicates that either there is a right-side iliosacral infl are (if the right thumb moved during the standing fl exion test), or there is a left-side iliosacral outfl are (if the left thumb moved during the standing fl exion test).

Rotations

1. The side of the positive standing flexion, or hip flexion test, is the dysfunctional side, and if that is the side which appears inferior (compared with its pair) it is assumed that the ilium on the inferior side has rotated *anteriorly* on the sacrum on that side.

   NOTE: Ipsilateral hip flexor shortness (e.g. psoas) might be responsible for apparent anterior rotation of the hemipelvis, and this should be assessed and if necessary treated before any attempt is made to correct the apparent IS restrictions (as described below).

2. The side of the positive standing flexion, or hip flexion test, is the dysfunctional side, and if the ASIS appears superior to its pair on that side, then the ilium has rotated *posteriorly* on the sacrum on that side (see Fig. 7.23Bi and Bii).

NOTE: Ipsilateral hip extensor shortness (e.g. hamstrings) might be responsible for apparent anterior rotation of the hemipelvis, and this should be assessed and if necessary treated before any attempt is made to correct the apparent IS restrictions (as described below).

Flares. While in the same position observing the ASIS positions, note is made of the relative positions of these landmarks in relation to the midline of the patient's abdomen, using either the linea alba or the umbilicus as a guide:

1. If one thumb is closer to the umbilicus than the other, it is necessary at this stage to once again refer to which side is dysfunctional.

2. Is the ASIS on the side which is further from the umbilicus outflared, or is the ASIS which is closer to the umbilicus indicative of that side being inflared?

The ASIS associated with the side on which the thumb moved superiorly during the standing flexion test is the dysfunctional side, and the decision as to whether there is an inflare (ASIS closer to umbilicus) or an outflare (ASIS further from umbilicus) is therefore obvious. Flare dysfunctions are usually treated prior to rotation dysfunctions (see Fig. 7.23 Biii and Biv).

NOTE: As with apparent rotational IS restrictions, there are likely to be particular muscular imbalances that directly influence such dysfunctional patterns; and these should receive attention prior to attempts to normalise hemipelvic flare restrictions.

MET Treatment of Iliac Inflare (Fig. 7.24A and B)

- The patient is supine and the practitioner stands on the dysfunctional side, with the cephalad hand stabilising the non-affected-side ASIS, and the caudad hand holding the ankle of the affected side (see Fig. 7.24A).
- The affected-side hip is flexed and abducted and full external rotation is introduced to the hip.
- The practitioner's forearm aligns with the lower leg, elbow stabilising the medial aspect of the knee.
- The patient is asked to lightly adduct the hip against the resistance offered by the restraining arm for 10 seconds.

- On complete relaxation, and on an exhalation, with the pelvis held stable by the cephalad hand, the flexed leg is taken into increased abduction and external rotation, as new 'slack' should now be available.
- This process is repeated once or twice, at which time the leg is slowly straightened while abduction and external rotation of the hip are maintained.
- The leg is then returned to the table.

NOTE: Care should be taken not to use the powerful leverage available from the flexed and abducted leg; its own weight and gravity provide adequate leverage, and the 'release' of tone achieved via isometric contractions will do the rest. It is very easy to turn an inflare into an outflare by overenthusiastic use of force. The degree of flare should be re-evaluated and any rotation then treated (see below).

MET Treatment of Iliac Outflare (Fig. 7.25)

- The patient is supine and the practitioner is on the same side as the dysfunctional ilium, supinated cephalad hand under the patient's buttocks with fingertips hooked into the sacral sulcus on the same side.
- The caudad hand holds the patient's foot on the treated side, with the forearm resting along the medial calf/shin area as the hand grasps the foot.

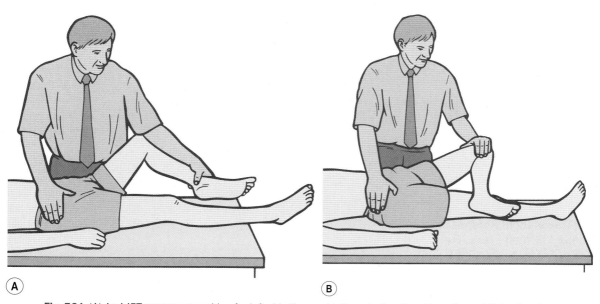

(A)   (B)

Fig. 7.24 (A) An MET treatment position for left-side iliosacral inflare dysfunction. Note the stabilising hand on the right anterior superior iliac spine (ASIS). (B) An alternative MET treatment position for left-side iliosacral inflare dysfunction. Note the stabilising hand on the right ASIS.

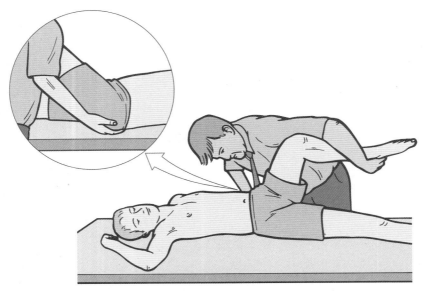

Fig. 7.25 MET treatment of iliosacral outflare on the left.

- The hip on the treated side is fully flexed and adducted and internally rotated, at which time the patient is asked to abduct the hip against resistance, using up to 50% of strength, for 10 seconds.
- Following this, and complete relaxation, slack is taken out and the exercise repeated once more.
- As the leg is taken into greater adduction and internal rotation, to take advantage of the release of muscular tone following the isometric contraction, the fingers in the sacral sulcus exert a traction towards the practitioner, effectively guiding the ilium into a more inflared position.
- After the final contraction, adduction and internal rotation are maintained as the leg is slowly returned to the table.
- The evaluation for flare dysfunction is then repeated, and if relative normality has been restored, any rotational dysfunction is then treated, using the methods described below.

MET Treatment of Anterior Iliac Rotation: Method 1 Patient Prone (Fig. 7.26A)

- The patient is prone. The practitioner stands at the side to be treated, at waist level.
- The affected leg and hip are flexed and brought over the edge of the table.
- The foot/ankle area is grasped between the practitioner's legs.

- The table-side hand stabilises the sacral area while the other hand supports the flexed knee and guides it into greater flexion, inducing posterior iliac rotation, until the restriction barrier is sensed:
  - By the palpating 'sacral contact' hand, or
  - By virtue of a sense of greater effort in guiding the flexed leg, and/or
  - By observation of pelvic movement as the barrier of resistance is passed.
- Once the barrier is engaged the patient is asked to attempt to straighten the leg against unyielding resistance, for 10 seconds using no more than 20% of available strength.
- On releasing the effort, and on complete relaxation, and on an exhalation, the leg/innominate is guided to its new barrier.
- Subsequent contractions can involve different directions of effort ('try to push your knee sideways', or 'try to bend your knee towards your shoulder', etc.) in order to bring into operation a variety of muscular factors to encourage release of the joint.[2]

---

[2]A supine position may also be used, or the same mechanics precisely can be incorporated into a side-lying position. The only disadvantage of side-lying is the relative instability of the pelvic region compared with that achieved in the prone and supine positions.

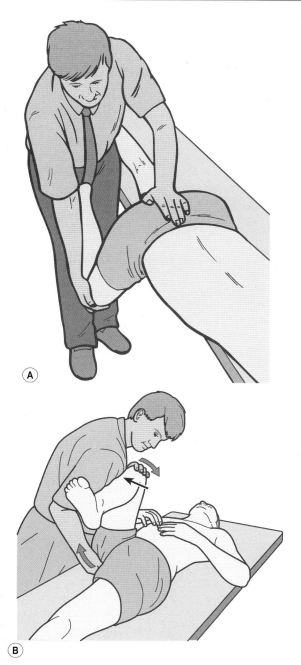

MET Treatment of Anterior Iliac Rotation: Method 2 Patient Supine (Fig. 7.26B)

- The practitioner stands at the side of the supine patient's anteriorly rotated innominate, facing the table.
- The knee and hip of the dysfunctional side should be flexed until the barrier is comfortably engaged – i.e. without undue force, with the practitioner's cephalad hand on the knee, maintaining its position.
- The practitioner places their caudad hand under the patient's pelvis so that the ischial tuberosity rests on their forearm and their hand palpates the SI joint (see Fig. 7.26B).
- The patient is requested to then extend the *hip* isometrically, against identical resistance, using less than 20% of available strength for 5 to 7 seconds.
- On cessation of the effort, and a full exhalation, the newly created 'slack' is taken up, as the hip is taken to a new flexion barrier.
- The sequence should then be repeated – possibly utilising a different direction of contraction – for example having the patient attempt to move the hip into flexion, or abduction, or adduction against resistance.
- Two to three repetitions are usually sufficient to achieve full and painless range of motion.

   Alternative: An alternative hand-hold (not illustrated) for this MET application would be to have the practitioner's cephalad hand underneath the patient's pelvis, palpating the SI/IS joint, while the caudad hand rested on the flexed knee, controlling the degree of hip flexion. This allows for a more sensitive identification of the restriction barrier than the method outlined above, but does not afford the same degree of control of isometric forces, particularly in the case of a very large patient and a smaller practitioner.

MET for Treatment of Posterior Iliac Rotation (Fig. 7.27)

- The patient is prone and the practitioner stands on the side opposite the dysfunctional IS joint.
- The table-side hand supports the anterior aspect of the patient's knee while the other rests on the SIJ of the affected side to evaluate bind.
- The affected leg is extended until free movement ceases, as evidenced by the following observations:
  - Bind is noted under the palpating hand, or
  - Sacral and pelvic motion are observed as the barrier is passed, or
  - A sense of effort is increased in the arm extending the leg.

Fig. 7.26 (A) MET treatment of an anterior iliosacral rotation restriction. (B) MET treatment of anterior iliosacral rotation restriction.

- The standing flexion test as described above should be performed again to establish whether the joint is now free.

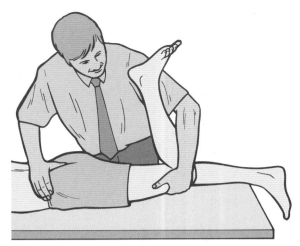

Fig. 7.27 MET treatment of a posterior iliosacral rotation restriction.

- With the practitioner holding the joint at its restriction barrier, the patient is asked, with no more than 20% of strength, to flex the hip against resistance for 10 seconds.
- After cessation of the effort, and completely relaxing, on an exhalation, the leg is extended further to its new barrier.
- No force should be used; the movement after the contraction simply takes advantage of whatever slack is then available.
- Variations in the direction of the contraction (perhaps involving abduction or adduction, or even attempted extension) are sometimes useful if no appreciable gain is achieved using hip and knee flexion.
- The standing flexion test is performed again to establish whether IS movement is now free, once a sense of 'release' has been noted following one of the contractions.

⏵ 'Shotgun' Method of Pelvic Stabilisation and Pubic Dysfunction

As a concluding element of any of the pelvic (SI or IS) approaches, a stabilisation method is recommended. As in a number of protocols described in this chapter (and the book as a whole) this remains a largely unvalidated approach with a long history of clinical use, and no negative reports or studies. The method has attracted a shorthand designation: 'shotgun method'.

This is also described in the osteopathic literature as appropriate for treatment of specific pubic symphysis dysfunctions (DeStefano, 2010) and in cases of advanced pregnancy, in relation to low-back pain (Petrie & Peck, 2000).

Experience suggests the methods are particularly useful during and following pregnancy when relaxin will have reduced stability in the pelvic articulations (Marnach et al., 2003; Daly et al., 1991).

Four variations of the 'shotgun' method are described below.

'Shotgun' method 1 (Fig. 7.28A)
- The patient is supine with knees and hips flexed, feet together.
- The practitioner stands at the patient's side and holds the knees together as the patient, using full strength (or less if this is uncomfortable) attempts to separate the knees.
- This effort is resisted for 3 to 4 seconds, and then repeated once more, before Method 2 (below) is employed.

'Shotgun' method 2 (Fig. 7.28B)
- The practitioner separates the knees, externally rotates the flexed hips, and places their forearm between them (palm on medial aspect of one knee and elbow on medial aspect of the other), as the patient, using full strength (or less if this is more comfortable) attempts to push the knees together for 3 to 4 seconds.
- After relaxation the method is repeated once more.

'Shotgun' method 3
- The patient's separated knees are slowly but forcefully adducted against the patient's attempts to maintain them in an abducted position (i.e. knees separated).
- This produces an isotonic eccentric stretch of the external hip rotator muscles, effectively toning these and producing a release in tone of the internal rotators, through RI.
- If the patient's leg strength is too great to easily overcome, a request should be made to allow the legs to slowly come together while maintaining resistance.

See discussion of slow eccentric isotonic stretches (SEIS) in Chapters 5 and also of their use in post-surgical settings, in Chapter 10.

'Shotgun' method 4
- The practitioner slowly but forcefully separates the patient's fully adducted thighs, which are touching each other at the outset.
- This forced abduction, against this resistance, involves an isotonic eccentric stretch of the internal hip rotator muscles, effectively toning these and producing a release in tone of the external rotators, through RI.

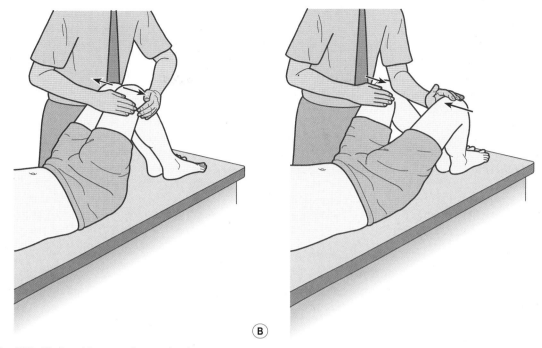

Fig. 7.28 (A) Practitioner resists patient's attempt to force knees apart. (B) Practitioner resists patient's attempt to force knees together.

- If the patient's leg strength is too great to easily over-come, a request should be made to allow the legs to slowly separate, while maintaining resistance.

See discussion of SEIS in Chapter 5 and also of their use in post-surgical settings, in Chapter 10.

This fourth variation of the 'shotgun' method has been found useful by Leon Chaitow as a final component of the 'shotgun' sequence, after the methods described above are completed.

❗ CAUTION

The myofascial forces created by these isometric and/or isotonic contractions, seem capable of resulting in a rapid normalisation of imbalances (possibly misalignment) at the symphysis, sometimes audibly. There may also be a loud 'popping' sound from the region of one or other inguinal ligament (which explains the use of '*shotgun*' as a nickname for the method). The patient should be forewarned that a harmless sound may be heard during the isometric contraction, but that is unlikely to be felt as anything other than a transient discomfort.

MET Treatment for Sacroiliac Dysfunction: Keeping It Simple

- It is well to remind ourselves – when considering the potential for complex confusion in analysis of sacral distortion patterns, and the possible influences on SI dysfunction, that there are only three pelvic bones – the two innominates and the sacrum.
- And there are only three pelvic joints – the right and left SI joint and the pubic symphysis.
- However, there are 45 muscles that attach to the pelvis – 16 to the ilium, 13 to the ischium and 16 to the pubes: transversus abdominis, quadratus lumborum, psoas, iliacus, rectus femoris, sartorius, piriformis, obturator internus and externus, quadratus femoris, inferior and superior gemelli, gluteus maximus, minimus and medius, hamstrings, gracilis, adductor longus, adductor brevis, adductor magnus, muscles of the pelvic floor, diaphragm.
- There are also numerous major ligaments: anterior and posterior SI, lesser and greater inguinal, sacrosciatic, iliolumbar, sacrotuberous, sacrospinous, iliofemoral, pubic, lumbosacral.

Clinical Questions When Confronted With Sacroiliac Dysfunction and Pain

- Are soft tissue dysfunctions (tightness, weakness, etc.) the cause of, or are they an effect of, pelvic and sacral dysfunctions? To some extent, the ASLR test can offer an answer. Further answers will be found if *all postural muscles* (see Chapters 2, 5 and 6) attaching to the pelvis, are evaluated for potential shortness, weakness, etc.
- Which muscle groups are most involved? Functional and other tests (see Chapter 5) can assist in identification of muscular imbalances.

It is suggested that it is logical to assess and treat these (using MET or other modalities) before focusing attention on apparent joint restrictions.

MET for Sacroiliac Dysfunction

This list of SI joint treatment methods utilising MET is not comprehensive, nor are the methods fully described. It is assumed that the brief descriptions and the illustrations are sufficient to guide clinicians towards adequate use of these safe, and frequently effective (personal experience) methods (Tigny, 2007; Lewit, 2010).

Method A (Fig. 7.29A)

- The SIJ rests on one hand while the ischium rests on practitioner's forearm.
- The other hand eases the flexed knee towards patient's ipsilateral axilla.
- SIJ mobilisation follows a 3- to 5-second isometric contraction after which new barriers are engaged as the knee is taken towards the axilla (various directions of isometric force should be attempted if an initial attempt fails to produce normalisation of SI dysfunction on that side).

Method B (Fig. 7.29B)

- The patient is supine, practitioner on side to be treated.
- One hand cups and holds the ipsilateral ischial tuberosity.
- The other hand is in contact with the anterior iliac crest.
- Following a 3- to 5-second isometric contraction (using the ipsilateral leg) – the ilium is directed caudally.

- Various directions of isometric force should be attempted if an initial attempt fails to produce normalisation of SI restriction on that side.

Method C (Fig. 7.29C)

The patient is hook-lying, with the practitioner at knee level, facing the head of the table.
- The practitioner's non-table-side arm is threaded under the ipsilateral knee, with the hand resting on the contralateral knee.
- Using the contralateral knee as a fulcrum, the ipsilateral thigh and pelvis are distracted, following an isometric contraction – for example: 'Lightly pull your knee towards your hip', OR 'Push your knee to the side – or towards the other knee' – always with light efforts, and with full resistance offered by the practitioner.
- Various directions of isometric force should be attempted if an initial attempt fails to produce normalisation.

Method D (Fig. 7.29D)

This method has been modified by the author from a protocol described by Lewit (2010, pp. 206–207) that derived from the original description by Stoddard (1962). The context of the modification – which involves use of an isometric contraction rather than active springing of the joint) can be best understood from the words of Lewit (2010, p. 206):

Neuromuscular techniques play virtually no role … because there are no muscles between the sacrum and ilium. [However] experience gleaned from chain reaction patterns has modified our thinking inasmuch as indirect connections apparently exist due to the sacrotuberous ligament and the attachment points of the ischiocrural muscles, pelvic floor, and piriformis, etc. As a result, the sacroiliac joint very often no longer requires treatment after the lower extremity, pelvic floor, and piriformis have been treated.

Not only does this accurate perspective confirm the broad theme of this chapter – and of Mitchell's direction to consider joint restrictions as potentially the result of myofascial changes – but it also opens the opportunity for the modification described below.

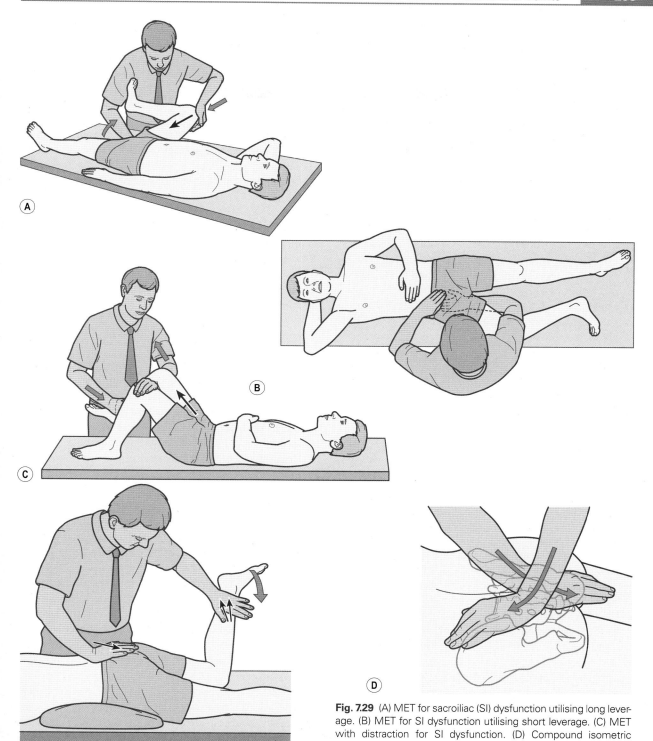

Fig. 7.29 (A) MET for sacroiliac (SI) dysfunction utilising long leverage. (B) MET for SI dysfunction utilising short leverage. (C) MET with distraction for SI dysfunction. (D) Compound isometric contraction of pelvic muscles for sacral and/or SI dysfunction. (E) Direct MET method for sacral dysfunction.

- The patient lies prone.
- In this example the practitioner stands on the patient's right and – with hands crossed – makes a pisiform contact, on the left posterior superior iliac spine (PSIS) with their left hand.
- The right hand makes a pisiform contact on the apex of the sacrum.
- The practitioner's arms should be straight in order to exert light but sustained pressure onto both contact points, easing them apart until a barrier is noted, as slack is removed from the skin and subcutaneous soft tissues.
- The patient is then requested to consciously contract pelvic muscles: 'Clench your buttocks, and simultaneously push your thighs together, for 3 to 4 seconds' OR 'Try to tighten your internal pelvic muscles by tightening these, as though attempting to stop yourself from urinating'.
- Following such a contraction, the contact hands ease the sacrum away from the contact point on the ilium (PSIS).
- If necessary the same procedure is repeated, and/or performed on the other SI joint.

Method E (Fig. 7.29E)

One hand palpates the SI joint while the other adds various directions of compression force, via contact on the flexed knee, while the patient offers resistance. Isometric or isokinetic or pulsed MET variables may be used, while the palpating hand assesses for motion/change at the SI joint.

- This method is designed to inhibit muscle tone at the lumbosacral junction and, in theory, allow correction of sacral torsion.
- The therapist stands at the side of the treatment table.
- The patient is prone with a pillow supporting the pelvis, and with the leg closest to the practitioner flexed at the knee.
- The heel of the practitioner's cranial hand is placed at the base of the patient's sacrum, in order to apply a caudally directed anterior force, to take out all slack.
- The practitioner uses their caudal hand to contact the inner aspect of the lower (flexed) leg in order to move the hip into medial rotation (see Fig. 7.29E).
- The patient is requested to introduce an external rotation at the hip, by pushing the lower leg medially, against the firm resistance of the practitioner's caudal hand, for 3 to 5 seconds.

- The cranial hand should sustain constant pressure directed anteriorly, on the base of the sacrum.
- The isometric contraction of the lateral rotators of the hip should apply traction to the ipsilateral aspect of the base of the sacrum, and should assist in mobilisation of the SIJ, and potentially normalise sacral torsion.
- The isometric contraction should be repeated three to four times with a brief rest between contractions, however the sacral pressure should be sustained throughout and between the isometric contractions.

MET Treatment for Temporomandibular Joint Dysfunction

Dysfunction of the TMJ is a vast subject, and the implications of such problems have been related to a variety of other areas of dysfunction, ranging from cranial lesions to spinal and general somatic alterations and endocrine imbalance (Gelb, 1977). The reader is referred to Janda's observations on postural influences on TMJ problems (see Chapter 5).

Diagnosis of the particular pattern of dysfunction is, of course, essential before safe therapeutic intervention is possible. There are many possible causes of TMJ dysfunction, and a cooperative relationship with a skilled dentist is an advantage in treating such problems, since many aspects relate to the presence of faults in the bite of the patient.

Inept manipulative measures can also traumatise the area, especially thrusting forces exerted onto the occiput while the head and neck are in extreme rotation.

Any situation in which the patient is required to maintain the mouth opened for lengthy periods, such as during dental work, or when a laryngoscope is being used, may induce strain, especially if the neck is extended at the time (Freshwater & Gosling, 2003).

All, or any, such patterns of injury should be sought when TMJ pain, or limitation of mouth opening is observed. Apart from correction of cranial dysfunction via skilled cranial osteopathic work, the muscular component invites attention, using MET methods and other appropriate measures. Gelb suggests a form of MET which he terms 'stretch against resistance' exercises.

Studies have supported the use of MET in treatment of TMJ dysfunction Delgado de la Serna et al., 2020. For example Rajadurai (2011) reports that 'MET is effective in reducing pain and improving mouth opening in patients with TMD [TMJ dysfunction]'.

MET TMJ Method 1 (Fig. 7.30A)

- RI is the objective when the patient is asked to open the mouth against resistance applied by the practitioner's, or the patient's own, hand (patient places elbow on table, chin in hand, and attempts to open mouth against resistance for ~10 seconds).
- The jaw would have been opened to a comfortable limit before attempting this, and after the attempt it would be taken to its new barrier before repeating.

- This MET method relaxes shortened muscles that may be inhibiting full opening of the mouth.

MET TMJ Method 2 (Fig. 7.30B)

- To relax short tight muscles using PIR, counterpressure would be required in order to prevent the open jaw from closing (using minimal force).
- This would require the thumbs (suitably protected) to be placed along the superior surface of the lower

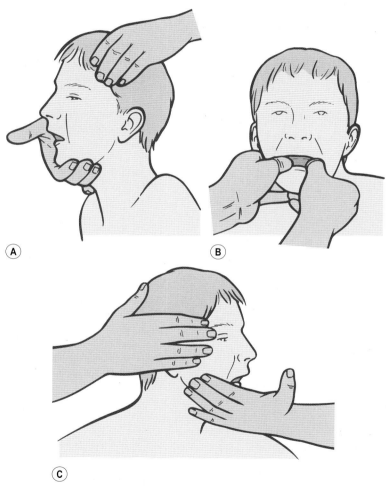

Fig. 7.30 (A) MET treatment of temporomandibular joint (TMJ) restriction, involving limited ability to open the mouth. The isometric contraction phase of treatment is illustrated as the patient attempts to open against self-applied resistance (see also Note in caption for Fig. 7.30B). (B) MET treatment of TMJ restriction, involving an isometric contraction in which the patient attempts to close the mouth against resistance. NOTE: Following both these procedures (A and B), the patient should be encouraged to gently stretch the muscles by opening the mouth widely. This can be assisted by the practitioner. (C) MET treatment of lateral restrictions of the TMJ. Following the isometric contraction as described, the lateral excursion is increased.

back teeth while an isometric contraction was performed by the patient.

- In this exercise the practitioner is directing force towards the barrier (practitioner-direct) rather than the patient (patient-direct).

MET TMJ Method 3 (Fig. 7.30C)

Lewit (1991), maintaining that laterolateral movements are important in TMJ treatment, has suggested the following method of treating TMJ problems:

- The patient sits with the head turned to one side (say the left in this example).
- The practitioner stands behind and stabilises the patient's head against their chest.
- The patient opens their mouth, allowing the chin to drop, and the practitioner cradles the mandible with their left hand, so that the fingers are curled under the jaw, away from him.
- The practitioner draws the jaw gently towards their chest, and when the slack has been taken up, the patient offers a degree of resistance to its being taken further, laterally.
- After a few seconds of gentle isometric contraction, the practitioner and patient relax simultaneously, and the jaw will usually have an increased lateral excursion.
- This is repeated several times.
- This procedure should be performed so that the lateral pull is away from the side to which the jaw deviates, on opening.

TMJ Self-Treatment Isometric Concentric Exercise

Gelb (1977) suggests a retrusive exercise be used in conjunction with the above, both methods being useful in eliminating 'clicks' on opening the mouth:

- The patient curls the tongue upwards, placing the tip as far back on the roof of the mouth as possible.
- While this is maintained in position, the patient is asked to slowly open and close the mouth (gently), to reactivate the suprahyoid, posterior temporalis and posterior digastric muscles (the retrusive group).
- The patient then places an elbow on a table, jaw resting on the clenched fist.
- This offers some resistance to the slow opening of the mouth – while the tongue is in the position as described above.
- This isometric concentric exercise should be performed five times with hand pressure, and then five

times without, ensuring that the lower jaw does not come forward.

- The lower teeth should always remain behind the upper teeth on closing.
- A total of 25 such movements should be performed, morning and evening.

In the next chapter the integrated use of MET with other soft tissue approaches is described, particularly in relation to treatment of myofascial (trigger-point) pain and dysfunction.

REFERENCES

Ali, A., Andrzejowski, P., Kanakaris, N.K., Giannoudis, P.V., 2020. Pelvic girdle pain, hypermobility spectrum disorder and hypermobility-type ehlers-danlos syndrome: a narrative literature review. J Clin Med 9 (12), 3992. doi:10.3390/jcm9123992.

Anggiat, L., Altavas, A.J., Budhyanti, W., 2020. Joint mobilization: theory and evidence review. Int. J. Sport Exer. Health Res. 4 (2), 86–90.

Awatani, T., Enoki, T., Morikita, I., 2018. Inter-rater reliability and validity of angle measurements using smartphone applications for weight-bearing ankle dorsiflexion range of motion measurements. Phys. Ther. Sport. 34, 113–120. doi:10.1016/j.ptsp.2018.09.002.

Bandy, W., Irion, J., Briggler, M., 1997. The effect of time and frequency of static stretching on flexibility of the hamstring muscles. Phys. Ther. 77, 1090–1096.

Barker, P., Briggs, C., Bogeski, G., 2004. Tensile transmission across the lumbar fasciae in unembalmed cadavers: effects of tension to various muscular attachments. Spine 29 (2), 129–138.

Bialosky, J.E., Beneciuk, J.M., Bishop, M.D., Coronado, R.A., Penza, C.W., Simon, C.B., et al., 2018. Unraveling the mechanisms of manual therapy: modeling an approach. J. Orthop. Sports Phys. Ther. 48 (1), 8–18. doi:10.2519/jospt.2018.7476.

Boudreau, P.A., Steiman, I., Mior, S., 2020. Clinical management of benign joint hypermobility syndrome: a case series. J. Can. Chiropr. Assoc. 64 (1), 43–54.

Brodin, H., 1982. Lumbar treatment using MET. Osteopath. Ann. 10, 23–24.

Brodin, H., 1987. Inhibition-facilitation technique for lumbar pain treatment. Man. Med. 3, 24–26.

Burns, D.K., Wells, M.R., 2006. Gross range of motion in the cervical spine: the effects of osteopathic Muscle Energy Technique in asymptomatic subjects. J. Am. Osteopath. Assoc. 106 (3), 137–142.

Carreiro, J., 2009a. Pediatric Manual Medicine: an Osteopathic Approach. Elsevier Health Sciences, pp. 1–12.

Carreiro, J., 2009b. Pediatric Manual Medicine: an Osteopathic Approach. Elsevier Health Sciences, pp. 155–192.

Cassidy, J., Lopes, A., Yong-Hing, K., 1992a. The immediate effect of manipulation, versus mobilization on pain and range of motion in the cervical spine: a randomized, controlled trial. J. Manipulative Physiol. Ther. 15, 570–575.

Cassidy, J.D., Quon, J.A., LaFrance, L.J., Yong-Hing, K., 1992b. The effect of manipulation on pain and range of motion in the cervical spine: a pilot study [published correction]. J. Manipulative Physiol. Ther. 15 (9), 495–500.

Chaitow, L., 2001. Muscle Energy Techniques, second ed. Churchill Livingstone, Edinburgh.

Chaitow, L., 2010. Positional Release Techniques, third ed. Churchill Livingstone, Edinburgh.

Chaitow, L., Bradley, D., Gilbert, C., 2002. Multidisciplinary Approaches to Breathing Pattern Disorders. Churchill Livingstone, Edinburgh.

Christensen, H.W., Vach, W., Vach, K., Manniche, C., Haghfelt, T., Hartvigsen, L., 2002. Palpation of the upper thoracic spine: an observer reliability study. J. Manipulative Physiol. Ther. 25 (5), 285–292.

Chopra, P., Tinkle, B., Hamonet, C., Brock, I., Gompel, A., Bulbena, A., et al., 2017. Pain management in the Ehlers–Danlos syndromes. Am. J. Med. Genet. Part C Semin. Med. Genet. 175 (1), 212–219.

Cibulka, M., Koldehoff, R., 1999. Clinical usefulness of a cluster of SIJ tests in patients with and without low back pain. J. Orthopaed. Sports Phys. Ther. 29 (2), 83–92.

Cook, C., Hegedus, E., Showalter, C., Sizer Jr., P.S., 2006. Coupling behavior of the cervical spine: a systematic review of the literature. J. Manipulative Physiol. Ther. 29 (7), 570–575.

Dabbs, V., Lauretti, W.J., 1995. A risk assessment of cervical manipulation vs. NSAIDs for the treatment of neck pain [review]. J. Manipulative Physiol. Ther. 18, 530–536.

Daly, J.M., Frame, P.S., Rapoza, P.A., 1991. Sacroiliac subluxation: a common treatable cause of low back pain in pregnancy. Fam. Pract. Res. J. 11, 149–159.

de las Penas, C.F., Cleland, J., Huijbregts, P., 2011. Neck and Arm Pain Syndromes: Evidence-informed Screening, Diagnosis and Management. Churchill Livingstone, Edinburgh, pp. 381–391.

Delgado de la Serna, P., Plaza-Manzano, G., Cleland, J., Fernández-de-Las-Peñas, C., Martín-Casas, P., Díaz-Arribas, M.J., 2020. Effects of Cervico-mandibular manual therapy in patients with temporomandibular pain disorders and associated somatic tinnitus: a randomized clinical trial. Pain Med 21 (3), 613–624. doi:10.1093/pm/pnz278.

DeStefano, L., 2010. Greenman's Principles of Manual Medicine. Lippincott Williams & Wilkins, Baltimore.

Tigny, D., 2007. Biomechanical analysis of SIJ & relevant kinesiology. In: Vleeming, A., Mooney, V., Dorman, T. et al. (Eds.), Movement, Stability and Low Back Pain. Churchill Livingstone, New York.

Dreyfuss, P., Dreyer, S., Griffen, J., Hoffman, J., Walsh, N., 1994. Positive SI screening tests in asymptomatic patients. Spine 19 (10), 1138–1143.

Egan, W.E., Flynn, T.W., Burns, S.A., et al., 2011. The thoracic spine: physical therapy patient management using current evidence. Current Concepts of Orthopedic Physical Therapy. APTA Orthopedic Section Home Study Course 2011.

Eccles, J.A., Davies, K.A., 2021. The challenges of chronic pain and fatigue. Clin. Med. 21 (1), 19–27.

Engelbert, R.H., Juul-Kristensen, B., Pacey, V., de Wandele, I., Smeenk, S., et al., 2017. The evidence-based rationale for physical therapy treatment of children, adolescents, and adults diagnosed with joint hypermobility syndrome/hypermobile Ehlers Danlos syndrome. Am. J. Med. Genet. C Semin. Med. Genet. 175 (1), 158–167. doi:10.1002/ajmg.c.31545.

Espejo, J.A., García-Escudero, M., Oltra, E., 2018. Unraveling the molecular determinants of manual therapy: an approach to integrative therapeutics for the treatment of fibromyalgia and chronic fatigue syndrome/myalgic encephalomyelitis. Int. J. Mol. Sci. 19 (9), 2673. doi:10.3390/ijms19092673.

Ewertowska, P., Trzaskoma, Z., Sitarski, D., Gromuł, B., Haponiuk, I., Czaprowski, D., 2020. Muscle strength, muscle power and body composition in college-aged young women and men with generalized joint hypermobility. PLoS One 15 (7), e0236266. doi:10.1371/journal.pone.0236266.

Exelby, L., 1996. Peripheral mobilisations with movement. Man Ther 1, 118–126.

Evjenth, O., Hamberg, J., 1984. Muscle Stretching in Manual Therapy. Alfta Rehab, Alfta, Sweden.

Feland, J., Myrer, J., Schulthies, S., Fellingham, G.W., Measom, G.W., 2001. The effect of duration of stretching of the hamstring muscle group for increasing range of motion in people aged 65 years or older. Phys. Ther. 81, 1100–1117.

Feldman, E.C.H., Hivick, D.P., Slepian, P.M., Tran, S.T., Chopra, P., Greenley, R.N., 2020. Pain symptomatology and management in pediatric Ehlers-Danlos syndrome: a review. Children (Basel) 7 (9), 146. doi:10.3390/children7090146.

Freshwater, Z., Gosling, C., 2003. The effect of specific isometric muscle energy technique on range of opening of the temporomandibular joint: a pilot study. J. Osteopath. Med. 6, 36.

Fryer, G., Morse, M., Johnson, J.C., 2009. Spinal and sacroiliac assessment and treatment techniques used by osteopathic physicians in the United States. Osteopath. Med. Prim. Care 3, 4. doi:10.1186/1750-4732-3-4.

Fryer, G., Ruskowski, W., 2004. Influence of contraction duration in MET applied to atlanto-axial joint. J. Osteopath. Med. 7 (2), 79–84.

Fryer, G., Fossum, C., 2009. Therapeutic mechanisms underlying muscle energy approaches. In: Fernández de las Peñas, C et al. (Ed.), Physical Therapy for Tension Type and Cervicogenic Headache. Jones & Bartlett, Boston.

Fryette, H., 1954. Principles of Osteopathic Technique. American Academy of Osteopathy Newark, Ohio.

Gelb, H., 1977. Clinical Management of Head, Neck and TMJ Pain and Dysfunction. W B Saunders, Philadelphia.

Ghibellini, G., Brancati, F., Castori, M., 2015. Neurodevelopmental attributes of joint hypermobility syndrome/Ehlers-Danlos syndrome, hypermobility type: update and perspectives. Am. J. Med. Genet. Part C Semin. Med. Genet. 169, 107–116. doi:10.1002/ajmg.c.31424.

Gibbons, P., Tehan, P., 1998. Muscle energy concepts and coupled motion of the spine. Man. Ther. 3 (2), 95–101.

Gibbons, P., Tehan, P., 2006. Manipulation of the Spine, Thorax and Pelvis: An Osteopathic Perspective, second ed. Elsevier Churchill Livingstone, Kidlington, UK.

Goodridge, J.P., 1981. Muscle energy technique: definition, explanation, methods of procedure. J. Am. Osteopath. Assoc. 81, 249–254.

Goodridge, J., Kuchera, W., 1997. Muscle energy techniques for specific areas. In: Ward, R. (Ed.), Foundations of Osteopathic Medicine. Williams and Wilkins, Baltimore.

Gray, J., Grimsby, O., 2004. Interrelationship of the spine, rib cage, and shoulder. In: Donatelli, R. (Ed.), Physical Therapy of the Shoulder, fourth ed. Churchill Livingstone, Edinburgh.

Greenman, P., 1996. Principles of Manual Medicine, second ed. Williams and Wilkins, Baltimore.

Grieve, G., 1984. Mobilisation of the Spine. Churchill Livingstone, Edinburgh.

Grimshaw, D.N., 2001. Cervicogenic headache: manual and manipulative therapies [review]. Curr. Pain Headache Rep. 5, 369–375.

Hakim, A.J., Grahame, R., 2003. A simple questionnaire to detect hypermobility: an adjunct to the assessment of patients with diffuse musculoskeletal pain. Int. J. Clin. Pract. 57, 163–166.

Harakal, J., 1975. An osteopathically integrated approach to whiplash complex. J. Am. Osteopath. Assoc. 74, 941–956.

Hardcastle, P., Nade, S., 1985. The significance of the Trendelenburg test. J. Bone Joint Surg. 67, 741–746.

Hartman, L., 1985. Handbook of Osteopathic Technique. Hutchinson, London.

Hasson, C.J., Miller, R.H., Caldwell, G.E., 2011. Contractile and elastic ankle joint muscular properties in young and older adults. PloS One 6 (1), e15953. doi:10.1371/journal.pone.0015953.

Hastings, J., Forster, J.E., Witzeman, K., 2019. Joint hypermobility among female patients presenting with chronic myofascial pelvic pain. PM R 11 (11), 1193–1199. doi:10.1002/pmrj.12131.

Heiderscheit, B., Boissonnault, W., 2008. Reliability of joint mobility and pain assessment of the thoracic spine and rib cage in asymptomatic individuals. J. Man. Manip. Ther. 16 (4), 210–216.

Hsieh, C.Y., Vicenzino, B., Yang, C.H., Hu, M.H., Yang, C., 2002. Mulligan's mobilization with movement for the thumb: a single case report using magnetic resonance imaging to evaluate the positional fault, hypothesis. Man. Ther. 7, 44–49.

Iqbal, M., Riaz, H., Ghous, M., Masood, K., 2020. Comparison of spencer muscle energy technique and passive stretching in adhesive capsulitis: a single blind randomized control trial. J. Pak. Med. Assoc. 70 (12(A)), 2113–2118. doi:10.5455/JPMA.23971.

Janda, V., 1988. In: Grant, R. (Ed.), Physical Therapy of the Cervical and Thoracic Spine. Churchill Livingstone, New York.

Johns, R.J., Wright, V., 1962. Relative importance of various tissues in joint stiffness. J. Appl. Physiol. 17, 824–828.

Jones, L., 1981. Strain and Counterstrain. Academy of Applied Osteopathy, Colorado Springs.

Kaltenborn, F., 1985. Mobilisation of Extremity Joints. Olaf Norlis Boekhandel, Norway.

Kaltenborn, F.M., Evjenth, O., Kaltenborn, T.B., Morgan, D., Vollowitz, E., 2008. Manual Mobilization of the Joints: Joint Examination and Basic Treatment. Vol. III: Traction-Manipulation of the Extremities and Spine, Basic Thrust Techniques. Norli, Oslo.

Kappler, R.E., Jones, J.M., 2003. Thrust (high-velocity/low-amplitude) techniques. In: Ward, R.C. (Ed.), Foundations for Osteopathic Medicine, second ed. Lippincott, Williams & Wilkins, Philadelphia, pp. 852–880.

Kirk, J.A., Ansell, B.M., Bywaters, E.G., 1967. The hypermobility syndrome. Musculoskeletal complaints associated with generalized joint hypermobility. Ann. Rheum. Dis. 26 (5), 419–425. doi:10.1136/ard.26.5.419.

Klingler, W., Schleip, R., Zorn, A., 2004, European Fascia Research Project Report. 5th World Congress Low Back and Pelvic Pain MelbourneNovember 2004.

Knebl, J.A., Shores, J.H., Gamber, R.G., et al., 2002. Improving functional ability in the elderly via the Spencer technique, an osteopathic manipulative treatment: a randomized, controlled trial. J. Am. Osteopath. Assoc. 102 (7), 387–396.

Kokmeyer, D., van der Wurff, P., 2002. The reliability of multitest regimens with specific SI pain provocation tests. J. Manipulative Physiol. Ther. 25 (1), 42–48.

Kuchera, W.A., Kuchera, M.L., 1994. Osteopathic Principles in Practice, second ed. Greyden Press, Columbus, Ohio.

Kwolek, A., 1989. Rehabilitation treatment with post-isometric muscle relaxation for haemophilia patients. J. Man. Med. 4, 55–57.

Lakhani, E., Nook, B., Haas, M., et al., 2009. Motion palpation used as a postmanipulation assessment tool for monitoring end-feel: a randomized controlled trial of test responsiveness. J. Manipulative Physiol. Ther. 32 (7), 549–555.

Lebiedowska, M.K., Fisk, J., 2009. Knee resistance during passive stretch in patients with hypertonia. J. Neurosci. Methods 179, 323–330.

Lederman, E., 1997. Fundamentals of Manual Therapy. Churchill Livingstone, London, p. 34.

Lederman, I., 2005. The Science and Practice of Manual Therapy, second ed. Churchill Livingstone, Edinburgh.

Lee, D., 1997. Treatment of pelvic instability. In: Vleeming, A., Mooney, V., Dorman, T. et al (Eds.), Movement, Stability and Low Back Pain. Churchill Livingstone, New York.

Lee, D., 2000. The Pelvic Girdle. An Approach to the Examination and Treatment of the Lumbo-Pelvic-Hip Region, second ed. Churchill Livingstone, Edinburgh.

Lee, D., 2010. The Pelvic Girdle. An Approach to the Examination and Treatment of the Lumbo-Pelvic-Hip Region, fourth ed. Churchill Livingstone, Edinburgh.

Lenehan, K., Fryer, G., McLaughlin, P., 2003. The effect of MET on gross trunk range of motion. J. Osteopath. Med. 6 (1), 13–18.

Levangie, P., 1999. Four clinical tests of SI joint dysfunction. Phys. Ther. 79 (11), 1043–1057.

Lewit, K., 1985. The muscular and articular factor in movement restriction. Man. Med. 1, 83–85.

Lewit, K., 1991. Manipulative Therapy in Rehabilitation of the Motor System. Butterworths, London.

Lewit, K., Rosina, A., 1999. Why yet another sign of SI joint restriction. J. Manipulative Physiol. Ther. 22 (3), 154–160.

Lewit, K., 2009. Manipulative Therapy: Musculoskeletal Medicine. Elsevier Health Sciences, Edinburgh, p. 33.

Lewit, K., 2010. Manipulative Therapy. Elsevier, Edinburgh pp. 206–207.

Liao, Z., Pu, T., Gu, H., Liu, W., 2015. Coupled motion of cervical spine in three level hybrid constructs. Biomed Mater Eng 26 (Suppl. 1), S637–S645. doi:10.3233/BME-151355.

Liebenson, C., Karpowicz, A., Brown, S., et al., 2009. The active straight leg raise test and lumbar spine stability. Phys. Med. Rehabil. 1, 530–535.

Lima, C.R., Martins, D.F., Reed, W.R., 2020. Physiological responses induced by manual therapy in animal models: a scoping review. Front. Neurosci. 14, 430. doi:10.3389/fnins.2020.00430.

Luckenbill-Edds, L., Bechill, G.B., 1995. Nerve compression syndromes as models, for research on osteopathic manipulative treatment [review]. J. Am. Osteopath. Assoc. 95, 319–326.

McAtee, R., Charland, J., 1999. Facilitated Stretching, second ed. Human Kinetics, Champaign, IL.

McPartland, J.M., 2008. Expression of the endocannabinoid system in fibroblasts and myofascial tissues. J. Bodyw. Mov. Ther. 12, 169–182.

Magnusson, S., Simonsen, E.B., Aagaard, P., Dyhre-Poulsen, P., McHugh, M.P., Kjaer, M., 1996. Mechanical and physiological responses to stretching with and without pre-isometric contraction in human skeletal muscle. Arch. Phys. Med. Rehabil. 77, 373–377.

Marnach, M., Ramin, K., Ramsey, P., Song, S.W., Stensland, J.J., An, K.N., 2003. Characterization of the relationship between joint laxity and maternal hormones in pregnancy. Obstet. Gynecol. 101, 331–335.

Meijne, W., van Neerbos, K., 1999. Intraexaminer and interexaminer reliability of the Gillet test. J. Manipulative Physiol. Ther. 22 (1), 4–9.

Mimura, M., Moriya, H., Watanabe, T., Takahashi, K.A., Yamagata, M.A, Tamaki, T.A., 1989. Three-dimensional motion analysis of the cervical spine with special reference to the axial rotation. Spine 14 (11), 1135–1139.

Mitchell Jr., F., 1998. Muscle Energy Manual, vol. 2. MET Press, East Lansing, p. 1.

Mitchell, F., Moran, P., Pruzzo, N., 1979. An Evaluation and Treatment Manual of Osteopathic Muscle Energy Procedures. MET Press, East Lansing, Michigan.

Mitchell Jr., F., 2009. Interview. In: Franke, H. (Ed.), The History of MET In: Muscle Energy Technique History-Model-Research. Verband der Osteopathen Deutschland, Wiesbaden.

Moore, S., Laudner, K., Mcloda, T., Shaffer, M.A., 2011. The immediate effects of muscle energy technique on posterior shoulder tightness: a randomized controlled trial. J. Orthopaed. Sports Phys. Ther. 41 (6), 400–407.

Mulligan, B., 2004. Manual Therapy: 'NAGS', 'SNAGS', 'MWMS' etc, fifth ed. Plane View Services Ltd, Wellington.

Olsén, M.F., Romberg, K., 2010. Reliability of the respiratory movement measuring instrument. Clin. Physiol. Funct. Imaging 30 (5), 349–353.

Onifer, S.M., Sozio, R.S., Long, C.R., 2019. Role for endocannabinoids in spinal manipulative therapy analgesia? Evid based complement. Altern. Med. 2019, Article ID 2878352, 5 pages doi:10.1155/2019/2878352 .

O'Sullivan, P.B., Beales, D.J., Beetham, J.A., Cripps, J., Graf, F., Lin, I.B., 2002. Altered motor control strategies in subjects with sacroiliac joint pain during the active straight-leg-raise test. Spine 27, E1–E8.

Patriquin, D., 1992. Evolution of osteopathic manipulative technique: the Spencer technique. J. Am. Osteopath. Assoc. 92, 1134–1146.

Peace, S., Fryer, G., 2004. Methods used by members of the Australian osteopathic profession to assess the sacroiliac joint. J. Osteopath. Med. 7 (1), 25–32.

Petrie, K., Peck, M., 2000. Alternative medicine, in maternity care: update in maternity care. Prim. Care 27 (1), 117–135.

Pfluegler, G., Kasper, J., Luedtke, K., 2020. The immediate effects of passive joint mobilisation on local muscle function. A systematic review of the literature. Musculoskelet. Sci. Pract. 45, 102106. doi:10.1016/j.msksp.2019.102106.

Qureshi, N.A., Alsubaie, H.A., Ali, G.I.M., 2019. Myofascial pain syndrome: a concise update on clinical, diagnostic and integrative and alternative therapeutic perspectives. Int. Neuropsychiatr. Dis. J. 13 (1), 1–14. https://doi.org/10.9734/indj/2019/v13i130100.

Rajadurai, V., 2011. The effect of muscle energy technique on temporomandibular joint dysfunction: a randomized clinical trail. Asian J. Sci. Res. 4, 71–77.

Ramos, M.M., Carnaz, L., Mattiello, S.M., Karduna, A.R., Zanca, G.G., 2019. Shoulder and elbow joint position sense assessment using a mobile app in subjects with and without shoulder pain-between-days reliability. Phys. Ther. Sport 37, 157–163.

Reed, M.L., Begalle, R.L., Laudner, K.G., 2018. Acute effects of muscle energy technique and joint mobilization on shoulder tightness in youth throwing athletes: a randomized controlled trial. Int. J. Sports Phys. Ther. 13 (6), 1024–1031.

Roussel, N., Nijs, J., Truijen, S., Smeuninx, L., Stassijns, G., 2007. Low back pain: clinimetric properties of the Trendelenburg test, active straight leg raise test, and breathing pattern during active, straight leg raising. J. Manipulative Physiol. Ther. 30, 270–278.

Ruddy, T.J., 1962. Osteopathic rhythmic resistive technic. Academy of Applied Osteopathy Yearbook, 1962, 23–31.

Sacks, H.A., Prabhakar, P., Wessel, L.E., Hettler, J., Strickland, S.M., Potter, H.G., et al., 2019. Generalized joint laxity in orthopaedic patients: clinical manifestations, radiographic correlates, and management. J. Bone Joint Surg. Am. 101 (6), 558–566. doi:10.2106/JBJS.18.00458.

Sathe, S.S., Rajandekar, T., Thodge, K., Gawande, V., 2020. Comparison between immediate effects of MET and passive stretching techniques on hamstring flexibility in patients with hamstring tightness: an experimental study. Indian J. Forensic Med. Toxicol. 14 (4), 6857–6862. doi:10.37506/ijfmt.v14i4.12701.

Schenk, R.J., Adelman, K., Rousselle, J., 1994. The effects of muscle energy technique on cervical range of motion. J. Man. Manipulative Ther. 2 (4), 149–155.

Schlager, A., Ahlqvist, K., Pingel, R., Nilsson-Wikmar, L., Olsson, C.B., Kristiansson, P., 2020. Validity of the self-reported five-part questionnaire as an assessment of generalized joint hypermobility in early pregnancy. BMC Musculoskelet. Disord. 21 (1), 514. doi:10.1186/s12891-020-03524-7.

Schleip, R., 2011. Strain hardening of fascia: static stretching of dense fibrous connective tissues can induce a temporary stiffness increase accompanied by enhanced matrix hydration. JBMT 16 (1), 94–100.

Scott-Dawkins, C., 1997. Comparative effectiveness of adjustments versus mobilizations in chronic mechanical neck pain. In: Proceedings of the Scientific Symposium. World Chiropractic Congress June 1997.

Seffinger, Hruby, R., 2007. Evidence-Based Manual Medicine. Elsevier, Philadelphia.

Selkow, N., Grindstaff, T., Cross, K., 2009. Short term effect of Muscle Energy Technique on pain in individuals with non-specific, lumbopelvic pain: a pilot study. J. Man. Manipulative Ther. 17 (1), E14–E18.

Shrier, I., Gossal, K., 2000. Myths and truths of stretching. Individualised recommendations for healthy muscles. Phys. Sports Med. 28 (8), 1–7.

Sirajudeen, M.S., 2020. Physical therapy management for child with generalized joint hypermobility. Majmaah J. Health Sci. 8 (1), 113–119.

Sizer Jr., P.S., Brismée, J.M., Cook, C., 2007. Coupling behavior of the thoracic spine: a systematic review of the literature. J. Manipulative Physiol. Ther. 30 (5), 390–399 10.1016/j.jmpt.2007.04.009.

Solecki, W., Błasiak, A., Laprus, H., Brzóska, R., 2020. Hyperlaxity and multidirectional shoulder instability. 360° Around Shoulder Instability. Springer, Berlin, Heidelberg, pp. 331–334.

Song, B., Yeh, P., Nguyen, D., Ikpeama, U., Epstein, M., Harrell, J., 2020. Ehlers-Danlos syndrome: an analysis of the current treatment options. Pain Phys 23 (4), 429–438.

Spencer, H., 1976. Shoulder technique. J. Am. Osteopath. Assoc. 15, 2118–2220.

Stanek, J.M., Parish, J., Rainville, R., Williams, J.G., 2020. Test–retest and intrarater reliability of assessing tibial rotation range of motion by two devices. Int. J. Athl. Ther. Train. 25 (5), 263–269. https://doi.org/10.1123/ijatt.2019-0080.

Steiner, C., 1994. Osteopathic manipulative treatment – what does it really do? J. Am. Osteopath. Assoc. 94 (1), 85–87.

Stiles, E., 1984a. Manipulation – a tool for your practice? Patient Care 18, 16–42.

Stiles, E., 1984b. Manipulation – a tool for your practice? Patient Care 45, 699–704.

Stoddard, A., 1962. Manual of Osteopathic Technique. Hutchinson, London.

Sturion, L.A., Nowotny, A.H., Barillec, F., Barette, G., Santos, G.K., Teixeira, F.A., et al., 2020. Comparison between high-velocity low-amplitude manipulation and muscle energy technique on pain and trunk neuromuscular postural control in male workers with chronic low back pain: a randomised crossover trial. S. Afr. J. Physiother. 76 (1), 1420. doi:10.4102/sajp.v76i1.1420.

Tewari, S., Madabushi, R., Agarwal, A., Gautam, S.K., Khuba, S., 2017. Chronic pain in a patient with Ehlers-Danlos syndrome (hypermobility type): the role of myofascial trigger point injections. J. Bodyw. Mov. Ther. 21 (1), 194–196. doi:10.1016/j.jbmt.2016.06.017.

Thomas, E., Cavallaro, A.R., Mani, D., Bianco, A., Palma, A., 2019. The efficacy of muscle energy techniques in symptomatic and asymptomatic subjects: a systematic review. Chiropr. Man. Therap. 27, 35. doi:10.1186/s12998-019-0258-7.

Timanin, E.M., Potekhina, Y.P., Mokhov, D.E., 2020. Studies of the viscoelastic characteristics of the muscles of the neck and upper thorax by the method of vibrational viscoelastometry. Biomed. Eng. 53, 332–336. doi:10.1007/s10527-020-09937-x.

Tinkle, B.T., 2020. Symptomatic joint hypermobility. Best Pract. Res. Clin. Rheumatol. 34 (3), 101508. doi:10.1016/j.berh.2020.101508.

Tinkle, B., Castori, M., Berglund, B., Cohen, H., Grahame, R., Kazkaz, H., 2017. Hypermobile Ehlers-Danlos syndrome (a.k.a. Ehlers-Danlos syndrome Type III and Ehlers-Danlos syndrome hypermobility type): clinical description and natural history. Am. J. Med. Genet. C Semin. Med. Genet. 175 (1), 48–69. doi:10.1002/ajmg.c.31538.

Uong, D., 2013. An experimental study comparing muscle energy technique versus high velocity low amplitude thrust at the cervical vertebra C2 and their effect on cervical range of rotation. Thesis, European School of Osteopathy, 2013. https://www.osteopathicresearch.org/s/orw/item/820.

Van Meulenbroek, T., Huijnen, I., Stappers, N., Engelbert, R., Verbunt, J., 2021. Generalized joint hypermobility and perceived harmfulness in healthy adolescents; impact on muscle strength, motor performance and physical activity level. Physiother. Theory Pract. 37 (12), 1438–1447. doi:10.1080/09593985.2019.1709231.

van Trijffel, E., van de Pol, R.J., Oostendorp, R.A.B., 2010. Inter-rater reliability for measurement of passive physiological movements in lower extremity joints is generally low: a systematic review. J. Physiother. 56 (4), 223–235.

Vleeming, A., Pool-Goudzwaard, A., Stoeckart, R., van Wingerden, J.P., Snijders, C.J., 1995. The posterior layer of the thoracolumbar fascia. Its function in load transfer from spine to legs. Spine 20 (7), 753–758.

Vleeming, A., Pool-Goudzwaard, A., Hammudoghlu, D., Stoeckart, R., Snijders, C.J., Mens, J.M., 1996. The function of the long dorsal sacroiliac ligament: its implication for understanding low back pain. Spine 21 (5), 556–562.

Vleeming, A., Snijders, C., Stoeckart, R., Mens, J., 1997. The role of the sacroiliac joints in coupling between spine, pelvis, legs and arms. In: Vleeming, A., Mooney, V., Dorman, T. et al (Eds.), Movement, Stability and Low Back Pain. Churchill Livingstone, New York.

Vleeming, A., Albert, H.B., Ostgaard, H.C., 2008. European guidelines for the diagnosis and treatment of pelvic girdle, pain. Eur. Spine J 17, 794–819.

Walkowski, S., Baker, R., 2011. Pain procedures in clinical practice. In: Lennard, T., Vivian, D., Walkowski, S. et al (Eds.), Osteopathic Manipulative Medicine: A Functional Approach to Pain, 155–171.

Ward, R., 1997. Foundations of Osteopathic Medicine. Williams and Wilkins, Baltimore.

Wilson, E., Payton, O., Donegan-Shoaf, L., Dec, K., 2003. Muscle energy technique in patients with acute low back pain: a pilot clinical trial. J. Orthopaed. Sports Phys. Ther. 33 (9), 502–512.

Wright, V., Johns, R.J., 1960a. Physical factors concerned with the stiffness of normal and disease joints. Bull. Johns Hopkins Hosp. 106, 215–231.

Wright, V., Johns, R.J., 1960b. Observations on the measurement of joint stiffness. Arthritis Rheum 3, 328–340.

Wu, J.Z., Li, Z.-M., Cutlip, R.G., 2009. A simulating analysis of the effects of increased joint stiffness on muscle loading in a thumb. BioMed. Eng. OnLine 8, 41. doi:10.1186/1475-925X-8-41.

Wurff, P., Van der Hagmeijer, R.H.M., Meyne, W., 2000. Clinical tests of the sacroiliac joint. A systematic methodological review. Parts 1, 2, 3: reliability. Man. Ther. 5, 30–36 89–96.

Yates, S., 1991. Muscle energy techniques. In: DiGiovanna, E. (Ed.), Principles of Osteopathic Manipulative Techniques. Lippincott, Philadelphia.

8

Muscle Energy Techniques in Complex or Challenging Spinal Cases

Donald R. Murphy

INTRODUCTION

Muscle energy techniques (METs) are widely applicable to a variety of patients and clinical situations. Practitioners trained in the application of manual therapies (and their patients) appreciate the benefits of MET. As emphasised in Chapters 1 and 4, and noted throughout the rest of this book, it is important that METs are applied in the context of the entire clinical picture, considering the biological, psychological and social factors that can contribute in each patient. Therefore the ability to apply the biopsychosocial (BPS) model in identifying the disparate clinical factors that may contribute in each patient, and to apply the most relevant method's that are more likely to positively impact each factor, is critical to practitioners of all types. General considerations and resources regarding application of the BPS model are provided in Chapters 1 and 4 of this book, while the volumes *Clinical Reasoning in Spine Pain Vol I and II* (Murphy, 2013, 2016) provide specifics regarding utilising Clinical Reasoning in Spine Pain (CRISP) in the application of the BPS model and an evidence-based approach in the diagnosis and management of patients with spine-related disorders. This approach to clinical reasoning is summarised in Box 8.1.

It is important for practitioners of manual therapy to have at their disposal a well-stocked toolbox of methods,

each of which can be applied in the situation for which it is most applicable. One manual method for which the literature and clinical experience have demonstrated effectiveness is high-velocity, low amplitude (HVLA) manipulation, applied to spinal joints in the treatment of spine-related disorders (Lawrence et al., 2008; Bronfort et al., 2010; Rubinstein et al., 2019). There are many patients for whom this type of joint manipulation is quite helpful as part of an overall management strategy designed to decrease pain and improve functional abilities.

As has been discussed throughout this book and particularly in Chapter 7, METs are also useful for joint manipulation, among other things (Thomas et al., 2019; Lerner-Lentz, 2021). They are particularly applicable in situations in which the practitioner might typically use HVLA but, for any of a variety of reasons to be discussed in this chapter, chooses not to. Evidence suggests that low-velocity techniques in general (Hurwitz et al., 2002; Gross et al., 2015) and MET in particular have equivalent effectiveness with HVLA. Clinical experience would suggest that there are individual patients or individual circumstances in which one method may be more effective than another, while growing evidence appears to support multimodal, personalised treatment approaches (Hidalgo et al., 2017; Coulter et al.,

2018; Plank et al., 2021). It is for this reason that it is important for any practitioner managing patients with spine-related disorders or other musculoskeletal problems to master a variety of manual treatments.

There are several patient characteristics in which the MET is particularly useful. These fall into the general categories of patient preference, acute radiculopathy, neurologic deficit, post-surgical patients, osteopenia or osteoporosis and nociplasticity (a definition and further discussion is provided later in this chapter on page 268).

PATIENT PREFERENCE

Perhaps the most common reason for choosing MET over HVLA for joint manipulation (or, conversely, HVLA over MET) is patient preference. There is a growing body of evidence that indicates that patient preference plays a strong role in the outcome of healthcare procedures in general (George & Robinson, 2010; DeLevry & Le, 2019). Evidence and practitioner feedback suggest this holds true for musculoskeletal conditions involving the spine as well (Plank et al., 2021). However, some studies have suggested that the question of patient preference may impact the therapeutic alliance on both sides more than the actual outcomes (Donaldson et al., 2013). The effect of patient preference on the outcome of spinal manipulation is particularly potent, given the intimate nature of this hands-on procedure and the important role that practitioner–patient interaction plays in the outcome of care that includes this treatment.

In this author's practice, the vast majority of patients are referred by medical doctors of various types as well as other healthcare practitioners. So, the bulk of this patient population does not seek consultation for the purpose of receiving spinal manipulation *per se*, but rather for relief of pain and restoration of function. However, these patients are all aware that they are being referred to a doctor of chiropractic who is a primary spine practitioner (Murphy et al., 2022). Because of the strong association that most lay people have between chiropractors and HVLA manipulation, many assume they are going to 'get cracked'. In addition, despite the well-established safety record of HVLA manipulation (Hurwitz et al., 2004; Oliphant, 2004; Rubinstein et al., 2007; Rubinstein, 2008; Stuber et al., 2012), many express great fear of this type of technique. Given the presence of fear among some patients, there is an increased likelihood that if HVLA is used in such patients (assuming manipulation in their particular case is indicated at all) their fear may negatively impact the outcome of care. It is with these patients that skills in the application of MET are most valuable. These patients usually express great relief when they discover that first, not everyone with a spine-related disorder requires joint manipulation and, second, in those for whom this treatment is indicated there is a wide variety of methods available to choose from, and it is likely that MET will be both helpful and well-tolerated in their case.

This is indirectly supported by a study by Hurwitz et al. (2004) in which they randomised patients with neck pain to receive HVLA manipulation or a low-velocity mobilisation technique (though this was not MET). They monitored the rate of transient adverse reactions to treatment in each group (transient increased pain is well documented to occur in 30% to 60% of patients treated with manipulation). It is usually mild or moderate and resolves in 24 to 48 hours (Senstad et al., 1996, 1997; Rubinstein, 2008; Gouveia et al., 2009; Goertz et al., 2016). The Hurwitz study found a lower incidence of adverse reaction in patients treated with low-velocity mobilisation compared to HVLA. Furthermore, patients with adverse reactions were generally less satisfied with care and less likely to have a positive outcome (Hurwitz et al., 2004). These researchers did not assess patient preference in this study, nor, indeed, was patient preference considered in a 2017 literature review synthesising the evidence regarding risks and benefits of this technique (Manitoba Health Professions Advisory Council, 2017) or more recent systematic reviews (Giacalone et al., 2020). However, it must be noted that in some regions HVLA therapy, or the osteopathic equivalent, osteopathic manipulation technique (OMT), constitutes a procedure; it is vital to acquire explicit patient informed consent before its application. There are legal implications for not doing so in some jurisdictions (Delany, 2002).

In contrast, in my experience some patients, particularly those with a previous history of a positive experience with HVLA, have a strong preference for HVLA rather than MET. The articular release that usually accompanies HVLA can be a powerful experience and these patients often express that they feel like 'nothing happened' if they do not experience this release (Demoulin et al., 2017). Having skill in providing HVLA manipulation is a great asset in these cases, provided that the practitioner is thoroughly trained and qualified to perform full clinical assessment and screening.

Box 8.2 provides a description of this author's clinical application of MET in this context.

Patients With Acute Radiculopathy

In this author's experience, most patients with cervical radiculopathy have painful joint dysfunction at the level and on the side of radiculopathy (Murphy, 2006; Murphy et al., 2006b), and a recent review of the literature suggests this to be a common presentation (Iyer & Kim, 2016). Thus, they have indications for manipulation at the involved level. There are those who have claimed that the presence of radiculopathy and/or herniated disc is a contraindication to manipulation (Saal et al., 1996; Rogers et al., 1998; Wolff & Levine, 2002; Haas et al., 2003). However, there is also evidence that patients with cervical or lumbar radiculopathy can be treated with an approach that includes manipulation without adverse reaction beyond occasional short-term increase in pain (Cassidy et al., 1993; BenEliyahu, 1994; BenEliyahu, 1996; Murphy et al., 2006a; Santilli et al., 2006; Zhu et al., 2015). Nonetheless, radiculopathy, particularly

---

BOX 8.2   The Application of MET in the Treatment of Painful Joint Dysfunction

My approach to using MET for the treatment of painful joint dysfunction is to set up the manoeuvre in a similar fashion as when I use high-velocity, low-amplitude (HVLA) manipulation, with the primary difference being the application of MET principles rather than a HVLA thrust.

So first the patient is positioned in a way that allows me to apply the therapeutic manoeuvre. A contact is taken that is identical to that taken when an HVLA manoeuvre is to be applied. The joint is moved in the desired direction (see below) until the 'barrier' is engaged, i.e. that point at which I initially perceive resistance to joint movement. At that point, the patient is asked to gently isometrically contract in the opposite direction as the one in which I am moving the joint. In the cervical spine, this can be done by simply having the patient look in the opposite direction of the one in which I am attempting to move the joint (in the case of rotation, flexion or extension) or to look straight up toward the forehead (in the case of lateral flexion). In the lumbar or thoracic spine, it can be done by having the patient gently attempt to move in the opposite direction of the one in which I am attempting to move the joint. This contraction should be minimal; just enough for me to sense the contraction. The patient is asked to hold this and to inhale, which generally creates increased muscle

activity. The patient is then asked to look into the direction of manipulation or to stop the isometric contraction and exhale, which causes relaxation of the muscles that would resist the movement I am attempting to create. At this point I continue to feel the barrier and wait for it to release. When it does, I slowly move with the joint until I engage another barrier, at which time the isometric contraction/relaxation and inhalation/exhalation process is repeated. Typically, three sequences are used, each time moving with the joint to a new barrier.

I have not seen any evidence that the direction in which the joint is moved is critical in terms of the outcome of joint manipulation. The exception is that a direction of movement that causes peripheralisation of symptoms (movement of symptoms into the extremity) during examination or while setting up the manipulative procedure up should be avoided. Thus, in choosing the desired direction of manipulation I focus on finding a position that is reasonably comfortable for the patient and does not cause peripheralisation of symptoms. It is important to note that there are times in which a certain amount of discomfort with manipulation is unavoidable or even necessary. However, this should be kept to a minimum if at all possible.

MET, Muscle energy techniques.

in the acute stage, can be volatile, with the pain easily provoked in response to any movement, including therapeutic manipulation for the purpose of addressing involved joint dysfunction. Therefore, in many cases of radiculopathy, MET is useful, as it is less likely to cause flare-up of pain in many cases compared to HVLA. In these cases, MET allows the practitioner to monitor the movement and the patient's symptoms more closely while he or she is applying the therapeutic manoeuvre.

One general principle that is useful when treating patients with radiculopathy (or any patient, for that matter) is that it is best not to move the patient in a direction that peripheralises the pain or neurologic symptoms. That is, the best direction to apply a mobilising manoeuvre is in a direction that is least likely to cause the patient's pain, paraesthesia or numbness to move distally in the extremity. Using MET in cases of radiculopathy allows the practitioner to carefully monitor the location, nature and severity of symptoms during the entire time in which the manoeuvre is being applied. This both provides the practitioner with immediate feedback from the patient and provides the patient with confidence that the symptoms are being carefully assessed during treatment. See Box 8.2 for more detail on this.

A study from this author's centre looked at the outcome of treatment of 35 consecutive patients with cervical radiculopathy (Murphy et al., 2006a). All were found to have painful joint dysfunction (Schneider et al., 2014) at the level and on the side of radiculopathy. Thus, all received manipulation. In 18 cases HVLA manipulation was used and in 13 MET was used. In the remainder both methods were used. The treatment was provided according to the CRISP principles (Murphy & Hurwitz, 2011) in which the multi-dimensional BPS nature of spine pain is considered. As such, treatment was multimodal and not limited only to manipulation. The outcome measures were: patient self-rating, Bournemouth Disability Index (BDI) and Numerical Pain Scale (NRS). Overall, the mean self-rated improvement was 75% at the end of treatment and 88% at long-term follow-up (mean 8 months). Mean percentage improvement in BDI score was 53% at the end of treatment and 78% at long-term follow-up and mean change in NRS was 4.3 at the end of treatment and 4.9 at long-term follow-up. No difference in outcome was found between patients whose treatment included HVLA and those whose treatment included MET. Of course, patients in this study were not randomised to receive either HVLA or

MET; the decision-making process discussed here was used in determining the technique to be used.

Patients With Neurologic Deficit

Particularly with patients who may have radiculopathy with neurologic deficit, or those who may have very mild symptoms or signs of cervical spondylotic myelopathy (Murphy et al., 2006a) it is important to move slowly and deliberately when applying manipulative procedures in the treatment of joint dysfunction. As in patients with painful radiculopathy, it is important for the practitioner to be able to carefully monitor any effect that the manual procedure has on symptoms so as to minimise the likelihood of exacerbating symptoms during or after the procedure. This applies to patients who may have sensory loss from radiculopathy or motor loss that greater than 3/5 (in patients with motor loss of 3/5 or worse, surgical consult should be strongly considered (Sharma et al., 2012; Overdevest et al., 2014; Petr et al., 2019)). It also applies to patients with mild, gradually developing signs or symptoms of cervical spondylotic myelopathy, such as hyper-reflexia with up-going toes, mild ataxia or early-onset difficulty with fine motor movements. Patients with more advanced myelopathy, such as those with moderate or severe spasticity or bowel/bladder involvement should be referred for surgical consultation.

In another study conducted at my centre we documented the clinical findings and outcomes of 27 patients with neck and/or arm pain and the finding of cervical spinal cord encroachment on MRI (Figs. 8.1 and 8.2). All had cervical joint dysfunction (Schneider et al., 2014); thus all were treated with some form of manipulation, 19 using HVLA, 9 using MET and 1 using both methods. Three of the patients had upper motor neuron signs. Of these, two had up-going toes and hyperreflexia in the extremities with normal jaw jerk; one of these two also had a sensory level to approximately C5. The third had equivocal toe response, hyperreflexia in the extremities and positive Hoffman's signs bilaterally with normal jaw jerk. None had bowel or bladder dysfunction. Also, none of the patients in this study had cord signal change on MRI. Clinically meaningful improvement (23.7-point improvement on the BDI, 3.9 points on the NRS) was found in pain and disability with no neurologic complications in any patient. Our conclusion was that the finding of spinal cord encroachment on MRI should not be considered an absolute contraindication

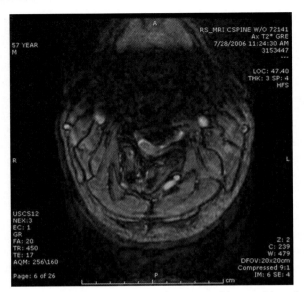

Fig. 8.1 Axial T2-weighed image of a 57-year-old man with neck pain who had cervical joint dysfunction. This was treated with muscle energy techniques without adverse reaction.

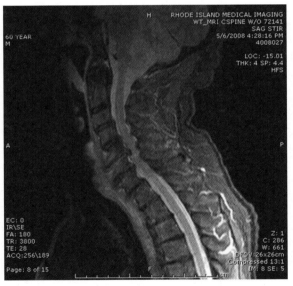

Fig. 8.2 Sagittal T2-weighted image of a 60-year-old man with neck and bilateral arm pain who had cervical joint dysfunction. This was treated with muscle energy techniques without adverse reaction.

for cervical manipulation. However, caution should always be used in all patients, and MET should be considered in cases in which neurologic deficit is found.

It must be noted that appropriate management of patients with neurologic deficit requires great manual skill as well as keen diagnostic acumen. Therefore it is essential that the practitioner only manage these patients if they have formal training, and sufficient experience and realistic confidence in their abilities in this regard.

Post-Surgical Patients

Manipulation is not typically a key element in the rehabilitation of patients immediately following spine surgery, but many patients who have had previous surgery have ongoing pain after surgery or develop new pain in the same area some time after having received it. In many of these patients, joint dysfunction is found to be at least one contributing factor, indicating the need for manipulation. In many cases, the pain involving an area of previous surgery can be volatile. Because of this, these patients are often best treated with a low-velocity approach such as MET. See Chapter 10 for more focused presentations of MET application in post-surgical rehabilitation.

Patients With Osteopenia or Osteoporosis

With the aging population, particularly in Western society, it can be expected that practitioners of all types will see a growing number of patients who have osteopenia or osteoporosis. The vertebrae in these patients may not be able to tolerate compression forces that normal vertebrae tolerate very well. The formula for force is well known: $F = ma$. So, the greater the acceleration involved in a manoeuvre the greater the force that is applied. In these patients, particularly those with significant osteoporosis, it is often advisable to use MET to keep the acceleration as low as necessary.

Patients With Nociplasticity

Nociplasticity is defined as 'pain that arises from altered nociception despite no clear evidence of actual or threatened tissue damage causing the activation of peripheral nociceptors or evidence for disease or lesion of the somatosensory system causing the pain' (Kosek et al., 2016; Kosek et al., 2021). It applies to changes that occur in the peripheral and/or central nervous system and result in a heightened or amplified experience of pain on the part of the patient. It is sometimes referred to as 'central sensitisation', although that is somewhat of a misnomer, as central sensitization is just one mechanism that can contribute to nociplasticity. For this reason, in

2021 the International Association for the Study of Pain updated the clinical criteria for central sensitisation and established fresh, more thorough and useful criteria for nociplastic pain (Nijs et al., 2021).

Nociplasticity is a common perpetuating factor in patients with chronic spinal pain (Murphy & Hurwitz, 2007; Murphy et al., 2008; Fitzcharles et al., 2021). It results from several peripheral and central nervous system changes such as hyperalgesic priming, central sensitisation (Latremoliere & Woolf, 2009), disruption of descending nociceptive modulation processes (Seaman & Winterstein, 1998) and alteration in brain structure and function that leads to a heightened pain experience (Wand et al., 2011). These neurophysiological processes are closely tied to the psychological factors that perpetuate spinal pain such as fear, catastrophising, passive coping, low self-efficacy and depressive symptoms (Seminowicz & Davis, 2006; Rhudy et al., 2009; Main et al., 2010). In these patients, peripheral stimuli that would normally be perceived as a mild discomfort, moderate pain or as not painful at all can be experienced as severely painful.

Gradual introduction of mobilising forces is necessary in many patients in whom nociplasticity is a prominent component of the clinical picture, and MET is ideal for this. First, MET allows for the treatment of joint dysfunction with lessened likelihood of flaring up pain. In addition, the best management strategy for nociplasticity is graded exposure, in which painful stimuli are introduced in a graded fashion, starting with the minimum stimulus necessary to mildly provoke pain and gradually increasing the stimulus as the patient's nociceptive system adapts and becomes desensitised (Bingel et al., 2007; Rennefeld et al., 2010; Nijs et al., 2015). MET is an excellent way to introduce graded exposure by using carefully controlled manual manoeuvres to provide stimuli that can easily be increased or decreased in intensity according to the level of habituation that is required.

CONCLUSION

It is essential for any practitioner who uses manual therapy to master a variety of methods of managing the various clinical entities that are amenable to such treatment, including joint dysfunction. HVLA manipulation is a well-established method of treating joint dysfunction that has abundant evidence of effectiveness in typical spine pain patients. However, to be well-rounded, practitioners will want to be able to handle complex or nuanced patients as well as the more typical ones. Many patients will have particular circumstances that will necessitate the use of a method other than HVLA manipulation. MET, which involves low-velocity manoeuvres and allows the practitioner to carefully monitor symptoms during the course of treatment, is an excellent tool for many complex patients.

REFERENCES

BenEliyahu, D.J., 1994. Chiropractic management and manipulative therapy for MRI documented cervical disk herniation. J. Manipulative Physiol. Ther. 17 (3), 177–185.

BenEliyahu, D.J., 1996. Magnetic resonance imaging and clinical follow-up: study of 27 patients receiving chiropractic care for cervical and lumbar disc herniations. J. Manipulative Physiol. Ther. 19 (9), 597–606.

Bingel, U., Schoell, E., Herken, W., Buchel, C., May, A., 2007. Habituation to painful stimulation involves the antinociceptive system. Pain 131 (1–2), 21–30.

Bronfort, G., Haas, M., Evans, R., Leininger, B., Triano, J., 2010. Effectiveness of manual therapies: the UK evidence report. Chiropr. Osteopat. 18, 3.

Cassidy, J.D., Thiel, H.W., Kirkaldy-Willis, W.H., 1993. Side posture manipulation for lumbar intervertebral disk herniation. J. Manipulative Physiol. Ther. 16 (2), 96–103.

Coulter, I.D., Crawford, C., Hurwitz, E.L., Vernon, H., Khorsan, R., Suttorp Booth, M., et al., 2018. Manipulation and mobilization for treating chronic low back pain: a systematic review and meta-analysis. Spine J. 18 (5), 866–879. doi:10.1016/j.spinee.2018.01.013.

Delany, C., 2002. Cervical manipulation—how might informed consent be obtained before treatment? J. Law Med. 10 (2), 174–186.

Delevry, D., Le, Q.A., 2019. Effect of treatment preference in randomized controlled trials: systematic review of the literature and meta-analysis. Patient 12 (6), 593–609. doi:10.1007/s40271-019-00379-6.

Demoulin, C., Baeri, D., Toussaint, G., Cagnie, B., Beernaert, A., Kaux, J.F., et al., 2017. Beliefs in the population about cracking sounds produced during spinal manipulation. Joint Bone Spine 85 (2), 239–242.

Donaldson, M., Learman, K., O'Halloran, B., Showalter, C., Cook, C., 2013. The role of patients' expectation of appropriate initial manual therapy treatment in outcomes for patients with low back pain. J. Manipulative Physiol. Ther. 36 (5), 276–283. doi:10.1016/j.jmpt.2013.05.016.

Fitzcharles, M.-A., Cohen, S.P., Clauw, D.J., Littlejohn, G., Usui, C., Häuser, W., 2021. Nociplastic pain: towards an understanding of prevalent pain conditions. Lancet 397 (10289), 2098–2110.

George, S.Z., Robinson, M.E., 2010. Preference, expectation, and satisfaction in a clinical trial of behavioral interventions for acute and sub-acute low back pain. J. Pain 11 (11), 1074–1082.

Giacalone, A., Febbi, M., Magnifica, F., Ruberti, E., 2020. The effect of high velocity low amplitude cervical manipulations on the musculoskeletal system: literature review. Cureus 12 (4), e7682. doi:10.7759/cureus.7682.

Goertz, C.M., Salsbury, S.A., Vining, R.D., Long, C.R., Pohlman, K.A., Weeks, W.B., et al., 2016. Effect of spinal manipulation of upper cervical vertebrae on blood pressure: results of a pilot sham-controlled trial. J. Manipulative Physiol. Ther. 39 (5), 369–380. doi:10.1016/j.jmpt.2016.04.002.

Gouveia, L.O., Castanho, P., Ferreira, J.J., 2009. Safety of chiropractic interventions: a systematic review. Spine 34 (11), E405–E413.

Gross, A., Langevin, P., Burnie, S.J., Bédard-Brochu, M.S., Empey, B., Dugas, E., et al., 2015. Manipulation and mobilisation for neck pain contrasted against an inactive control or another active treatment. Cochrane Database Syst. Rev. (9) Cd004249.

Haas, M., Groupp, E., Panzer, D., Partna, L., Lumsden, S., Aickin, M., 2003. Efficacy of cervical endplay assessment as an indicator for spinal manipulation. Spine 28 (11), 1091–1095.

Hidalgo, B., Hall, T., Bossert, J., Dugeny, A., Cagnie, B., Pitance, L., 2017. The efficacy of manual therapy and exercise for treating non-specific neck pain: a systematic review. J. Back Musculoskelet. Rehabil. 30 (6), 1149–1169. doi:10.3233/BMR-169615.

Hurwitz, E.L., Morgenstern, H., Harber, P., Kominski, G.F., Yu, F., Adams, A.H., 2002. A randomized trial of chiropractic manipulation and mobilization for patients with neck pain: clinical outcomes from the UCLA Neck-Pain Study. Am. J. Public Health 92 (10), 1634–1641.

Hurwitz, E.L., Morgenstern, H., Vassilaki, M., Chiang, L.M., 2004. Adverse reactions to chiropractic treatment and their effects on satisfaction and clinical outcomes among patients enrolled in the UCLA Neck Pain Study. J. Manipulative Physiol. Ther. 27 (1), 16–25.

Iyer, S., Kim, H.J., 2016. Cervical radiculopathy. Curr. Rev. Musculoskelet. Med. 9 (3), 272–280. doi:10.1007/s12178-016-9349-4.

Kosek, E., Clauw, D., Nijs, J., Baron, R., Gilron, I., Harris, R.E., et al., 2021. Chronic nociplastic pain affecting the musculoskeletal system: clinical criteria and grading system. Pain 162 (11), 2629–2634.

Kosek, E., Cohen, M., Baron, R., Gebhart, G.F., Mico, J.A., Rice, A.S.C., et al., 2016. Do we need a third

mechanistic descriptor for chronic pain states? Pain 157, 1382–1386.

Latremoliere, A., Woolf, C.J., 2009. Central sensitization: a generator of pain hypersensitivity by central neural plasticity. J. Pain 10 (9), 895–926.

Lawrence, D.J., Meeker, W., Branson, R., Bronfort, G., Cates, J.R., Haas, M., et al., 2008. Chiropractic management of low back pain and low back-related leg complaints: a literature synthesis. J. Manipulative Physiol. Ther. 31 (9), 659–674.

Lerner-Lentz, A., O'Halloran, B., Donaldson, M., Cleland, J.A., 2021. Pragmatic application of manipulation versus mobilization to the upper segments of the cervical spine plus exercise for treatment of cervicogenic headache: a randomized clinical trial. J. Man. Manip. Ther. 29 (5), 267–275.

Main, C.J., Foster, N., Buchbinder, R., 2010. How important are back pain beliefs and expectations for satisfactory recovery from back pain? Best Pract. Res. Clin. Rheumatol. 24 (2), 205–217.

Manitoba Health Professions Advisory Council., 2017. Cervical spine manipulation: a rapid literature review. https://www.gov.mb.ca/health/rhpa/docs/appendix_c.pdf

Murphy, D.R., 2006. Herniated disc with radiculopathy following cervical manipulation: nonsurgical management. Spine J, 6, 459–463.

Murphy, D.R., 2013. Clinical Reasoning in Spine Pain Volume I: Primary Management of Low Back Disorders.

Murphy, D.R., 2016. Clinical Reasoning in Spine Pain Volume II: Primary Management of Cervical Disorders and Case Studies in Primary Spine Care.

Murphy, D.R., Hurwitz, E.L., 2007. A theoretical model for the development of a diagnosis-based clinical decision rule for the management of patients with spinal pain. BMC Musculoskelet. Disord. 8, 75.

Murphy, D.R., Hurwitz, E.L., 2011. Application of a diagnosis-based clinical decision guide in patients with neck pain. Chiropr. Man. Therap. 19 (1), 19.

Murphy, D.R., Hurwitz, E.L., Gregory, A.A., 2006a. Manipulation in the presence of cervical spinal cord compression: a case series. J. Manipulative Physiol. Ther. 29 (3), 236–244.

Murphy, D.R., Hurwitz, E.L., Gregory, A.A., Clary, R., 2006b. A nonsurgical approach to the management of patients with cervical radiculopathy: a prospective observational cohort study. J. Manipulative Physiol. Ther. 29 (4), 279–287.

Murphy, D.R., Hurwitz, E.L., Nelson, C.F., 2008. A diagnosis-based clinical decision rule for patients with spinal pain part 2: review of the literature. Chiropr. Osteopat. 16, 8.

Murphy, D.R., Justice, B., Bise, C.G., Timko, M., Stevans, J.M., Schneider, M.J., 2022. The primary spine practitioner as a new role in healthcare systems in North America. Chiropr. Man. Therap. 30 (1), 6.

Nijs, J., Lahousse, A., Kapreli, E., Bilika, P., Saraçoğlu, I., Malfliet, A., et al., 2021. Nociplastic pain criteria or recognition of central sensitization? Pain phenotyping in the past, present and future. J. Clin. Med. 10, 3203. doi:10.3390/jcm10153203.

Nijs, J., Lluch Girbés, E., Lundberg, M., Malfliet, A., Sterling, M., 2015. Exercise therapy for chronic musculoskeletal pain: innovation by altering pain memories. Man. Ther. 20 (1), 216–220.

Oliphant, D., 2004. Safety of spinal manipulation in the treatment of lumbar disk herniations: a systematic review and risk assessment. J. Manipulative Physiol. Ther. 27, 197–210.

Overdevest, G.M., Vleggeert-Lankamp, C.L., Jacobs, W.C., Brand, R., Koes, B.W., Peul, W.C., et al., 2014. Recovery of motor deficit accompanying sciatica – subgroup analysis of a randomized controlled trial. Spine J 14 (9), 1817–1824.

Petr, O., Glodny, B., Brawanski, K., Kerschbaumer, J., Freyschlag, C., Pinggera, D., et al., 2019. Immediate versus delayed surgical treatment of lumbar disc herniation for acute motor deficits: the impact of surgical timing on functional outcome. Spine 44 (7), 454–463.

Plank, A., Rushton, A., Ping, Y., Mei, R., Falla, D., Heneghan, N.R., 2021. Exploring expectations and perceptions of different manual therapy techniques in chronic low back pain: a qualitative study. BMC Musculoskelet. Disord. 22 (1), 444. doi:10.1186/s12891-021-04251-3.

Rennefeld, C., Wiech, K., Schoell, E.D., Lorenz, J., Bingel, U., 2010. Habituation to pain: further support for a central component. Pain 148 (3), 503–508.

Rhudy, J.L., France, C.R., Bartley, E.J., Williams, A.E., McCabe, K.M., Russell, J.L., 2009. Does pain catastrophizing moderate the relationship between spinal nociceptive processes and pain sensitivity? J. Pain 10 (8), 860–869.

Rogers, C., Joshi, A., Dreyfuss, P., 1998. Cervical intrinsic disc pain and radiculopathy. In: Malanga GA, (Ed.), Cervical Flexion-Extension/Whiplash Injuries Spine: State of the Art Reviews, Philadelphia: Hanley and Belfus, vol. 12, chapter 2, pp. 323–356.

Rubinstein, S.M., 2008. Adverse events following chiropractic care for subjects with neck or low-back pain: do the benefits outweigh the risks? J. Manipulative Physiol. Ther. 31 (6), 461–464.

Rubinstein, S.M., de Zoete, A., van Middelkoop, M., Assendelft, W.J.J., de Boer, M.R., van Tulder, M.W., 2019. Benefits and harms of spinal manipulative therapy for the treatment of chronic low back pain: systematic review and meta-analysis of randomised controlled trials. BMJ 364, l689.

Rubinstein, S.M., Leboeuf-Yde, C., Knol, D.L., de Koekkoek, T.E., Pfeifle, C.E., van Tulder, M.W., 2007. The benefits outweigh the risks for patients undergoing chiropractic care for neck pain: a prospective, multicenter, cohort study. J. Manipulative Physiol. Ther. 30 (6), 408–418.

Saal, J.S., Saal, J.A., Yurth, E.F., 1996. Nonoperative management of herniated cervical intervertebral disc with radiculopathy. Spine 21 (16), 1877–1883.

Santilli, V., Beghi, E., Finucci, S., 2006. Chiropractic manipulation in the treatment of acute back pain and sciatica with disc protrusion: a randomized double-blind clinical trial of active and simulated spinal manipulations. Spine J. 6 (2), 131–137.

Schneider, G.M., Jull, G., Thomas, K., Smith, A., Emery, C., Faris, P., et al., 2014. Derivation of a clinical decision guide in the diagnosis of cervical facet joint pain. Arch. Phys. Med. Rehabil. 95 (9), 1695–1701.

Scott-Dawkins, C., 1997. The comparative effectiveness of adjustments versus mobilisation in chronic mechanical neck pain, Proceedings of the Scientific Symposium. World Chiropractic CongressWorld Federation of Chiropractic, Tokyo.

Seaman, D.R., Cleveland, 3rd, C., 1999. Spinal pain syndromes: nociceptive, neuropathic, and psychologic mechanisms. J Manipulative Physiol Ther 22 (7), 458–472.

Seaman, D.R., Winterstein, J.F., 1998. Dysafferentation: a novel term to describe the neuropathophysiological effects of joint complex dysfunction. A look at likely mechanisms of symptom generation. J. Manipulative Physiol. Ther. 21 (4), 267–280.

Seminowicz, D.A., Davis, K.D., 2006. Cortical responses to pain in healthy individuals depends on pain catastrophising. Pain 120 (3), 297–306.

Senstad, O., Leboeuf-Yde, C., Borchgrevink, C.F., 1996. Side-effects of chiropractic spinal manipulation: types frequency, discomfort and course. Scand. J. Prim. Health Care 14, 50–53.

Senstad, O., Leboeuf-Yde, C., Borchgrevink, C., 1997. Frequency and characteristics of side effects of spinal manipulative therapy. Spine 22 (4), 435–441.

Sharma, H., Lee, S.W., Cole, A.A., 2012. The management of weakness caused by lumbar and lumbosacral nerve root compression. J. Bone Joint Surg. Br. 94 (11), 1442–1447.

Stuber, K.J., Wynd, S., Weis, C.A., 2012. Adverse events from spinal manipulation in the pregnant and postpartum periods: a critical review of the literature. Chiropr. Man. Therap. 20, 8.

Thomas, E., Cavallaro, A.R., Mani, D., Bianco, A., Palma, A., 2019. The efficacy of muscle energy techniques in symptomatic and asymptomatic subjects: a systematic review. Chiropr. Man. Therap. 27, 35.

Wand, B.M., Parkitny, L., O'Connell, N.E., Luomajoki, H., McAuley, J.H., Thacker, M., et al., 2011. Cortical changes in chronic low back pain: current state of the art and implications for clinical practice. Man. Ther. 16 (1), 15–20.

Wolff, M.W., Levine, L.A., 2002. Cervical radiculopathies: conservative approaches to management. Phys. Med. Rehabil. Clin. N. Am. 13, 589–608.

Zhang, Y.Q., Tang, J.S., Yuan, B., Jia, H., 1997. Inhibitory effects of electrically evoked activation of ventrolateral orbital cortex on the tail-flick reflex are mediated by periaqueductal gray in rats. Pain 72 (1-2), 127–135.

Zhu, L., Wei, X., Wang, S., 2015. Does cervical spine manipulation reduce pain in people with degenerative cervical radiculopathy? A systematic review of the evidence, and a meta-analysis. Clin. Rehabil. 30 (2), 145–155.

9

Manual Resistance Techniques in Rehabilitation

Craig Liebenson, Curtis Thor Rigney

CHAPTER CONTENTS

The goal of rehabilitation as viewed in this chapter is to restore function in the locomotor system. Manual resistance techniques (MRTs) – of which muscle energy technique (MET) variations form a major part – are excellent bridges between passive and active care. When applying MRTs/METs, the practitioner controls the direction, magnitude, velocity and timing of each force generated by the patient. Indications for MRTs include the inhibition of overactive muscles, the facilitation of underactive muscles, and the mobilisation of joints with restricted motion. They are also an ideal method for introducing the practice of self-care. See Boxes 9.1 and 9.2 at the end of the chapter for summaries of common clinical applications of MET as well as questions relating to MET usage.

DESCRIPTION OF REHABILITATION

Rehabilitation as defined by the World Health Organization is 'a set of interventions designed to optimise functioning and reduce disability in individuals with health conditions in interaction with their environment' (World Health Organization (WHO), 2021). There are different approaches to achieve these rehabilitation goals. One is to focus on a tissue in a lesion or the pain generating structure (Geffen, 2003). Another is to view an individual's musculoskeletal condition from a body-wide perspective with an appreciation of kinematic chains under the control of the sensory-motor nervous system (Kobesova & Osborne, 2012). In this chapter, the body-wide approach to rehabilitation will be the focus with significant attention paid to the primary role of motor control. MRTs have an important role regardless of the healthcare practitioners' rehabilitation paradigm.

CLINICAL PROGRESSION OF CARE

Once diagnosis of the main site of tissue injury or pain generation has been made, treatment matched to the main goal of acute care – namely pain relief – can be initiated. As the patient's acute pain subsides, the recovery phase starts. During this phase the healthcare provider should attempt to identify the potential sources of biomechanical overload that may have led to tissue injury or pain in the first place. When these often-distant sources are identified, and linked to the pain generator, rehabilitation efforts can be used to improve function in the relevant dysfunctional kinetic chain pattern. MRTs are valuable interventions that assist in the restoration of locomotor function and can be used during both the acute and recovery phases. The gentle isometric contractions of Postisometric Relaxation (PIR) technique are an example method that is well suited for acute care. Facilitation methods, such as the diagonal patterns of proprioceptive neuromuscular facilitation (PNF), described later in this chapter, are more applicable in the recovery phase.

POSTISOMETRIC RELAXATION (PIR) TECHNIQUES

The use of isometric contractions is an excellent technique for treating the neuromuscular component of a stiff, shortened or tight muscle (Lewit, 1986; Liebenson, 1989, 1990; Liebenson & Murphy, 1998; Agrawal, 2016). If trigger points are present, PIR is particularly effective as a major part of their deactivation (for more on trigger points and MET methodology, see also Chapter 14) (Lewit & Simons, 1984; Sharma, 2010; Buchmann et al., 2014).

The physiological and theoretical influences of isometric contractions are fully discussed in Chapters 2, 4 and 5, and while such contractions may not fully explain the clinical benefits of MET, to the extent previously considered, it appears that they may be involved in enhanced stretch tolerance, which is now thought to offer a more likely explanation, as explained in Chapter 4 (Sterling et al., 2001; Wilson et al., 2003).

Method

1. The clinician's first priority is to identify the pathological barrier (Fig. 9.1). See Chapter 2, p. 19 and Box 2.2, p. 36, and Chapter 5, Box 5.1. This is noted the moment resistance starts when taking out the slack. The location of the barrier is confirmed by sensing a lack of normal resilience, or 'spring', at the end of range.
2. Tension is held at the barrier without letting go of the slack while waiting for a release of tissue tension (release phenomenon). There should be no stretch or bounce.
3. If, after a brief latency, no release phenomenon occurs, the patient can be requested to gently push away from the barrier against matched resistance

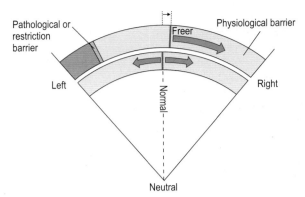

Fig. 9.1 The barrier phenomenon.

– using up to 10% of maximum effort – to create an isometric contraction.
4. Once the isometric contraction is achieved, the patient can be requested to take a deep breath in and to hold both the contraction and breath for 7 to 10 seconds.
5. The patient then releases first the effort, then the breath.
6. The clinician **waits** to feel a sense of 'release' of the tissue tension.
7. Only after feeling the release should slack be taken up and the tissues gently lengthened to the new barrier.
8. This process is repeated up to five times.
9. At the conclusion, a reciprocal inhibition contraction can be usefully introduced by having the patient contract the antagonist muscles attempting to move towards the barrier against resistance.

If, however, no release occurs using the above method, the following modifications may be attempted individually or in combination:

- Utilise respiratory synkinesis (e.g. breathe in and hold during the contraction phase then exhale during the release/relaxation phase).
- Have the patient increase time of the contraction phase for up to 30 seconds.
- Have the patient use more force (i.e. 'as little as possible or as much as necessary').
- Add visual synkinesis if appropriate (look in the direction of contraction and then the direction of release – see also Chapters 5, 6 and 7).
- It may be useful to vary the method of muscle isolation. For example, when lengthening the anterior fibres of upper trapezius, slack is taken out with the upper cervical spine in flexion, together with

contralateral lateral flexion of the neck ipsilateral rotation of the neck and shoulder depression. Altering the order in which the slack is taken out can isolate tension to that component of the muscle that needs attention.

- Other related tissues may need to be treated before use of MET (e.g. joint mobilisation or facilitation of antagonists with reciprocal inhibition).

According to Lewit (personal communication 1999), because muscle is contractile tissue, if a muscle has decreased in length, 90% of the time this is due to it being contracted. The treatment in these cases is therefore relaxation. He estimates that in approximately 10% of cases, it is due to connective tissue changes whose treatment is stretching. It is not, however, wise to stretch a muscle containing an active trigger point until it has been inhibited (see Box 9.2, Figs 9.23A, B and 9.24A, B).

PROPRIOCEPTIVE NEUROMUSCULAR FACILITATION (SEE ALSO CHAPTER 2)

Proprioceptive neuromuscular facilitation (PNF) was originally utilised for neuromuscular re-education in stroke patients (Kabot, 1950). Later it was discovered that it was clinically useful in rehabilitating children with cerebral palsy (CP) (Levine et al., 1954). This led to its use for a wide range of orthopaedic conditions.

PNF is associated with a philosophy of care that treats the whole body through the stimulation of proprioceptors (Adler et al., 2021). The use of basis movement patterns is a key area of focus as they are of neurodevelopmental origin and are incorporated in functional activities such as swimming, running, climbing, throwing, etc. Therefore, in contrast to most isotonic training approaches that are uniplanar, PNF activation methods resist movement in multiple planes simultaneously. For instance, a diagonal pattern of movement will be resisted at the same time as a flexion/extension and abduction/adduction of an extremity (see Chapter 7, Fig. 7.6A and B).

The shoulder girdle is a good example of the clinical utility of PNF principles in rehabilitation of physical performance capacity. Once pain and inflammation begin to subside, PNF patterns can be utilised to restore function in the shoulder (Figs 9.2 and 9.3). Such exercises can be combined with muscle balancing approaches, joint mobilisation/manipulation and closed chain stabilisation procedures.

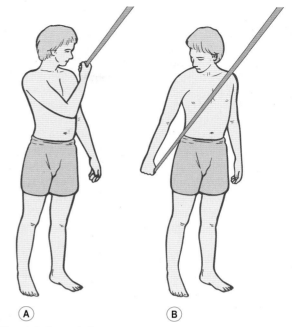

Fig. 9.2 (A and B) Upper extremity extension technique ('seatbelt').

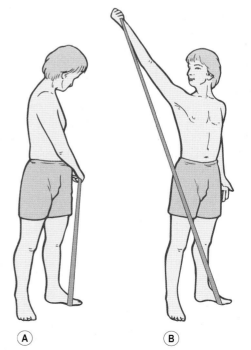

Fig. 9.3 (A and B) Upper extremity flexion technique ('drawing a sword').

THE ENVIRONMENTAL BASIS FOR MUSCLE IMBALANCE

Janda et al.'s (2006) model of muscle imbalance drives much of our clinical decision-making. Certain muscles active during static postures tend to become overactive or even shorten due to prolonged use of constrained postures (Lewit, 1999a). Other muscles active during dynamic activities tend to become inhibited or even weak from disuse. Static postural muscle overactivity is a natural result of modern society's emphasis on constrained postures. Dynamic muscle underactivity is predictable because modern lifestyles are predominantly sedentary. Sedentarism has been reported to be present in approximately 80% of the adult population (Bernstein et al., 1999). In simple terms, sedentarism can be attributed to persons if they do not engage in activities like walking, jogging, dancing or calisthenics at least five times per week (Ricciardi, 2005).

- The static muscle system typically involves superficial muscles such as upper trapezius, sternocleidomastoid, erector spinae and the hamstrings.
- In contrast, the dynamic muscle system utilises more of the deep stabilisers such as transversus abdominus, multifidus and the deep neck flexors.

The development of these predictable muscle imbalances is further spurred by the diminished afferent flow of sensory information from the periphery, in particular the soles of the feet, due to footwear, walking on flat surfaces and a lack of variety in foot movements. It is believed that prolonged reduction of proprioceptive stimulation results in an increase in fatigue-ability and an alteration of normal movement patterns. The motor control system becomes less able to adapt to various biomechanical sources of repetitive strain (Page, 2006).

The goal of neurodevelopment of the locomotor system is to achieve the upright posture and gait (Janda et al., 2006). Since 85% of gait involves single leg stance, posture should be defined in single rather than double leg stance (Janda, 1983; Janda et al., 2006). Brügger and Janda have shown how deleterious sedentarism is (Lewit, 1999a). For example, Brügger describes typical sedentary posture via a linkage system. He has shown how approximation of the sternum to the symphysis pubis increases both end-range loading, and muscular tension (Lewit, 1999a; Liebenson, 1999). It is possible, however, to demonstrate that postural correction can immediately improve joint function and muscle tone.

Experiment in Postural Correction (Figs 9.4 and 9.5)

- Check upper trapezius tension/trigger points in slump position (see also Fig. 9.23A).
- Perform the Brügger relief position, and then recheck (see Fig. 9.5 and description below).
- Check cervical rotation in the slump position; perform the Brügger relief position and recheck.
- Check arm abduction in slump; perform the Brügger relief position and recheck.

Brügger's relief position facilitates dynamic phasic muscles (muscles which tend toward inhibition – see Chapter 2 discussion on phasic and tonic/postural muscles) – and reciprocally inhibits postural muscles (muscles which tend toward shortening). His demonstrable advice is very effective in improving patient compliance with home exercises. It is also an excellent way to increase awareness of the value of postural correction (Lewit, 1999a).

Brügger's Relief Position

To perform Brügger's postural relief exercise:
1. The individual is asked to sit perched in an upright position at the edge of a chair (see Fig. 9.5). The hips are abducted with the feet shoulder width apart.
2. The elbows are extended, forearms supinated and finger abducted while the cervical spine is lengthened (carefully avoiding chin-poking).
3. When in this position actively held, forceful exhalation is performed using the abdominal musculature.

Developmental Influences

The similarities between muscles with the tendency toward *hypertonicity,* as Janda suggests, to many of those muscles which are held short while in the foetal position are noteworthy. These include in the upper quarter:
- The finger, hand and wrist flexors
- The shoulder internal rotators and adductors
- The shoulder girdle elevators (Kolár, 1999).
  In the lower quarter, they include:
- The ankle plantar flexors and invertors
- The hip flexors, internal rotators and adductors.

As the infant's motor control system develops, the antagonists of these hypertonic prone muscles become facilitated. Which, in turn, leads to their reflexive inhibition.

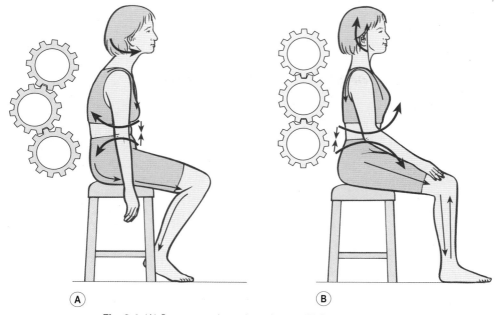

Fig. 9.4 (A) Sternosymphyseal syndrome. (B) Brügger relief position.

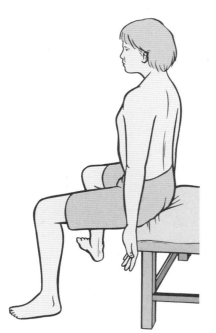

Fig. 9.5 Brügger relief position.

In contrast, those muscles *inhibited* (weakened) in the upper extremity of the infant include:

- Finger, wrist, elbow and shoulder extensors
- Forearm supinators
- Shoulder external rotators and abductors.
  Those in the lower extremity include:
- Toe extensors
- Ankle dorsiflexors and pronators
- Hip abductors and external rotators.

The parallel between the postural muscles that tend to overactivity in adults as a result of sedentarism, and the muscles that are used to maintain the foetal position, appears obvious.

Similarly, Janda's phasic (also known as dynamic) muscles are almost identical to the muscles whose activation during neurodevelopment brings about an upright posture. That there is a central neurological programme for these different types of muscles is further reinforced by noting which muscles become spastic in children with CP, and which muscles are paralysed in people who have suffered a stroke. It becomes clear that balance between agonist and antagonist muscles is essential for a proper functional motor control system (Cholewicki & McGill, 1996; Kolár, 1999; Oliveira et al., 2015).

Certain landmark stages exist in the transition from a tonic, reflex motor system (spinal and brain stem control) to a balanced postural control system, capable of volitional control locomotion (cortical control) (Kobesova &

Kolár, 2014). Each stage of the neurodevelopment of posture depends upon a set of specific conditions being met. Specific points of body support, centration of key joints and agonist-antagonist muscular coactivation are all necessary for development of each landmark of neurodevelopment of the postural control system (Kolár, 1999).

Agonist-antagonist coactivation patterns evolve as neurodevelopment progresses to take the infant from a foetal position at birth, to a stable upright posture at approximately 3 years of age. In the first month after birth, the infant's muscles move its entire body in primitive general movements lacking specific purpose. At the end of the first month, in response to emotional motivations, the child begins to orient its head. This is not a reflex movement, but under higher motor control (Kobesova & Kolár, 2014).

As posture develops, the reflexively based tonic contractions begin to relax, thus reducing reciprocal inhibition and facilitating the coactivation patterns necessary for joint centration and load bearing. For instance, at the end of the first month, coactivation of antagonists at the cervicocranial junction centrates C0–C1:

- Deep neck flexors are facilitated.
- Short cervical extensors are no longer tonically active.

If the tonic contraction of the upper cervical extensors does not relax, then joint centration of C0–C1 is not possible, and the infant will be less able to control its head movements for successful orientation.

Coactivation of antagonists occurs proximally at the shoulder and hip by the third month as a prerequisite for weightbearing on all fours (i.e. creeping and crawling):

- Activation of lower scapular fixators, shoulder external rotators, trunk extensors, hip abductors external rotators
- Reduction in tonic activity of scapular elevators, shoulder internal rotators, trunk hip adductors and internal rotators.

Failure of coactivation due to persistent tonic activity results in faulty neurodevelopment of the motor system. This allows a persistence of trunk flexion, eventually promoting both the lower crossed and upper crossed syndromes (Figs 9.6 and 9.7). To address this muscle imbalance, Kolár utilises treatments that include the stimulation of reflex trigger zones at key areas of postural support in the infant, such as the symphysis pubis, sternum or occiput to facilitate coactivation patterns (Kolár, 1999).

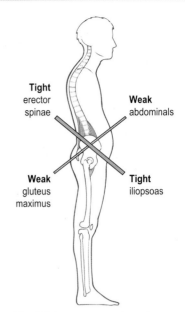

Fig. 9.6 Lower crossed syndrome.

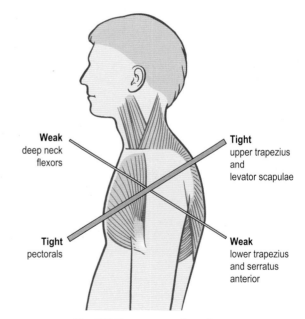

Fig. 9.7 Upper crossed syndrome.

The Key Role of Coactivation of Antagonists in Producing and Maintaining Upright Posture

Equilibrium is a result of co-contraction of antagonists. This co-activation typically develops in the second through to the fourth months of life. This second stage of motor control occurs at the subcortical level. At 4 to 6 weeks, emotional motivation (such as orientation to the mother) initiates the desire to purposefully turn the head. Trunk stability is required before any purposeful movement of the head, neck or extremities can be performed. This is the birth of posture and motor control. Postural reactions are supraspinal. The coactivation of antagonists creates maximum congruence of joints, thus promoting equilibrium and joint loading (Kobesova & Kolár, 2014).

During development of upright posture, the upper extremity tonic activity (flexion, internal rotation, adduction and pronation) is joined with phasic activity (extension, external rotation, abduction and supination). In the lower extremity, tonic activity (ankle plantar flexion and inversion, hip flexion, internal rotation and adduction) is joined with phasic activity (ankle dorsiflexion and eversion, hip external rotation and abduction).

Development from one stage to another requires that balanced muscle contraction of antagonists replaces dominance of tonic muscular activity. This coactivation centrates or aligns joints to maximum congruence. Such coactivation is not reflex (brain stem), but supraspinal, and is the beginning point of postural-motor activity in the human (Kolár, 1999).

Sedentarism reduces afferent input – particularly from the sole of the foot – and promotes tension in postural (anti-gravity) muscles while leading to inhibition in dynamic phasic muscles. Janda's muscle imbalances are a predictable result of this with their typical associated faulty movement patterns and repetitive microtrauma to joints. Brügger has developed a systematic approach to improving posture complementing that evolved by Janda (Lewit, 1999a).

Functional Screening Tests

Certain screening tests have been developed by Janda for identifying agonist–antagonist–synergist relationships during stereotypical movement patterns (Liebenson & Chapman, 1998; Liebenson et al., 1998; Lewit, 1999a; Frank et al., 2020). These kinesiological relationships – simply described as muscle imbalances – alter joint stress by changing movement patterns, or the axis of rotation, during movement. The screening tests

illustrated in Figs 9.8 to 9.14 include hip extension, hip abduction, trunk flexion, scapular fixation during arm abduction, upper cervical flexion, trunk lowering from a push-up, and respiration.

When faulty movement patterns are present, they are key perpetuating factors of myofascial or joint pain (Watson & Trott, 1993; Treleaven et al., 1994; Babyar, 1996; Barton & Hayes, 1996; Edgerton et al., 1996). A modern term for the relationship of such movement patterns to symptoms is *regional interdependence* (Wainner et al., 2007).

The knee is an excellent example of this. Athletes with decreased neuromuscular control of the body's core, measured during sudden force release tasks and trunk repositioning, are at increased risk of knee injury. Impaired trunk proprioception and deficits in trunk control have been shown to be predictors of knee injury (Zazulak et al., 2007a, 2007b).

When it comes to an example of the shoulder, the function of the glenohumeral joint is clearly dependent on the stability offered by the shoulder girdle (Assila, 2021). This is further demonstrated by increased hand strength resulting from improved shoulder girdle stability (Kobesova et al., 2015).

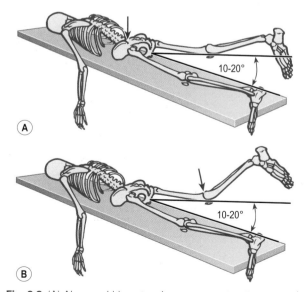

Fig. 9.8 (A) Abnormal hip extension movement pattern associated with shortened psoas. Leg raising is initiated with an anterior pelvic tilt. (B) Abnormal hip extension movement pattern associated with excessive substitution of the hamstrings. Leg raising is initiated with knee flexion.

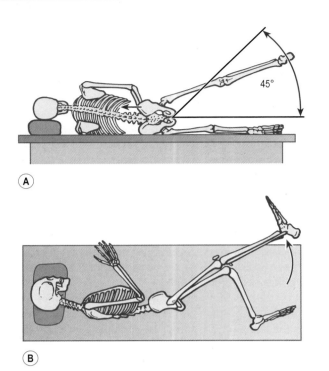

Fig. 9.9 (A) Abnormal hip abduction movement pattern associated with excessive substitution of the quadratus lumborum. Leg raising is initiated with a cephalad shift of the pelvis. (B) Abnormal hip abduction movement pattern associated with excessive substitution of the tensor fascia lata. Leg raising is initiated with flexion of the hip joint.

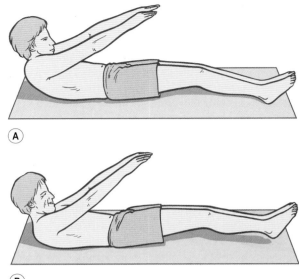

Fig. 9.10 (A) Normal trunk flexion movement pattern. (B) Abnormal trunk flexion movement pattern associated with excessive substitution of the psoas. Heels rise up off the table before the shoulder blades are lifted.

The lumbar spine is another good example where it has been shown that hip dysfunction (in particular stiffness) is correlated with disabling low-back pain (McGill et al., 2003).

It has also been shown that decreased mobility of the thoracic spine is correlated with neck pain (Norlander & Nordgren (1998); Cleland et al., 2005, 2007; Masaracchio et al., 2019), and shoulder impingement syndrome (Bang & Deyle, 2000; Bergman et al., 2004; Boyles et al., 2009; Land et al., 2019).

Unless movement patterns are improved during performance of activities of daily life so that joint stability is maintained, soft tissue or mobilisation/manipulation treatments will fail to achieve lasting results. Additionally, exercises performed without proper form will reinforce muscle imbalances due to the use of 'trick' movement patterns that substitute

synergists for inhibited agonists (Parnianpour et al., 1988; Grabiner et al., 1992; Arendt-Nielson et al., 1995; Edgerton et al., 1996; Hodges & Richardson, 1996; O'Sullivan et al., 1997; Sparto et al., 1997; Hodges & Richardson, 1998, 1999).

Experiment in Facilitation of an Inhibited Muscle Chain

Eccentric facilitation of a chain of inhibited muscles brings about reciprocal inhibition of the tonic muscle chain. The tonic muscle chain is typically over-activated in individuals with sterno-symphyseal syndrome (Lewit, 1999a, 1999b).

The typical muscle imbalance involves over-activity in the muscles described by Kolár as tonic together with inhibition of those responsible for co-activation during development from a kyphotic to upright posture (Kolár, 1999). Such hypertonic muscle chains often involve trigger or tender points in both inhibited and overactive muscle groups (Lewit, 1999b). These hypertonic muscle chains are the rule rather than the exception in chronic pain states because of the body's attempt to immobilise the region (Lewit, 1999b).

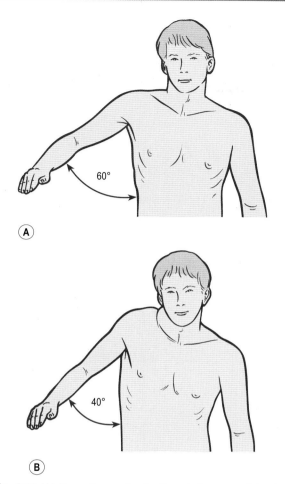

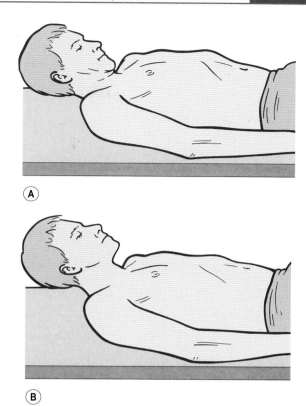

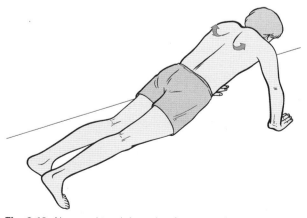

Fig. 9.11 (A) Normal scapular fixation during arm abduction movement pattern. (B) Abnormal scapular fixation during arm abduction movement pattern associated with excessive substitution of the upper trapezius and levator scapulae. Scapulae or shoulder girdle elevates before the arm has abducted 45 degrees.

Fig. 9.12 (A) Normal upper cervical flexion movement pattern. (B) Abnormal upper cervical flexion movement pattern associated with excessive substitution of the sternocleidomastoid and/or shortening of the suboccipitals. Head is raised towards the chest with chin poking (i.e. upper cervical extension) occurring.

Investigation

To identify a hypertonic muscle chain in the upper extremity it is useful to identify one-sided predominance of the following dysfunctions:

- Restricted wrist extension mobility
- Trigger points in upper trapezius, pectoralis major
- Tender attachment points in upper ribs 1 to 3, and the lateral or medial epicondyle.

In the lower extremity one-sided predominance may be evident in relation to the following dysfunctions:

- Restricted hamstring length

Fig. 9.13 Abnormal trunk lowering from a push-up movement pattern associated with inhibition/weakness of the serratus anterior. Winging of the right scapula.

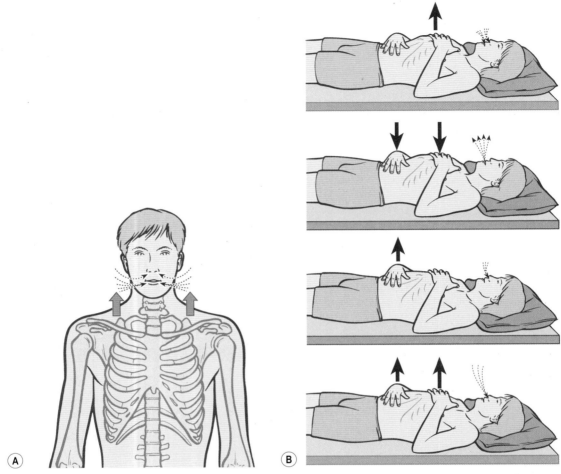

Fig. 9.14 (A) Abnormal respiration associated with elevation of the clavicle(s) during relaxed inhalation. (B) The most severe dysfunction occurs when the belly moves inwards during inhalation ('paradoxical breathing').

- Trigger points in adductor longus and magnus, pectineus, gluteus medius, gluteus maximus and/or the longitudinal arch of the foot.

Brügger's Facilitation Method for Inhibited Muscle Chains in the Extremities

Indications:
- Any time it is appropriate to release tension in multiple muscles simultaneously
- When a one-sided chain is present, especially in chronic pain patients.

Once a predominantly one-sided chain has been identified in either the upper or the lower extremity, treatment involves a strong contraction (40% to 80% of maximum effort) of the inhibited muscle chain in a sequence of movements that bring about reciprocal inhibition of the chain of hypertonic muscles. An eccentric MET is used to maximise reciprocal inhibition of the hypertonic muscle chain. More force is utilised in these eccentric contractions than in the typical PIR methods. Each of the following movements is resisted individually, one after the other. Approximately three repetitions of each movement are performed.

Note: The description above involving strong (up to 80% available strength) isometric contractions, indicates that this protocol relates to PNF, more than to MET methodology.

- The patient contracts against the clinician's resistance while allowing motion in the opposite direction.
- The clinician then slowly stretches the muscle while the patient maintains resistance, thus achieving an eccentric contraction. (**Note:** Slow eccentric isotonic stretching (SEIS) is described, in an MET context, in Chapter 6 in relation to musculoskeletal dysfunction, and also Chapter 10, in post-surgical rehabilitation use.)

The purpose is to facilitate these muscles being stretched and reciprocally inhibit the antagonistic muscles.

In the upper quarter eccentrically resist:

- Finger and thumb abduction (Fig. 9.15A and B)
- Wrist and finger extension and thumb abduction (Fig. 9.16A and B)
- Forearm supination (Fig. 9.17A and B)
- Shoulder external rotation (Fig. 9.18A and B)

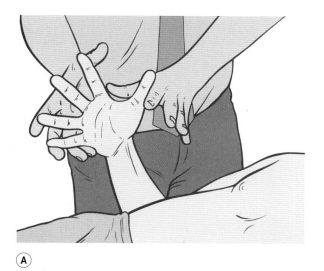
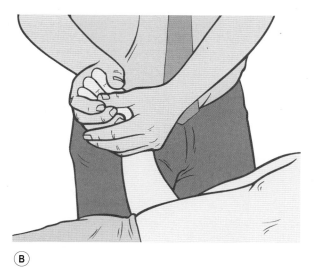

Fig. 9.15 (A and B) Eccentric resistance of finger and thumb abduction.

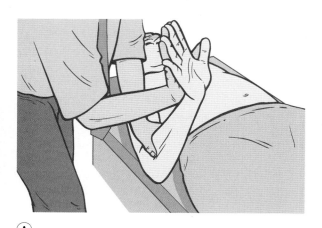
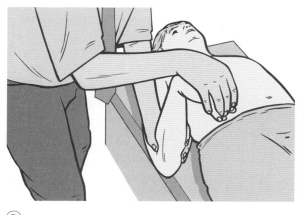

Fig. 9.16 (A and B) Eccentric resistance of wrist and finger extension and thumb abduction.

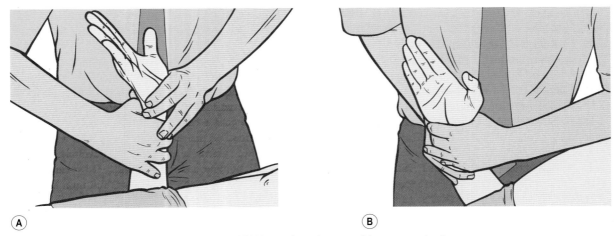

A   **B**

Fig. 9.17 (A and B) Eccentric resistance of forearm supination.

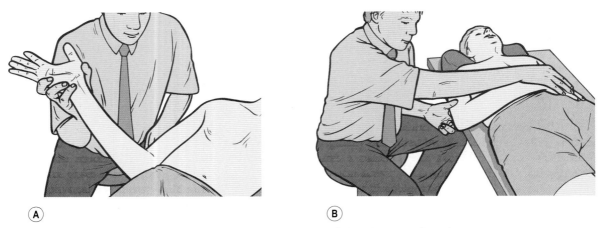

A   **B**

Fig. 9.18 (A and B) Eccentric resistance of shoulder external rotation.

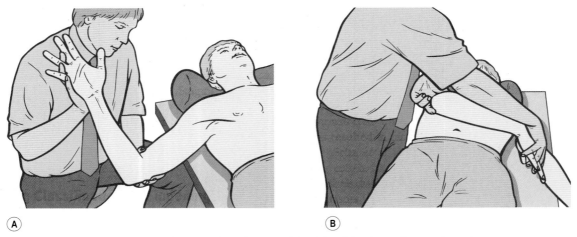

A   **B**

Fig. 9.19 (A and B) Eccentric resistance of shoulder abduction and external rotation.

- Shoulder abduction and external rotation (Fig. 9.19A and B).
  In the lower quarter eccentrically resist:
- Toe extension, ankle dorsiflexion and eversion (Fig. 9.20A and B)
- Hip abduction (Fig. 9.21A and B)
- Hip external rotation (Fig. 9.22A and B).

It is notable that the resistance to shoulder abduction and external rotation is almost identical to the final position of the PNF D2 upper extremity flexion – 'drawing a sword' position (see Fig. 9.3).

CONCLUSION

This chapter has presented a functional approach to rehabilitation of the motor system. The identification and treatment of nociceptive kinematic chains involving agonist/antagonist muscles containing trigger points enhance our ability to restore muscle balance and improve joint stability. It is within this context that MET methods may be usefully employed. That is to eliminate trigger points, reduce hypertension in muscles, lengthen short muscles and facilitate inhibited muscles.

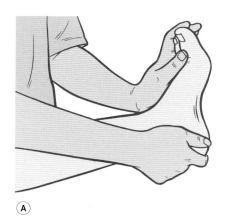
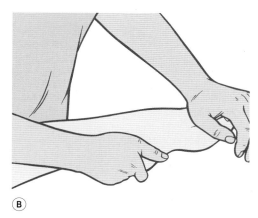

(A) (B)

Fig. 9.20 (A and B) Eccentric resistance of toe extension, ankle dorsiflexion and eversion.

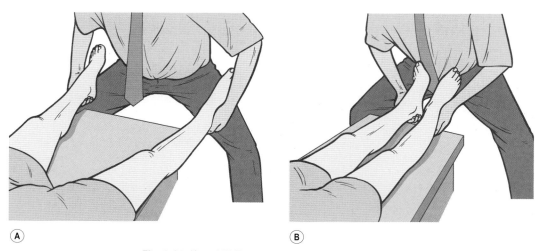

(A) (B)

Fig. 9.21 (A and B) Eccentric resistance of hip abduction.

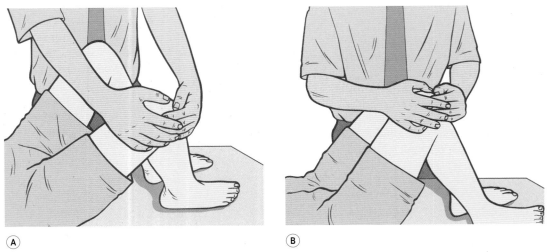

(A)   (B)

Fig. 9.22 (A and B) Eccentric resistance of hip external rotation.

BOX 9.1   Common Questions About Manual Resistance Techniques (MRTs) Such as MET

Q1. Should muscles be lengthened gently or firmly?
A: Gently.
Q2. Is the 'barrier phenomenon' similar in MRTs and in thrust techniques?
A: See discussion of barriers in Chapters 2, 6 and 7.
Q3. How long does it take to perform MRT/MET on a muscle?
A: Less than a minute.
Q4. If MRT is unsuccessful, what does that suggest?
A: The problem may be in the connective tissue.
Q5. Are these techniques arduous for the healthcare provider to perform?
A: Not typically.
Q6. Besides relaxing a muscle, MRT can be used for what other purposes?
A: To mobilise joints or prepare a muscle for more aggressive stretching techniques.
Q7. What are the indications for MRT?
A: Increased muscle tension, treatment of trigger points (see Chapter 14 and Box 9.2) and joint restriction (see Chapter 7).

BOX 9.2   Common Clinical Applications of Manual Resistance Techniques (Including MET) (Figs 9.23A, B and 9.24A, B)

A. Trigger Point (Semi-Active)
Indication: palpation of taut band in muscle, with twitch sign and referred pain phenomenon.
Treatment: this is primarily a neuromuscular phenomenon, not a connective tissue problem. Treatment therefore requires a minimum of force. Use MRTs (isometric contractions). Light ischaemic compression can also be used, especially for trigger points on the surface. The pressure should be just enough to engage a barrier to resistance and, following a latency, should achieve a release phenomenon. Greater force risks facilitating a contraction in the muscle as it 'defends' the barrier (see also Chapter 14).
   Experiment: try to find a trigger point in the upper trapezius (using a light flat pincer grip). Hold the taut band between your fingers. Then roll the taut band through your fingers as you search the length of the muscle for a motor response in the trigger point (i.e. local twitch response (LTR), see Fig. 9.23). Once you have found an LTR, try to release the trigger point with MRTs (isometric contractions) and then repalpate.

BOX 9.2   Common Clinical Applications of Manual Resistance Techniques (Including MET)—cont'd

B. Shortened Muscle (Passive or Semi-Active)

Indication: positive length test for decreased range of motion.

Treatment: start with MRTs. If MRT is unsuccessful, it is likely that there are connective tissue changes since mere relaxation alone did not result in a release of the muscle to a new resting length. There are two options:

1. Perform myofascial release by folding the muscle perpendicularly against itself and hold until release is 'sensed' (see Fig. 9.24). Then take out slack. This avoids the stretch reflex and is ideal for superficial muscles such as the pectoralis major.
2. If muscle is deep (e.g. iliopsoas), treat with a more forceful technique such as contract–relax antagonist contract (CRAC) or postfacilitation stretch (PFS). PFS is similar to MRT as described earlier except that a greater contraction force (25%–100% of a patient's maximum) is used, after which a fast stretch is applied (Liebenson, 2006). **Note:** if you are using PFS, certain safety rules should be observed. These include the following: stretch over the largest, most stable, least painful joint; joints should be 'loose packed'; avoid uncoupled movements; and do not stretch nerves if they are irritated. **Note:** *Use of strong contractions relates to PNF usage, not to MET.*

Experiment: Test the length of the iliopsoas and adductors (see Figs 9.8A, B and 9.9A, B) and then perform a muscle energy procedure and re-evaluate.

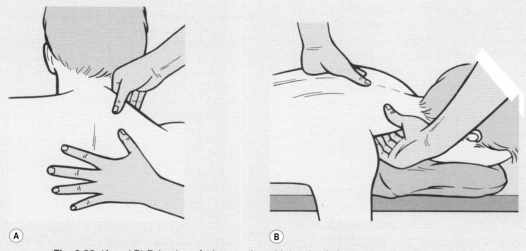

Fig. 9.23 (A and B) Palpation of trigger point with local twitch response in upper trapezius.

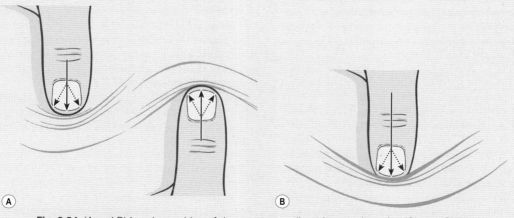

Fig. 9.24 (A and B) Local stretching of tissues surrounding trigger point using 'S' and 'C' bends.

MET, Muscle energy technique; *MRT,* manual resistance technique; *PNF,* proprioceptive neuromuscular facilitation.

The investigation of chains that form in our patients are invaluable aids in troubleshooting. It is not enough simply to identify a muscle imbalance and treat those muscles. The dysfunctional chain must also be identified and treatment of a key link given. The concept of muscle imbalance is reinforced by knowledge of neurodevelopment of the upright posture. Developmental kinesiology gives us a blueprint of movement stereotypes as well as terms of functional joint centration. Supraspinal control, which begins after 3 weeks of life, is the beginning of voluntary motor control. If chains of agonist–antagonist muscle incoordination that are hypothetically related to various stages of neurodevelopment of the upright posture are improved, significant advances in the treatment of motor system problems will likely result. In fact, functional joint centration at different stages of development gives us a model upon which to identify correct or faulty movement patterns. For instance, just as C0–C1 centrates by 6 weeks of life, it should not be de-centrated in adults. Similarly, the scapula moves caudally after 3 months; triple flexion of hips/knees/ankles occurs by 4 months, etc.

Continued research into agonist–antagonist coactivation, joint congruence, equilibrium, maximisation of joint load handling ability and neurological programmes in the adult, representative of neuro-developmental stages, is eagerly anticipated.

REFERENCES

Adler, S.S., Beckers, D., Buck, M., 2021. PNF in Practice – An Illustrated Guide, fifth ed. Springer-Verlag, Berlin.

Agrawal, S., 2016. Comparison between post isometric relaxation and reciprocal inhibition maneuvers on hamstring flexibility in young healthy adults: randomized clinical trial. Int. J. Med. Res. Health Sci. 5 (1), 33–37. doi:10.5958/2319-5886.2016.00008.4.

Arendt-Nielson, L., Graven-Nielson, T., Svarrer, H., Svensson, P., 1995. The influence of low back pain on muscle activity and coordination during gait. Pain 64, 231–240.

Assila, N., Duprey, S., Begon, M., 2021. Glenohumeral joint and muscles functions during a lifting task. J. Biomech. 126, 110641.

Babyar, S.R., 1996. Excessive scapular motion in individuals recovering from painful and stiff shoulders: causes and treatment strategies. Phys. Ther. 76, 226–238.

Bang, M.D., Deyle, G.D., 2000. Comparison of supervised exercise with and without manual physical therapy for patients with shoulder impingement syndrome. J. Orthop. Sports Phys. Ther. 30, 126–137.

Barton, P.M., Hayes, K.C., 1996. Neck flexor muscle strength, and relaxation times in normal subjects and subjects with unilateral neck pain and headache. Arch. Phys. Med. Rehabil. 77, 680–687.

Bergman, G.J., Winters, J.C., Groenier, K.H., et al., 2004. Manipulative therapy in addition to usual medical care for patients with shoulder dysfunction and pain: a randomized, controlled trial. Ann. Intern. Med. 141, 432–439.

Bernstein, M., Morabia, A., Sloutskis, D., 1999. Definition and prevalence of sedentarism in an urban population. Am. J. Public Health. 89 (6), 862–867. doi:10.2105/ajph.89.6.862.

Boyles, R.E., Ritland, B.M., Mirale, B.M., et al., 2009. The short-term effects of thoracic spine thrust manipulation on patients with shoulder impingement syndrome. Man. Ther. 14, 375–380.

Buchmann., J., Neustadt, B., Buchmann-Barthel, K., et al., 2014. Objective measurement of tissue tension in myofascial trigger point areas before and during the administration of anesthesia with complete blocking of neuromuscular transmission. Clin. J. Pain 30 (3), 191–198.

Cholewicki, J., McGill, S.M., 1996. Mechanical stability of the in vivo lumbar spine: implications for injury and chronic low back pain. Clin. Biomech. 11 (1), 1–15.

Cleland, J.A., Childs, J.D., Fritz, J.M., Whitman, J.M., Eberhart, S.L., 2007. Development of a clinical prediction rule for guiding treatment of a subgroup of patients with neck pain: use of thoracic spine manipulation, exercise, and patient education. Phys. Ther. 87, 9–23.

Cleland, J.A., Childs, J.D., McRae, M., Palmer, J.A., Stowell, T., 2005. Immediate effects of thoracic manipulation in patients with neck pain: a randomized clinical trial. Man. Ther. 10, 127–135.

de Oliveira, L.C., de Oliveira, R.G., Pires-Oliveira, de Almeida Pires-Oliveira, D.A., 2015. The Pilates method improves the relationship agonist-antagonist flexor and extensor knee in elderly: a randomized controlled trial. Man. Ther. Posturol. Rehabil. J. 13, 1–7. doi:10.17784/mtprehabJournal.2015.13.278.

Edgerton, V.R., Wolf, S.L., Levendowski, D.J., Roy, R.R., 1996. Theoretical basis for patterning EMG amplitudes to assess muscle dysfunction. Med. Sci. Sports Exerc. 28, 744–751.

Frank, C., Liebenson, C., Veverkovaf, M., 2020. Evaluation of muscular imbalance. In: Liebenson, C. (Ed.), Rehabilitation of the Spine: A Patient Centered Approach. Wolters Kluwer, Philadelphia, pp. 339–359.

Geffen, S., 2003. 3: Rehabilitation principles for treating chronic musculoskeletal injuries. Med. J. Aust. 178 (5), 238–243.

Grabiner, M.D., Koh, T.J., Ghazawi, A.E., 1992. Decoupling of bilateral paraspinal excitation in subjects with low back pain. Spine 17, 1219.

Hodges, P.W., Richardson, C.A., 1996. Inefficient muscular stabilization of the lumbar spine associated with low back pain. Spine 21, 2640–2650.

Hodges, P.W., Richardson, C.A., 1998. Delayed postural contraction of the transverse abdominis associated with movement of the lower limb in people with low back pain. J. Spinal Disord. 11, 46–56.

Hodges, P.W., Richardson, C.A., 1999. Altered trunk muscle recruitment in people with low back pain with upper limb movements at different speeds. Arch. Phys. Med. Rehabil. 80, 1005–1012.

Janda, V., 1983. On the concept of postural muscles and posture in man. Aust. J. Physiother. 29, 83–84.

Janda, V., Frank, C., Liebenson, C., 2006. Evaluation of muscle imbalances. In: Liebenson, C. (Ed.), Rehabilitation of the Spine: A Practitioner's Manual, second ed. Lippincott Williams and Wilkins, Baltimore.

Kabot, H., 1950. Studies on neuromuscular dysfunction XIII: new concepts and techniques of neuromuscular reeducation for paralysis. Perm. Found. Med. Bull. 8, 121–143.

Kobesova, A., Dzvonik, J., Kolar, P., Sardina, A., Andel, R., 2015. Effects of shoulder girdle dynamic stabilization exercise on hand muscle strength. Isokinet. Exerc. Sci. 23 (1), 21–32. doi:10.3233/IES-140560.

Kobesova, A., Kolar, P., 2014. Developmental kinesiology: three levels of motor control in the assessment and treatment of the motor system. J. Bodyw. Mov. Ther. 18 (1), 23–33. doi:10.1016/j.jbmt.2013.04.002.

Kobesova, A., Osborne, N., 2012. The Prague School of rehabilitation. Int. Musculoskelet. Med. 34 (2), 39–41. doi:10.1179/1753614612Z.00000000014.

Kolár, P., 1999. The sensomotor nature of postural functions, its fundamental role in rehabilitation. J. Orthop. Med. 21 (2), 40–45.

Land, H., Gordon, S., Watt, K., 2019. Effect of manual physiotherapy in homogeneous individuals with subacromial shoulder impingement: a randomized controlled trial. Physiother. Res. Int. 24 (2), e1768. doi:10.1002/pri.1768.

Levine, M.G., Kabot, H., Knott, M., Voss, D.E., 1954. Relaxation of spasticity by physiological techniques. Arch. Phys. Med. Rehabil. 35, 214–223.

Lewit, K., 1986. Postisometric relaxation in combination with other methods of muscular facilitation and inhibition. Man. Med. 2, 101–104.

Lewit, K., 1999a. Manipulative Therapy in Rehabilitation of the Motor System, third ed. Butterworths, London.

Lewit, K., 1999b. Chain reactions in the locomotor system in the light of coactivation patterns based on developmental neurology. J. Orthop. Med. 21 (2), 52–58.

Lewit, K., Simons, D.G., 1984. Myofascial pain: relief by postisometric relaxation. Arch. Phys. Med. Rehabil. 65, 452–456.

Liebenson, C.S., 1989. Active muscular relaxation techniques, part one. Basic principles and methods. J. Manipulative Physiol. Ther. 12, 6.

Liebenson, C.S., 1990. Active muscular relaxation techniques, part two. Clinical application. J. Manipulative Physiol. Ther. 13, 1.

Liebenson, C., 1999. Advice for the clinician. J. Bodyw. Mov. Ther. 3, 147–149.

Liebenson, C., 2006. Manual resistance techniques. In: Liebenson, C. (Ed.), Rehabilitation of the Spine: A Practitioner's Manual, second ed. Lippincott Williams and Wilkins, Baltimore.

Liebenson, C., Chapman, S., 1998. Rehabilitation of the Spine: Functional Evaluation of the Lumbar Spine. Williams and Wilkins, Baltimore [videotape].

Liebenson, C., DeFranca, C., Lefebvre, R., 1998. Rehabilitation of the Spine: Functional Evaluation of the Cervical Spine. Williams and Wilkins, Baltimore [videotape].

Liebenson, C., Murphy, D., 1998. Rehabilitation of the Spine: Post-isometric Relaxation Techniques – Low Back and Lower Extremities. Williams and Wilkins, Baltimore [videotape].

Masaracchio, M., Kirker, K., States, R., Hanney, W.J., Liu, X., Kolber, M., 2019. Thoracic spine manipulation for the management of mechanical neck pain: a systematic review and meta-analysis. PLoS ONE 14 (2), e0211877. doi:10.1371/journal.pone.0211877.

McGill, S., Grenier, S., Bluhm, M., Preuss, R., Brown, S., Russell, C., 2003. Previous history of LBP with work loss is related to lingering deficits in biomechanical, physiological, personal, psychosocial and motor control characteristics. Ergonomics 46, 731–746.

Norlander, S., Nordgren, B., 1998. Clinical symptoms related to musculoskeletal neck-shoulder pain and mobility in the cervico-thoracic spine. Scand. J. Rehabil. Med. 30, 243–251.

O'Sullivan, P., Twomey, L., Allison, G., Sinclair, J., Miller, K., Knox, J., 1997. Altered patterns of abdominal muscle activation in patients with chronic low back pain. Aust. J. Physiother. 43, 91–98.

Page, P., 2006. Sensorimotor training: a 'global' approach for balance training. J. Bodyw. Mov. Ther. 10 (1), 77–84. doi:10.1016/j.jbmt.2005.04.006.

Parnianpour, M., Nordin, M., Kahanovitz, N., Frankel, V., 1988. The triaxial coupling of torque generation of trunk muscles during isometric exertions and the effect of fatiguing isoinertial movements on the motor output and movement patterns. Spine 13, 982–992.

Ricciardi, R., 2005. Sedentarism: a concept analysis. Nurs. Forum. 40 (3), 79–87. doi:10.1111/j.1744-6198.2005.00021.x.

Sharma, A., Angusamy, R., Kalra, S., Singh, S., 2010. Efficacy of post-isometric relaxation versus integrated neuromuscular ischaemic technique in the treatment of upper trapezius trigger points. Indian J. Physiother. Occup. Ther. 4 (3), 1–10.

Sparto, P.J., Parnianpour, M., Marras, W.S., Granata, K.P., Reinsel, T.E., Simon, S., 1997. Neuromuscular trunk performance and spinal loading during a fatiguing isometric trunk extension with varying torque requirements. Clin. Spine Surg. 10 (2), 145–156.

Sterling, M., Jull, G.A., Wright, A., 2001. Cervical mobilisation: concurrent effects on pain, sympathetic nervous system activity and motor activity. Man. Ther. 6 (2), 72–81.

Treleaven, J., Jull, G., Atkinson, L., 1994. Cervical musculoskeletal dysfunction in post-concussional headache. Cephalgia 14, 273–279.

Wainner, R.S., Whitman, J.M., Cleland, J.A., Flynn, T.W., 2007. Regional interdependence: a musculoskeletal examination model whose time has come. J. Orthop. Sports Phys. Ther. 37 (11), 658–660.

Watson, D.H., Trott, P.H., 1993. Cervical headache: an investigation of natural head posture and upper cervical flexor muscle performance. Cephalgia 13, 272–284.

Wilson, E., Payton, O., Donegan-Shoaf, L., Dec, K., 2003. Muscle energy technique in patients with acute low back pain: a pilot clinical trial. J. Orthop. Sports Phys. Ther. 33, 502–512.

World Health Organization. (2021). Rehabilitation. 23 September 2021. https://www.who.int/news-room/fact-sheets/detail/rehabilitation.

Zazulak, B.T., Hewett, T.E., Reeves, N.P., et al., 2007a. Deficits in neuro-muscular control of the trunk predict knee injury risk: a prospective biomechanical-epidemiologic study. Am. J. Sports Med. 35, 1123–1130.

Zazulak, B.T., Hewett, T.E., Reeves, N.P., Goldberg, B., Cholewicki, J., 2007b. The effects of core proprioception on knee injury: a prospective biomechanical-epidemiological study. Am. J. Sports Med. 35, 368–373.

10

MET in Post-Surgical Rehabilitation

Shraddha Parmar Pradhan, Ashok Shyam, Sasha Chaitow

CHAPTER CONTENTS

INTRODUCTION

Rehabilitation forms a very important part of musculoskeletal surgery; however, postoperative rehabilitation poses special problems. Postoperative pain is one of the most important factors that prevents cooperation in many patients. In this situation, more often than not, patients do not allow the therapist to perform optimal joint and muscle mobilisation. In addition, overzealous passive rehabilitation may lead to injury to fragile tissue in the postoperative period. During the early stages of postoperative rehabilitation, slow eccentric isotonic stretching (SEIS)/isolytic contraction (ILC) may play an important role by virtue of its two important properties, that is, relative pain-free mobilisation and relative mobilisation within patients' capacity to bear pain. Although in the literature on muscle energy techniques (MET), use in a postoperative setting is sparse (indicatively Faqih et al., 2019; Thomas et al., 2020), we have found that when cautiously applied, the principles of MET provide definite benefits. We have been using these techniques in our postoperative patients for the last 13 years, including during both early and delayed postoperative situations. This chapter describes our growing understanding of the underlying principles of SEIS and its successful application in post-surgical patients.

CLINICAL POST-SURGICAL SITUATIONS

Once the orthopaedic operative management is over, further management is directed towards the rehabilitation of the patient. Immediate and late post-surgical periods are distinct, because musculoskeletal physiology differs in these periods. These can be roughly divided into the initial 3 weeks after surgery, the acute period, followed by the subacute period, up until 6 weeks. In the acute period, the tissues are inflamed and fragile and the patient experiences relatively more pain. Pain will cause reflex muscle guarding and resulting hypomobility. During the acute phase, attempts should be made to identify the potential sources of biomechanical overload or imbalance that may have occurred during the primary injury, and/or that may occur secondarily during the postoperative period due to surgically induced trauma (such as debridement of injured muscle mass, resection of tendons, soft tissue handling during surgery). These factors not only cause biomechanical imbalance but are also a source of pain. Muscle imbalance/weakness and pain play a role in restricting joint mobility in the acute postoperative period. In addition, in the acute phase, an injured joint will assume a loose-packed position to accommodate the increased volume of fluid within the joint space. This helps to decrease pain and provides comfort to the patient; however, it leads to relative adaptive shortening of the soft tissue component in the surroundings among other potential complications (Pujol et al., 2015). Thus, in the acute phase, more emphasis is placed on muscle re-education than on stretching, and SEIS is our preferred modality in this period.

Patients who present in the subacute phase are those who had unstable fracture geometry or who required immobilisation in the acute phase. Immobilisation after surgery often leads to the shortening of connective tissue, the formation of adhesions, scar tissue, keloids and fibrotic contracture of muscles, tendons and other connective tissue (Konno et al., 2021, 2022). Any process or event that disturbs the normal functioning of a specific joint structure will set up a chain of events that eventually affects not only every part of the joint but also its surrounding joints and soft tissues (De Andrade et al., 1965; Spencer et al., 1984) and results in joint stiffness. Restriction of normal joint mobility depends on the joint type and surrounding tissues. Restriction in the wrist joint has been estimated at 47% joint capsule involvement, 41% surrounding muscles and intermuscular fasciae, 10% tendons and 2% skin tissue (Johns & Wright, 1962). That is very different from the elbow joint, as muscles and tendons have accounted for 84% of the variance in elbow stiffness (Chleboun et al., 1997). In such cases, stretching caused by normal movements may cause severe pain, and mobility may not spontaneously return without specific stretching treatment (Ylinen, 2008). Stretching during the repair process is important, especially in older people. With restricted mobility for an extended period of time, elastic connective tissue is gradually replaced by fibrous tissue. Extensive infiltration of less elastic fibrous tissue will result in permanent restriction of mobility. Thus, in this phase, more emphasis is on stretching using isolytic contractions (i.e. rapid eccentric stretching – see below) that have the ability to break down tight, shortened tissue and the replacement of these with superior material.

The different phases of pathology associated with the different stages of the postoperative period demand quite different interventions. In the acute and subacute phases, pain and reflex muscle spasms are major issues – conditions that are more responsive to SEIS. Here, the stretch force is slow and gradual, resulting in less pain, and easing any reflex spasm. As the tissues are still elastic, slow and gradual stretching can easily overcome soft tissue resistance, thus preventing stiffness. In chronic phases, as the immobilisation period increases, the elasticity of the tissues decreases and pain is relatively reduced. In such cases, a more rapid isotonic eccentric stretch in the form of ILC has been found to be more useful to break down the infiltrating fibrosis and adhesions. Thus, although SEIS and ILC are both forms of eccentric isotonic contractions (see Chapters 2, 5 and 7), the major difference between them relates to the speed of stretching. SEIS can therefore be equated to ILC performed at a far slower speed.

MUSCLE PHYSIOLOGY RELEVANT TO THE POST-SURGICAL ENVIRONMENT

Muscle immobilised in a lengthened or neutral position maintains muscle weight and fibre cross-sectional area better than muscle immobilised in a shortened position (see Chapters 2, 5 and 7). In the postoperative period, reflex muscle guarding, muscle inhibition due to pain, relative limb immobility, limb positioning because of pain, etc., often leads to adaptive shortening (Johns & Wright, 1962; William & Goldspink, 1978). Immobilisation in a relatively shortened position causes the length of the fibre to decrease, leading to an increase in connective tissue deposition and decreased muscle extensibility, in turn causing loss of its contractile function (Bloomfield, 1997). Lewit (1985) directed attention to a balanced view when he stated:

The naive conception that movement restriction in passive mobility is necessarily due to articular lesion has to be abandoned. We know that taut muscles alone can limit passive movement and that articular lesions are regularly associated with increased muscular tension.

This can be one of the factors responsible for restricted joint mobility (Konno et al., 2021, 2022).

Muscle length is known to affect the contractile properties of the muscle as a whole. Alteration in the resting length of the muscle affects its functioning capacity and causes relative muscle weakness (Gossman et al., 1982; Bloomfield, 1997; Bogdanis, 2012). Thus, a vicious cycle of postoperative pain and reflex muscle contraction leads to stiffness and also weakness of the muscle (secondary to direct injury to muscles) which in turn leads to more immobility and a decrease in muscle extensibility. The purpose of stretching is to increase joint mobility, muscle length and flexibility as well as to relax the muscle in general. Metabolism is less efficient in stiff muscles because of increased intramuscular pressure and decreased circulation of fluids. Stretching increases the elasticity of muscles, tendon, fascia, joint ligaments and joint capsules. An increase in muscle tone will often lead to pain caused by the irritation of nerve endings or the increase in pressure in and between muscles, which causes a slowing of the metabolism. Symptoms of pain can be reduced with the relaxation of muscles by stretching (Kisner & Colby, 2002; Pujol et al., 2015). Thus early mobilisation has become a common practice after surgery and trauma.

NEED FOR FUNCTIONAL MUSCLE RE-EDUCATION AFTER SURGERY IN THE IMMEDIATE AND LATE POST-SURGICAL PERIOD

Just as strength and endurance exercises are essential interventions to improve impaired muscle performance in the acute phase, when restricted mobility adversely affects function in the subacute phase, stretching interventions become an integral component of the individualised rehabilitation programme (Bloomfield, 1997; Cação-Benedini et al., 2014; Kay, 2020).

Active exercises and stretching will promote the orientation of fibres along the direction of movement, limit the infiltration of cross fibres between collagen fibres and prevent excessive collagen formation (Kisner & Colby, 2002). According to Kisner and Colby, when a muscle is stretched or elongated the stretch force is transmitted to the whole muscle fibre through the connective tissue around it. During the stretch, both longitudinal and lateral force transmission occurs. After repeated stretches there is mechanical disruption of cross bridges as the filaments slide apart, leading to abrupt lengthening of the

sarcomere ('sarcomere give') (Magnusson et al., 1996; Klotz et al., 2021).

Stretching has an impact on both contractile and non-contractile tissues. As the muscle is stretched in the absence of a contraction, there is a point at which the muscle begins to resist that stretch. This pull is attributed to the elastic recoil of the passive structures within the muscles, i.e. intervening connective tissues. Interfascial and fascial release occurs following stretching, which plays an important role in maintaining the muscle's length and extensibility (Magnusson et al., 1996; Cação-Benedini et al., 2014). Harrelson et al state that joint and surrounding soft tissues respond favourably to mechanical stimuli and that structural modifications are noted soon after exercise (Harrelson, 1991).

Rehabilitation thus requires the patient to exercise the injured as well as the surrounding joint(s) and soft tissues (David, 1999). Joint disease and injury involve a decrease in the elasticity of connective tissue. The goals of soft tissue therapy include reduction of pain, relaxation of hypertonic muscles, lengthening of restricted tissues, improvement of local circulation, promotion of wound healing and restoration of normal joint and soft tissue functioning (Donatelli & Owens-Burkhart, 1981). Donatelli and Owens-Burkhart supply evidence that movement maintains joint lubrication and critical fibre distance within the matrix and ensures an orderly deposition of collagen fibrils. It is generally accepted that stretching improves the effectiveness of the rehabilitation programme even if the precise mechanisms remain unclear (Freitas et al., 2018; Andrade et al., 2020). Thus, both strengthening (re-education) of the muscle and stretching are essential for postoperative rehabilitation of the patients, while the choice of optimum techniques lies with the therapist, the surgeon, and the patient (see Chapters 1 and 8).

WHY MET IN THE POST-SURGICAL CONDITION/REHABILITATION?

Muscle balance is important for normal joint function. An imbalance between agonist and antagonist muscles of a joint can disturb joint function (Hertling & Kessler, 2006; Gorkovenko et al., 2012; Latash, 2018). In post-surgical situations, the surgical approach is through one of these muscles (either agonist or antagonist). This leads to a direct imbalance between them due to relative weakness of the affected muscle group and relative tightness of the opposing muscle group. MET is an approach that can make a major contribution toward joint mobilisation and achievement of muscle balance. MET is a product of a variety of schools, although its origin may be found in osteopathic, orthopaedic and physiotherapy techniques (see Chapter 3). This technique is used in clinical practice to restore mobility of joints, retrain global movement patterns, reduce tissue oedema, stretch fibrotic tissue, reduce muscle spasms and retrain stabilising function of the intersegmentally connected muscles (Malliaropoulos et al., 2004; Askling, 2014). All these factors play an important role in rehabilitation in the postoperative period. The main physiological basis of MET appears to rest on an understanding of the viscoelastic properties of the muscle-tendon unit and the Golgi Tendon Apparatus (GTA). See Chapter 4 for current research evidence relative to the mechanisms of MET.

Viscoelasticity: Viscoelastic properties involve the hysteresis response of the muscle-tendon unit (Garrett et al., 1988; Mlyniec et al., 2021). It has been proposed that stretching exercises may alter the viscoelastic behaviour of the muscle-tendon unit (Garrett et al., 1988; Kubo, 2018). Instantaneous changes within muscle also result in large but temporary responses in its bio-physiological and biomechanical properties (Parmar et al., 2011; Freitas et al., 2018; Konno et al., 2021). Passive stretching to the elastic limit can allow these tissues to resume the original resting length. Passive stretching beyond the elastic limit, into plasticity, will lead to a greater soft tissue length compared to the original resting length when the stretch is removed. Prolonged lengthening of the contractile units of muscle, the sarcomeres, into the plastic range of motion (ROM), progressively leads to increased soft tissue length due to an increased number of sarcomeres in series. Non-contractile units of soft tissues include ligaments, joint capsule and fascia, which all consist of collagen and elastin fibres. Prolonged lengthening of collagen, up to its yield point, leads to tissue lengthening due to permanent tissue deformation. Elastin fails without deformation, with high loads. The more elastin the tissues contain, the more flexible the tissues. To avoid damaging soft tissues, healing and remodelling time must be allowed between periods of stretching. The serial elastic component (SEC) and parallel elastic component (PEC) represent the elastic structures of the muscle. Tendons and connective tissues within the contractile proteins are a major part of the SEC. It has been

suggested that the active components, the cross bridges themselves, are elastic structures (Ylinen, 2008). The PEC component consists of muscle fascia, membrane, sarcolemma and sarcoplasm. These tissues are passive elastic structures of the muscle. During stretching of a tight muscle, tension will increase in both SEC and PEC. During contraction, actin and myosin draw over each other, increasing the number of transverse bridges. They store energy during the stretching of contracting muscles (eccentric contraction). With an increase in length, elastic energy is stored in all parts of a tense muscle. It is freed either quickly or slowly, with stretch release, depending on the speed of movement. Stretching becomes important to recovery after treatment of the acute post-surgical stage. Stretching can begin carefully, and within pain tolerance, following the prescribed immobilisation period usually after 2 to 3 days.

Early mobilisation has been shown to improve connective tissue and capillary circulation in the area of trauma. Repair fibres form in the same direction as the original fibres and the overproduction of the fibrous connective tissue with fibres running in all directions is prevented. Connective tissue in muscles should form in the same direction as contractile muscle fibres to improve force. Proposed mechanisms are thought to be either (1) a direct decrease in muscle stiffness via passive viscoelastic changes or (2) an indirect decrease due to reflex inhibition and consequent viscoelasticity changes from decreased actin-myosin cross bridging. Decreased muscle stiffness would then allow for increased joint ROM (Garrett et al., 1988; Mlyniec et al., 2021).

Golgi Tendon Apparatus: Garrett et al. (1988) found actively contracted muscles can withstand 15% more stretching force than passive, relaxed muscles. Similarly, the energy absorption capacity of active muscles is 100% more than relaxed muscles (Parmar et al., 2011). Therefore muscles endure far more stress while active than when passively stretched. It has been suggested that muscle contraction, prior to stretching, will activate the Golgi tendon organs (GTO), which encourage muscle relaxation by causing inhibition of motor neurons via activation of the Renshaw cells to reduce muscle sensitivity to contraction. According to the theory of neuromuscular relaxation, muscle contraction prior to stretching activates muscle spindle receptors, which decreases their sensitivity, reducing muscle tension and resistance to stretch, and decreases motor neuron activity owing to autogenic inhibition (Karatzaferi et al., 2003, 2008; Ylinen, 2008; Aagaard, 2018; Osama, 2021). Thus, the muscle-tendon system can be stretched further when active muscle resistance is reduced via the nervous system. However, it has also been claimed that active muscle contraction before stretching may be harmful because it activates motor nerves and increases muscle tension (Ylinen, 2008). This may limit the use of MET in the immediate, acute postoperative phase.

Active muscle contraction has been shown to have neurophysiological effects (Herzog, 2015). Active muscle contraction causes pain inhibition. Muscles can be stretched further due to the rise in pain tolerance levels which has shown to be a reason for improved ROM after stretching (Koltyn et al., 1996; Kosek et al., 1996; Lannersten & Kosek, 2010; Freitas et al., 2018). It most likely causes elastic and plastic changes in muscles as well, which vary in relation to the intensity of contraction. ROM has been found to improve even further when combined with active contraction of the agonist muscles (Nagano et al., 2019). It has been supposed that this is because of the decrease in the electrical activity of the antagonist muscles due to reciprocal inhibition caused by the contraction of the agonist muscles during stretching.

The scientific rationale of stretching is based on the effect of the technique on the muscle receptors. The GTO which is one of the receptors, is a protective mechanism that inhibits the contraction of the muscle in which it lies. It has a very low threshold for firing (i.e. it fires easily) after an active muscle contraction and has a high threshold for firing with passive stretch (Blum et al., 2017; Lyle & Nichols, 2019). Moreover, after the use of the MET procedure on the previously contracted tissues, there exists a latency period of anything from 15 to 30 seconds during which the muscle can be taken to its new resting length or stretched more easily than would have been the case before contraction (Guissard, 1988; Blum et al., 2017). During stretching, circulation will actually decrease due to blood vessels becoming narrower, while intramuscular pressure increases. Increased activity of the sympathetic nervous system causes constriction of the small arterioles, further decreasing circulation. There will be a rebound following the stretch, and circulation will respond by increasing acutely. This helps flush away metabolites and reduce pain.

The justification for the employment of soft tissue manipulation techniques on post-surgical patients was suggested by Janda (1991) who pointed out, that since clinical evidence abounds that joint mobilisation (thrust or gentle mobilisation) influences the muscles which are in anatomic or functional relationships with the joint, it may well be that normalisation of the excessive tone of the muscles alongside its proprioceptive implications are providing the benefit. By implication, normalisation of the muscle tone by other means (such as MET) would provide an equally useful basis for a beneficial outcome and joint normalisation. Since a reduction in muscle spasm/contraction commonly results in a reduction in joint pain, the answer to many such problems would seem to lie in appropriate soft tissue attention. To explain how MET would be able to influence this situation Van Buskirk (1990) states:

> In indirect muscle energy, the skeletal muscles in the shortened area are initially stretched to the maximum extent allowed by the somatic dysfunction (to the barrier). With the tissues held in this position, the patient is instructed to contract the affected muscle voluntarily. This isometric activation of the muscle will stretch the internal connective tissues. Voluntary activation of the motor neurons to the same muscles also blocks transmission in spinal nociceptive pathways. Immediately following the isometric phase, passive extrinsic stretch is imposed, further lengthening the tissues towards the normal easy neutral.

SEIS/ILC AS A FORM OF ACTIVE STRETCHING TECHNIQUE IN THE POSTOPERATIVE PHASE

Forms of active stretching technique used in the postoperative phase are:
- SEIS (when the stretch force is slow and gradual)
- ILC (when the stretch is more rapid).

Isotonic Eccentric MET: This is a type of MET where a direct contraction of a muscle is resisted and overcome by the therapist. An isotonic eccentric contraction involves the origins and insertions of the muscles involved becoming further separated as they contract, despite the patient's effort (20% to 30% effort) to approximate them.

Since in the immediate postoperative phase the muscles in and around the involved area are in a state of reflex muscle spasm or guarding, the use of SEIS technique appears to help prevention of muscle atrophy, starts early retraining, and helps to reduce pain while involving the patient's own muscular effort in gaining ROM. When performed slowly an isotonic eccentric stretch has the effect of toning the muscles involved, and of inhibiting the antagonists to those muscles, with minimal or no tissue damage.

However, in the later postoperative period, when there are adhesions expected to occur after the immobilisation period, the stretch force needed to gain ROM has to be more rapid and of a higher intensity than SEIS. This rapid force used is expected to cause tissue lysis and breaking of adhesions, thereby assisting in gaining joint ROM (Hody et al., 2019). Hence ILC technique is the preferred choice in the late postoperative period (Gerber et al., 2009).

CLINICAL EVIDENCE AND CLINICAL CASE SETTINGS

With the above understanding of MET, we started our study on the application of MET in a post-surgical situation. This was planned as a Level I study, a prospective double-blinded randomised controlled trial that compared the effects of MET and passive manual stretch (PMS) in postoperative hip fracture fixation patients (Parmar et al., 2011; Vilchez-Barrera & Hernán-Santana, 2020).

Methodology

We included subjects with proximal femur fractures treated with a standard lateral approach with fixation using a four-hole dynamic hip screw-plate system. We excluded subjects with pathological fractures, revision surgeries, associated ipsilateral injuries and subjects with a neurological and vascular disorder or subjects treated with an extended approach or fixation. We also excluded subjects with previous or concurrent knee pain. Eligibility criteria were met and subjects were accepted for the study with prior written consent and an explanation of the study to each subject. A total of 61 subjects were selected for the study as per inclusion criteria. Excluding the 9 dropouts, a total of 52 subjects completed the entire study. Subjects were randomly allotted to the two groups, a SEIS group and a PMS group. A double-blind

study was conducted to minimise bias. A pre-intervention assessment was carried out by the assessment therapist for pain assessment (on the VAS) and knee ROM measurements (in degrees with a universal 360 degrees goniometer). The SEIS group received the slow eccentric isotonic stretch to the knee extensors, in the side-lying position; while the PMS group received passive manual stretching to the knee extensors in the side-lying position, by the same interventional therapist. The intervention common to both groups included ankle pumping exercises, static quadriceps exercises, static hamstring exercises, assisted active heel drags, assisted active straight leg raising exercises, assisted active abduction exercises in a supine position to the affected extremity, and free active ROM exercises to the opposite unaffected extremity and both upper extremities as well as unilateral bridging exercises. Frequency of treatment for both the groups was once a day for the morning session. Duration of the entire treatment session for both groups was 20 to 25 minutes. Intervention (SEIS or PMS) was started from postoperative day 3 up to postoperative day 12 by the interventional therapist. A post-intervention assessment was carried out by the assessment therapist for pain and knee ROM measurements. Final readings were noted in the assessment form, a master chart was prepared and data were analysed.

Results: In the PMS group, there was a significant improvement in the VAS scores, knee ROM and knee ROM deficit after the treatment period ($P < .001$). On the other hand, the SEIS group also demonstrated significant improvement in all of these outcomes; however, pain relief was greater in the SEIS group ($P < .001$).

Clinical Application

With encouraging results in one particular postoperative setting, we started applying MET to various postoperative patients. In general, patients were referred to us at two stages: early postoperative or the acute phase (within 3 weeks of surgery) and delayed postoperative or the subacute to chronic phase (more than 3 weeks up to 3 months). We used different techniques of MET as per the presentation. Again, the application of different MET techniques also depended on the stability and location of the fractures. A periarticular fracture (metaphyseal or intra-articular) may require postoperative immobilisation and thus presents late for treatment with ILC. A stable fracture in the shaft of long bones, which had been internally fixed, might be taken up for earlier therapy using SEIS techniques. With the advancement in the orthopaedic field and new technologies of fracture fixation, more fractures come into the stable category, requiring early mobilisation.

In immediate post-surgery groups, we used SEIS in order to prevent excessive pain and to also allow gradual gentle lengthening, thereby assisting in the remodelling of the injured, as well as the surrounding, soft tissue. In the later presented cases (i.e. chronic phase) we used ILC which is more vigorous, in order to assist in breaking the fibrotic adhesions by controlled microtrauma, thus allowing improvement in elasticity and circulation during remodelling.

For the purpose of mobilising a joint, the joint is put in a specific position to facilitate optimum contraction of a particular muscle or muscle group. The patient is asked to contract the muscle against counter-pressure that is greater than the patient's force, thus causing the muscle to contract eccentrically. This causes the muscle to elongate, thus moving one bone in relation to its articulating counterpart, helping to restore normal to near-normal joint ROM.

Clinical Examples
Scenario 1

Distal end radius. We treated seven patients in 2011 with distal radius fracture treated with open reduction and internal fixation (ORIF). When the patient arrived, the standard preliminary assessment was carried out and there was a discussion with the operating surgeon. Following this, the treatment was initiated for the wrist joint as well as the surrounding joints (fingers, elbow and shoulder).

Case 1 (Fig. 10.1A and B): A 35-year-old male diagnosed with closed fracture lower end radius, displaced, extra-articular, treated with ORIF with locking Ellis plate, without DNVC, presented on outpatient department basis 2 weeks postoperatively. Initial wrist ROM prior to initiation of any exercises was: flexion: 0 to 10 degrees, extension: 0 to 15 degrees, radial deviation: 0 to 5 degrees, ulnar deviation: 0 to 5 degrees, pronation: 0 to 20 degrees, supination: 0 to 15 degrees. MET in the form of SEIS was applied for 5 to 7 repetitions, once a day for 14 sessions, 6 days a week. After 14 sessions the wrist ROM was: flexion: 0 to 80 degrees, extension: 0 to 75 degrees, radial deviation: 0 to 15 degrees, ulnar deviation: 0 to 20 degrees, pronation: 0 to 80 degrees, supination: 0 to 75 degrees.

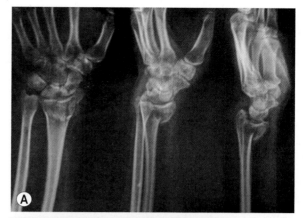

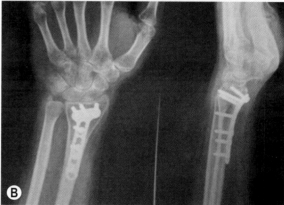

Fig. 10.1 (A) Preoperative radiograph of 35-year-old male with fractured distal end radius. (B) Postoperative radiograph showing open reduction internal fixation using locking plate. Rehabilitation using muscle energy techniques (MET) was started 2 weeks post-surgery.

Case 2 (Fig. 10.2A and B): A 23-year-old female diagnosed with closed right fracture lower end radius, displaced, extra-articular, treated with ORIF with locking Ellis plate, without DNVC, presented on outpatient department basis 5 weeks postoperatively. Initial wrist ROM prior to initiation of any exercises was: flexion: 0 to 30 degrees, extension: 0 to 25 degrees, radial deviation: 0 to 15 degrees, ulnar deviation: 0 to 20 degrees, pronation: 0 to 40 degrees, supination: 0 to 35 degrees. MET in the form of ILC was applied for 5 to 7 repetitions, once a day for 10 sessions, 6 days a week. After 10 sessions the wrist ROM was: flexion: 0 to 90 degrees, extension: 0 to 85 degrees, radial deviation: 0 to 15 degrees, ulnar deviation: 0 to 25 degrees, pronation: 0 to 90 degrees, supination: 0 to 90 degrees.

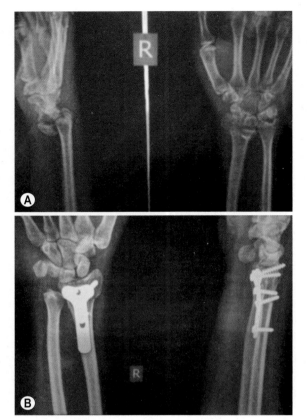

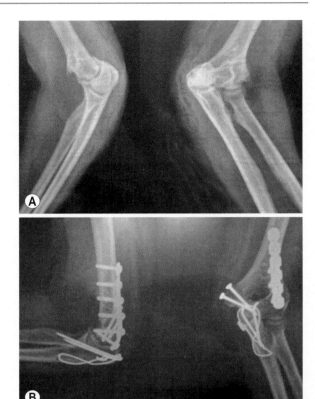

Fig. 10.2 (A) Preoperative radiograph of 23-year-old female with fractured distal end radius. (B) Postoperative radiograph showing open reduction internal fixation using locking plate. Rehabilitation using muscle energy techniques (MET) was started 5 weeks post-surgery.

Fig. 10.3 (A) Preoperative radiograph of 50-year-old female with fractured supracondylar humerus. (B) Postoperative radiograph showing open reduction internal fixation using plating. Rehabilitation using muscle energy techniques (MET) was started 7 weeks post-surgery.

Scenario 2

Supracondylar humerus. We treated 18 patients in 2011 with supracondylar humerus fracture treated with ORIF. When the patient arrived, the standard preliminary assessment was carried out and there was a discussion with the operating surgeon. Following this, the treatment was initiated for the elbow joint as well as the surrounding joints (fingers, wrist and shoulder).

Case 1 (Fig. 10.3A and B): A 50-year-old female diagnosed with left supracondylar humerus with intra-articular extension, treated with ORIF with two screws and a plate, presented on an outpatient department basis 7 weeks postoperatively. Initial elbow ROM prior to initiation of any exercises was from 30 degrees of extension to 70 degrees of flexion, pronation: 0 to 10 degrees, supination: 0 to 50 degrees. MET in the form

of ILC was applied for 8 to 10 repetitions, once a day for 40 sessions, 6 days a week. After 40 sessions the elbow ROM was 0 degrees of extension to 135 degrees of flexion, pronation: 0 to 90 degrees, supination: 0 to 90 degrees.

Case 2 (Fig. 10.4A and B): A 48-year-old male diagnosed with closed fracture right supracondylar humerus with intra-articular extension, without DNVC, treated with ORIF with elbow link control protocol, presented on outpatient department basis 3 weeks postoperatively. Initial elbow ROM prior to initiation of any exercises was from 40 degrees of extension to 90 degrees of flexion, pronation: 0 to 30 degrees, supination: 0 to 25 degrees. MET in the form of SEIS was applied for 8 to 10 repetitions, once a day for 30 sessions, 6 days a week. After 30 sessions the elbow ROM was 0 degrees

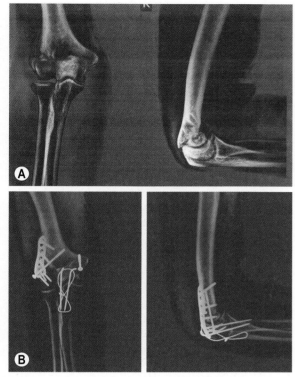

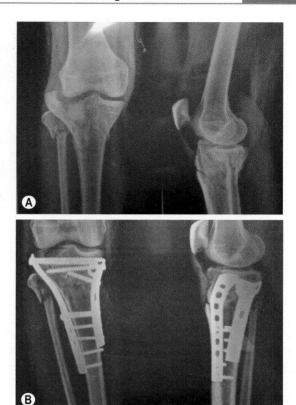

Fig. 10.4 (A) Preoperative radiograph of 48-year-old male with fractured supracondylar humerus. (B) Postoperative radiograph showing open reduction internal fixation using locking plate. Rehabilitation using muscle energy techniques (MET) was started 3 weeks post-surgery.

Fig. 10.5 (A) Preoperative radiograph of 58-year-old male with fractured upper end tibia. (B) Postoperative radiograph showing open reduction internal fixation using bicondylar plating. Rehabilitation using muscle energy techniques (MET) was started 1 week post-surgery.

of extension to 140 degrees of flexion, pronation: 0 to 90 degrees, supination: 0 to 90 degrees.

Scenario 3

Upper end tibia. We treated 23 patients in 2011 with distal radius fracture treated with ORIF. When the patient arrived, the standard preliminary assessment was carried out and there was a discussion with the operating surgeon. Following this, the treatment was initiated for the knee joint as well as the surrounding joints (ankle and hip).

Case 1 (Fig. 10.5A and B): A 58-year-old male diagnosed with closed left upper-end tibia with bicondylar split, without DNVC, treated with ORIF with bicondylar plating, presented in an outpatient department basis 1 week postoperatively. Initial knee ROM prior to

initiation of any exercises was from 0 degrees of extension to 20 degrees of flexion. MET in the form of SEIS was applied for 5 to 7 repetitions, once a day for 55 sessions, 6 days a week. After 55 sessions the knee ROM was 0 degrees of extension to 135 degrees of flexion.

Case 2 (Fig. 10.6A and B): A 45-year-old male diagnosed with closed right upper-end tibia with medial condylar split and depression, without DNVC, with old healed lower third tibia with an implant in situ, treated with ORIF with medial buttress plating, presented on outpatient department basis 4 weeks postoperatively. Initial knee ROM prior to initiation of any exercises was from 10 degrees of extension to 50 degrees of flexion. MET in the form of ILC was applied for 8 to 10 repetitions, once a day for 45 sessions, 6 days a week. After 45 sessions the knee ROM was 0 degrees of extension to 150 degrees of flexion.

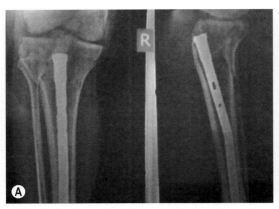 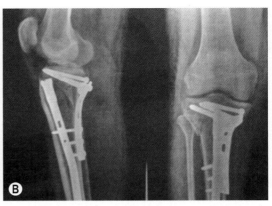

Fig. 10.6 (A) Preoperative radiograph of 45-year-old male with fractured upper end tibia. (B) Postoperative radiograph showing open reduction internal fixation using medial buttress plating. Rehabilitation using muscle energy techniques (MET) was started 4 weeks post-surgery.

Scenario 4

A single case study of arthroscopic single row repair for supraspinatus + infraspinatus with long head of biceps tenotomy with acromioplasty. Fig. 10.7A and B: A 50-year-old male, a businessman by profession, had a history of jerk to the shoulder and presented with difficulty in shoulder movements. Following an MRI report, the above surgery was performed.

Physiotherapy rehabilitation protocol as per the operating surgeon's advice was carried out, starting at 3 weeks postoperatively. Regular physiotherapy and progressively graded exercises were administered. Five months after the surgery, he presented with almost full ROM for all movements except external rotation which was restricted terminally.

After consulting with the operating surgeon, permission for the application of MET was given.

The patient was positioned supine with pillow support under the neck. The operated side glenohumeral joint was placed in 45 degrees abduction and 90 degrees of elbow flexion. The hand was taken into external rotation till the first resistance barrier was met. MET in the form of ILC was applied for 7 to 8 repetitions. After a break of 2 to 3 minutes, the glenohumeral joint was taken into 90 degrees abduction and 90 degrees elbow flexion and the same procedure was followed. MET was applied for 7 to 8 repetitions once a day for 3 weeks (18 sessions). Appropriate care was taken to ensure that the patient's pain tolerance threshold was not crossed.

Elbow ranges pre- and post- MET were as follows:

1. In the 45 to 90 degrees position, external rotation range improved from 50 to 95 degrees (Fig. 10.7A and B)

2. In the 90 to 90 degrees position, external rotation range improved from 40 to 90 degrees (Fig. 10.8A and B).

Scenario 5

Two cases of post-traumatic elbow stiffness undergoing open adhesiolysis. The first case was a capitulum fracture treated with ORIF with two Herbert's screws. One year postoperatively, the elbow went into stiffness with restricted ranges. The second case was a conserved radial neck fracture which at the end of 8 months postoperatively went into stiffness.

Open adhesiolysis was performed and on table ranges achieved were discussed with the operating surgeon. CPM and regular rehabilitation protocols were initiated. End ranges were not achieved during the follow-up that happened at 8 weeks. Permission to apply MET was received.

MET for improving flexion (Fig. 10. 9A and B) and extension (Fig. 10.10A and B) was applied as follows: Patient was positioned supine with shoulder placed at 45 degrees abduction. Elbow joint was taken into flexion to reach the first resistance barrier. Isolytic MET was applied and the joint was taken into a new range till the second resistance barrier was achieved. Similarly, the elbow joint was taken into extension in the same position to reach the first resistance barrier. Isolytic MET was applied for 5 to 8 repetitions once a day for 3 to 4 weeks (22 sessions).

To achieve end ranges of supination and pronation (Fig. 10.11A and B), the patient's position was seated, with a neutral shoulder position and 90 degrees of elbow flexion and mid-prone. MET was applied for 5 to

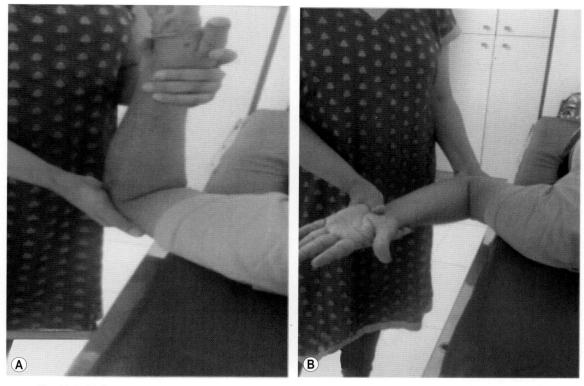

Fig. 10.7 (A) Starting position of 45 to 90 degrees position for muscle energy techniques (MET) application. (B) Post MET application in the 45 to 90 degrees position to achieve the end range.

8 repetitions once a day for 2 to 3 weeks (15 sessions). At the end of these 15 sessions, end-range restrictions were released and full ROM was achieved.

Scenario 6

Application of MET in the prehabilitation phase. A 21-year-old male presented with a history of twisting injury to the knee while football. MRI confirmed a complete ACL tear along with a grade 1 medial meniscus tear. He was advised to undergo prehabilitation training and an ACL reconstruction surgery was planned 3 weeks later.

On clinical examination, knee joint effusion was present. It was also observed that his quadriceps had gone into reflex myogenic inhibition because of which the flexion ROM of the knee joint was restricted.

Placing the patient in a prone position, the knee was taken into flexion to reach the first resistance barrier. Post-isometric relaxation form of MET was applied for 8 to 10 repetitions once a day for 10 sessions, achieving full flexion range before surgery which was planned at 3 weeks.

PRECAUTIONS AND CONTRAINDICATIONS

Using MET in the correct manner is very safe with no side effects. The most important precaution is using the correct force and leverage, especially when dealing with acute and subacute conditions. When applied to a previously injured or healing tissue, forces of contraction or stretch should be matched to the stage of healing and repair of the injury to avoid further tissue damage and to promote optimal healing (Lederman, 2005). ILC MET should be applied slowly and carefully with a request for patient feedback at all necessary times.

Situations where ILC MET cannot be applied:
- When the operating surgeon has not given permission to use MET.
- Compound fractures, open injuries and possibility of infection.
- Associated head injuries and poor general condition of the patient.

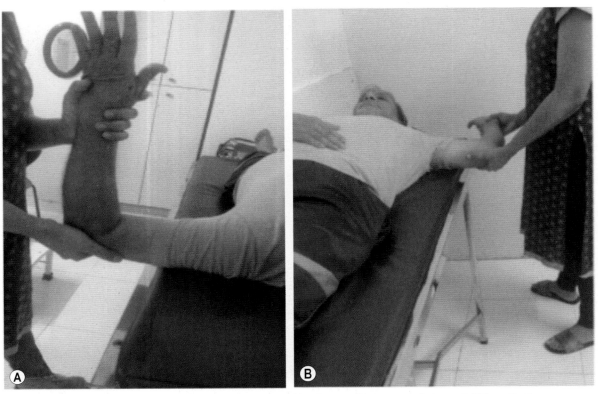

Fig. 10.8 (A) Starting position of 90 to 90 degrees position for muscle energy techniques (MET) application. (B) Post MET application in the 90 to 90 degrees position to achieve the end range.

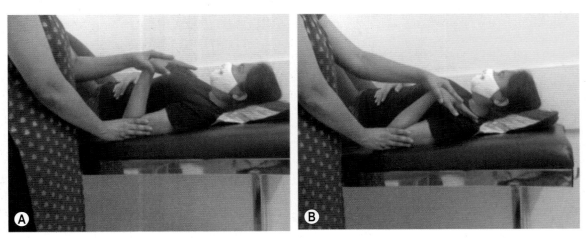

Fig. 10.9 (A) Flexion range of motion (ROM) in the first session was 100 degrees. (B) Flexion ROM which improved to 140 degrees after 3 weeks.

- Critically ill patients, conditions where metastasis is suspected.
- Osteoporosis, marked hypermobility/laxity.

- Children or individuals who are not able to actively participate in understanding the force-counterforce concept to generate a desired controlled contraction.

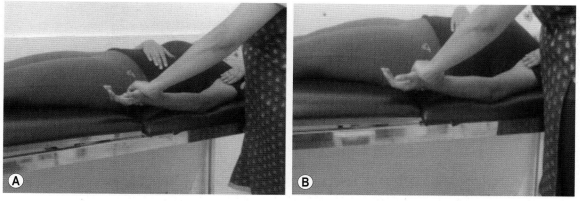

Fig. 10.10 (A) Extension range of motion (ROM) in the first session was 25 degrees. (B) Extension ROM which improved to 0 degrees after 4 weeks.

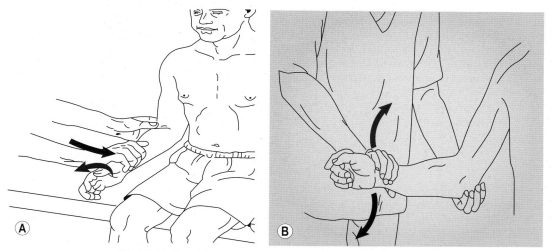

Fig. 10.11 (A and B) RED – patient force, BLACK – therapist force.

Complications can arise in situations when the patient is not compliant or does not understand the instructions given, thereby causing harm to the injured or repaired bony and/or soft tissues. Hence ILC MET needs to be applied with the utmost precautions, with simultaneous monitoring and constant feedback, during and post MET application.

FURTHER SCOPE

From the above few clinical application studies, it is relatively clear that the use of isotonic eccentric forms of MET (both ILC and SEIS) helped in gaining joint ROM, especially in the soft tissue changes had occurred in the treated as well as the surrounding joint areas. However, the gains in the joint ROM are measured clinically. Statistical analysis and further research would actually help quantify these clinically achieved gains in the joint ROM and give us consolidated data for the application of the technique in postoperative cases, thereby helping to replace or combine with the standard methods of gaining joint ROM. Subjectively, we would like to comment that pain tolerance is significantly better and there is an early recovery of ROM of the joints when these methods are used.

CONCLUSION

Isotonic eccentric forms of MET (both ILC and SEIS) are extremely useful in achieving joint ROM in post-operative case settings. Its application is not restricted to soft tissue dysfunctions but is advantageous over the standard stretching methods used in gaining early joint ROM in a surgically treated bone fracture. It has also been observed that ILC MET has proven beneficial in achieving end-range ROM restrictions in the late post-operative phase. Its scope in prehabilitation requires more clinical application to establish its benefits.

REFERENCES

Aagaard, P., 2018. Autogenic recurrent Renshaw inhibition is elevated in human spinal motor neurones during maximal eccentric muscle contraction in vivo. Acta Physiol. (Oxf.). 223 (4), e13107. doi:10.1111/apha.13107.

Andrade, R.J., Freitas, S.R., Hug, F., Le Sant, G., Lacourpaille, L., Gross, R., Quillard, J.-B., McNair, P.J., Nordez, A., 2020. Chronic effects of muscle and nerve-directed stretching on tissue mechanics. J. Appl. Physiol. 129 (5), 1011–1023.

Askling, C.M., Tengvar, M., Tarassova, O., Thorstensson, A., 2014. Acute hamstring injuries in Swedish elite sprinters and jumpers: a prospective randomised controlled clinical trial comparing two rehabilitation protocols. Br. J. Sports Med. 48 (7), 532–539. doi:10.1136/bjsports-2013-093214.

Bloomfield, S.A., 1997. Changes in musculoskeletal structure and function with prolonged bed rest. Med. Sci. Sports Exerc. 29 (2), 197–206.

Blum, K.P., Lamotte D'Incamps, B., Zytnicki, D., Ting, L.H., 2017. Force encoding in muscle spindles during stretch of passive muscle. PLoS Comput. Biol. 13 (9), e1005767. doi:10.1371/journal.pcbi.1005767.

Bogdanis, G.C., 2012. Effects of physical activity and inactivity on muscle fatigue. Front. Physiol. 3, 142. doi:10.3389/fphys.2012.00142

Cação-Benedini, L.O., Ribeiro, P.G., Prado, C.M., Chesca, D.L., Mattiello-Sverzut, A.C., 2014. Immobilization and therapeutic passive stretching generate thickening and increase the expression of laminin and dystrophin in skeletal muscle. Braz. J. Med. Biol. Res. 47 (6), 483–491. doi:10.1590/1414-431x20143521.

Chleboun, G.S., Howell, J.N., Conatser, R.R., Giesey, J.J., 1997. The relationship between elbow flexor volume and angular stiffness at the elbow. Clin. Biomech. (Bristol, Avon) 12, 383–392.

David, H., 1999. Osteopathic Approach to Soft Tissue Therapy. Hemme Approach Publications, Florida.

De Andrade, J.R., Grant, C., Dixon, A.S., 1965. Joint distension and reflex inhibition in the knee. J. Bone Joint Surg. Am. 47, 313–322.

Donatelli, R., Owens-Burkhart, A., 1981. Effects of immobilization on the extensibility of periarticular connective tissue. J. Orthopaed. Sports Phys. Ther. 3, 67–72.

Faqih, A.I., Bedekar, N., Shyam, A., Sancheti, P., 2019. Effects of muscle energy technique on pain, range of motion and function in patients with post-surgical elbow stiffness: a randomised controlled trial. Hong Kong Physiother. J. 39 (1), 25–33. doi:10.1142/S1013702519500033.

Freitas, S.R., Mendes, B., Le Sant, G., Andrade, R.J., Nordez, A., Milanovic, Z., 2018. Can chronic stretching change the muscle-tendon mechanical properties? A review . Scand. J. Med. Sci. Sports 28, 794–806. doi:10.1111/sms.12957.

Garrett, W.E., Nikolaou, P.K., Ribbeck, B.M., Glisson, R.R., Seaber, A.V., 1988. The effect of muscle architecture on the biomechanical failure properties of skeletal muscles under passive extension. Am. J. Sports Med. 16, 7–12.

Gerber, J.P., Marcus, R.L., Dibble, L.E., Greis, P.E., Burks, R.T., LaStayo, P.C., 2009. Effects of early progressive eccentric exercise on muscle size and function after anterior cruciate ligament reconstruction: a 1-year follow-up study of a randomized clinical trial. Phys. Ther. 89, 51–59. doi:10.2522/ptj.20070189.

Gorkovenko, A.V., Sawczyn, S., Bulgakova, N.V., Jasczur-Nowicki, J., Mishchenko, V.S., Kostyukov, A.I., 2012. Muscle agonist-antagonist interactions in an experimental joint model . Exp. Brain Res. 222 (4), 399–414. doi:10.1007/s00221-012-3227-0.

Gossman, M.R., Sarhmann, S.A., Rose, S.J., 1982. Review of length associated changes in muscles-experimental evidence and clinical implication. Phys. Ther. 62, 1799–1808.

Guissard, N., 1988. Muscle stretching and motor neurone excitability. Eur. J. Appl. Physiol. 58, 47–52.

Harrelson, G.L., 1991. Physiologic Factors of Rehabilitation. Physical Rehabilitation of the Injured Athlete. W.B Saunders, Philadelphia, pp. 13–34.

Hertling, D., Kessler, R., 2006. Management of Common Musculoskeletal Disorders – Physical Therapy Principles and Methods, third ed. Lippincott, Philadelphia, New York.

Herzog, W., Powers, K., Johnston, K., Duvall, M., 2015. A new paradigm for muscle contraction. Front. Physiol. 6, 174. doi:10.3389/fphys.2015.00174.

Hody, S., Croisier, J.L., Bury, T., Rogister, B., Leprince, P., 2019. Eccentric muscle contractions: risks and benefits. Front. Physiol. 10, 536. doi:10.3389/fphys.2019.00536.

Janda, V., 1991. Muscle spasm – a proposed procedure for differential diagnosis. Man. Med. 1001, 6136–6139.

Johns, R.J., Wright, V., 1962. Relative importance of various tissues in joint stiffness. J. Appl. Physiol. 17, 824–828.

Karatzaferi, C., Franks-Skiba, K., Cooke, R., 2008. Inhibition of shortening velocity of skinned skeletal muscle fibers in conditions that mimic fatigue. Am. J. Physiol. Regul. Integr. Comp. Physiol. 294, R948–R955. doi:10.1152/ajpregu.00541.2007.

Karatzaferi, C., Myburgh, K.H., Chinn, M.K., Franks-Skiba, K., Cooke, R., 2003. Effect of an ADP analog on isometric force and ATPase activity of active muscle fibers. Am. J. Physiol. Cell Physiol. 284, C816–C825. doi:10.1152/ajpcell.00291.2002.

Kay, A.D., Blazevich, A.J., Fraser, M., Ashmore, L., Hill, M.W., 2020. Isokinetic eccentric exercise substantially improves mobility, muscle strength and size, but not postural sway metrics in older adults, with limited regression observed following a detraining period. Eur. J. Appl. Physiol. 120 (11), 2383–2395. doi:10.1007/s00421-020-04466-7.

Kisner, C., Colby, L., 2002. Therapeutic Exercises Foundation and Techniques, fourth ed. Jaypee Brothers, New Delhi, India, pp. 171–180.

Klotz, T., Bleiler, C., Röhrle, O., 2021. A physiology-guided classification of active-stress and active-strain approaches for continuum-mechanical modeling of skeletal muscle tissue. Front. Physiol. 12, 685531. doi:10.3389/fphys.2021.685531

Koltyn, K.F., Garvin, A.W., Gardiner, R.L., Nelson, T.F., 1996. Perception of pain following aerobic exercise. Med. Sci. Sports Exerc. 28, 1418–1421.

Konno, R.N., Nigam, N., Wakeling, J.M., 2021. Modelling extracellular matrix and cellular contributions to whole muscle mechanics. PLoS One 16 (4), e0249601. doi:10.1371/journal.pone.0249601.

Konno, R.N., Nigam, N., Wakeling, J.M., Ross, S.A., 2022. The contributions of extracellular matrix and sarcomere properties to passive muscle stiffness in cerebral palsy. Front. Physiol. 12, 804188. doi:10.3389/fphys.2021.804188.

Kosek, E., Ekholm, J., Hansson, P., 1996. Modulation of pressure pain thresholds during and following isometric contraction in patients with fibromyalgia and in healthy controls. Pain 64, 415–423.

Kubo, K., 2018. Effects of static stretching on mechanical properties and collagen fiber orientation of the Achilles tendon in vivo. Clin. Biomech. 60, 115–120. https://pubmed.ncbi.nlm.nih.gov/30342379/.

Lannersten, L., Kosek, E., 2010. Dysfunction of endogenous pain inhibition during exercise with painful muscles in patients with shoulder myalgia and fibromyalgia. Pain 151, 77–86.

Latash, M.L., 2018. Muscle coactivation: definitions, mechanisms, and functions. J. Neurophysiol. 120 (1), 88–104.

Lederman, E., 2005. The Science and Practice of Manual Therapy, second ed. Elsevier Churchill Livingstone, Edinburgh.

Lewit, K., 1985. The muscular and articular factor in movement restriction. Man. Med. 1, 83–85.

Lyle, M.A., Nichols, T.R., 2019. Evaluating intermuscular Golgi tendon organ feedback with twitch contractions. J. Physiol. 597 (17), 4627–4642. doi:10.1113/JP277363.

Magnusson, S.P., Simonsen, E.B., Aagaard, P., 1996. Biomechanical responses to repeated stretches in human hamstring muscle in vivo. Am. J. Sports Med. 24, 622–628.

Malliaropoulos, N., Papalexandris, S., Papalada, A., Papacostas, E., 2004. The role of stretching in rehabilitation of hamstring injuries: 80 athletes follow-up. Med. Sci. Sports Exerc. 36, 756–759.

Mlyniec, A., Dabrowska, S., Heljak, M., Weglarz, W.P., Wojcik, K., Ekiert-Radecka, M., Obuchowicz, R., Swieszkowski, W., 2021. The dispersion of viscoelastic properties of fascicle bundles within the tendon results from the presence of interfascicular matrix and flow of body fluids. Mater. Sci. Eng. C 130.

Nagano, K., Uoya, S., Nagano, Y., 2019. Effects of antagonistic muscle contraction exercises on ankle joint range of motion. J. Phys. Ther. Sci. 31 (7), 526–529. doi:10.1589/jpts.31.526.

Osama, M., 2021. Effects of autogenic and reciprocal inhibition muscle energy techniques on isometric muscle strength in neck pain: a randomized controlled trial. J. Back Musculoskelet. Rehabil. 34 (4), 555–564. doi:10.3233/BMR-200002.

Parmar, S., Shyam, A., Sabnis, S., Sancheti, P., 2011. The effect of isolytic contraction and passive manual stretching on pain and knee range of motion after hip surgery: a prospective, double-blinded, randomized study. Hongkong Physiother. J. 29, 25–30.

Pujol, N., Boisrenoult, P., Beaufils, P., 2015. Post-traumatic knee stiffness: surgical techniques. Orthop. Traumatol. Surg. Res. 101 (1), S179–S186.

Spencer, J.D., Hayes, K.C., Alexander, I.J., 1984. Knee joint effusion and quadriceps reflex inhibition in man. Arch. Phys. Med. Rehabil. 65, 171.

Thomas, A., D'Silva, C., Mohandas, L., Pais, S.M.J., Samuel, S.R., 2020. Effect of muscle energy techniques V/S active range of motion exercises on shoulder function post modified radical neck dissection in patients with head and neck cancer – a randomized clinical trial . Asian Pac. J. Cancer Prev. 21 (8), 2389–2393. doi:10.31557/APJCP.2020.21.8.2389.

Van Buskirk, R.L., 1990. Nociceptive reflexes and the somatic dysfunction. J. Am. Osteopath. Assoc. 90 (9), 792–809.

Vilchez-Barrera, M.E., Hernán-Santana, G., 2020. Eficacia de las técnicas de energía muscular en síndromes dolorosos musculoesqueléticos: una revisión sistemática. Fisioterapia 42 (3), 145–156. https://doi.org/10.1016/j.ft.2020.01.003.

William, P.E., Goldspink, G., 1978. Changes in sarcomere length and physiological properties in immobilized muscle. J. Anat. 127, 459–468.

Ylinen, J., 2008. Stretching Therapy for Sports and Manual Therapies. Section 1 – Stretching Theory, English edition. Churchill Livingstone, Elsevier, Philadelphia.

11

MET in the Physical Therapy Setting

Eric Wilson

CHAPTER CONTENTS

Low-back pain (LBP) is managed with a diverse assortment of treatments that run the spectrum from well-constructed theories to ridiculous gadgets, and all points in between. Perhaps the reason there are so many different 'treatments' for LBP is that none of them seems to work all of the time. This is an unsettling thought. Instead, it may be that 'low-back pain' is not a single entity but a vast array of impairments whose consequences can be summed up with three letters – LBP. One of the problems inherent in treating patients with LBP is the difficulty of determining which interventions to apply to which patients. Why does *manipulation* work for some patients but not others? Why does *traction* resolve some patients' symptoms but exacerbate others?

The medical model tells us that 'diagnosis drives treatment'. This is true in most cases: a patient with 'knee pain', for example, would receive a different course of treatment if the source of the pain was diagnosed as patellar tendinopathy, versus an iliotibial band syndrome. Unfortunately, trying to apply this medical model to LBP is akin to attempting to force a square peg into a round hole because LBP is not homogenous. While often portrayed as homogenous, a pathoanatomical diagnosis is only available in approximately 2.99%

of all LBP cases (Henschke et al., 2009). Therefore, the identification of subgroups of patients with LBP who respond favourably to specific interventions has been deemed a research priority (Borkan et al., 1998; Pransky et al., 2011).

CLASSIFICATION MODELS

This mandate has produced numerous classification models, most of which have not withstood the attention of repeated testing via randomised controlled trials. One classification model, originally reported by Delitto et al. (1995) has weathered the rigours of repeated testing and, as a result, has been refined over the past two and a half decades into a valid and clinically useful tool. Some people may confuse the term *classification model* with that of *cookbook therapy*. A cookbook approach requires all patients receive the same treatment, regardless of their clinical presentation. This would be akin to providing McKenzie's extension exercises to all patients with LBP regardless of their signs and symptoms. While some patients would improve from this treatment, most would not. A classification model, on the other hand, attempts to group patients into categories based on the treatment that will provide them with the most benefit. Consider a cookbook approach to be like a hammer – everything gets treated like a nail regardless of its individual characteristics, whereas a classification model makes the hammer more efficient (by finding it more nails and fewer screws to hit).

A classification model also allows the physical therapist to work outside of the often-limiting confines of a diagnosis. The difference between a *diagnosis* and a *classification* is striking. Diagnosis can be defined as *the means of establishing the source of a patient's impairment or symptoms,* while classification is *a method of arranging clinical data into predetermined categories of impairments or diagnoses in order to make informed decisions regarding treatment.* Classification systems are beneficial in the treatment of LBP because most patients with LBP have no attributable pathology, the population comprises numerous heterogenous subgroups, and the use of a classification-based scheme may allow clinicians to treat their patients more effectively (Riddle, 1998; Fritz et al., 2003; Fritz & Brennan, 2007a; Fritz et al., 2007b, 2007c). In addition, these attributes of the classification system allow closer adherence to the model of whole-person healthcare, as discussed in Chapter 1.

An additional benefit of using a classification-based model is that it does not rely on the acuity of a patient's symptoms to drive the treatment process. A symptom acuity or time model often relies on time since injury, or time since onset of symptoms. If the time model was adequate, physical therapists would rarely treat patients with severe symptoms and/or inflammation, months or years after an injury occurred. Using the time model, all patients should be completely healed within 12 weeks of the initial injury, barring the effects of infection, etc. The vast majority of patients who present for physical therapy do not fit into this category.

Instead, the classification-based model uses 'staging' (Delitto et al., 1995; Fritz et al., 2003; Alrwaily et al., 2016) in an attempt to classify patients into one of several categories during the initial evaluation. Staging also advocates the continuous reassessment of patients in order to determine if they warrant reclassification. This component of a classification-based model is ideal since patients typically see their physical therapist more frequently than they do other healthcare providers.

Staging Classification and Indexing

Staging is based on patient symptoms and functional disability (measured with disability indexes) in order to 'classify' patients. The use of patient-reported measures of disability (disability indexes) is a key component of the classification model and as such warrants further discussion. While there are numerous disability indexes available to clinicians, we will focus on two of the more clinician-friendly in classifying and treating patients with LBP – the Oswestry (ODI) and the Fear Avoidance Belief Questionnaire (FABQ).

The Oswestry Disability Index (Fairbank et al., 1980) is one of the best-known disability indexes for use with patients with LBP. The ODI is a 10-item, 100-point index in which higher scores equate to more disability. It has been reported as reliable, valid and sensitive to change, and is universally accepted as the gold standard for LBP research (Kopec et al., 1996; Deyo et al., 1998) with over 6900 results in PubMed. Moreover, it has a reported minimal clinically important difference (MCID) of six points (Fritz & Irrgang, 2001), which allows the clinician to measure a true change in a patient's status. Research has demonstrated that patients with a score of 12% or less are capable of returning to full occupational or recreational activities. The ODI takes approximately 3 to 5 minutes for a patient to complete and requires less than 30 seconds to score.

The Fear Avoidance Belief Questionnaire (FABQ) was originally described by Waddell et al. (1993) and measures a patient's fear avoidance using two subscales: physical activity and work. The FABQ has been shown to predict disability and work loss, as well as future disability (Waddell et al., 1993; Hadijistavropoulos & Craig, 1994; Klenerman et al., 1995; Crombez et al., 1999). The FABQ has also been shown to be a key component of the clinical prediction rule (CPR) for thrust joint manipulation (TJM) and LBP (Flynn et al., 2002; Childs et al., 2004; Hicks et al., 2005; Cleland et al., 2009).

Both the ODI and FABQ are powerful tools that are appropriate for use in almost all orthopaedic physical therapy settings.

The original treatment-based classification (TBC) approach for the treatment of LBP (Delitto et al., 1995) demonstrated that matching treatments to classifications resulted in faster, more efficient and cost-effective care (Fritz et al., 2003; Fritz & Brennan, 2007a; Fritz et al., 2007b, 2007c). The classification system is divided into three distinct stages:

1. Patients in Stage 1 are unable to perform basic functions (walk <1/4 mile, stand <15 minutes, sit <30 minutes) and typically have an ODI score between 40%

and 60%. The primary goal of physical therapy during this stage is *pain modulation.*

2. Patients in Stage 2 are able to accomplish basic functions but are limited in their activities of daily living (ADLs). Their ODI scores typically fall between 20% and 40%. Physical therapy goals are to *continue to modulate pain and to begin addressing impairments.*

3. The third and final stage pertains to a patient's *inability to return to high-demand activity* such as manual labour or athletic competition. The ODI scores for patients in this stage are typically below 20% and the goal of physical therapy should be to facilitate their return to their previous activity level. It has been this author's experience that MET is a very effective intervention for patients in both Stages 1 and 2.

Further Refinement of the Treatment-Based Classification
TBC 2.0

Fritz et al. (2003) modified the classification scheme originally described by Delitto and compared it with the *Agency for Healthcare Research and Quality* (AHCPR) guidelines. The authors randomised 76 subjects with work-related LBP of less than 3 weeks' duration into either the AHCPR group or the Classification group. Patients in the Classification group were placed into one of four categories: mobilisation, specific exercise, stabilisation or traction based upon the most current physical examination criteria in the peer-reviewed literature at that time (Table 11.1). Criteria for the mobilisation category included unilateral symptoms without signs of nerve root compression, asymmetrical lumbar side-bending restrictions, lumbar hypomobility and sacroiliac dysfunction. Patients in the AHCPR group received treatment based upon AHCPR guidelines (staying active, reassurance, low-stress aerobics, general muscle conditioning). ODI measures taken at intake and at 4 weeks demonstrated a statistically significant difference ($P = .031$) in favour of the Classification group. Return to work status was also measured at the 4-week mark demonstrating a statistically significant difference ($P = .017$) in favour of the Classification group.

TBC 3.0

Alrwaily and colleagues (2016) further refined the TBC in 2016 by dividing the classification into three primary classifications that more reflects the rehabilitation continuum: Symptom Modulation, Movement Control and Functional Optimisation (Fig. 11.1). When compared to TBC 2.0, this refinement moves *Stabilisation Exercises* from Symptom Modulation to Movement Control under the *motor control* subclassification while adding the *active rest* subclassification to Symptom Modulation. Restoring motion is the bridge between Symptom Modulation and Movement Control, whereas muscle endurance training is the bridge between Movement Control and Functional Optimisation.

In order for this TBC scheme to be successful, the subclassification criteria for each of the three classifications must be as evidence-based as possible. Flynn et al. (2002) investigated the factors that favoured success with SI joint TJM in 75 patients with LBP. The authors developed a CPR based upon five factors:
- Duration of symptoms less than 16 days
- FABQ work subscale less than 19 points
- Symptoms not distal to the knee
- At least one hip with internal rotation greater than 35 degrees
- Hypomobility and pain at one or more lumbar levels with posterior-anterior (PA) spring testing.

Flynn reported that the more factors present, the greater the chance of success with TJM. For example, a patient with four out of five factors present would have a 95% chance of success as opposed to 68% for a patient

TABLE 11.1	Classification Criteria for Mobilisation Category	
Category	**Examination Findings**
Mobilisation category	Unilateral symptoms without signs of nerve root compression
Sacroiliac joint pattern	Positive findings for SI joint dysfunction using pelvic symmetry and standing and seated forward flexion tests
	Unilateral symptoms without signs of nerve root compression
Lumbar pattern	Assessment of lumbar side-bending asymmetry lumbar hypomobility

Adapted from Fritz et al. (2007a).

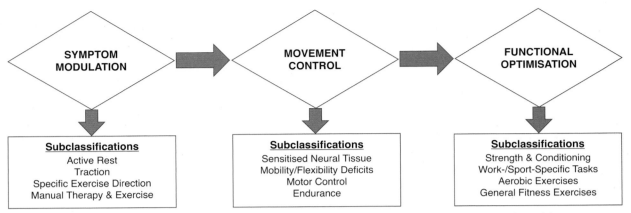

Fig. 11.1 Modified treatment-based classification system for patients with low-back pain. (Adapted from Alrwaily et al., 2016.)

with only three factors present. While the CPR holds true regardless of which factors are present, the authors reported the most important factor for success was 'duration of symptoms less than 16 days' with a positive likelihood ratio of 4.3. Note these criteria differ significantly from the physical examination criteria used by Fritz et al. (2003). This CPR was a critical step in establishing valid examination findings in order to sub-classify patients with LBP into the mobilisation category.

The next step in validating this CPR was performed by Childs et al. (2004). The authors randomised 131 patients into either a TJM and exercise group or an exercise-only group. Each group received five treatments and follow-ups at 1 week, 4 weeks and 6 months. The TJM/exercise group ($n = 70$) received TJM and range of motion exercises for just the first two treatments, and then stabilisation exercises for the last three treatments. The exercise group received stabilisation exercises only. Childs reported that a patient with four of the five factors reported by Flynn et al., had a 92% chance of success (+LR 13.2) with TJM. Moreover, the authors reported that a patient with less than three factors present only had a 7% chance of success (−LR 0.10) with manipulation.

While the research by Flynn et al. (2002) and Childs et al. (2004) is encouraging for the relative weight it adds to the literature regarding the effectiveness of 'manual therapy', newer evidence forces us to proceed cautiously in extrapolating the results of TJM interventions to muscle energy technique (MET). Cleland et al. (2009) compared two different TJM interventions with prone PA mobilisations utilising the same study design as Childs et al. (2004). The authors randomised 112 subjects into

one of three groups. Those that received the prone PA mobilisations received two bouts of 60-second Maitland Grade IV PA mobilisations over the spinous processes of two lumbar segments. The other two groups either received either a supine or side-lying TJM intervention. While there was no statistically significant difference between the two groups receiving TJM, the two TJM groups did demonstrate a statistically significant difference over the PA mobilisation group at the 1-week ($P < .001$), 4-week ($P < .001$) and 6-month ($P = .009$) follow-ups. The authors believe that the difference found between the outcomes of the TJM and mobilisation groups was due to the 'thrust', although the group that received PA mobilisations did exceed the MCID of the ODI after 1 week. However, as we will see later in this chapter, MET has several neurophysiologic mechanisms in its favour – even without the thrust.

MET STUDIES

The direct effects of MET have been examined in few studies. Wilson et al. (2003) published the first randomised controlled trial to investigate the efficacy of MET at the lumbar spine in symptomatic populations. Sixteen subjects (8 males, 8 females; ages 19 to 44) with LBP (duration 2 to 9 weeks) were randomised with stratification (age, gender, ODI score) into the control group ($n = 8$) or the experimental group ($n = 8$). Each group received identical supervised neuromuscular re-education and strengthening exercises with the experimental group receiving the independent variable (MET, five isometric repetitions utilising post-contraction relaxation phenomena). Each group received physical therapy twice a week for 4 weeks for a total of eight visits. ODI scores were obtained at the first and eighth visits. A two-tailed t-test revealed a statistically significant difference ($P > .05$) in favour of the experimental group. The mean number of muscle energy interventions required for the experimental group was 3.3 (range 2 to 4). This data supports what many clinicians have known for years: MET is a reliable means to return patients to full activity in a quick and efficient manner.

Unfortunately, there is a paucity of literature supporting the reliability of determining which spinal level(s) a clinician should direct the MET towards. Three systematic reviews have addressed the reliability of spinal palpatory diagnostics. Hestbaek and Leboeuf-Yde (2000) determined that while motion palpation was valid, the overall reliability was 'poor'. Huijbregts (2002) stated there were too many flaws in the methods and statistics of the studies he reviewed to demonstrate the value of spinal palpation. Finally, Seffinger et al. (2004) concluded that the results for motion palpation were 'poor' regardless of the examiner's experience. Moreover, the only study to report the reliability of detecting somatic dysfunctions by palpating positional asymmetry at the spine as reported by Greenman demonstrated 'poor' reliability ($\kappa = .34$) (Degenhardt et al., 2005).

However, all is not lost. Careful examination of the literature clearly shows us that studies that demonstrate poor diagnostic reliability have focused on the palpation of end-feels (Boline et al., 1988; Mootz et al., 1989; Keating et al., 1990), the assessment of joint play (Gonnella et al., 1982; Jull & Bullock, 1987) and passive range of motion (Bergstrom & Courtis, 1986; Jull & Bullock, 1987; Leboeuf et al., 1989). In fact, only Leboeuf and colleagues studied symptomatic subjects.

Positive Reliability Study

Only one study to date (Wilson, 2008) has addressed the reliability of detecting a mobility restriction in the lumbar spine via static palpation and position assessment in symptomatic subjects. While the results of this study are favourable, some limitations should be stated from the start. This study addressed intra-rater reliability only, and it has only been published as an abstract. It has been presented in the United States at state and national forums, including the 2008 American Academy of

Orthopedic Manual Physical Therapists National Convention where it garnered 'Best Platform Presentation' honours. While promising, the results must be generalised with caution.

A total of 750 patients were screened for inclusion over an 18-month period by a single clinician. Inclusion criteria included an initial ODI score between 30% and 60%, a chief complaint of pain in the lumbar spine, only one lumbar somatic dysfunction present, and at least four of five clinical predictors for success with manipulation as described by Flynn et al. (2002). Exclusion criteria were identical to those used in the studies published by Flynn et al. (2002) and Childs et al. (2004). Subject demographics (mean and standard deviation) were as follows: age 32 (9.1), duration of symptoms 35.4 days (11.1) and ODI 50.18 (6.3). 34.5% of the subjects were female. Fifty-five subjects met the criteria for inclusion and each subject underwent three sessions that were 2 to 3 days apart:

- Session 1: Initial ODI and palpatory assessment 1 using a second person as a recorder
- Session 2: Palpatory assessment 2 and treatment with muscle energy (treating the named dysfunction from Session 2)
- Session 3: Final ODI

In order to have agreement, the palpatory assessments from Sessions 1 and 2 had to match and there had to be at least a 12% improvement in the ODI from Session 3. Twelve percent improvement reflects twice the MCID for the ODI as reported by Fritz and Irrgang (2001). If both criteria were met, agreement occurred. If either (or both) criteria were not met, agreement did not occur. Regardless of the outcome, the patients were then discharged from the study and treatment continued.

The operational definition for making the assessment varied from previous methods in two important ways. First, the author placed their thumbs over the area of the laminae and applied an anteriorly directed force *while observing for equal nailbed blanching*. This prevents a common mistake: palpating harder with your dominant hand. When this occurs, the examiner will almost always observe an 'asymmetry' in the transverse plane towards their non-dominant hand. The second variation required the examiner to observe for the asymmetry by placing their eyes on the same plane as the vertebral segment of interest (Fig. 11.2A and B) and looking at a point between the segments (area of the spinous process) with their dominant eye. This does two things:

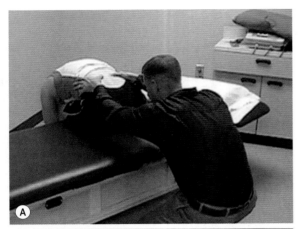

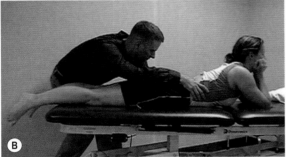

Fig. 11.2 Assessment for dysfunction by placing eyes in the same plane as the spine. (A) ERS dysfunction. (B) FRS dysfunction.

(1) it prevents the examiner from staring at one side versus the other. If the examiner stares at one side, they will typically be fooled into thinking that is the side of the asymmetry; (2) by placing their eyes on the same plane as the vertebral segment the examiner does not rely on depth perception to make their assessment. The author also standardised the patient positions in flexion, neutral and extension in order to further improve the reliability of the assessment.

The author made an identical assessment on Sessions 1 and 2 on 51 of 55 patients. Those same 51 patients

met or exceeded the 12% improvement in the ODI and had a mean percent-change score of 31.8%. The author's assessments between Sessions 1 and 2 did not agree on four patients. The mean percent-change score for these four patients was only 11.7%. The lack of agreement predicted less success with the MET intervention. The percent agreement and Kappa statistics can be found in Table 11.2. This research provides some preliminary support for a revised operational definition for performing the palpatory assessment prior to the use of MET.

Misconceptions in the Literature

Physical therapists treat appendicular musculoskeletal impairments with a diverse and vast array of interventions and techniques. Yet, some clinicians treat spinal impairments as if they were an entity separate from the rest of the body. However, not all fault lies with the individual practitioners. Several prominent articles in the peer-reviewed literature have perpetuated the belief that the treatment of 'low-back pain' has its own set of rules, regardless of their contradictions to basic rehabilitative science. Some have even gone as far as to discredit the efficacy of physical therapy for patients with spinal pain. Therefore, a brief discussion of a few articles that have been detrimental to the use of physical therapy to combat LBP is warranted. An understanding of each article's limitations is important for educating referral sources and patients alike.

The primary concern with the following two articles is that they perpetuate the belief that physical therapy is either not indicated for patients with LBP or that it should only be tried after standard care by a general practitioner has failed. There is evidence in the literature supporting manual therapy and other physical therapy interventions in the treatment of LBP (Hadler et al., 1987; MacDonald & Bell, 1990; Spratt et al., 1993; Stankovic & Johnell, 1995; O'Sullivan et al., 1997; Hides et al., 2001; Flynn et al., 2002; Wilson et al., 2003; Childs et al., 2004; Cleland et al., 2006, 2009; Hicks et al., 2005;

TABLE 11.2	**Reliability of Lumbar Palpatory Assessment**			
Restriction	Agreement	% Agreement	Kappa	Significance
Right flexion	12/14	85.7%	0.714	P < .001
Left flexion	14/15	93.3%	0.867	P < .001
Right extension	8/9	88.8%	0.778	P < .01
Left extension	17/17	100%	1.0	P < .001

Browder et al., 2007; Fritz & Brennan, 2007a; Fritz et al., 2007b, 2007c; Franke et al., 2014; Hidalgo et al., 2014; Paige et al., 2017; Shekelle et al., 2017).

Unfortunately, earlier clinical trials investigating their efficacy have not sought to determine which patients might benefit from a specific treatment (Dettori et al., 1995; Faas et al., 1995; Cherkin et al., 1998). As one might expect, the results of these trials are usually not strong enough to advocate one intervention over another. This has led to the argument that physical therapy offers no advantage over standard care provided by general practitioners. This line of thought may skew the referral practice of general practitioners who would otherwise refer their patients with spinal pain to physical therapy. This causes two problems. First, delaying physical therapy care can impede the patients' recovery (Wilson et al., 2003; Childs et al., 2004; Wand et al., 2004; Nordeman et al., 2006). As is true of most medical conditions, whether a bacterial infection or an acute onset of LBP, the sooner the patient receives appropriate treatment, the greater the likelihood of that treatment's success. Finally, recent findings in the literature suggest that the societal increase of chronic LBP can be linked to improperly managed acute LBP (Hides et al., 1994, 1996, 2001).

Some authors have reported that 80% to 90% of patients with LBP will 'spontaneously' recover within 3 months (Faas et al., 1993; Malanga & Nadler, 1999). In light of this statement, it is necessary to question the odds of the 'spontaneous' recovery of a ruptured anterior cruciate ligament or of a flexor tendon tear in the same time period. While the over-generalisation is obvious, the validity of such statements should be questioned rather than being accepted at face value.

Faas et al. (1993) randomised 473 patients with acute, nonspecific LBP of less than 3 weeks' duration into one of three treatment groups: placebo, usual care by a general practitioner, and physical therapy. The authors concluded that 'patients who are referred to a physiotherapist for exercise therapy or to a back school in this way receive a lot of needless, expensive attention for complaints that in most cases would have disappeared spontaneously anyway'. A critical review of this study identified limitations in the use of the Nottingham Health Profile Questionnaire as an outcome measure, assessment of patient compliance, and in the authors' rationale for their choice of physical therapy intervention – Williams' flexion exercises. The results of this study are limited to the lack of demonstrated efficacy of Williams' flexion exercises, and should not be extrapolated to the profession of physical therapy in the treatment of LBP. Unfortunately, this article has made many healthcare providers sceptical regarding physical therapy's efficacy in treating this impairment.

Cherkin et al. (1998) compared the efficacy of physical therapy, chiropractic care and an educational booklet in patients with acute LBP. Three hundred and twenty-one patients were randomised without stratification into three treatment groups as follows: McKenzie treatment by physical therapists, high-velocity/low-amplitude (HVLA) thrust spinal manipulation by chiropractors, and an educational booklet provided by general practitioners. Patients who sought care from a primary care physician who continued to have pain 7 days after consultation were eligible for inclusion in this study. These potential subjects were screened by research assistants utilising the SF-36 health survey questionnaire and a list of exclusion criteria that included sciatica. The authors reported that patients receiving physical therapy and chiropractic care had only slightly better outcomes than patients in the booklet group that only neared significance ($P = .05$) at the 1-year follow-up. A critical review of this study revealed limitations in the use of a 'bothersome' scale as an outcome measure, discrepancies between the number of treatments in the McKenzie and chiropractic groups and the lack of control for exercise in the chiropractic and booklet groups. The limitations in this study's design weaken the authors' conclusions that physical therapy and spinal manipulation are no better than an educational booklet for patients with acute LBP.

CLINICAL UTILISATION OF MUSCLE ENERGY TECHNIQUE

Traditionally, MET has been utilised to break the pain/spasm cycle as described by Roland (1986), restore normal structure and function to a joint or motion segment (often overlapping with breaking the pain/spasm cycle), and to strengthen previously inhibited and/or weakened muscles. This paradigm can be easily shifted to follow the classification model previously reported by Alrwaily and colleagues (2016). Recall that the stages of the classification system (TBC 3.0) involve (1) Symptom Modulation, (2) Movement Control and (3) Functional

Optimisation. MET is an exceptional intervention for patients in the first two of these stages.

Staging

Clinical Correlation: LBP and Ankle Sprains

Most physical therapists who work in an outpatient orthopaedic setting feel comfortable treating a patient with an ankle sprain. The same principles used to treat an ankle sprain can be used to treat a patient with a spinal impairment. Let's quickly compare the two injuries and their treatments. When a patient sustains an acute ankle injury, the physical therapist will typically utilise the PRICE mnemonic (protect, rest, ice, compression, elevation) during the initial treatment in order to limit the effects of the injury and to reduce pain. This coincides with the Symptom Modulation stage of Alrwaily's classification model.

Stage 1: Symptom Modulation

We typically modulate pain at the injured ankle by placing the patient on a partial or non-weight-bearing status, as well as the using either tape or a brace. These treatments serve to keep stresses off of the injured tissues, primarily the ligaments and joint capsule. When a patient injures the back, we can use MET to protect the area by restoring normal structure and function to the joint (taking the stresses off the soft tissues) and by decreasing pain. MET is an excellent intervention for breaking the pain/spasm cycle. Passive manual therapy techniques (e.g. joint mobilisations, HVLA thrust techniques) assist in breaking the pain/spasm cycle by inhibiting alpha motor-neuron activity via a stretch reflex (Indahl et al., 1997; Dishman & Bulbulian, 2000). This inhibition has been shown to last from 2 seconds to 6 minutes (Dishman & Bulbulian, 2000). MET not only inhibits the alpha motor neuron, but the technique's gentle stretching also inhibits Ia afferent nerves via post-activation depression. This is due to MET's ability to decrease the sensitivity of muscle spindles to stretch. This effect has been shown to last for more than 2 days (Avela et al., 1999a, 1999b). This evidence fortifies the argument for the use of MET over other techniques in that the effects are not only longer lasting, but also because MET resolves the pain/spasm cycle by acting locally as well as at the dorsal horn on both the efferent and afferent nerves. This is particularly true in the lumbar spine where afferents from nociceptors synapse with alpha motor neurons of the spinal extensors.

A common question in the use of MET centres around the *direction of force application*. Many practitioners advocate applying the force to the hypertonic muscles in order to achieve a post-contraction relaxation effect (e.g. ERS Right – the patient is placed on their right side and contraction of the extensors, right rotators and right sidebenders is resisted). Others believe it is better to apply the force to the weakened side in order to obtain a reciprocal inhibition effect on the hypertonic muscles (e.g. ERS Right – the patient is placed on their left side and contraction of the flexors, left rotators and left sidebenders is resisted). Both are valid and effective techniques for restoring normal structure and function to the motion segment. The use of the *reciprocal inhibition* method is very useful when patients have signs of muscle spasm or muscle guarding and a high 'SINSS'. SINSS stands for Severity, Irritability, Nature, Stage and Stability. Severity correlates to a patient's VAS rating of their pain, whereas Irritability correlates to the magnitude of their pain increasing with provocative movements. Nature relates to the source of the patient's pain whereas Stage relates to the acuity of their pain. Finally, Stability relates to the amount of time and/or activities required to return symptoms to baseline following a provocative movement. A patient with high SINSS may do better with the *reciprocal inhibition* method. Moreover, directly recruiting these muscles will invariably cause pain to the patient thus reducing compliance and impeding the practitioner-patient relationship. A patient with low SINSS will do well with a *post-contraction relaxation* method. Therefore, it is this author's opinion that the patient's SINSS should inform the direction of force at each session versus adherence to one approach over the other.

One of the concerns many practitioners have regarding MET is that it can be time-consuming to apply to a patient with multiple segmental levels of dysfunction. During the Symptom Modulation stage, MET can be viewed as the follow-on treatment of choice after utilising a general/nonspecific TJM technique at the spinal region of interest, such as those described in the works of Flynn et al. (2002), Childs et al. (2004) and Cleland et al. (2009).

Example. An example would be a patient with right-sided LBP without symptoms distal to the knee. The practitioner could perform a right sacroiliac joint gapping TJM in order to modify the compensatory spinal and/or SI joint impairment, and upon reassessment, discover the location of the primary dysfunction and treat it with MET. A point should be made that MET is not the ancillary intervention in this scenario. The nonspecific TJM is being used as a primary intervention to 'clean up' the clinical picture so that the physical therapist can more rapidly identify the location of the underlying impairment. The TJM will also provide a critical 2 seconds to a 6-minute window of analgesia in which the segmental-specific assessment and immediate application of the MET intervention can be applied. Once identified, the impairment can be more effectively treated with MET because the adjacent spinal segments will not act as a 'dirty lever' throughout the treatment.

Other interventions can be applied beforehand to prepare for the MET instead of TJM. Non-irritating PA joint mobilisations can be applied over the spinous processes or the facet joints of the spinal region. These reduce alpha motor-neuron activity via the stretch reflex as previously discussed. If PA mobilisations are not well tolerated by the patient, a transverse glide directed above or below the irritable segments can be applied. A steady, rhythmic transverse glide, properly applied, can relax the patient and provide a critical window for continued interventions. The practitioner can also use several modalities as a pre-treatment such as ice packs, ice massage or brief/intense transcutaneous electrical nerve stimulation (TENS). Ice massage is one of the favoured pre-treatments in the sports medicine setting since it can decrease C fibre activity, decrease local inflammation and modulate pain via the gate control theory, and the time to maximum effect is considerably less than that of an ice pack. For these reasons, an ice massage is also an excellent choice for a post- MET intervention (if it was not already used during the pre-treatment). Finally, dry needling (applied by a properly trained clinician) along the deep paraspinals can also provide pain relief prior to MET.

Post-treatment interventions allow the practitioner to obtain longer-lasting results from the primary intervention, especially if a patient must return to occupational activities immediately following the treatment session. Particular focus should be paid to interventions that inhibit pain and/or spasm. Examples include TENS, ice and analgesic balms. Finally, the benefits of MET can be prolonged by prescribing a specific home exercise programme (HEP). A HEP specific to the patient's dysfunction can decrease the number of MET sessions required to return the patient to full activity (Wilson et al., 2003).

Stage 2: Movement Control

Movement Control has four sub-classifications that should be assessed for and treated in order. They are (1) *sensitised neural tissue*, (2) *mobility and/or flexibility deficits*, (3) *motor control* and (4) *endurance*. *Motor Control* is further subdivided *into activation, acquisition and assimilation. Activation* is the patient's ability to isolate and contract specific muscles/muscle groups such as the lumbar multifidus or the deep abdominals. The lumbar multifidi can be reliably assessed using the Lift-Off Test (Hebert et al., 2015) while the deep abdominals can be assessed using the Drawing-in Manoeuvre (Moghadam et al., 2019). *Acquisition* assesses the patient's ability to move the body in a single plane with gravity reduced with dissociation of adjacent regions. An example of this is the Pelvic Clock exercise performed from 12 o'clock to 6 o'clock. Finally, *assimilation* assesses the patient's ability to move in multiple planes with the full effects of gravity.

Returning to the analogy of the ankle sprain, most physical therapists will attempt to promote and facilitate the proliferation phase of tissue healing by applying gentle, controlled forces to the soft tissues, in a pain-free range, once the inflammation has subsided and symptoms are well controlled. The practitioner can provide the same treatment to a patient with spinal dysfunction by utilising MET in a segment-specific strengthening role. It is important to consider that most patients with an ankle sprain will continue to report slight to moderate pain during this time (VAS 2 to 4/10), and we should expect the same from our patients with spinal pain at the onset of this stage.

While MET is highly effective in treating spinal impairments by restoring normal structure and function to a joint and/or motion segment, there are numerous theories as to how such 'joint dysfunctions' occur. Let's take a quick tangent to discuss two of the more credible theories: dysfunction of the spine's intersegmental muscles or the facet joint/capsule. These two theories overlap in numerous ways thus creating a 'chicken or egg' question. Understanding the basics of these theories and their underlying biomechanical and neurological principles can be helpful in the treatment of patients with spinal pain.

Intersegmental muscles: An alteration in the length and/or tone of the intersegmental muscles (e.g. intertransversarii, rotatores and multifidi) can cause numerous compounding problems. These 'short restrictors' can act as a biomechanical tether (Greenman, 1996) at a motion segment. This shifts the motion segment's axis of rotation posteriorly from the vertebral body to the facet joint. Therefore, the means by which the motion segment attenuates and distributes forces across the joint surfaces becomes altered. This 'tethering' also places prolonged strain on the static restraints of the motion segment. These structures are richly innervated, primarily by the major and lesser descending branches of the sinovertebral nerve, and thus can become a major contributor to the patient's pain. The primary role of the intersegmental muscles is proprioception, as they lack both the size and the biomechanical advantage of the prime movers of the spine. Dysfunction of these muscles can lead to incorrect afferent input to the central nervous system, resulting in a distorted view of the spatial relationships of the motion segments. This can lead to an ineffective use and/or disuse of the primary dynamic stabilisers of the spine (Hides et al., 2001).

Facet joint: The facet joint and its capsule can cause significant pain and dysfunction. When the axis of rotation of a dysfunctional segment moves posteriorly to the facet joint, the entire motion segment must pivot upon the now-engaged facet joint surfaces. In the lumbar spine, the facet joints are accustomed to accepting only 15% (Porterfield & DeRosa, 1998a) of the axial load placed upon the motion segment. When the axis of rotation shifts, the facet joint surfaces become maximally engaged. As loads continue to increase, shear forces develop across the joint surfaces. This shearing can cause damage to the cartilage of these synovial joints, thus creating another pain mechanism. This continued loading can also lead to stresses at the facet joint capsule which can cause altered afferent input to the central nervous system from the Type 1 mechanoreceptors within the capsule. The effects of this mechanism are similar to that of the intersegmental muscles.

The application of MET can reverse the effects of both of these theoretical causes of joint dysfunction. The contract-relax mechanism of MET on intersegmental muscles unbinds the motion segment, thus relieving the stresses on the joint capsule and other static restraints. The ability of MET to mobilise a motion segment within a pain-free range causes a stretch reflex to occur at the facet joint capsule. This results in an inhibition of alpha motor-neuron activity which effectively relaxes the dynamic 'tetherers' of the motion segment. MET effectively utilises the biomechanical and neurological

components of the motion segment to reverse the effects of joint dysfunction by treating the cause, not the symptoms, of the impairment.

MET is the intervention of choice to continue to improve symptoms and motion during the Movement Control stage. Patients will typically present with only a few, mild mobility impairments, so the treatment is not as time-consuming as it would have been in Stage 1 (Symptom Modulation). The use of MET will also allow the patient to be more active since its effects typically last longer than passive treatments. This is an important consideration. As patients increase their activity levels, they also increase the loading and the stress to the injured tissues. MET can often keep an active (or even an overactive) patient in Movement Control, whereas they might regress back to Symptom Modulation if a passive technique were used instead.

Addressing Impairments: Segmental-Specific Strengthening

There are numerous ways in which strength training can be incorporated into the rehabilitation of patients with joint and/or motion segment dysfunctions. While many practitioners view strength training as a separate approach, many clinicians and researchers alike, advocate the importance of a seamless transition from manual therapy interventions to resistance exercise prescription (Hides et al., 1996, 2001; O'Sullivan et al., 1997; Wilson, 2001; Wilson et al., 2003; Childs et al., 2004; Cleland et al., 2009) as well as the use of precision strength training exercises focused at specific levels of spinal segment dysfunction (Hides, 2004).

Danneels et al. (2001) demonstrated that multifidus atrophy occurred in patients with chronic LBP, compared with asymptomatic controls. Patients with acute, unilateral LBP have multifidus atrophy correlated to the segment and side of their lumbar pain (Hides et al., 1994, 1996). The authors also reported that the multifidus muscle's recovery is not 'automatic' after acute LBP. A longitudinal study conducted by Hides et al. (2001) investigated the difference between patients with first-episode, acute LBP who received standard medical management versus instruction on exercises focused on retraining the multifidus muscle. One- and 3-year follow-ups demonstrated that the patients who received standard medical management had an 84% and 75% chance of an insidious recurrence of their pain at 1 and 3 years, respectively. Compare this to the 30% and 35% chance of recurrence

(1- and 3-year follow-up) with the exercise group, and it is clear that multifidus muscle re-education is an important component in the successful long-term management of LBP. MET offers physical therapists a unique tool for the initial management of this problem.

Utilising MET as an initial means of strength training is a vital bridge between manual therapy and resistance exercise prescription. The technique should be used only after the patient has progressed from the Symptom Modulation to the Movement Control classification and the corrective MET (or other manual therapy intervention) has successfully broken the pain/spasm cycle and/or restored normal mobility to the motion segment. Wilson et al. (2003) reported that patients with acute LBP required a mean of only three MET sessions for normality to be restored to the motion segments of the lumbar spine.

The need for segmental-specific strengthening is based on the neurological process of reciprocal innervation. Reciprocal innervation is a process, controlled at the spinal cord level, in which the activation of an agonist muscle causes immediate inhibition of its antagonist muscle(s). As previously stated, a dysfunction at a spinal motion segment can be explained by several theories. However, a common underlying component of these theories involves the inhibition of muscles due to either a tethering/tightening effect on their antagonists or via inhibition from the stretch reflex at a facet capsule or both (Gordon, 1991; Greenman, 1996; Indahl et al., 1997).

Research has demonstrated a need for segmental-specific re-education in order for the lumbar multifidus musculature to recover from an acute injury (Hides, 2004). Using MET provides an excellent, albeit sometimes time-consuming, method of selectively targeting and strengthening previously inhibited muscles. The physical therapy setting is the ideal environment to utilise this intervention, especially in areas where physicians are hit hard by managed care and third-party payer restrictions. Performing segmental-specific strength training requires the same skills needed to perform the corrective manual therapy technique. Therefore, it should not be delegated to an assistant or a technician, nor should it be provided as a HEP.

It is important to repeat some critical elements of incorporating MET as an intervention during the *motor control* component of the Movement Control stage. First, any sensitised neural tissues must be addressed and resolved followed by any flexibility and/or mobility impairments. Impairments from either (or both) of

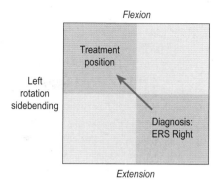

Fig. 11.3 Quadrant method for segment-specific strength training.

these elements of the Movement Control classification will, more often than not, impair motor recruitment, thus any testing of motor control prior to their resolution will often provide data of questionable utility. To review, the subsets of *motor control* are *activation, acquisition* and *assimilation*.

To reduce confusion, the quadrant method is a simple and effective technique for remembering how to treat a patient with segmental-specific strengthening exercises. An example of the quadrant method can be found in Fig. 11.3. By using this technique, the patient is placed in the opposite position to that in which they received the corrective MET procedure. Therefore, if a patient had a flexed, left-rotated, left side-bent (FRS Left) restriction at L4, and was treated in left side-lying to correct the dysfunction, he/she would be placed in right side-lying, as if being treated for an extended, right-rotated, right side-bent (ERS Right) restriction at L4 (Fig. 11.4B–E).

The rationale for this is simple. A patient with an FRS left at L4 has a tightness or hypertonicity of the flexors, left rotators and left side-benders at the L4 motion segment. This hypertonicity causes an inhibition (via the reciprocal inhibition mechanism) of the extensors, right rotators and right side-benders at L4. If allowed to persist, this inhibition can quickly lead to disuse atrophy. Placing the patient in right side-lying, as if treating an ERS Right, allows the practitioner to isolate the extensors, right rotators and right side-benders with the MET procedure. The only difference between the *corrective* technique and the *strengthening* technique is that the practitioner does not take the slack out of the motion segment after each contraction. The practitioner should be careful not to have the patient exert too great

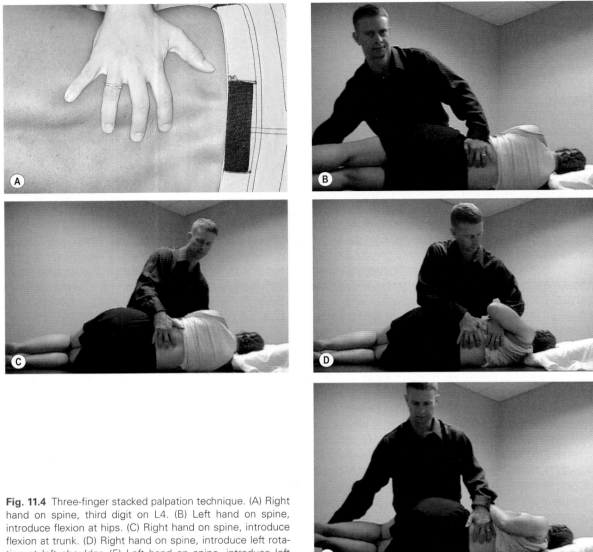

Fig. 11.4 Three-finger stacked palpation technique. (A) Right hand on spine, third digit on L4. (B) Left hand on spine, introduce flexion at hips. (C) Right hand on spine, introduce flexion at trunk. (D) Right hand on spine, introduce left rotation at left shoulder. (E) Left hand on spine, introduce left side-bending at hip.

a force during these contractions. Contractions should be pain-free, but a mild to moderate amount of discomfort during and immediately after the contraction can be tolerated (recall the ankle sprain analogy).

During the *activation* component of *motor control*, the practitioner can elicit slow, progressively stronger contractions in the position mentioned above. This will allow recruitment of intersegmental muscles, followed by deep then superficial multifidi. Care should be used

to not 'overexert' these muscles. Even this relatively low-level muscle contraction could be perceived as highly intense so the volume should be low and rest intervals should be fairly long.

During the *acquisition* component, the practitioner can be a bit more aggressive with their exercise prescription. Using MET in the position described above with a slow, small amplitude of movement can set the patient up for success during more global movement patterns such as the pelvic clock. The practitioner should also consider progressing from long lever arms (legs) to short lever arms (pelvis) with MET during this component of rehab.

Positioning for Segmental-Specific Strengthening

Patient positioning is an important consideration during this procedure. While MET can be performed in numerous positions, it is advantageous to have the patient lie on the same side as the inhibited muscles (right side-lying for an 'ERS Right'). This position will require the clinician to hold the patient's lower extremity against gravity. If the technique were performed with the patient on the left side, the patient would have to assist the clinician in holding the leg against gravity and an over-riding contraction of the prime mover muscles would be elicited.

Isolation of effort: three-finger stacking. It is very important to isolate the motion segment in question while performing this technique. To do this, the practitioner should incorporate a three-finger 'stacked' palpation method (see Fig. 11.4). This is done by placing the pad of the third digit lightly over the spinous process of the segment in question and the pads of the second and fourth digits over the spinous processes of the segments above and below. This will allow the practitioner to quickly determine whether the motion has been isolated to the motion segment. This principle is based on Fryette's third law of spinal motion: the more motion you introduce into a motion segment from one plane, the less motion you will be able to introduce from other planes. The three-finger stacked method allows the clinician to feel the motion coming to the segment with the first finger, feel the motion at the segment of interest with the middle finger, and determine if any motion has 'spilled over' with the third finger.

For example, using the above illustration of an ERS Right at L4, the patient lies on the right side facing the practitioner.

Finger placement: The practitioner would place the pad of the left third finger over the spinous process of L4 with the second finger over the spinous process of L5 and the fourth finger over the spinous process of L3 (Fig. 11.4A).

Introduction of flexion: The practitioner would then fully extend the patient's hips and then slowly move them into flexion (Fig. 11.4B). Since motion (flexion) is being introduced from the 'bottom up', the examiner's second

finger (over the spinous process of L5) would be the first to palpate the motion, followed by the third finger at L4. When the examiner begins to palpate the initial motion at L3 (fourth finger), the process is stopped and a slight amount of extension at the hips is introduced until the motion is felt moving inferior to L3 and back into the L4 motion segment. The examiner would then begin to introduce motion from the 'top down' by flexing the patient's trunk. Some practitioners will continue to palpate with the right hand and reach across with the left arm in order to extend the patient's trunk. This is bad tradecraft as the position does not allow the practitioner the degree of fine control required to isolate the motion segment, especially in a highly symptomatic patient.

The examiner should switch hands, placing the third finger of the right hand over the spinous process of L4 and the fourth and second fingers over the spinous processes of L5 and L3, respectively. The examiner would then flex the patient's trunk until motion is palpated under the second finger at L3, and continue as described above until L4 is isolated (Fig. 11.4C).

Introduction of left rotation: The examiner can now use the left hand to introduce left rotation down to L4 by rotating the patient at the shoulder (Fig. 11.4D). It is important to ensure the patient's shoulders are 'stacked': that is, in-line along the vertical axis, prior to initiating rotation. In this manner, the examiner ensures no rotation has 'leaked' into the motion segment prior. The examiner would first sense the motion under the second finger of the right hand (L3) and then under the third finger as the motion entered the L4 motion segment. Many practitioners advocate introducing rotation prior to introducing the sagittal plane motion; however, it is much more difficult to isolate the motion segment this way. The sagittal plane motion (flexion in this example) provides a natural stopping point for the rotation, making the isolation of the motion segment easier.

Introduction of left side-bending: The practitioner then switches hands once and places the left hand over the spinous processes of interest, as described above. The patient's legs should be grasped at the ankles and the legs lifted towards the ceiling (left side-bending) using the knees as the pivot point (Fig. 11.4E). Recall that Fryette's third law stipulates that very little motion will be required to finish isolating the motion segment since two planes of motion have already been introduced into the motion segment. As the legs are elevated, the examiner will feel the motion (coming from 'bottom up') first under the second finger (L5) as it moves up to L4. The motion segment is now isolated and is ready for the first isometric contraction.

Muscle activation: It is important for the patient to provide a very small contraction. The focus is to strengthen the small intersegmental muscles. These will quickly become overpowered by the larger prime mover muscles if too great a contraction is elicited. The clinician should bear in mind that the core musculature will activate before the periphery, therefore the muscle contraction should be measured in 'ounces' (grams) instead of 'pounds' (kilos). The following are some examples of useful instructions to give to the patient:

- 'Meet my force as I pull your leg towards the ceiling, but do not overpower me'.
- 'Push into my hand as if you were pushing on an egg you did not want to break'.

The practitioner should be careful to note the location of the muscle contraction in relation to the spinal segment. Any contraction felt along the paraspinal musculature is indicative of too strong a contraction. It is important that the clinician observes for compensatory movements or muscle activation, during these exercises. Typically, patients will attempt to compensate at a region other than their back (legs, chest, neck, shoulders). A patient that is unable to cease this compensatory activity is no longer receiving a benefit, and the exercise set should be concluded.

Progressing the Process

There are numerous ways to progress this exercise programme. While individual tastes will vary, it is important to keep several factors in mind. Segmental-specific strengthening should have two distinct focuses or phases:

1. Motor Control (activation, acquisition, assimilation)
2. Endurance.

The focus of the exercise can be changed by manipulating some basic parameters of exercise prescription: number of sets, duration of each set, total time of each contraction, type of contraction, rest intervals between sets (Table 11.3). The clinician should focus on training the fast glycolysis and oxidative energy systems since these muscles need to be active in all anti-gravity positions (Porterfield & DeRosa, 1998b). The following contains an overview of the process. An example with detailed step-by-step instructions can be found in Appendix A.

The importance of rest. Rest intervals are easily overlooked, but their importance is critical, especially during the *motor control* focus. These prolonged rest periods will allow an almost, if not a complete, recovery of the muscles' energy system before the next set is performed (Komi, 1986; Stone & Conley, 1994). It is imperative to avoid overworking these muscles during the *motor control* phase of this programme and submaximal efforts have been advocated in the literature for the larger stabilising muscles (Hicks, 2005). The intersegmental muscles will fatigue quickly and this may lessen their ability to prevent the impairment from returning. Appropriate follow-ups should be scheduled to ensure the patient does not have a reoccurrence of their dysfunction during this period. Progression criteria from *motor control* to the *endurance* phase should be based on the patient's ability to perform all contractions without pain or fatigue.

The *endurance* phase consists of isometric, concentric and/or eccentric exercises with two to three sets of greater than 12 repetitions each. This phase will focus on both the fast glycolytic and oxidative energy systems with a recommended rest period of at least 30 seconds between sets.

TABLE 11.3	**Segmental Strengthening Progression: Basic Exercise Parameters**				
Phase	**Contraction Type**	**Contraction Duration (s)**	**Reps**	**Sets**	**Rest Interval Between Sets**
Activation	Isometric	3–5	3–5	2–3/day	25–45 s
Acquisition	Isometric Concentric	~11	3–5	2–3/day	11–33 s
Endurance	Isometric Concentric Eccentric	5	>12	2–3	30 s

Parameters. There are three independent parameters that should be included as well:

1. Patient position
2. Surface stability
3. Motion resisted

These parameters (Fig. 11.5) are progressed independently of one another with the patient's desired return to activity as a primary determining force.

- *Patient positioning* progresses from long to short lever-arms, and from an unloaded to a loaded spine. Utilising long lever-arms (legs) that the clinician supports against gravity makes it easier for weakened muscles to fire without fatigue. It is imperative the patient be trained with their spine in a loaded position in order to decrease the likelihood of their impairment becoming a chronic condition (Hides, 2004). These can occur in the *assimilation* phase of *motor control*. Examples of these positions can be found in Table 11.4.
- *Patient surfaces* should progress from stable to unstable once the patient is capable of performing the exercise in the seated position (see Table 11.3). Unstable surfaces should progress from uniplanar (foam rolls, bolsters) to multiplanar (trampoline, Dyna-Disc, exercise ball) and uniplanar surfaces should be used in multiple axes, especially the oblique. Adding a

change to the surface should be done on a set-by-set basis depending on the individual patient's tolerance.
- Finally, the *motion being resisted* (side-bending, rotation, flexion, extension) can be manipulated. The programme should begin by resisting single-plane motions, primarily side-bending and rotation. The spinal flexors and extensors have an incredible mechanical advantage over the intersegmental muscles, and they will most likely override any initial attempts to isolate the intersegmental muscles. For this reason, resisting the sagittal plane muscles should not be incorporated into the programme until the patient has progressed to the standing positions (*assimilation*). As the patient advances through the seated progression the therapist can begin having the patient resist motions from two or more planes simultaneously.

SUMMARY AND CONCLUSION

Physical therapists and other appropriately trained manual therapy practitioners, as a general rule, are able to treat patients more frequently and for longer durations than many other medical practitioners. For that reason, PTs tend to have a larger array of treatment options at their disposal. This also affords PTs the opportunity to use multiple

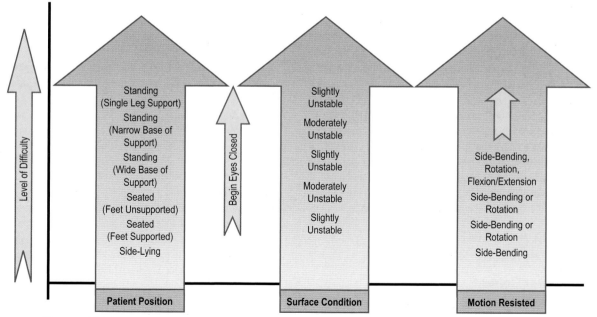

Fig. 11.5 Three independent parameters for the segmental strengthening programme. Slightly unstable: foam roll, bolster, Dyna-Disc, trampoline, etc. Moderately unstable: exercise ball, foam wedge, etc.

TABLE 11.4   Patient Positions and Surfaces Combined

	Foam Roll FP	Foam Roll OP	Dyna-Disc	Swiss Ball	Mini-Tramp
Sidelying	Simple	Simple	Simple	N/A	N/A
Seated	Moderate	Moderate	Moderate	Difficult	N/A
Standing Wide Base	Difficult	Advanced	Difficult	N/A	Difficult
Standing Narrow Base	Difficult	Advanced	Difficult	N/A	Difficult
Standing Tandem	Advanced	Advanced	Advanced	N/A	Advanced
Standing Single Leg	Advanced	Advanced	Advanced	N/A	Advanced

FP, Frontal plane; OP, oblique plane.

techniques and/or interventions in their treatments and to use specific interventions in multiple ways. This is especially true of MET; it is extremely malleable to the environment and it can be adjusted to work with different types of therapists, patients, clinical settings and stages of pain or impairment. A benefit of MET is that once the underlying principles are learned, techniques can be immediately and easily modified by the practitioner.

This chapter has attempted to place MET's role in the physical therapy clinic within the context of the current peer-reviewed literature, in order to make a powerful clinical tool even more effective. To do this, a paradigm shift has been advocated to begin classifying patients into subgroups utilising a classification model (Alrwaily, 2016) and CPRs (Flynn et al., 2002; Childs et al., 2004) as well as a modified operational definition for static palpation and position assessment (Wilson, 2008). A new role for MET has been discussed in segment-specific strengthening programmes and appropriate exercise prescription principles have been outlined. MET is one of the most practical, safe and user-friendly interventions available to physical therapists. It allows clinicians to make an immediate impact on their patients' pain and disability and can be utilised when other interventions may be contraindicated.

APPENDIX A: SEGMENTAL STRENGTHENING PROGRAMME

Part 1: Motor Control

Part 1a: Activation

In this example, the patient has been treated for an ERS Right at L4:

- Patient treated with segmental strengthening in FRS left (L4) position.
- Isolate motion segment as previously described.
- First set:
  - Instruct the patient to perform a gentle, isometric contraction for 3 to 5 seconds.
  - Rest for 5 to 10 seconds (between contractions) and ask the patient to produce another contraction.
  - Continue for a total of 3 to 5 reps
- Rest period:
  - Rest for approximately 25 to 45 seconds between sets.
  - Perform a total of 2 to 3 sets per day.

*NOTE: If exercise technique falters, stop/have the patient stop the set at that point. Double the rest time between sets and attempt the next set. If the technique continues to degrade, stop and wait several hours prior to attempting again. Otherwise, there is a risk of reinforcing poor movement patterns.

Part 1b: Acquisition

Very similar to Part 1a (Activation) with the following modifications:

- Allow small amplitudes of motion to occur within the motion segment
- Contraction strength should slowly increase throughout the course of the contraction until superficial paraspinal muscles are firing
- Increase contraction time to about 11 seconds (5 seconds concentric, 1 second hold, 5 seconds gentle eccentric).

*NOTE: If exercise technique falters, stop/have the patient stop the set at that point. Double the rest time between sets and attempt the next set. If the technique continues to degrade, stop and wait several hours prior to attempting again. You do not want to reinforce poor movement patterns.

- The assimilation phase can be performed with the patient in standing and the examiner resisting through at least two planes of motion
- Criteria to progress to *endurance* phase:
  - Perform all reps and sets without pain or fatigue.

Part 2: Endurance Phase

- Isolate motion segment:
  - Motion segment isolation for eccentric contraction. Place motion segment at 'bottom' of available motion.
- In the example of treating a patient in left side-lying (FRS left) position:
  - Feel for motion entering the L5 motion segment (second finger of right hand).
  - Slowly add motion until the initial motion is palpated at L4: do not continue past this point.
  - First set more than 12 reps.
  - Instruct patient to perform gentle isometric, concentric or eccentric contraction (Box 11.1) for 5 seconds.
  - Rest for 1 second and ask the patient to perform another contraction.
  - Continue for 2 to 3 sets with approximately 30 seconds of rest between sets.

BOX 11.1 Concentric and Eccentric Contractions

Concentric Contractions
- Remember the muscles being trained are very small, therefore they do not require a lot of motion.
- Use the three-finger stacked technique to determine when the concentric contraction has left the motion segment. Stop at this time and use the brief interlude between repetitions to reposition the patient.

Eccentric Contractions
- Begin with the motion segment isolated at the 'bottom' of the available motion.
- Instruct the patient to 'gently resist' your force: 'I am going to slowly raise your leg to the ceiling. I want you to gently resist this motion. I am going to slightly overpower your force.' This will produce an eccentric contraction.

Instruct the patient to walk around the clinic during the rest period in order to increase blood flow to the area. Box 11.1

REFERENCES

Alrwaily, M., Timko, M., Schneider, M., Stevans, J., Bise, C., Hariharan, K., et al., 2016. Treatment-based classification system for low back pain: revision and update. Phys. Ther. 96, 1057–1066.

Avela, J., Kyröläinen, H., Komi, P.V., Rama, D., 1999a. Reduced reflex sensitivity persists several days after long-lasting stretch-shortening cycle exercise. J. Appl. Physiol. 86, 1292–1300.

Avela, J., Kyröläinen, H., Komi, P.V., 1999b. Altered reflex sensitivity after repeated and prolonged passive muscle stretching. J. Appl. Physiol. 86, 1283–1291.

Bergstrom, E., Courtis, G., 1986. An inter- and intra-examiner reliability study of motion palpation of the lumbar spine in lateral flexion in the seated position. Eur. J. Chiropr. 34, 121–141.

Boline, P.D., Keating, J.C., Brist, J., Denver, G., 1988. Interexaminer reliability of palpatory evaluations of the lumbar spine. Am. J. Chiropr. Med. 1, 5–11.

Borkan, J.M., Koes, B., Reis, S., Cherkin, D.C., 1998. A report from the second international forum for primary care research on low back pain. Reexamining priorities. Spine 23, 1992–1996.

Browder, D.A., Childs, J.D., Cleland, J.A., Fritz, J.M., 2007. Effectiveness of an extension-oriented treatment approach in a subgroup of subjects with low back pain: a randomized clinical trial. Phys. Ther. 87, 1–11.

Cherkin, D.C., Deyo, R.A., Battié, M., Street, J., Barlow, W., 1998. A comparison of physical therapy, chiropractic manipulation, and provision of an educational booklet for the treatment of patients with low back pain. N. Engl. J. Med. 339 (15), 1021–1029.

Childs, J.D., Fritz, J., Flynn, T.W., Irrgang, J.J., Johnson, K.K., Majkowski, G.R., et al., 2004. A clinical prediction rule to identify patients with low back pain most likely to benefit from spinal manipulation: a validation study. Ann. Internal Med. 141, 920–928.

Cleland, J.A., Childs, J.D., Palmer, J.A., Eberhart, S., 2006. Slump stretching in the management of non-radicular low back pain: a pilot clinical trial. Man. Ther. 11 (4), 279–286.

Cleland, J.A., Fritz, J.M., Kulig, K., Davenport, T.E., Eberhart, S., Magel, J., et al., 2009. Comparison of the effectiveness of three manual physical therapy techniques in a subgroup of patients with low back pain who satisfy a clinical prediction rule: a randomized clinical trial. Spine 34 (25), 2720–2729.

Crombez, G., Vlaeyen, J.W., Heuts, P.H., Lysens, R., 1999. Pain-related fear is more disabling than pain itself: evidence on the role of pain-related fear in chronic back pain disability. Pain 80, 329–339.

Danneels, L.A., Vanderstraeten, G.G., Cambier, D.C., Witvrouw, E.E., Bourgois, J., Dankaerts, W., et al., 2001. Effects of three different training modalities on the cross sectional area of the lumbar multifidus muscle in patients with chronic low back pain. Br. J. Sports Med. 35, 186–194.

Degenhardt, B.F., Snider, K.T., Snider, E.J., Johnson, J.C., 2005. Interobserver reliability of osteopathic palpatory diagnostic tests of the lumbar spine: improvements from consensus training. J. Am. Osteopath. Assoc. 105 (10), 465–473.

Delitto, A., Erhard, R.E., Bowling, R.W., 1995. A treatment-based classification approach to low back syndrome: identifying and staging patients for conservative treatment. Phys. Ther. 75, 470–479.

Dettori, J.R., Bulock, S.H., Sutlive, T.G., Franklin, R.J., Patience, T., 1995. The effects of spinal flexion and extension exercises and their associated postures in patients with acute low back pain. Spine 20, 2303–2312.

Deyo, R.A., Battie, M., Beurskens, A.J., Bombardier, C., Croft, P., Koes, B., et al., 1998. Outcome measures for low back pain research. A proposal for standardized use. Spine 23, 2003–2013.

Dishman, J.D., Bulbulian, R., 2000. Spinal reflex attenuation associated with spinal manipulation. Spine 25, 2519–2525.

Faas, A., Chavannes, A., van Eijk, J.T., Gubbels, J.W., 1993. A randomized, placebo-controlled trial of exercise therapy in patients with acute low back pain. Spine 18, 1388–1395.

Faas, A., van Eijk, J.T., Chavannes, A.W., Gubbels, J.W., 1995. A randomized trial of exercise therapy in patients with acute low back pain: efficacy on sickness absence. Spine 20, 941–947.

Fairbank, J.C., Couper, J., Davies, J.B., O'Brien, J.P., 1980. The Oswestry low back pain disability questionnaire. Physiotherapy 66, 271–273.

Flynn, T., Fritz, J., Whitman, J., Wainner, R., Magel, J., Rendeiro, D., et al., 2002. A clinical prediction rule for classifying patients with low back pain who demonstrate short-term improvement with spinal manipulation. Spine 27, 2835–2843.

Franke, H., Franke, J.D., Fryer, G., 2014. Osteopathic manipulative treatment for nonspecific low back pain: a systematic review and meta-analysis. BMC Musculoskelet. Disord. 15, 1–18.

Fritz, J.M., Brennan, G.P., 2007a. Preliminary examination of a proposed treatment-based classification system for patients receiving physical therapy for neck pain. Phys. Ther. 87 (5), 513–524.

Fritz, J.M., Cleland, J.A., Brennan, G.P., 2007c. Does adherence to the guideline recommendation for active treatments improve the quality of care for patients with acute low back pain delivered by physical therapists? Med. Care. 45, 973–980.

Fritz, J.M., Cleland, J.A., Childs, J.D., 2007b. Subgrouping patients with low back pain: evolution of a classification approach to physical therapy. J. Orthop. Sports Phys. Ther. 37, 290–302.

Fritz, J.M., Delitto, A., Erhard, R.E., 2003. Comparison of classification-based physical therapy with therapy based on clinical practice guidelines for patients with acute low back pain: a randomized clinical trial. Spine 28, 1363–1372.

Fritz, J.M., Irrgang, J.J., 2001. A comparison of a modified Oswestry low back pain disability questionnaire and the Quebec back pain disability scale. Phys. Ther. 81, 766–788.

Gonnella, C., Paris, S.V., Kutner, M., 1982. Reliability in evaluating passive intervertebral motion. Phys. Ther. 62, 436–444.

Gordon, J., 1991. Spinal mechanisms of motor coordination. In: Kandel, E., Schwartz, J., Jessell, T. (Eds.), Principles of Neural Science, third ed. Appleton & Lange, Norwalk, pp. 581–595.

Greenman, P., 1996. Principles of Manual Medicine, second ed. Williams & Wilkins, Baltimore, pp. 65–73.

Hadijistavropoulos, H.D., Craig, K.D., 1994. Acute and chronic low back pain: cognitive, affective, and behavioral dimensions. J. Consult. Clin. Psychology 62, 341–349.

Hadler, N.M., Curtis, P., Gillings, D.B., Stinnett, S., 1987. A benefit of spinal manipulation as adjunctive therapy for acute low-back pain: a stratified controlled trial. Spine 12, 703–705.

Hebert, J.J., Koppenhaver, S.L., Teyhen, D.S., Walker, B.F., Fritz, J.M., 2015. The evaluation of lumbar multifidus muscle function via palpation: reliability and validity of a new clinical test. Spine J. 15, 1196–1202.

Henschke, N., Maher, C.G., Refshauge, K.M., Herbert, R.D., Cumming, R.G., Bleasel, J., et al., 2009. Prevalence of and screening for serious spinal pathology in patients presenting to primary care settings with acute low back pain. Arthritis Rheum. 60, 3072–3080.

Hestbaek, L., Leboeuf-Yde, C., 2000. Are chiropractic tests for the lumbo-pelvic spine reliable and valid? A systematic critical literature review. J. Manip. Physiol. Ther. 23 (4), 258–275.

Hicks, G.E., Fritz, J.M., Delitto, A., McGill, S.M., 2005. Preliminary development of a clinical prediction rule for determining which patients with low back pain will respond to a stabilization exercise program. Arch. Phys. Med. Rehabil. 86, 1753–1762.

Hidalgo, B., Detrembleur, C., Hall, T., Mahaudens, P., Nielens, H., 2014. The efficacy of manual therapy and exercise for different stages of non-specific low back pain: an update of systematic reviews. J. Man. Manip. Ther. 22, 59–74.

Hides, J.A., 2004. Paraspinal mechanism in low back pain. In: Richardson, C.A., Hodges, P., Hides, J.A. (Eds.), Therapeutic Exercise for Lumbopelvic Stabilization: A Motor Control Approach for the Treatment and Prevention of Low Back Pain. Churchill Livingstone, Edinburgh, pp. 149–161.

Hides, J.A., Jull, G.A., Richardson, C.A., 2001. Long-term effects of specific stabilizing exercises for first-episode low back pain. Spine 26, E243–E248.

Hides, J.A., Richardson, C.A., Jull, G.A., 1996. Multifidus muscle recovery is not automatic after resolution of acute, first-episode low back pain. Spine 21, 2763–2769.

Hides, J.A., Stokes, M.J., Saide, M., Jull, G.A., Cooper, D.H., 1994. Evidence of lumbar multifidus muscle wasting ipsilateral to symptoms in patients with acute/subacute low back pain. Spine 19, 165–172.

Huijbregts, P.A., 2002. Spinal motion palpation: a review of reliability studies. J. Man. Manip. Ther. 10 (1), 24–39.

Indahl, A., Kaigle, A.M., Reikerås, O., Holm, S.H., 1997. Interaction between the porcine lumbar intervertebral disc, zygapophysial joints, and paraspinal muscles. Spine 22, 2834–2840.

Jull, G., Bullock, M., 1987. The influence of segmental level and direction of movement on age changes in lumbar motion as assessed by manual examination. Physiother. Pract. 3 (3), 107–116.

Keating Jr., J.C., Bergmann, T.F., Jacobs, G.E., Finer, B.A., Larson, K., et al., 1990. Interexaminer reliability of eight evaluative dimensions of lumbar segmental abnormality. J Manip. Physiol. Ther. 13, 463–470.

Klenerman, L., Slade, P.D., Stanley, I.M., Pennie, B., Reilly, J.P., Atchison, L.E., et al., 1995. The prediction of chronicity in patients with an acute attack of low back pain in a general practice setting. Spine 20, 478–484.

Komi, P.V., 1986. Training of muscle strength and power: interaction of neuromotoric, hypertrophic, and mechanical factors. Int. J. Sports Med. 7 (Suppl. 1), 10–15.

Kopec, J.A., Esdaile, J.M., Abrahamowicz, M., Abenhaim, L., Wood-Dauphinee, S., Lamping, D.L., et al., 1996. The Quebec back pain disability scale: conceptualization and development. J. Clin. Epidemiol. 49, 151–161.

Leboeuf, C., Gardner, V., Carter, A., Scott, T.A., 1989. Chiropractic examination procedures: a reliability and consistency study. J. Aust. Chiropr. Assoc. 19, 101–104.

MacDonald, R.S., Bell, C.M.J., 1990. An open controlled assessment of osteopathic manipulation in nonspecific low-back pain. Spine 15, 364–370.

Malanga, G.A., Nadler, S.F., 1999. Nonoperative treatment of low back pain. Mayo Clin. Proc. 74, 1135–1148.

Moghadam, N., Ghaffari, M.S., Noormohammadpour, P., Rostami, M., Zarei, M., Moosavi, M., Kordi, R., 2019.

Comparison of the recruitment of transverse abdominis through drawing-in and bracing in different core stability training positions. J. Exerc. Rehabil. 15, 819–825.

Mootz, R.D., Keating Jr., J.C., Kontz, H.P., Milus, T.B., Jacobs, G.E., 1989. Intra- and interobserver reliability of passive motion palpation of the lumbar spine. J. Manipulative Physiol. Ther. 12, 440–445.

Nordeman, L., Nilsson, B., Moller, M., Gunnarsson, R., 2006. Early access to physical therapy treatment for subacute low back pain in primary health care: a prospective randomized clinical trial. Clin. J. Pain 22, 505–511.

O'Sullivan, P.B., Phyty, G.D., Twomey, L.T., Allison, G.T., 1997. Evaluation of specific stabilizing exercise in the treatment of chronic low back pain with radiologic diagnosis of spondylolysis or spondylolisthesis. Spine 22, 2959–2967.

Paige, N.M., Miake-Lye, I.M., Booth, M.S., Beroes, J.M., Mardian, A.S., Dougherty, P., et al., 2017. Association of spinal manipulative therapy with clinical benefit and harm for acute low back pain: systematic review and meta-analysis. JAMA 317, 1451–1460.

Porterfield, J., DeRosa, C., 1998. Mechanical Low Back Pain: Perspectives in Functional Anatomy, second ed. W.B. Saunders, Philadelphia, pp. 121–168.

Porterfield, J., DeRosa, C., 1998. Mechanical Low Back Pain: Perspectives in Functional Anatomy, second ed. W.B. Saunders, Philadelphia, pp. 81.

Pransky, G., Borkan, J.M., Young, A.E., Cherkin, D.C., 2011. Are we making progress?: the tenth international forum for primary care research on low back pain. Spine 36, 1608–1614.

Riddle, D.L., 1998. Classification and low back pain: a review of the literature and critical analysis of selected systems. Phys. Ther. 78, 708–737.

Roland, M.O., 1986. A critical review of the evidence for a pain-spasm-pain cycle in spinal disorders. Clin. Biomech. 1, 102–109.

Seffinger, M.A., Najm, W.I., Mishra, S.I., Adams, A., Dickerson, V.M., Murphy, L.S., et al., 2004. Reliability of spinal palpation for diagnosis of back and neck pain: a systematic review of the literature. Spine 29 (19), E413–E425.

Shekelle, P.G., Paige, N.M., Miake-Lye, I.M., Beroes, J.M., Booth, M.S., Shanman, R., 2017. The Effectiveness and Harms of Spinal Manipulative Therapy for the Treatment of Acute Neck and Lower Back Pain: A Systematic Review.

Spratt, K.F., Weinstein, J.N., Lehmann, T.R., Woody, J., Sayre, H., 1993. Efficacy of flexion and extension treatments incorporating braces for low-back pain patients with retrodisplacement, spondylolisthesis, or normal sagittal translation. Spine 18, 1839–1849.

Stankovic, R., Johnell, O., 1995. Conservative treatment of acute low back pain. A 5-year follow-up study of two methods of treatment. Spine 20, 469–472.

Stone, M.H., Conley, M.S., 1994. Bioenergetics. In: Baechle, T. (Ed.), Essentials of Strength Training and Conditioning. Human Kinetics. Champaign, pp. 67–85.

Waddell, G., Newton, M., Henderson, I., Somerville, D., Main, C.J., 1993. A fear-avoidance beliefs questionnaire (FABQ) and the role of fear-avoidance beliefs in chronic low back pain and disability. Pain 52, 157–168.

Wand, B.M., Bird, C., McAuley, J.H., Doré, C.J., MacDowell, M., De Souza, L.H., 2004. Early intervention for the management of acute low back pain: a single-blind randomized controlled trial of biopsychosocial education, manual therapy, and exercise. Spine 29, 2350–2356.

Wilson, E., 2001. Neuromuscular reeducation and strengthening of the lumbar stabilizers. J. Strength Condition. 24, 72–74.

Wilson, E., 2008. The intra-rater reliability of detecting a mobility restriction in the lumbar spine by static palpation and position assessment [Abstract]. J. Man. Manip. Ther. 16 (3), 167.

Wilson, E., Payton, O., Donegan-Shoaf, L., Dec, K., 2003. Muscle energy technique in patients with acute low back pain: a pilot clinical trial. J. Orthop. Sports Phys. Ther. 33, 502–512.

12

MET in a Massage Therapy Setting

Luke Allen Fritz

CHAPTER CONTENTS

Massage, massage therapy and massage therapy practice can be defined as:

- **Massage**: Massage is a patterned and purposeful soft tissue manipulation accomplished by the use of digits, hands, forearms, elbows, knees and/or feet, with or without the use of emollients, liniments, heat and cold, hand-held tools or other external apparatus, for the intent of therapeutic change.
- **Massage therapy**: Massage therapy consists of the application of massage and non-hands-on components including health promotion and education messages for self-care and health maintenance. Therapy, as well as outcomes, can be influenced by therapeutic relationships and communication; the therapist's education, skill level, and experience; and the therapeutic setting.
- **Massage therapy practice**: Massage therapy practice is a client-centred framework for providing massage therapy through a process of assessment and evaluation, plan of care, treatment, reassessment and reevaluation, health messages, documentation, and closure in an effort to improve health and/or

well-being. Massage therapy practice is influenced by the scope of practice and professional standards and ethics (Kennedy et al., 2016).

The advancement of massage therapy research, together with enhanced levels of education for massage therapists, has resulted in the inclusion of muscle energy techniques (MET) and other manual modalities in massage therapy practice. A typical massage protocol may involve manual gliding, kneading, compressing, percussion (pounding, tapping, slapping, etc.) and oscillating (rocking, vibrating, shaking) of soft tissues but is not limited to these methods (Box 12.1). Additional variations on the nomenclature of these methods are found in Box 12.2.

Other than the typical soft tissue approaches listed above, therapeutic massage therapy includes passive and active movement of the joints as part of assessment and/or treatment, and it is in these instances that MET methods readily integrate into massage therapy.

Applied massage therapy methods create a range of stimuli that positively influence bodily functions including neuro-endocrine processes, fluid (blood and lymph)

BOX 12.1   Massage Therapy Foundations

In the practice of massage therapy, the massage session is a blended and integrated combination of the methods adapted by various modifiers to achieve the session outcomes (relaxation/well-being, stress management, pain management, functional mobility). Massage therapy is often provided as an integrated session over the body using multiple methods in an application sequence over an extended period of time (30–90 min). The session is typically done with a client/patient lying on a table with minimal clothing and draped modestly using various positioning (prone, supine, side-lying). However, massage can also be provided over clothing, on a mat on the floor, and seated. Massage can also be provided as a local treatment.

Four main evidence-informed outcomes for massage therapy:

- Relaxation/well-being
- Stress management
- Pain management
- Functional mobility

Four main approaches to care:

- Palliative
- Restorative
- Condition management
- Therapeutic change

Massage application is mechanical force generated by two actions:

- Pushing
- Pulling

Nine primary massage methods are used to create mechanical force:

- Static methods/holding
- Compression
- Gliding
- Torsion, twisting (kneading)
- Shearing (friction)
- Elongation
- Oscillation
- Percussion
- Movement

Methods are adapted by the following 12 modifiers:

- Pressure
- Point of application (location and broadness of contact)
- Magnitude (intensity)
- Direction
- Drag
- Speed
- Pacing
- Rhythm
- Sequencing and transitioning
- Frequency
- Duration
- Intention for outcome

Adapted methods generate appropriate force to load the body tissue to create the following five stresses to which the physiology must adapt:

- Compression stress
- Tension stress
- Shear stress
- Torsion stress
- Bending stress

BOX 12.2   Massage Therapy Variations

An issue in the massage therapy community, as well as other manual therapy disciplines, is an abundance of naming/nomenclature terms. The various forms and styles are variations of the foundational concepts presented in Box 12.1. This box provides only a small sample of the names of massage therapy methods. When compared and contrasted the named forms and styles are much more alike than different. Often found in a form or style of massage are movement methods that are similar to Muscle Energy Techniques.

Common

Classical massage

Western massage

Swedish massage

Myotherapy massage

Neuromuscular massage

Deep tissue massage

Connective tissue massage

Myofascial release

Reflexology

Cultural systems, i.e. Shiatsu, Ashiatsu, Amma, Tui Na, Thai, Lomi Lomi, Ayurvedic Massage

Population based: pre-/post-natal, sports, geriatric

Condition based: oncology massage, lymphatic massage, etc.

movement through the tissues, as well as improved pliability of connective tissue and other soft tissue structures (Gasibat & Suwehli, 2017; Alves et al., 2019; Case et al., 2021; Espí-López et al., 2020).

A common goal of massage is to support mobility. Optimal mobility allows an individual to move with ease during their daily activities as well as undertake a variety of leisure and exercise-related physical activities. Most often the approach used to increase mobility involves stretching (elongation) methods to improve flexibility. Stretching might involve the movement of a joint to bring the soft tissues into a state of tension, or mechanical force application that directly addresses the soft tissues. Both methods involve a variety of mechanisms that appear to change the pliability of the associated connective tissues and influence the tone of the muscle, thereby encouraging a more normal resting length. Massage therapists can use either approach or a combination of both to support functional mobility (Gao et al., 2011; Samukawa et al., 2011; Tozzi et al., 2011; Matsuo et al., 2019; Vieira et al., 2021).

Both excessive, as well as limited flexibility of soft tissues are undesirable, and if either are noted, MET use during massage may be appropriate. Massage targeting myofascial trigger points is effective in treating hypomobility and the incorporation of MET supports a beneficial outcome (Huang et al., 2010; Trampas et al., 2010; Ransone et al., 2019; Clarke & Allen, 2021).

Massage is much less effective in addressing excessive flexibility or hypermobility. Aspects of MET application can be used to increase the motor tone of the muscle structures, thus offering support for hypermobile structures.

When MET is used to facilitate stretching, this should be based on the assessed presence of a hypomobile joint, or local soft tissue dysfunction. When an increase in range of motion is the therapeutic objective, MET facilitation stretching programmes have been shown to be most effective. The mechanisms associated with MET have been explained as involving an increase in stretch tolerance following isometric contractions (Mahieu et al., 2009; Sharman et al., 2009; Michaeli et al., 2017).

Based on such research, as well as on clinical experience, the following recommendations are presented for the various forms of MET-facilitated stretching in the context of therapeutic massage:

- Each jointed area should be assessed during the massage for available range of motion.
- Only joints that test as hypomobile should attract MET-related stretching of associated soft tissues, with the stretch targeting restoration of normal joint function, while not seeking to increase joint range beyond normal parameters.
- Stretching should not be used in association with joints that are hypermobile, or that appear to move beyond their normal physiological range.
- If for any reason, increased flexibility is considered beneficial, for example, when an athlete participates in a sport that mandates joint movement beyond normal parameters, soft-tissue stretching may be cautiously used to support an ideal increased range of motion related to performance-based demands.

MARRYING ASSESSMENT AND TREATMENT

Most massage methods can be used for both assessment and treatment. Palpation assessment includes typical massage movements such as gliding, kneading and compressing in order to assess for temperature changes, tissue texture, tissue pliability, fluid status and tissue congestion. These same methods can then be used to introduce a variety of mechanical forces, including tension, shear, bend and torsion in order to affect the structure and function of the soft tissues being treated.

Various mechanical forces are also applied, again using the same methods, to influence neural and endocrine functions that affect mood, pain perception and proprioception to produce functional benefits (Lederman, 1997, 2010; King et al., 2010; Zadkhosh et al., 2018; Li et al., 2019; Chen et al., 2020; Field, 2021).

Soft Tissues

Assessment of joints for ranges of motion offers evidence as to the relative length of attaching soft tissue structures. Lengthened or shortened soft tissues identified during such assessment may be the result of modifications of neural control (e.g. increased motor tone), myofascial trigger points, viscoelastic connective tissue changes and/or fluid congestion, all of which would modify the degree of stiffness (Lederman, 1997, 2010; Simons & Mense, 1998).

Joints

Alteration in joint structure can lead to changes in movement potential, as noted in Chapters 7 and 10. A joint may be diseased (as in degenerative joint disease), there may be changes in joint play or the joint may have effusion which influences its ability to move freely. Joint alterations often affect the firing sequences of attaching muscles. Joint stability may also be influenced by the relative tightness or laxity of ligaments, as well as by the tone and tightness of attaching musculature. Both form stability (shape and structure of the joint surfaces, capsule and ligaments) and force stability (action of muscles, and other soft tissues, associated with the joint) may be affected, something particularly true of the sacroiliac joint with its complex musculo-ligamentous support system (Neumann, 2002). By influencing the muscles that form the force-couples at the joint, its stability and movement potential can be altered (Neumann, 2002, 2009, 2017).

When there is joint dysfunction there are almost always changes in the muscle function associated with the joint, resulting in a combination of imbalance between agonists, synergists, fixators and antagonists, some of which may be hypertonic and short, while others may be inhibited and possibly lengthened (Lederman, 1997; Chaitow & DeLany, 2011). It is in such situations that MET methods are particularly useful to introduce changes in muscle behaviour.

In general, therapeutic massage application targets shortened and abnormally tight structures, with the objective of restoring structural balance by lengthening and softening these areas in order to balance pulling forces in the soft tissues (Kassolik et al., 2007; Huang et al., 2010). MET can be an effective addition to the massage protocol to address such changes by modifying stretch perception, increasing stretch tolerance or tissue pliability.

Laxity

Experience indicates that massage is not particularly effective in addressing lax or inhibited soft tissue structures. Some form of therapeutic exercise is usually required to re-establish strength and tone in weakened or lax tissues. Muscle energy methods can be used to treat these conditions (see Chapters 5, 6 and 9). MET applied to over-shortened, hypertonic muscles will automatically result in improved tone and function in their weak/inhibited antagonists (Lewit, 1999).

Additional exercise, possibly using isotonic forms of MET, can be introduced to enhance function in the inhibited structures. MET methods that are most effective for the stimulation of inhibited muscles include pulsed MET and isotonic eccentric methods.

Summary

- Massage comprises methods that affect the soft tissue and the joints.
- Optimising joint movement is part of the objectives of massage.
- Movement is a primary assessment tool.
- Movement dysfunction can be addressed during the application of massage, using muscle energy methods.

INTEGRATING MUSCLE ENERGY METHODS INTO THE MASSAGE SESSION

Previously there existed an opinion among many massage therapists that therapeutic massage required a flowing, rhythmically integrated quality, the intention being to provide a relaxation experience (Tappan & Benjamin, 1998; Salvo & Anderson, 2004; Nicholls, 2008). As a result, many who perform massage seem hesitant to move the client around, to 'change the position of the client', or to ask the client to participate actively in the massage session. While passive rhythmic application certainly has value, such an approach represents only one aspect of therapeutic massage. Currently, it is increasingly common for massage therapists to incorporate a variety of additional, more active methods (such as MET) into treatment sessions. Massage therapy involves many outcome objectives, including those that result in increases in range of motion and more optimal neuromuscular function. MET is an appropriate and efficient addition to massage methodology to achieve these goals.

The question really is not *whether* MET should be part of the massage system, but *how* to incorporate MET into the typical massage session, so that the general impression of massage as rhythmic and soothing is not lost.

'Wellness' and Therapeutic (Clinical) Modes of Massage

The typical massage application is often a general (constitutional, 'wellness') whole body approach, with the results being an increase in well-being and normalisation of nonspecific homeostatic body functioning. All massage, including relaxation, restorative or wellness massage (different names – similar outcomes), can be classified as therapeutic, in the sense that the aim is to provide benefit to the client. The term increasingly used to describe focused, outcome-based massage, which is targeting a pathology or dysfunction, is clinical massage. MET can be incorporated into both massage styles.

It is necessary to determine if the massage approach is wellness, restorative and relaxation based, or whether the massage is addressing a specific outcome, such as pain reduction or increased mobility. If a client's goal for the massage is to be pampered, to sleep, to be soothed, and other such goals, then any method, including MET, that requires active client participation, might be inappropriate. If the massage has an outcome objective of pain relief and increased mobility or the targeting of some other specific result, then adaptive methods, including MET – are appropriate, and indeed probably essential.

There are some myths about massage that need to be challenged in order to justify the inclusion of MET methods into the massage setting:

1. *The client should be passive during the massage.* The client does not have to be passive during the massage. Unless the goal of the massage is sleep, the client should be actively involved, even if only to provide feedback during assessment and intervention processes.
2. *Massage must be provided with rhythmic flowing strokes.* Massage does not have to follow a set protocol, where one stroke flows into the next. This is only one form of massage.

It is important to acknowledge that one of the strengths of full body massage is an interconnected approach to the body allowing all areas to be addressed. This 'interconnected approach' supports the integration of the body to the stimuli and forces imposed upon it during the massage. Therefore, massage provides an excellent platform for not only integration of MET methods into the session, but generally supports the body in adapting to the changes provided by such methods, be it strengthening weak muscles (by removing inhibitory influences from antagonists, as well as the use of toning methods), or lengthening shortened muscles.

The question arises as to whether it is possible to provide a soothing integrated rhythmic massage that also integrates the use of MET. The answer is affirmative and the rest of this chapter will describe how this can be accomplished.

Earlier in the chapter, an explanation of massage was offered that included gliding, kneading, compressing, oscillating and movement methods. In therapeutic massage, passive and active movement of the joints are included, and MET is easily integrated into massage at this point. An example follows as to how this may be achieved.

Example: Massage Including MET to Stretch the Hip Flexor Tissues

Imagine that the client is in the prone position and that the leg is being treated. The massage therapist might use passive joint movement to flex and extend the knee to assess the range and quality of movement. Let's assume that knee flexion is found to be limited as a result of soft tissue changes rather than joint restriction (a judgement based on the quality of end-feel as the knee is flexed) and that the quadriceps muscle is shortened (Fig. 12.1).

- The massage therapist uses passive joint movement to position the muscle just short of bind (see definition of bind, and discussion of barriers, in Chapter 2, p. 19, and Box 2.2, p. 36).
- The client is asked to move the heel gently towards the buttocks while an equal resistance force is applied by the massage therapist, and the hamstring isometrically contracts for about 7 seconds.
- After the contraction, the massage therapist stretches the soft tissues of the anterior thigh by easing the foot towards the buttocks.

The contraction of the antagonists to the shortened quadriceps (hamstrings) would result in an improved ability to stretch the anterior thigh.

An alternative to waiting until the contraction ceases before stretching would be to introduce a stretch of the hamstrings while they were being contracted. This is accomplished by slowly applying a resistance force to the leg that is greater than the contraction force created by the hamstrings obliging the knee to extend. This application is an eccentric isotonic stretch (Fig. 12.2), and the effect would be to tone the hamstrings while simultaneously inhibiting the quadriceps so that the area is more easily stretched (see Chapters 2, 5, 6, 9, 10 and 14 for further examples of isotonic eccentric MET).

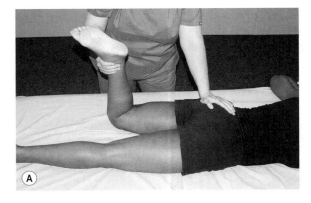

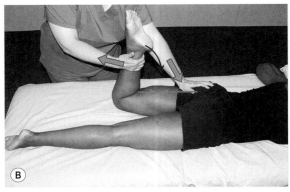

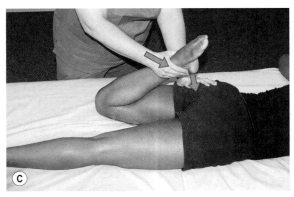

Fig. 12.1 (A) Range of motion of the knee. (B) Isometric contraction of hamstrings. (C) Stretch of anterior thigh soft tissue.

This example describes how MET can be integrated into massage. Using other massage methods to gain the same degree of release achievable by MET procedures could take far longer and would possibly be less effective.

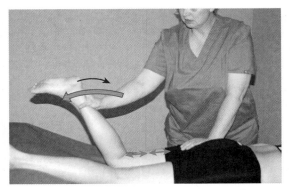

Fig. 12.2 Eccentric isotonic stretch of hamstrings.

The following section provides sample protocols for the effective integration of MET into the massage treatment.

MET IN A TYPICAL MASSAGE SETTING

Two scenarios are presented as examples of how to incorporate MET into the massage session. The first describes the general inclusion of MET into the massage of an area (arm). The second is a hypothetical case involving how massage, including MET, could be used to address low-back pain.

The description of the massage is provided as though the reader is watching the massage as it occurs. It would be helpful for the reader to visualise the examples, or to actually perform them as they are described.

It is assumed that the reader understands the basic methods of gliding (effleurage), kneading (petrissage), compression, oscillation (rocking and shaking) and percussion (Fig. 12.3). These are the main methods of massage that introduce various stimuli and force into the soft tissues, with the objective of eliciting a beneficial response. It is necessary to clarify the meaning of the terms that describe various joint movements.

- *Passive:* Therapist performs the action, client does nothing.
- *Active:* Client performs the action.
- *Active assisted:* Client performs the action but is partially assisted by the therapist.
- *Active resisted:* Client performs the action but is partially resisted by the therapist.

The total movement pattern of any jointed area is its range of motion. During all types of joint movement, the soft tissue (i.e. muscle-connective tissue unit) is being addressed.

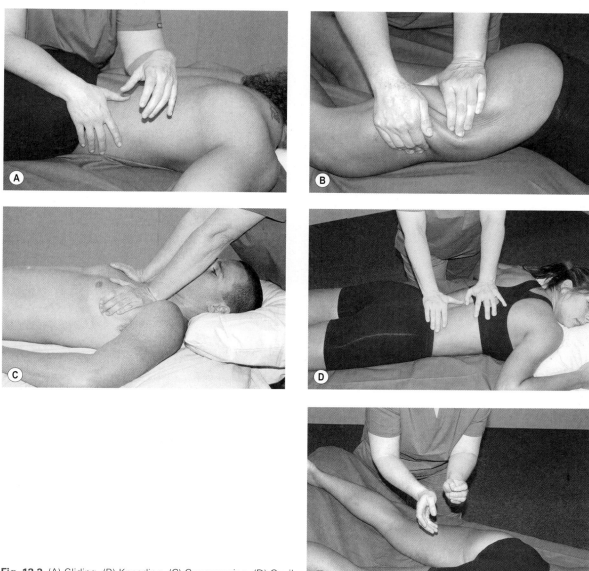

Fig. 12.3 (A) Gliding. (B) Kneading. (C) Compression. (D) Oscillation (rocking). (E) Percussion.

MET as Part of a General Massage Application

The client wishes to receive a full-body restorative massage with a specific focus on elbow discomfort. The following description targets the aspect of the full body massage relating to the upper limb on the affected side.

- The client is supine and the upper limb is being massaged. It is assumed that the posterior torso and shoulder have already been massaged.

- When beginning to massage an area, passive joint movement is used to identify the condition of the range of motion in the area. The massage practitioner gently and rhythmically moves the joints being assessed through the available ranges of motion.

- Let us assume that the initial assessment of the elbow and wrist using passive joint movement identifies a decreased range of motion in elbow extension of 15 degrees, with wrist extension being slightly limited. There is moderate pain reported and apprehension exhibited, during elbow extension.

- Once the area has been assessed passively, and limits in motion identified, the client actively moves the area and the massage therapist compares the results with the passive assessment. In this example let us assume that during the active joint movement the wrist limitation was normal, but the elbow motion remained limited, as described above.
- Massage addresses the arm as the next area in the general massage application.
- Let us assume that, during this massage application, palpation assessment identifies the presence of a trigger point in the brachialis and brachioradialis that is associated with the increased muscle tension in the forearm.
- Compression is applied to the trigger point while passive joint movement positions the tissues so that the pain sensation is reduced – thereby employing a form of positional release technique, known as strain–counterstrain, as discussed in Chapter 14 (Fig. 12.4).
- When the area is returned to the neutral position (i.e. the elbow is straightened), kneading is applied to the area of the trigger point with the intention of lengthening and stretching the local tissue (Fig. 12.5).
- At this time the elbow would be moved through passive ranges of motion, in order to identify any remaining restrictions.
- The area is again massaged and then positioned so that the elbow is slightly flexed. A muscle contraction is introduced to activate the flexors by having the client lightly push against the massage therapist's restraining hand for 5 to 7 seconds. After this, the elbow is extended to stretch the tight soft tissues (Fig. 12.6).

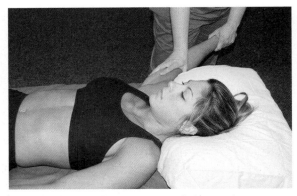

Fig. 12.5 Stretching area of trigger point.

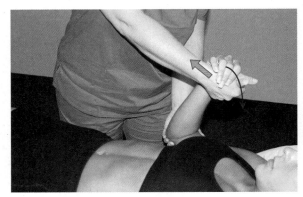

Fig. 12.6 An isometric contraction of elbow flexors.

- General massage and passive joint movement are used to reassess the area.
- Attention then shifts to the forearm and the wrist, and the forearm is massaged.
- The wrist flexors are positioned at slight tension, and the client resists against counterpressure provided by the massage therapist, to assess muscle strength.
- After this, the wrist extensors are positioned at slight tension and again the client resists a counterpressure provided by the massage therapist, to assess muscle strength.
- Let us assume that the flexor muscles test as strong, and the wrist extensors test weak.
- The wrist flexors are massaged to reduce muscle tension and then MET methods prepare the wrist flexors for stretching.
- It would be appropriate to use MET in some integrated combination (see Chapters 2, 5 and 14). The massage therapist then stretches the wrist flexors.

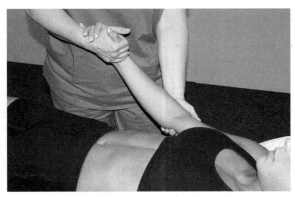

Fig. 12.4 Positional release of brachialis.

- Next, the wrist extensors are isolated and the client is instructed to pulse rhythmically against the massage therapist's resisting hand, with the intention of activating (toning, facilitating) the weak extensor muscles (see notes on Ruddy's pulsed MET in Chapters 2, 3, 6, 7 and 14).
- After 20 pulses the client is asked to again contract the wrist extensors against a counterpressure applied by the massage therapist. In this example let us assume that the wrist extensors now test strong and the area is generally massaged again to integrate the response.
- The hand is next to be massaged.
- The entire area is again taken through passive joint movement to reassess the range of motion. Any changes would be noted and charted.
- The massage then continues in the typical full body massage style, with MET being incorporated wherever indicated by what is identified during the massage, as in the example of the arm.

Case Study

A 48-year-old female has been referred for massage as part of a management programme for low-back pain. The client has been diagnosed with reduced disc space at L 3, 4, 5 with slight disc bulging at L5. Surgery is not indicated and conservative treatment has been prescribed. The main source of pain and disability appears to be muscular, both as a result of protective guarding and intermittent nerve impingement involving shortened soft tissue structures. The forms of treatment being received include physical therapy, osteopathic care, massage and muscle relaxing medication, to be used as needed.

The treatment plan for the massage is to provide general restorative massage, with the objectives of pain relief, enhancement of sleep, reduction of fascial stiffness (especially lumbodorsal fascia), as well as offering attention to shortened latissimus dorsi, hamstrings, psoas, paraspinal muscles and quadratus lumborum and associated connective tissues.

The general treatment plan for massage involves 60 minutes, twice a week, for 12 weeks. The massage follows a relatively classic style using gliding, kneading, compression, etc. in a relaxing and rhythmic manner.

Active and passive joint movement and palpation assess the current condition of tissue shortening at each session. Methods are adapted to target shortened fascial areas, and MET is used to address muscles that have shortened due to increased motor tone.

The following describes a typical massage session as part of the prescribed treatment plan.

Patient Prone

- Massage begins with the patient prone.
- When the tissues are warm and more pliable, deep slow gliding along the paraspinal muscles commences.
- When an area is identified by the client as contributing to the back pain, the glide stops, and ischaemic compression is used.
- As this is being done the client is asked to extend the spine and rotate towards the pain to create an isolated contraction at the point of the compressed tissue.
- The contraction is held for 7 to 10 seconds and then the client is asked to rotate away from the pain and to push down into the table with the anterior torso, and to draw the abdominals in, thereby contracting the anterior torso muscles to create reciprocal inhibition of spinal muscles.
- At the same time, the massage therapist slightly increases the compressive force and again begins to use gliding strokes through the tissues, which effectively produces isolated stretching of the shortened symptomatic area.
- This process continues until about 50% of the muscle's increased motor tone is reduced. Since a possible reason for the muscle shortening is the protection of the spine, the goal should be to modify the excessive muscle tension, rather than trying to eliminate it.
- The massage then becomes more general to increase fluid movement (i.e. enhanced circulation, and lymphatic drainage) in the area, and to assist in the integration of the changes.
- While the client remains prone the massage application addresses the gluteals, hamstrings and calves.
- General massage application is used to assess and warm the area.

Since the hamstrings are one of the areas to be specifically addressed in the treatment plan, MET methods may well be useful.

- In the prone position it is difficult to lengthen the hamstrings, however gradually applied compressive gliding, from the distal attachments to the proximal attachments, while the client slowly actively flexes and extends the knee, is likely to result in a more relaxed, and lengthened hamstring group. This type of application also addresses the connective tissue shortening.
- The massage then becomes general again.

Patient Side-Lying

- The client is placed in the side-lying position to more easily access latissimus dorsi and quadratus lumborum, and the general massage application resumes.
- Gliding over the latissimus dorsi begins at the hip and progresses to the shoulder.
- To lengthen the latissimus dorsi the client's arm is positioned with the arm placed over the client's head, with the lateral aspect of the arm against the side of her face (Fig. 12.7).
- A resistance force is applied by the massage therapist at the medial aspect of the arm near the elbow, and the client is asked to move the arm away from her face and back towards her side, resulting in an isometric contraction of the latissimus dorsi.
- The amount of effort asked for would be about 10% of maximal strength for a duration of approximately 7 to 10 seconds.
- The massage therapist then reverses the focus of the resistance force and the client attempts to move the arm towards her head, resulting in an isometric contraction of the deltoid and inhibition of the latissimus dorsi.
- This alternating contraction application is repeated two or three times after which the client is asked to take the arm through the resistance barrier in order to stretch the shortened muscle while the massage therapist assists in the lengthening process.
- When the new barrier is identified, the client repeats the sequence of resisted contractions and assisted stretching. This is an example of a muscle energy procedure that can be summarised as contract-relax antagonist contract – lengthen and then stretch.

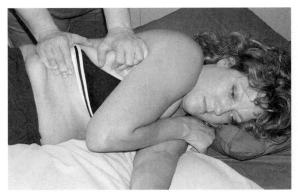

Fig. 12.8 Massage of area for direct tissue stretching.

- The tissues would subsequently be gently returned to a neutral position.
- The soft tissue is massaged again, both to palpate for changes and to support adaptation of the soft tissue to the new length.
- If additional areas of bind are identified then the massage therapist uses kneading to create bend and torsion loading on the short binding tissue to directly stretch it (Fig. 12.8).
- When sufficient length has been achieved, the area is then generally massaged to help integrate the changes.
- While the client is in the side-lying position, the quadratus lumborum and adjacent soft tissue can be lengthened by stabilising the iliac crest and having the client tilt (hike) the hip, activating the muscle.
- The tissues are then lengthened by having the client lower the leg behind the trunk, coupled with stretching by the massage therapist.
- MET can also be used to address the psoas while the client is in the side-lying position.
- The client is positioned so that while lying on her side both hips are flexed to about 90 degrees with one leg on top of the other. The knees are also flexed to about 90 degrees.
- The massage therapist stands behind the client, grasps the upper leg, and extends the hip to 0 degrees, while the knee remains flexed. The massage therapist then grasps the client's anterior thigh, just above the flexed knee, and stabilises the client in the lumbar area.
- The massage therapist applies a resistance force to the anterior thigh as the client attempts to move the hip into flexion, resulting in isometric contraction of the

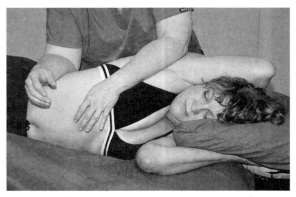

Fig. 12.7 Position of arm, side-lying.

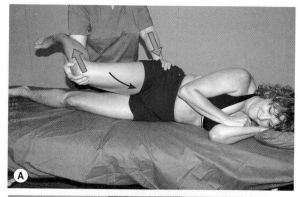

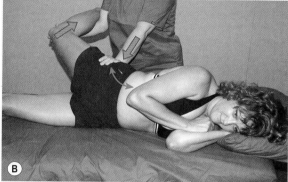

Fig. 12.9 (A) Isometric contraction for psoas, side-lying. (B) Post-isometric psoas stretch, side-lying.

psoas. The contraction force only needs to be 15% to 20% of maximal strength and held for about 10 seconds (Fig. 12.9A).
- The client relaxes and then attempts to move the hip into hyperextension while assisted by the massage therapist, resulting in stretching of the psoas. This procedure is repeated two or three times (Fig. 12.9B).
- The massage application continues to generally address the rest of the body in the side-lying position.
- The client is positioned on the other side and the process is repeated.

Patient Supine
- The client is positioned supine. Massage continues, beginning at the feet and progressing towards the hips.
- The leg is flexed at the hip and the knee is extended (straight leg raise) to assess for the shortening of the hamstrings.
- When the barrier is identified the client contracts against a resistance force applied by the massage

therapist on the gastrocnemius, near the knee, by bringing the leg down towards the table using 10% to 20% contraction force, for about 7 seconds.
- The hamstrings are then stretched by raising the leg.
- The knee remains extended while the massage therapist slowly flexes the hip until the barrier is again identified. The procedure is then repeated.
- The process is repeated on the other side.

At this point in the massage session, all target areas have been addressed using MET, and the therapist can generally massage the rest of the body in the supine position.

This case study example provides suggestions for integrating MET into massage to address a specific condition.

SUMMARY

The flow of the massage session involves the skilled weaving of MET elements into a full body rhythmic, soothing, effective massage experience. Based on the examples provided, it is easy to see how muscle energy methods can be integrated into the massage session. It is difficult for this author to imagine performing a massage session without incorporating MET methods as an intervention tool.

MET methods are generally safe and well accepted by clients. It may be prudent to explain MET methods to clients prior to the massage session.

To effectively integrate MET methods into the massage, the massage therapist needs to be knowledgeable regarding joint movement patterns and normal ranges of motion. With practice and a shift in perception, the massage professional should be able to introduce these methods, and the underlying concepts, into the massage session, resulting in greater benefits to the client.

REFERENCES

Alves, M., Jardim, M.H.D.A.G., Gomes, B.P., 2017. Effect of massage therapy in cancer patients. Int. J. Clin. Med. 8 (2), 111–121.

Case, L.K., Liljencrantz, J., McCall, M.V., Bradson, M., Necaise, A., Tubbs, J., et al., 2021. Pleasant deep pressure: expanding the social touch hypothesis. Neuroscience 464, 3–11. doi:10.1016/j.neuroscience.2020.07.050.

Chaitow, L., DeLany, J., 2011. Clinical Application of Neuromuscular Techniques. The Lower Body 2. Churchill Livingstone, Edinburgh, pp. 35–37.

Chen, Y., Li, Q., Zhang, Q., Kou, J., Zhang, Y., Cui, H., et al., 2020. The effects of intranasal oxytocin on neural and behavioral responses to social touch in the form of massage. Front. Neurosci. 14, 589878. doi:10.3389/fnins.2020.589878.

Clarke, J., Allen, L., 2021. The effect of muscle energy techniques on latent trigger points of the gastrocnemius muscle. Sport J. Published online 12 Feb 2021, https://thesportjournal.org/article/the-effect-of-muscle-energy-techniques-on-latent-trigger-points-of-the-gastrocnemius-muscle/.

Espí-López, G.V., Serra-Añó, P., Cuenca-Martínez, F., Suso-Martí, L., Inglés, M., 2020. Comparison between classic and light touch massage on psychological and physical functional variables in athletes: a randomized pilot trial. Int. J. Ther. Massage Bodywork. 13 (3), 30–37.

Field, T., 2021. Massage Therapy Research Review. Int. J. Psychol. Res. Rev. 4, 45 –45.

Gao, F., Ren, Y., Roth, E.J., Harvey, R., Zhang, L.Q., 2011. Effects of repeated ankle stretching on calf muscle-tendon and ankle biomechanical properties in stroke survivors. Clin. Biomech. 26 (5), 516–522.

Gasibat, Q., Suwehli, W., 2017. Determining the benefits of massage mechanisms: a review of literature. Rehabil. Sci. 2 (3), 58–67.

Huang, S.Y., Di Santo, M., Wadden, K.P., Cappa, D.F., Alkanani, T., Behm, D.G., 2010. Short-duration massage at the hamstrings musculotendinous junction induces greater range of motion. J. Strength Cond. Res. 24 (7), 1917–1924.

Kassolik, K., Andrzejewski, W., Brzozowski, M., Trzesicka, E., Apoznanski, W., Szydelko, T., et al., 2007. Medical massage as a physiotherapeutic method in benign prostatic hyperplasia in men. J. Bodyw. Mov. Ther. 11, 121–128.

Kennedy, A.B., Cambron, J.A., Sharpe, P.A., Travillian, R.S., Saunders, R.P., 2016. Clarifying definitions for the massage therapy profession: the results of the best practices symposium. Int. J. Ther. Massage Bodywork 9 (3), 15–26. https://doi.org/10.3822/ijtmb.v9i3.312.

King, H.H., Janig, W., Patterson, M.M., 2010. The Science and Clinical Application of Manual Therapy. Churchill Livingstone, Edinburgh.

Lederman, E., 1997. Fundamentals of Manual Therapy, Physiology, Neurology and Psychology. Churchill Livingstone, Edinburgh, pp. 7–8, 23–25, 39–40, 55–56, 66–67, 95–96, 126, 133–137, 213–221.

Lederman, E., 2010. The myth of core stability. J. Bodyw. Mov. Ther. 14 (1), 84–98.

Lewit, K., 1999. Manipulation in Rehabilitation of the Locomotor System, third ed. Butterworths, London.

Li, Q., Becker, B., Wernicke, J., Chen, Y., Zhang, Y., Li, R., et al., 2019. Foot massage evokes oxytocin release and activation of orbitofrontal cortex and superior temporal sulcus. Psychoneuroendocrinology 101, 193–203. doi:10.1016/j.psyneuen.2018.11.016.

Mahieu, N.N., Cools, A., De Wilde, B., Witvrouw, E., 2009. Effect of proprioceptive neuromuscular facilitation stretching on the plantar flexor muscle-tendon tissue properties. Scand. J. Med. Sci. Sports 19 (4), 553–560.

Matsuo, S., Iwata, M., Miyazaki, M., Fukaya, T., Yamanaka, E., Nagata, K., et al., 2019. Changes in flexibility and force are not different after static versus dynamic stretching. Sports Med. Int. Open. 3 (3), E89–E95. doi:10.1055/a-1001-1993.

Michaeli, A., Tee, J.C., Stewart, A., 2017. Dynamic oscillatory stretching efficacy on hamstring extensibility and stretch tolerance: a randomized controlled trial. Int. J. Sports Phys. Ther. 12 (3), 305–313.

Neumann, D.A., 2002, 2009, 2017. Kinesiology of the Musculoskeletal System Foundations for Physical Rehabilitation. Mosby, St Louis, MO, pp. 18–19 1641, 308.

Nicholls, D., 2008. Beard's Massage: Principles and Practice of Soft Tissue Manipulation. New Zealand J. Physiother. 36 (3), 173–174.

Ransone, J.W., Schmidt, J., Crawford, S.K., Walker, J., 2019. Effect of manual compressive therapy on latent myofascial trigger point pressure pain thresholds. J. Bodyw. Mov. Ther. 23 (4), 792–798. doi:10.1016/j.jbmt.2019.06.011.

Salvo, S.G., Anderson, S.K., 2004. Mosby's Pathology for Massage Therapists. Mosby, St Louis, MO, pp. 423.

Samukawa, M., Hattori, M., Sugama, N., Takeda, N., 2011. The effects of dynamic stretching on plantar flexor muscle-tendon tissue properties. Man. Ther. 16 (6), 618–622.

Sharman, M.J., Cresswell, A.G., Riek, S., 2009. Proprioceptive neuromuscular facilitation stretching: mechanisms and clinical implications. Scand. J. Med. Sci. Sports 19 (4), 553–560.

Simons, D., Mense, S., 1998. Understanding and measurement of muscle tone as related to clinical muscle pain. Pain 75 (1), 1–17.

Tappan, F.M., Benjamin, P.J., 1998. Tappan's Handbook of Healing Massage Techniques, Holistic, Classic, and Emerging Methods, third ed. Appleton and Lange, Norwalk, CN, pp. 147.

Tozzi, P., Bongiorno, D., Vitturini, C., 2011. Fascial release effects on patients with non-specific cervical or lumbar pain. J. Bodyw. Mov. Ther. 15 (4), 405–416.

Trampas, A., Kitsios, A., Sykaras, E., Symeonidis, S., Lazarou, L., 2010. Clinical massage and modified proprioceptive neuromuscular facilitation stretching in males with latent myofascial trigger points. Phys. Ther. Sport 11 (3), 91–98.

Vieira, D.C.L., Opplert, J., Babault, N., 2021. Acute effects of dynamic stretching on neuromechanical properties: an interaction between stretching, contraction, and movement. Eur. J. Appl. Physiol. 121, 957–967. https://doi.org/10.1007/s00421-020-04583-3.

Zadkhosh, S.M., Ariaee, E., Zandi, H.G., 2018. The effect of massage therapy on aggression in youth wrestlers. J. Phys. Educ. Health Sport 5 (1), 6–13.

13

MET in Treatment of Athletic Injuries

Ken Crenshaw, Nathan Shaw, Derek Somerville, Ryan DiPanfilo

CHAPTER CONTENTS

Active participation in competitive athletics by its nature carries inherent risks of physical injury and dysfunction. Each sport creates the possibility of unique injuries and specific physical adaptations as a result of the particular physical demands of the sport and the position played within it. As competitive athletics (especially when involving one-sport specialisation) continue to increase in popularity, the risk of injury and/or dysfunction can increase as well. Specialised healthcare providers for athletes are essential for the prevention, recognition, assessment, management and rehabilitation of sports injuries.

The very special nature of returning athletes to sport after injury, or prevention of injury is very complex. Understanding that injury and dysfunction go hand in hand, as one may be causative of the other, creates the need for in-depth knowledge of human tissue function. The elite competitive athlete is highly pressured by multiple social, physical, economic and emotional demands. These pressures, combined with increasing demands from team management and their own economic concerns, place an enormous responsibility on the sports medicine team to keep athletes fit and participating.

This chapter will:

1. Discuss the adaptation, function and dysfunction of athletes in competitive sports.
2. Provide sound assessment techniques, classification systems, treatment and rehabilitation options for the most common musculoskeletal problems.
3. Explain how muscle energy techniques (MET) are used within the total healthcare system for athletes.
4. Explain specific injury/dysfunction scenarios and give systematic therapy options utilising MET and other adjunct modalities.

It is not the intention of the authors, nor within the scope of this chapter, to provide all-inclusive details of every possible sport-related musculoskeletal problem. Rather, the objective is to suggest ways in which MET, in combination with other therapies, might be used in the treatment of the most common athletic injuries and/or dysfunctions. The authors concur that it is not currently mainstream practice for most Western sports medicine providers to use neuromuscular therapy that includes the use of MET in the prevention, management and rehabilitation of athletic injuries. The principles and methods outlined in this chapter represent the combined experience of its authors and are presented in the hope that they will stimulate interest in others whose work involves helping injured athletes and/or who aim to prevent athletic injuries.

ADAPTATION OF ATHLETES

Sport, in general, requires high levels of repetitive physical activity and training to achieve specific performance objectives. In addition, exercise regimens are utilised to improve athletic qualities through physical adaptation. The combining of these two components requires tactful planning and constant assessment to avoid overload of the musculotendinous and neuromuscular systems. Athletes will inherently adapt to the imposed demands of their sport, the physical requirements of the position played within the sport and their exercise regimens, or else they will become prone to injury or inadequate performance. This philosophy is based on the specific adaptation to imposed demands (SAID) principle discussed by Kraemer and Gomez (2001). Specific tissue (be it joint, muscular, tendinous, fascial, osseous or ligamentous/capsular) will accommodate uniquely in each athlete. For example, generalised patterns of adaptation are recognised in the overhead-throwing athlete (Box 13.1).

BOX 13.1 Personal View on Adaptation in the Athlete

Age seems to be a key feature in the adaptation process. As discussed, humeral retroversion occurs in overhead throwers, and the authors are currently researching the influence of age on this process. Presumably, the process occurs between 12 and 13 years of age, prior to growth plate closure and is dependent upon the amount of throwing involved (Meister, 2005).

Any repetitive activity produces specific demands for adaptation. In sports, trainers along with coaches and therapists/practitioners are responsible for the encouragement of healthy adaptation. It is essential for a certain level of adaptation to occur for athletes to compete at elite levels, for without specific adaptation to the imposed demands, the musculoskeletal system would almost certainly fail to function efficiently. In essence, the adaptation helps to pre-position the body for the sport's demands. There seems to be a fine line as to the degree of adaptation that is desirable, beyond which deleterious effects such as injury (shoulder laxity for example) become more likely (Pieper, 1998).

Following injury, the musculoskeletal system is required to adapt to the new situation and function with injured or healing tissue. It is in this state that care is required to prevent re-injury and reduce dysfunctional patterns of use so that appropriate and functional adaptation can occur. Following further injury, multiple injuries or extreme injury, functional adaptation may not be possible, so that decompensation and dysfunction become almost inevitable. In elite athletes, a minute degree of dysfunction makes the difference between winning and losing, whereas in the non-athlete, incurring the same degree of dysfunction may create no more than a minor inconvenience.

Excluding injuries, the consequences of specialised adaptation required to compete at elite levels of sport do not seem to affect the athlete's lifestyle.

Overhead sports that require highly repetitive actions tend to demand multiple adaptations throughout the shoulder and its kinetic chain. While such functional adaptational changes might be considered injuries in non-overhead athletes, they could be considered useful and even necessary in the overhead athlete. If function determines form, and form determines function, it could be argued that the resulting dysfunctions are functional adaptations in a healthy stress-resistant athlete.

Moreover, variables such as left-right symmetry and flexibility, often associated with an injury-free state, might be undesirable in a one-side dominant, high-stress, repetitive situation. However, precisely a particular tissue or tissues may have adapted in relation to such activities remains controversial. Various experts (Pieper, 1998; Crockett et al., 2002; Osbahr et al., 2002; Reagan et al., 2002; Wilk et al., 2002; Borsa et al., 2006) have described a variety of adaptational possibilities in the throwing shoulder. The common pattern of the throwing shoulder to develop an increased range of external

rotation and decreased internal rotation is one of many adaptations (Fig. 13.1A–C).

Borsa et al. (2005, 2006) assessed professional baseball players and concluded that no correlation exists between the loss of shoulder internal rotation and capsular tightness, whereas others feel that the loss of shoulder internal rotation may be capsular in nature (Burkhart et al., 2000, 2003).

If a more global view of the body is taken, both scapular resting position and mobility have been identified as areas of altered adaptation in the overhead athlete

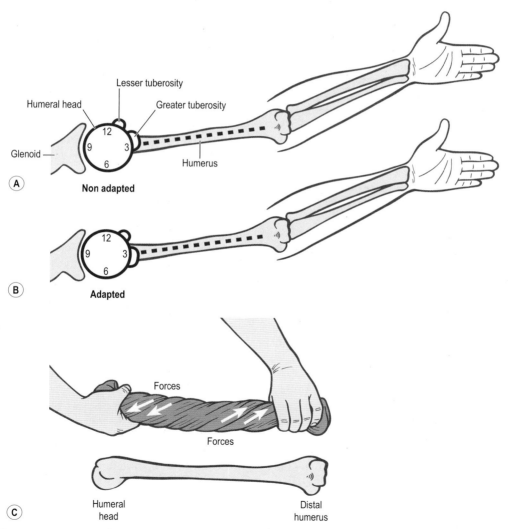

Fig. 13.1 (A–C) Osseous adaptation of the humerus from repetitive overhead throwing (humeral retroversion) is one of several adaptations in athletes.

(Gibson et al., 1995; Myers et al., 2005). More specifically, the function of the scapula relates to the health of the glenohumeral joint and thus should be assessed. It appears that insufficient scapular stabilisation could contribute to overuse injuries of the shoulder (Warner et al., 1992; Kebaetse et al., 1999; Lukasiewicz et al., 1999; Ludewig & Cook, 2000; Johnson et al., 2001; Cools et al., 2004, 2005).

Continuing with the global perspective, an even more anatomically distant relationship can be observed between the scapula and rib cage. As the scapula sits on the rib cage, the orientation of the scapula is somewhat dictated by the rib cage position. For example, a neutrally oriented scapula on a malpositioned ribcage may present as a malpositioned scapula. Therefore, it is important to assess all the interconnected constituent parts of a collective whole to be able to identify the probable causes or mechanisms of a pathomechanical pattern.

Another common finding in the throwing athlete is the presence of increased tone in the bicep, as it is under extreme eccentric force demand during deceleration of the elbow after the release of the thrown object. Additionally, the rotator cuff muscles (supraspinatus, subscapularis, teres minor, infraspinatus) seem to demonstrate muscular weakness post-throwing, which, if not managed, could lead to dysfunction (Mullaney et al., 2005; Dale et al., 2007).

Managing stress resistance is critical in athletic performance. The lack of stress resistance in the overhead athlete may lead to injury, while control of stress may lead to adequate adaptation. One of the most notable local problems affecting the overhead athlete are glenoid labrum tears and specifically superior labral tears that extend from anterior to posterior (SLAP tears). The mechanisms associated with SLAP tears are maximal shoulder external rotation and/or rapid elbow extension, which causes forceful contraction of the biceps brachii with shoulder deceleration after ball release (Andrews et al., 1991; Wilk et al., 2005). Still, the question remains, is a slight SLAP tear a necessary adaptation to allow the extreme throwing shoulder motions? Or is it a chronic overload that is countered by a high-stress resistance? Hence, once the stress resistance decreases, the athlete presents with a symptomatic and possibly disabling SLAP tear. It is the authors' experience that there are 'symptomatic' and 'asymptomatic' SLAP tears, and that they may be a common or necessary adaptation if not excessive.

Debate is ongoing as to what structures are adjusting and it is the authors' thought that each athlete adapts differently. To what extent and what structures adapt in the overhead athlete appears to be individual, depending on the relationship between the nature and degree of stress applied and stress resistance. Given this information, the clinician should assess each athlete and not assume that all are the same. Assessment may give unique insights that allow for the creation of specialised treatment plans for injured athletes in addition to preventative programmes, based on individual findings.

The ability of an athlete to adapt adequately seems to be what permits sustained competition at the top levels of a chosen sport. However, it is crucial to differentiate between dysfunction/injury and sport-specific or functional adaptation when assessing an injury situation in the athlete. As adaptations from sport occur, it is necessary to consider an athlete's daily living habits. Any repetitive or prolonged activity will create an adaptation that may negatively affect function and performance. Greenfield et al. (1995), demonstrated that poor posture involving a forward head position can affect the shoulder of the throwing athlete. Postural adaptive changes can be observed in the upper and lower crossed syndromes, as described by Janda (1987, 1988) (see Box 5.2, Chapter 5). To ensure optimal function athletes should always be assessed for such postural adaptations, and for more specialised training adaptations.

Psychological, emotional, social, environmental, as well as nutritional stressors combined with ageing, competition requirements, travel and sleep-pattern disruption all add to the professional athlete's adaptation burden. General health depends on more than the absence of disease, and it is critical to keep stressors to a minimum and/or use strategies such as recovery and relaxation techniques to improve the management of adaptive demands (Selye, 1956).

DYSFUNCTION IN SPORTS

Optimal physical function is critical for the success of the elite athlete. Strength, balance, power, speed, agility, coordination, endurance and mobility are important elements in most sports (Kraemer & Gomez, 2001). These elements will almost certainly be hindered by the presence of neuro-muscular dysfunction. Whether postural imbalance, local tissue disturbance, psychosocial/psychosomatic influences or some other factor is involved, the sports medicine team needs to be able to recognise and address the problem to retain optimal performance.

Identifying compensatory movement patterns in the elite athlete is highly individualistic. Understanding the general concepts of adaptation is inevitably useful in managing acquired dysfunctional patterns. Postural deviations, such as those described by the upper and lower crossed syndromes, can be compared with an idealised postural norm. The resulting variations of overactive versus inhibited muscles generally compared by agonist and antagonist muscular relationships can change ideal joint positions. This change can increase biomechanical distress and repetitive microtrauma across the decentrated joint structures.

Developmental kinesiology provides uniform stages of functional movement patterns established at a young age. These autonomic motor patterns are predictable in the first year of life and represent the purest of functional movement patterns for an individual. The developmental stages demonstrate ideal joint centration and functional movement patterns that can also be utilised as a postural norm. Deviations from the individual's postural norm create biomechanical distress across joints.

The concept of functional centration is essential in understanding the relationship between joints and muscles. The terms 'centration', 'decentration', 'subluxation', and 'luxation' used mainly in orthopaedics (and chiropractic) describe the morphological and/or pathological conditions of joints. Functional joint centration implies maximum load bearing capability (i.e. the best and possible distribution of the load at the articular surfaces). In other words, it implies maximum contact of articular surfaces during each position during movement, allowing for ideal proprioceptive input.

Dysfunctional neuromuscular patterns may involve changes in respiration, possibly due to improper function or position of the diaphragm. Such patterns can be the result of the central nervous system (CNS) prioritising respiration over postural stabilisation (Hodges, 2001). This in part encourages the development of compensatory patterns in the global kinetic chain by destabilising abdominal pressure which negatively affects core stabilisation. Consequently, bilateral rib flares can develop, changing joint position in the thoracic rib cage. Destabilisation of the core accelerates undesirable adaptive patterns that predispose the body to injury by affecting muscular length-tension relationships across joints in multiple planes. Overactivity of accessory breathing musculature reinforces the poor respiratory pattern. This resultant maladaptive compensatory activity can contribute to or exacerbate dysfunction throughout the kinetic chain.

As competitive seasons wear on, athletes may demonstrate the cumulative effects of the many stressors encountered. These effects range from the development of spinal dysfunction to digestive disturbances and specific inflexibility/mobility patterns, which may lead to a decrease in performance and increased susceptibility to injury.

Training methods that focus on achieving strength and power that, according to Kraemer and Gomez (2001), require using Type II fibres (fast twitch, fatigue-sensitive fibres) are widely used in many sports See Chapter 2, p. 26-7, and Chapter 5, p. 117. When performed inappropriately or within a poorly balanced programme, many of these training variations promote faulty movement patterns. Therefore, faulty training approaches may be as much to blame for injury as overtraining or overuse. Furthermore, specific neuromuscular firing patterns described by Fritz and Grosenbach (2004) can be altered by daily living habits or adaptation to sports demands. Muscles that are required to undergo strength training to improve athletic qualities may become dysfunctional and/or prone to inappropriate firing patterns. According to Chaitow and DeLany (2002):

Excessive strength training frequently results in muscular imbalances between opposing muscle groups, as those which are being strengthened inhibit and overwhelm their antagonists ... This effect is not inevitable but reflects poorly designed training programmes.

Norris (2004) mentions that 'to strengthen a muscle for a specific movement, an exercise must mimic the movement as closely as possible'.

Traditionally strength and power training has utilised bilateral extremity exercises, such as barbell squats or bench press exercises. Most training regimens were developed towards anterior musculature or accelerator-dominant exercises. The posterior dominant chain decelerators and stabilisers were an afterthought. This method of training is another factor that may lead to increases in injury and dysfunction of the athlete, as it may train muscles and not the actual movement patterns required in a particular sport.

According to Myrland (2004), athletes must be able to produce and reduce force with balance and control on one leg. Proficiency in reciprocal movements is paramount to athletic development as most athletic motions are done in multi-planar and contralateral movements (Fig. 13.2A–C).

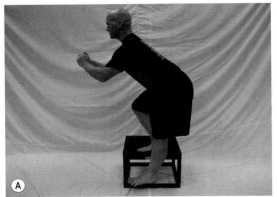

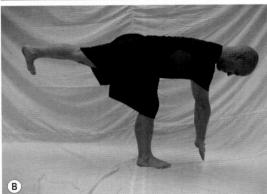

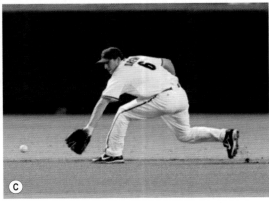

Fig. 13.2 (A–C) Exercises that utilise unilateral movements may be more advantageous than bilateral movements.

Boyle (2004) states that conditioning programmes should include acceleration, deceleration and change of direction as most injuries occur during these phases of movement.

It is also important to develop both muscle specificity and movement specificity. Fritz and Grosenbach (2004) and Riley and Bommarito (2004) described the cross extensor and flexor reflexes that many athletes utilise in sports. Their views show the need to train in an ipsilateral manner for proper neural firing patterns. These concepts can be programmed into a corrective/preventative plan for each athlete (Fig. 13.3A–C).

It is the authors' experience that strategies to counteract postural misalignment, faulty training programmes and other promoters of dysfunction will minimise potential damage, or potential damage, to tissues. These strategies may include MET, other manual soft tissue work, corrective exercise programmes, biomechanical adjustments, appropriate exercise selection and modification of training volume/recovery.

SCREENING FOR DYSFUNCTION

A meticulous and thorough screening for dysfunction is imperative as it may identify and help correct any problems before they cause irreparable tissue damage. The screening should look for overall gross movement dysfunction, postural abnormalities, flexibility, bilateral functional symmetry and muscle and joint function. It is the authors' view that in the presence of altered muscular length-tension relationships, optimum movement may not be anatomically possible. There are many general and specific tests that can help in determining dysfunction. Since many have been explained in detail previously in Chapters 6 and 9, the authors have chosen to describe several specific tests that work well in the sports environment, in addition to the previously mentioned tests. The combination of these test options should give the practitioner a reasonable picture of an athlete's current state of functionality. The relevance of these assessments to MET is explained later in this chapter.

Pre-Season Screen

An orthopaedic exam (of joint, ligamentous, cartilage and general neuromuscular function) should be coupled with a general well-being exam (internal organ, optical, dental, urinalysis, blood work) by a general medical physician.

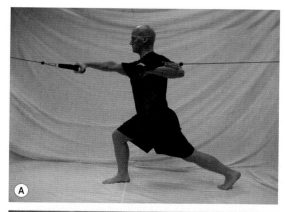

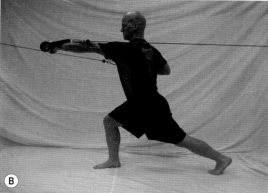

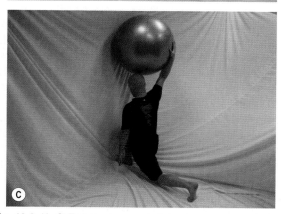

Fig. 13.3 (A–C) Training in a contralateral manner may help to activate the cross-extensor or cross-flexor reflexes, therefore aiding motor control in sport-specific movements.

A six-category screen should include these exams:
1. Static posture
2. Dynamic postures
3. Spine angle symmetry assessment

4. Breathing and abdominal function/strength
5. Overall flexibility/mobility
6. Manual assessment/muscle testing.

Static posture is the position from which all movement begins and ends. Therefore, the initial assessment of length–tension relationships begins here. Each athlete should have a static photograph taken in anatomical position from an anterior view, posterior view and lateral views, both right and left. The photographs ideally should be taken with reference to a plumb line or grid chart, offering a baseline for future comparison. The static abnormalities are noted and compared with further screening data.

Assessment of dynamic posture should be made with the same four views, utilising digital video as the recording device. The initial dynamic test is the overhead squat test. The athlete should be instructed to keep a dowel or foam roll overhead with arms extended. Two complete, full squats in each of the four directions should be completed (Fig. 13.4A and B). A single leg squat will increase the load and decrease stability providing a more specific test (Fig. 13.5). Dynamic scapulothoracic motion is noted by the athlete abducting his/her arms into a palm-touching position overhead and/or horizontally abducting (rowing) the arms with elbows bent to 90 degrees of flexion. These tests look for general kinetic chain movement patterns. They can help identify both quality of movement and segmental stabilisation in the scapulothoracic and scapulohumeral musculature (Fig. 13.6A–C).

Spine Measurements

After all posture, video and dynamic movement tests are compiled, a battery of goniometric/inclinometer measurements can be taken. This will allow specific variances to be noted in specific joints or joint segments and give detail for corrective strategies.

It is important to have a fundamental understanding of the spine and joint movements available prior to analysing the data. In all sports, the spine plays a central role in accomplishing the objectives of the sport (Farfan, 1996). Therefore, proximal stability, or 'punctum fixum' (fixed end/fixed point/starting point), will help promote distal mobility (Kolar, 2007).

According to Chek (2003), the standing curvature of the lumbar spine and the thoracic spine can be assessed via a dual inclinometer in the following manner. To assess static thoracic curvature and thoracic extension,

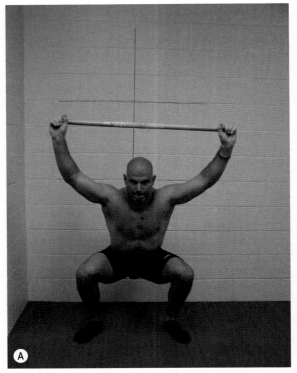
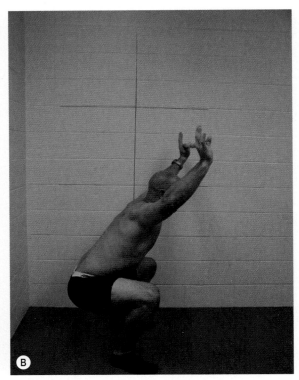

Fig. 13.4 (A and B) Screening for dynamic dysfunction should include the overhead squat assessment in all directions.

the practitioner should place the superior inclinometer on a central point between the C7–T1 spine junction and the inferior inclinometer on a central point between the T12–L1 junction before obtaining readings in neutral and extended positions. Another measurement of thoracic extension can be performed with the shoulders fully flexed overhead, elbows extended and palms in a neutral position. This measurement allows the practitioner to see how the upper extremities and thoracic extension function together (Fig. 13.7A and B).

Lumbar curvature can be measured in neutral, extended and flexed positions by placing the superior inclinometer between the T12–L1 junction and the inferior inclinometer between the L5 (or L6)–S1 junction and obtaining angles in the three different positions (Fig. 13.8A and B).

The normal range for static thoracic and lumbar curvature is 30 to 35 degrees according to Chek (2003). The available thoracic extension motion should be equal to the same degree as its measurement (e.g. a 30-degree

thoracic curve should have 30 degrees of extension). With the arms overhead, the thoracic extension in the spine should allow for at least 14 degrees of movement (Chek, 2003).

Hip Region Measurements

General assessment of the medial hamstring/hip adductors, rectus femoris/iliopsoas, hamstring, tensor fascia lata and quadratus lumborum have been described in Chapter 6. In addition, goniometric measurements of hip flexion/extension/internal rotation/external rotation and pelvic tilt should be performed.

Abdominal Strength and Coordination

Optimal core stabilisation is dependent on proper intercoordination of abdominal and respiratory musculature. Inspiration begins as the diaphragm contracts and draws caudally while creating a natural vacuum in the pleural cavity. The thoracic rib cage moves in a cephalad direction only as an accessory motion to normal intercostal

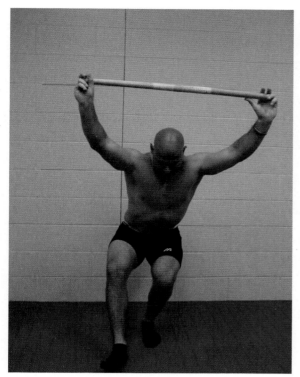

Fig. 13.5 A single-leg squat will increase load, decrease stability and show faulty movement patterns more specifically than the overhead squat.

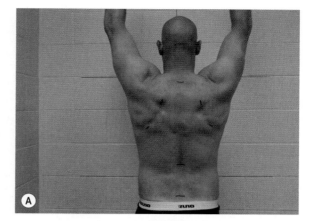

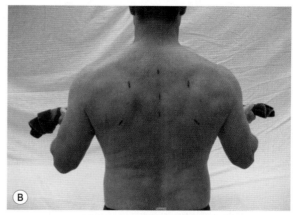

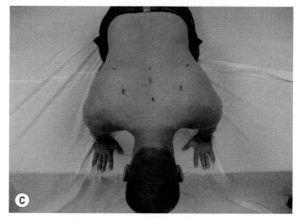

Fig. 13.6 (A–C) The practitioner should assess movement in both scapulospinal and scapulohumeral musculature for proper firing sequences and quality of motion. (A) Normal scapular overhead motion. (B) Scapular motion and control with muscular resistance. (C) Scapular control in a quadruped loaded position.

expansion. Contents of the abdominal viscera are compressed into the lower abdominal cavity and pelvic floor. The increase in intra-abdominal pressure through diaphragmatic activation, along with proper opposition via contractions of the surrounding abdominal musculature, results in 360 degrees of stiffness or 'bracing' of the outer wall (Liebenson, 2007) (Fig. 13.9).

Core function requires an individual to be able to create three-dimensional pressure of the abdominal wall when full caudal positioning of the ribs is achieved during exhalation. Then, the individual must maintain enough core pressure to control the relative caudal positioning of the ribs while allowing three-dimensional expansion of the abdominal wall and rib cage throughout the inhalation process. Abdominal coordination and strength may be tested by observing the athlete's ability to breathe optimally and correctly utilise his diaphragm as described above. This ability to generate 360-degree stiffness can be evaluated and assigned a simple manual

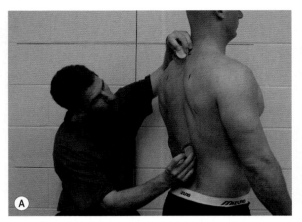
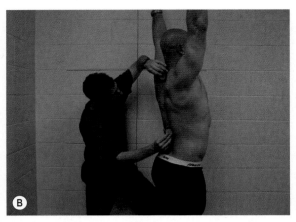

Fig. 13.7 (A and B) Thoracic spine measurements will give the practitioner an objective measurement of spine function. (Chek, 2003; Magee, 2008).

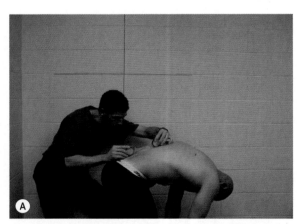

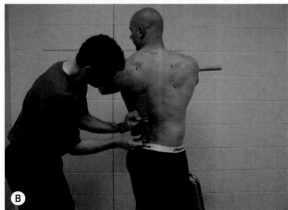

Fig. 13.8 (A and B) Lumbar spine measurements to assess curvature and movement will help the practitioner with screening (Chek, 2003; Magee, 2008).

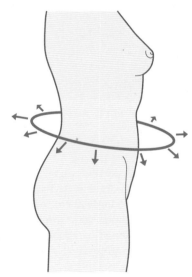

Fig. 13.9 360 degrees of stiffness or 'bracing' in the outer abdominal wall. (Reprinted with permission from Liebenson, 2007.)

muscle test value via palpation. Poor core stabilisation results in global adaptation patterns throughout the kinetic chain. Such dysfunction leads to compensatory over-activity of distal and proximal segments at the extremities. The pattern is commonly observed with over-active paraspinal musculature, leading to anterior pelvic rotation and elevation of the thoracic rib cage. This faulty 'scissor-like' position results in decentration of the spine, causing abnormal length-tension relationships across distal joints (Kolar, 2010).

Dynamic neuromuscular stabilisation (DNS) is a rehabilitative approach described by Kolar (2010) that achieves functional stabilisation by activating the 'integrated stabilising system of the spine' (ISSS). During purposeful (dynamic) movement, stabilisation of the spine and torso is achieved through muscular activation of 'short intersegmental spinal muscles (multifidi), deep neck flexors, the diaphragm, the abdominal wall and the pelvic floor' (Kolar, 2010). Functional stabilisation is achieved when the spinal musculature works as one unit and the quality of movement is undisturbed by dysfunction or pathology.

Diaphragmatic Control

The patient lies supine with the ribs in an exhaled position. The knees are bent with the feet on the table. Instruction is given for the patient to use diaphragmatic activation to create intra-abdominal pressure in caudal and three-dimensional directions around the core during exhalation. Attention is given by the practitioner to providing external cues to guide the ribs in a caudal direction while palpating the abdominal wall to maintain 'stiffness' of the oblique musculature (Fig. 13.10).

Function

Training of sagittal spine stabilisation continues with maintaining the position of the thoracic ribs in an exhaled position and continued expansion of the abdominal wall. The hips and knees are bent to 110 and 90 degrees of flexion respectively. Attention is given to training respiration and rib positioning while maintaining intra-abdominal pressure during a static supine hip flexion position (3-month developmental position) (Fig. 13.11A and B).

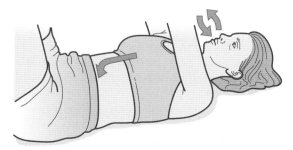

Fig. 13.10 Abdominal stiffness with ribs in caudal position. (Reprinted with permission from Liebenson, 2007.)

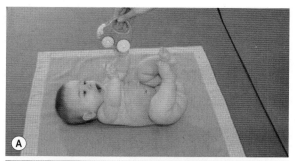

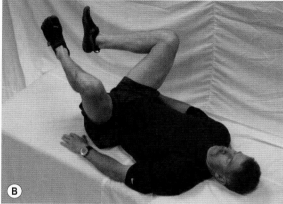

Fig. 13.11 (A and B) The 3-month developmental stage creates the ideal positioning for diaphragm and deep neck flexor activation.

Strengthening. Developing functional strength continues with the ability to maintain sagittal spine stabilisation during functional movement patterns. The exercise increases in difficulty by alternating the hips in a reciprocal flexion and extension direction for specified sets and repetitions (Fig. 13.12).

Endurance training. Retraining of the respiratory and abdominal function is dependent on achieving endurance of the stabilising spine musculature. The patient is directed to maintain rib positioning and intra-abdominal pressure while progressing through more difficult reciprocating movements for up to 2 minutes per set for a total of four sets.

Lower Extremity Measurements

Knee and ankle movements can be assessed via goniometric measurements. A navicular drop test of the foot can assess pronation and its possible effects up the kinetic chain (DeLany, personal communication, 2004). Finding the neutral position for the subtalar joint is

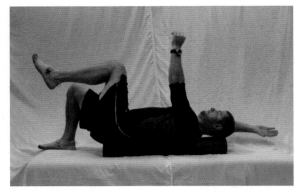

Fig. 13.12 Gradually increase loads on stabilisation system by moving extremities, or decrease stability, or both.

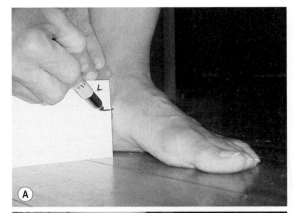

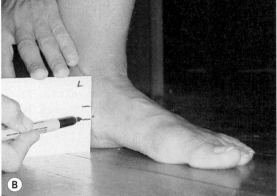

Fig. 13.13 (A and B) The navicular drop test can help determine dysfunction beginning in the foot and being transferred up the kinetic chain. (Reprinted with permission from Thompson, 2005.)

achieved by noting the medial prominence of the navicular bone in a non-weightbearing position. The athlete is then asked to weight-bear and the drop in navicular height is measured, as described as a navicular drop test by Thompson (2005). Also to be considered as significant is the degree of elevation (off the floor) of the first metatarsal when the foot is placed in the subtalar neutral position. The presence of an elevated position of the first metatarsal has been described as primus metatarsus elevatus by Rothbart (2002), which he hypothesises has significant whole-body postural implications (Fig. 13.13A and B).

Upper Extremities

In the throwing athlete, special attention should be given to the shoulder and elbow. All joint movements should be assessed and compared bilaterally. Values will frequently differ between dominant and non-dominant sides; however, these measurements may still be within the normal range, comparatively speaking. Wilk (2004) presented an example in professional baseball pitchers of the norm (external rotation at 90 degrees abduction: dominant side 129 ± 9 degrees, non-dominant side 122 ± 10 degrees; internal rotation at 90 degrees abduction: dominant side 62 ± 9 degrees, non-dominant side 70 ± 10 degrees) (Fig. 13.14).

Manual Assessment of Connective Tissues

The last screening component is a thorough manual assessment of the connective tissue structures to confirm identified dysfunctions from the previous assessment. Restrictions identified in the superficial subcutaneous tissue are often indicative of underlying pathology.

Deeper connective tissue restrictions can be the result of adaptive changes in the global system. Tissue restriction is assessed for its ability of multi-directional ease and pliability. According to Stecco and Stecco (2009): 'once the fascial afferents are normal, that is, no longer nociceptive, then the muscle tone normalises itself'. Treatment of these fascial afferent points should be 'dissolved completely before proceeding'. It is the authors' experience that optimal non-compensatory movement cannot be achieved in the presence of soft tissue dysfunction, emphasising the importance of manual assessment.

CORRECTIVE/PREVENTATIVE STRATEGIES

After a careful and comprehensive screening for dysfunction, an individualised corrective/preventative programme should be developed from the data collected.

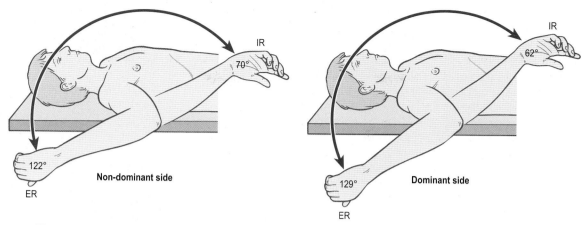

Fig. 13.14 The total motion concept discussed by Wilk (2004) shows the adaptation of the throwing shoulder in the professional baseball pitcher. (Reprinted with permission from Wilk, 2004.)

The programme may include stretching, strengthening, inhibition, repositioning or some other form of correcting identified musculoskeletal imbalances and dysfunction. Clearly, within such a corrective/preventative programme, the use of MET, in treatment or rehabilitation, may be relevant (see Chapters 6, 7, 9, 10, 11, 12 and 14). To identify movement pathology within the global kinetic chain, observation is vital as every test is an exercise and every exercise is a test. The relevance of these assessments to MET is explained later in this chapter.

Dynamic Flexibility Versus Static Stretching

Magee (2008) describes flexibility as the range of motion available in one or more joints, which is a function of contractile tissue resistance primarily, as well as ligament and joint capsule resistance. Whereas mobility refers to the ability of an individual to move any part of their body, using their joints and muscles, without pain or restriction (Frederick & Frederick, 2006). Both flexibility and mobility in the athlete are important for athletic performance if the motions are to be dynamically controlled. Any individual (athlete or not) will compensate for a lack of flexibility/mobility by using alternate movement patterns. It is possible for an athlete to perform well even when poor biomechanical motions are used, but eventually, a decrease in optimal tissue function will be experienced. It is therefore important to discuss what type of range of motion programme to use and when to use it.

There are many variations of stretching including proprioceptive neuromuscular facilitation (PNF), static stretching, MET and dynamic methods. These methods have been discussed by McAtee (1993), Kurz (1994) and Chaitow (2001), as well as in Chapters 2 and 4. Although the optimal method for improving athletic performance and decreasing injury may be debatable, the authors of this chapter advocate a systematic choice based on research evidence, clinical experience and athlete needs. Gleim and McHugh (1997) and Thacker et al. (2004) have shown evidence that stretching does not prevent sports injury. The most critical component of injury prevention appears to be an active warm-up. Young and Behm (2002) indicated that static stretching may inhibit maximal force production if performed within 1 hour prior to competition. This may reduce an athlete's ability to succeed in his/her competition. These findings support a more dynamic or active form of stretching/warm-up prior to competition. Static stretching, PNF, MET and other methods appear to be more beneficial post-competition, or at least 3 to 4 hours pre-competition, and/or during the rehabilitation process. Moore et al. (2011) noted that MET may help in lengthening soft tissues of the posterior shoulder, which has been a prominent point of debate in recent years.

Warm-Up

As Gleim and McHugh (1997) and Thacker et al. (2004) have demonstrated, warm-up is critical to injury prevention. A general increase in blood flow will aid in any mobility programme. An adequate dynamic warm-up may consist of 5 to 10 minutes of cardiovascular activity at 40% to 50% maximum heart rate along with sport-specific movements. It is the authors' preference to have all athletes do a general warm-up prior to any flexibility/corrective exercise session.

Recovery Techniques

As in any sport, the determinant of good function resides not only in the amount of targeted training work that an athlete does but also in the quality of recovery that takes place between exercise and/or athletic competition. Stress is simply a stimulus that interacts with the physiology of the body. Depending on the intensity of the stress, it can either injure or improve the athlete's functionality. To improve, there must be a balance between stress and recovery. According to Calder (1990), the following techniques can help athletes with their recovery from exercise or competition:

1. Proper nutrition and hydration
2. Hot/cold hydrotherapy techniques
3. General sports massage
4. Relaxation techniques (breathing, meditation, visualisation, flotation tank, music, etc.)
5. Rest or sleep.

In the presence of good general body conditioning and adequate recovery techniques, injury recovery will be optimal.

MUSCLE ENERGY TECHNIQUES (MET) AND INTEGRATED NEUROMUSCULAR INHIBITION TECHNIQUES (INIT) IN SPORTS INJURIES

As has been discussed, athletes may be injured or develop a variety of biomechanical dysfunctions. Prevention, treatment, rehabilitation and return to activity are critical components of an athlete's and a team's success. MET can be usefully and easily integrated into the total care of each athlete. However, it is important to understand that MET is only one element of the many available modalities. MET and its use in athletic settings will be described below in combination with other therapies. Emphasis on managing everyone's well-being and symptoms are the primary objectives.

Prevention of Injury Using MET, INIT and Other Techniques

The authors feel that the many acute dysfunctions that are described daily by athletes as 'general stiffness' or 'general soreness' can be managed by the following sequence:

1. Assessment of movement limitations
2. Assessment of skin mobility for underlying pathology
3. Assessment of myofascial trigger points
4. Assessment of breathing patterns and core dysfunction
5. General body warm-up or localised warm-up using moist heat or hydrotherapy
6. General massage (gliding primary application)
7. Modified version of INIT
8. MET for shortened structures
9. Functional range conditioning (FRC)
10. Isotonic/isometric/isokinetic corrective exercise programme
11. Post-exercise or post-competition recovery techniques
12. Appropriate nutrition and hydration.

The INIT used in this sequence was first described by Chaitow (1994), although the method described here is a variation. Palpate the trigger point:

> by direct finger or thumb pressure. The local tissues in which the trigger point lies should then be positioned in such a way as to reduce reported pain (entirely or at least to a great extent). At that time most (dis) stressed fibres in which the trigger point is housed would be in a position of relative ease [see Chapter 14 for a description of strain/counterstrain]. The trigger point would then be receiving both direct inhibitory pressure (mild or perhaps intermittent) and would have been positioned so that the tissues surrounding it are relaxed (relatively or completely).
>
> *Nagrale et al. (2010)*

It is the view of the authors of this chapter that this position should be maintained for 20 to 40 seconds, or until muscle release occurs.

Following this initial stage MET, utilising an isometric contraction of shortened musculature, with a post-facilitation stretch would then be initiated.

Isometric contractions should commence from the 'easy' resistance barrier (as described in Chapter 2). The shortened muscles (agonists) are isometrically contracted for 5 to 10 seconds using approximately 20% of their maximal contraction strength with the practitioner meeting and matching the athlete's effort. The athlete is requested to inhale diaphragmatically at the start of the contraction and to exhale, relax and to then breathe normally. As the contraction effort ends, the shortened muscle is stretched to its new barrier, slightly beyond and held for at least 10 seconds and up to 60 seconds. This process is repeated several times, with a 5-second break between repetitions. Each isometric contraction begins from the new barrier position. (See Chapter 2 for full discussion of barriers.)

In combination with the effects of MET and INIT, the principles of the FRC system can be applied to help solidify newly acquired articular ranges of motion. The FRC System was founded on two main principles: (1) The principle of progressive adaptation, which involves improving the load absorption capacity of any tissue by imparting progressively incremental loads on that tissue resulting in eventual sufficient adaption to the load demands and (2) the principle of specificity which encompasses training the nervous system how to adequately control specific and progressively increasing ranges of motion. Utilising a host of various methods, the FRC system aims in general to (1) simultaneously increase and strengthen articular ranges of motion (Expand), (2) condition the nervous system to reach full active articular capacity (Control) and (3) maximise movement fluidity through training practice (Create) (Spina, 2013a). Simply put, the FRC system of training aims to maximally enhance articular mobility (aka active, usable ROM). For the purposes of the scope of this chapter, the FRC-specific methods of progressive angular isometric loading (PAILs) and regressive angular isometric loading (RAILs) will be selected and described.

The PAILs method combines stretching with isometric loading at *progressive* articular angles while the RAILs method involves the same stretching yet using isometric loading at *regressive* articular angles. Both methodologies are used sequentially with one another to both expand range of motion (overriding the stretch reflex) and strengthen (maximal motor unit recruitment during isometric tissue contraction) within those expanded ranges in the effort to invoke eventual tissue adaptation which will prepare the tissue to function adequately in the new ranges of motion (Spina, 2013b; Spina, 2013c). PAILs/RAILs method includes three different levels of progressing intensity that can be chosen depending on the target goals. Level I PAILs/RAILs sequencing is utilised primarily in the acute injury setting when early

signs/symptoms are a limiting factor in function. The purpose involves communicating through force applied from low-level contractions within tissue to correctly influence how the cells produce and lay down collagen during the healing process. Levels II and III PAILs/RAILs are mainly employed in the subacute/chronic injury settings when healing has advanced and/or in asymptomatic preventative cases to enhance, train and solidify articular mobility.

Indications

- Stretching contracted soft tissue (fascia, muscle) or tissues housing active trigger points
- To optimise length-tension relationships
- To maximise neuromuscular function, thus increasing biomechanical efficiency.

Acute Injury Care With MET and Other Therapies

From a practitioner's perspective, the acute injury is the most fragile of all cases. Care to prevent further damage, while helping set up the optimal healing environment, is important and requires precise protocols.

The authors prefer the following treatment sequence in most acute muscle injuries. Joint, ligament, cartilage or bone damage may alter the sequence. The guidelines described below may usefully be applied in a variety of injury settings, where possible and appropriate.

1. Immediate cryotherapy, compression and elevation to moderate inflammation
2. Within 24 hours of injury, tissue oscillation therapy for lymphatic drainage and/or frequency-specific microcurrent therapy are used concurrently with cryotherapy for pain and control of inflammation
3. Deactivation of surrounding kinetic chain trigger points
4. Skin release or gliding techniques to assist the free motion of underlying fascia
5. Neural mobilisation if indicated
6. Correction of breathing patterns and any core dysfunction
7. 24 to 48 hours post-injury, INIT/MET/FRC in injured tissue and/or surrounding tissues
8. Proprioception exercises as tolerated
9. Corrective exercise programme
10. Any other acute therapies and progression to rehabilitation.

INIT/MET in Acute Settings

The following INIT/MET sequence is used in the acute injury:

- Identify any trigger points in the injured muscle or surrounding muscles with direct finger or thumb pressure.
- Gently compress the trigger points, either intermittently or persistently (as discussed fully in Chapter 14)
- Take the muscle into a position of ease that does not violate injured tissue, and hold for 20 to 40 seconds, after which a contraction in the antagonist muscle is initiated.
- The contraction should involve 20% or less of maximum contraction strength and should be held for 5 to 10 seconds.
- The practitioner's force should meet and match the athlete's force.
- This is thought to create reciprocal inhibition (RI) in the injured muscle (Lewit, 1999), however, see further discussion of the debate regarding RI (and PIR) in Chapters 2 and 5.
- The athlete should inhale prior to the contraction, and exhale and relax after the contraction.
- Within 5 seconds of relaxation, a very gentle movement of the injured muscle *to its new barrier (without any stretching effort)* should be initiated, provided there is no pain.
- Repeat once or twice more.
- This technique may be modified for sub-acute injuries, by adding an isometric contraction of the injured tissue itself, followed by post-isometric relaxation and mild stretch.

Indications

- Relaxation of acute muscle spasms or trigger points.
- Stimulation of neuromuscular firing to prevent muscle shutdown.
- A further alternative of the use of a MET variation in sub-acute settings (see Chapter 9 for more detail), involves the use of slowly performed isotonic eccentric stretches to encourage coherent remodelling (Parmar et al., 2011).

FRC in Acute Settings

The following FRC sequence (Level 1) is used in the acute injury (Spina, 2013d; Spina, 2013e):

- Identify injured tissue and corresponding target movement to influence
- Assume first perceived barrier of non-painful tension in the stretched position of target injured tissue (agonist)
- Passively maintain the position for 10 to 30 seconds
- Inhale and gradually build light, non-painful tension isometrically (20% of maximum contraction) in the stretched agonist tissue (PAILs) against the resistance of the practitioner
- The athlete's force should meet and match the practitioner's force
- Hold the isometric contraction for 10 seconds while maintaining normal breath sequencing and abdominal bracing
- Upon relaxation, the athlete gently increases the stretch depth so as not to violate the injured agonist tissue
- Inhale again and gradually build light tension isometrically (20% of maximum contraction) in the opposing antagonist tissue (RAILs) against the resistance of the practitioner
- Hold the isometric contraction for 10 seconds while maintaining normal breath sequencing and abdominal bracing
- Upon relaxation, re-establish the passive hold
- Repeat the procedure two or three times more staying within a non-painful range of motion

Indications

- Relaxation of acute muscle spasm and/or neurological guarding mechanism post-injury (2013d).
- Stimulation of neuromuscular firing for motor unit recruitment to prevent muscle deconditioning and improve neural drive.
- Applying progressive internal loads (without joint shearing) over time into damaged tissue to beneficially influence cells in the production and deposition of collagen during the early-stage healing process (2013d).
- The sub-acute PAILs/RAILs variation (Level 2) involves increased ramping of the maximum contraction percentages (50% to 80%) at each non-painful stretch barrier while holding each passive stretch for a 2-minute minimum. The increased ramping of contraction percentage allows for stronger potential influence on collagen deposition in addition to enhanced neural drive and motor unit recruitment within the targeted tissues for strength/movement control gains (2013d). The 2-minute minimum stretch time will create the best opportunity for the CNS to move beyond the temporary analgesic effect of stretching and instead invoke actual neural adaptation in stretch tolerance which ultimately governs the range of motion capability.

Chronic Injury and Long-Term Rehabilitation Using MET

Although chronic injuries are not particularly delicate, they are often the most difficult to treat because they may be perpetuated by deep-seated dysfunction. Adequate time and therapy are required to correct this type of injury. Rehabilitation from an injury that may have required surgery or immobilisation can be managed in a similar fashion to the chronic injury. Both cases require a thorough assessment of the entire kinetic chain for possible contributors to the injury. Once dysfunctions are identified, specific manual therapies, modalities and other techniques can be applied.

MET, INIT and a corrective isometric/isotonic/isokinetic exercise programme can be implemented in the following sequence:

1. General body warm-up
2. Specific modality treatment to increase blood flow
3. Specific modality treatment to promote lymphatic drainage, decrease pain/spasm if indicated
4. General massage to loosen overlying and surrounding tissues
5. Correction of breathing patterns and core dysfunction
6. INIT and MET (including pulsed MET – see Chapters 5 and 7) as noted in the MET/INIT sequences described above in relation to acute injury. The only difference between this approach (MET/INIT) in acute and chronic settings is that – following an isometric contraction – tissues are taken to their new barrier if the condition is acute, and beyond the barrier into stretch, if chronic
7. Corrective exercise programme
8. Recovery techniques – mentioned previously.

Indications

- Stretching of chronic shortened tissues (myofascial, muscle, fibrotic).
- Stretching tissues with active trigger points.

FRC in Chronic Settings

The following FRC sequence (Level 3) is used in the advanced injury setting (Spina, 2013e):

- Identify injured tissue and corresponding target movement to influence
- Assume first perceived barrier of non-painful tension in the stretched position of target injured tissue (agonist)
- Passively maintain the position for 2 minutes

- Inhale and gradually build light, non-painful tension isometrically (80% or greater of maximum contraction) in the stretched agonist tissue (PAILs) against the resistance of the practitioner
- The athlete's force should meet and match the practitioner's force
- Hold the isometric contraction for 30 seconds while maintaining normal breath sequencing and abdominal bracing
- Upon relaxation, the athlete gently increases the stretch depth so as not to violate the injured agonist tissue
- Inhale again and gradually build light tension isometrically (80% or greater of maximum contraction) in the opposing antagonist tissue (RAILs) against the resistance of the practitioner
- Hold the isometric contraction for 30 seconds while maintaining normal breath sequencing and abdominal bracing
- Upon relaxation, re-establish the passive hold
- Repeat the procedure two or three times more staying within a non-painful range of motion

Indications

- Relaxation of any muscle spasm and/or neurological guarding mechanism remaining from the initial injury
- Stimulation of neuromuscular firing for motor unit recruitment to prevent muscle deconditioning and improve neural drive
- Applying high-level internal loads (without joint shearing) over time to maximise the load-bearing capacity of targeted tissues while creating lasting neural adaptation to solidify the control of newly acquired ranges of motion around a specific joint(s) (Spina, 2013c).

MET USING ISOTONIC, ISOMETRIC AND ISOKINETIC CONTRACTIONS FOR STRENGTHENING WEAK POSTURAL MUSCLES

As explained in Chapters 6 and 10, these MET procedures are used in various aspects of injury rehabilitation, preventative and corrective programmes. Their use is dependent on the athlete's needs and the injury assessment.

Injured athletes are usually treated daily, leaving little requirement for instruction as to home/self-care exercises. However, if athletes are not available for treatment daily then a home programme should be implemented frequently involving self-stretching, mobilisation and strengthening exercises.

The following are some specific athletic injuries and useful management options using MET or INIT.

Case A: Sub-Acute Low-Back Strain

An athlete reports low-back pain. His subjective pain score is a 6/10, 10 being the most intense. His activity level is compromised. He states that he first felt the pain following a series of flexion movements during skills practice, 7 days prior. His chief complaint is generalised low back pain that is in the L4/L5/S1 area and, as the pain increases with an activity, it migrates laterally to both PSIS regions. The orthopaedic physician exam revealed no remarkable findings, with negative x-ray findings for spondylolysis/spondylolisthesis, and the neurologic exam was normal. The athlete had no previous history of back injury.

The diagnosis was a low-back strain. Objective evaluation information was as follows:

Test/Measurement	Finding	Norms (Chek, 2003; Magee, 2008)
1st rib angle (degrees)	31	25
SCM (degrees)	75	45–60
Thoracic curve (degrees)	57	30–35
Thoracic extension (degrees)	20	57 (reverse of T-curve)
Thoracic rotation (L/R)	35/40	35–50
Lumbar curve (degrees)	15	30–35
Lumbar extension (degrees)	15	20–35
Lumbar flexion (degrees)	24	40–60
Lumbar rotation (L/R)	6/8	3–18
Pelvic tilt: ASIS to PSIS (degrees)	13L, 12R	4–7
Hip rotation IR (L/R) Hip rotation ER (L/R)	25L, 35R 50L, 41R	30–40 IR 40–60 ER
Abdominal/breathing function	Poor/weak	

General testing demonstrated bilateral rectus femoris, psoas and spinal erector tightness. Bilateral foot pronation was evident together with the general internal orientation of the femurs, as well as genu recurvatum.

Manual assessment indicated bilateral skin restriction paraspinals, suggesting possible fascial restriction. Several trigger points were identified in the quadratus lumborum and erector spinae musculature. There was also bilateral psoas hypertonicity with tender points localised in the iliacus muscles. Both adductor muscle groups as well as piriformis were hypertonic.

Treatment

Treatment was initiated with a 5-minute stationary bicycle ride, followed by tissue oscillation modalities and tissue manipulation to the skin, underlying fascia and musculature in the thoracolumbar region. Trigger point areas previously identified were addressed with INIT (as described earlier in this chapter). MET using isometric contraction of agonist/post facilitation stretch (also described earlier in the chapter) was applied bilaterally to iliopsoas, rectus femoris and the right hip adductors. Self-mobilisation of the thoracic spine was performed with the use of a foam roller. Corrective exercises were implemented as follows:

1. Appropriate abdominal function exercise progressions focusing on correct rib position and diaphragm function were started. These progressions follow a sequence that begins with appropriate function, progressing to strength and finally endurance features.
2. Hip alignment exercises were utilised to specifically target the restoration of symmetry to goniometric measures in all three planes of motion. These isometric positional exercises encourage innominate, as well as acetabular femoral alignment (Fig. 13.15A and B).
3. Posterior kinetic chain exercises were initiated to promote strength and endurance in the gluteals and thoracic extensor/lower trapezius musculature. The optimum function requires strength as well as correct positioning of the scapulae. Time under tension is a key variable. See Chapter 5 for a discussion of isotonic eccentric and isokinetic variations of MET.
4. Exercises were prescribed to strengthen the deep neck flexors and to restore ideal spinal positioning. These exercises are based on developmental positions identified in the first year of life. These specific positions enable innate motor programmes to use appropriate firing patterns to facilitate the desired musculature and promote joint centration (Fig. 13.16).

Following this corrective programme, the athlete tolerated light skills activity well. After skills practice, a

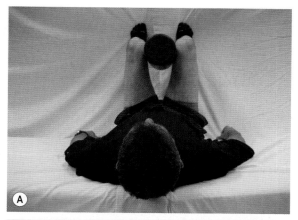

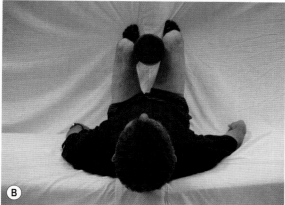

Fig. 13.15 (A and B) Exercises promoting reciprocal adduction/internal rotation and abduction/external rotation of the acetabular femoral joints on the right and left sides.

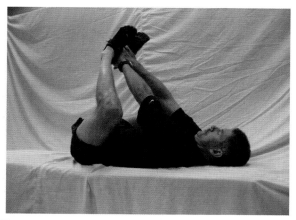

Fig. 13.16 The 5 to 6 months developmental stage creates a more advanced position for diaphragm and deep neck flexor activation.

second session of treatment excluding soft tissue work and trigger point deactivation was conducted. The second session ended with recovery-hydrotherapy techniques and cryotherapy. Return to full activity was based on symptoms and tolerance.

Case B: Shoulder Tendonitis (Subacromial Long Head of Biceps)

An overhead-throwing athlete reported right anterior shoulder soreness following a game. He had previously been experiencing periodic soreness in the anterior shoulder in the subacromial region. The athlete stated that his initial soreness started after a biomechanical change in throwing 2 weeks prior and that the soreness is tolerable when he gets warmed up. He has had no previous history of shoulder injury/pain. A subsequent examination by an orthopaedic physician, and MRI, revealed subacromial inflammation in the long head of the biceps.

The diagnosis was subacromial impingement/tendonitis. Objective evaluation prior to injury was as follows:

Test/Measurement	Finding	Norms (Chek, 2003; Magee, 2008)
1st rib angle (degrees)	37	25
SCM (degrees)	82	45–60
Thoracic curve (degrees)	52	30–35
Thoracic extension (degrees)	20	52 (reverse of T-curve)
Thoracic rotation (L/R)	35/40	35–50
Lumbar curve (degrees)	38	30–35
Lumbar extension (degrees)	20	20–35
Lumbar flexion (degrees)	15	40–60
Lumbar rotation (L/R)	2/7	3–18
Pelvic tilt: ASIS to PSIS (degrees)	13L, 12R	4–7
Hip rotation IR (L/R)	20L/33R	30–40
Hip rotation ER (L/R)	61L/50R	40–60
Abdominal/breathing function	Poor/weak	

General evaluation demonstrated that the athlete had pronounced bilateral protraction of both shoulders and internal rotation of the arms. A decrease in internal rotation and an increase in external rotation was noted in the right shoulder when compared with the left. Tests showed tightness of the pectorals and latissimus dorsi. Manual muscle testing revealed weakness (of the injured arm) in flexion of the shoulder (4/5), prone horizontal abduction with the thumb pointing upward (3/5) and external rotation at 0 degrees abduction. Manual assessment indicated bilateral pectoral tightness as well as hypertonic levator scapula, upper trapezius, subscapularis and infraspinatus.

Treatment

Initial treatment included a deep tissue oscillation modality, moist heat and general body warm-up – in conjunction with anti-inflammatory medications prescribed by a physician and general massage of the pectoral and latissimus dorsi muscles. Hypertonic or trigger point tissues were treated with the chronic injury version of INIT technique. MET using an isometric contraction of antagonist (Method 2), (Fig. 13.17A and B) as explained previously, was applied to the hypertonic muscles.

Corrective exercises were implemented as follows:

1. Appropriate abdominal function exercise progressions were started, beginning with the initiation of correct rib and diaphragm positioning. These progressions started with appropriate function, progressing to strengthening and finally endurance.
2. Posterior kinetic chain exercises to promote improved rib and shoulder girdle positioning were introduced. Length/tension relationships play a key role in position and in the establishment of correct motor sequences. Normal length/tension relationships equate to improved function, which are prerequisites to the existence of optimal strength and endurance.
3. Exercises to strengthen the deep neck flexors and restore ideal spinal positioning were commenced. These exercises are based on developmental positions identified in the first year of life. These specific positions enable innate motor programmes to use correct firing patterns to facilitate the desired musculature and promote joint centration (Fig. 13.18).
4. Thoracic mobilisation was initiated via the use of foam rollers.
5. Specific isotonic/isokinetic/reactive stabilisation exercises for the rotator cuff and scapular muscles were

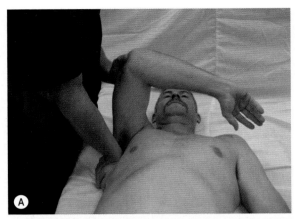
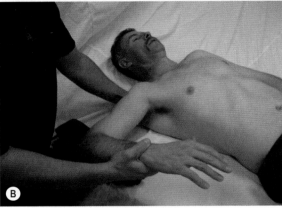

Fig. 13.17 (A and B) Many overhead-throwing athletes are limited in shoulder horizontal adduction and internal rotation which can be improved by muscle energy techniques (MET).

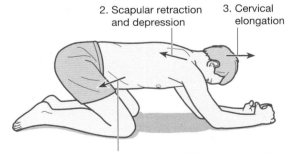

2. Scapular retraction and depression

3. Cervical elongation

1. Diaphragm '360 degree' inflation

Fig. 13.18 This developmental position is a corrective technique to facilitate proper scapular/thoracic, deep neck flexor and diaphragm activation.

used. See Chapter 5 for a discussion of isotonic eccentric and isokinetic variations of MET.

Following the corrective exercise programme, the athlete could participate in any skills activity that did not produce pain. After skills practice, recovery hydrotherapy techniques, cryotherapy and microcurrent treatment concluded the session. Return to full activity was based on symptoms and tolerance of functional activities.

Case C: Shoulder Subscapularis Strain and Anterior Capsule Sprain

An overhead-throwing athlete was removed from his start in the fourth inning after reporting right shoulder discomfort and an eventual decrease in fastball velocity. He reported that the symptoms initially occurred while warming up in the bullpen prior to his start that day. He had no previous symptoms leading up to the injury. A subsequent examination by an orthopaedic physician, and MRI, revealed a high-grade subscapularis strain with mild anterior capsule sprain.

Objective evaluation prior to injury was as follows:

Test/Measurement	Finding	Norms (Kapandji, 1982; Chek, 2003; Magee, 2008)
Thoracic curve (degrees)	31	30–35
Shoulder flexion (L/R)	176L/171R	180
Shoulder horizontal abduction	38L/41R	30–40
Shoulder horizontal adduction	40L/21R	30–45
Shoulder rotation IR (L/R)	85L/76R	90
Shoulder rotation ER (L/R)	113L/113R	90
Lumbar curve (degrees)	26	30–35
Pelvic tilt: ASIS to PSIS (degrees)	10L, 6R	4–7
Straight leg raise	61L/65L	90
Hip abduction	35L/28L	45
Hip rotation IR (L/R)	43L/32R	30–40
Hip rotation ER (L/R)	32L/33R	40–60
Abdominal/breathing function	Poor/weak	

General evaluation demonstrated that the athlete had increased external rotation with concomitant reduced internal rotation of shoulders. The decrease in internal rotation was more pronounced in the right shoulder when compared with the left. Tests also showed motion limitations in right horizontal adduction and bilateral flexion. Manual muscle testing revealed weakness (of the injured arm) in external rotation with arm at this side (4/5). Special testing showed mild discomfort with a posterior labral shear test only. Manual assessment indicated bilateral pectoral tightness as well as hypertonic levator scapula, upper trapezius and infraspinatus. Palpation revealed only mild tenderness along the posterior humeral head.

Treatment

Early phase treatment included a combination of several modalities (i.e. contrast hydrotherapy, microcurrent, pneumatic compression and prolonged low frequency electrical muscle stimulation) to aid the healing process both locally and systemically. In conjunction with the modalities, the continuation of effective warm-up, heart-rate-based conditioning and lower body/modified upper body resistance training splits was performed for the purpose of maintaining and improving upon in-season baseball work capacity. Manual myofascial work of identified areas of aberrant tissue tension and hypertonic or trigger point tissues was also prioritised. In addition, specialised manual rib cage mobilisations and targeted breathing work to improve scapula and shoulder position were carried out. To positively influence fibroblastic activity and reduce the local neurological guarding post-injury, the acute injury version (Level I) of FRC's PAILs/RAILs technique was selected and utilised on a daily basis. As the healing progressed and pain-free function returned, the more advanced versions (Levels II and III) of FRC's PAILs/RAILs were utilised at a frequency of 2 to 3 days per week to strengthen and enhance the load-bearing capacity of the previously injured tissue while solidifying neurologic control of newly acquired ranges of shoulder motion post-injury.

A comprehensive strengthening and reconditioning programme was implemented as follows:
1. Appropriate breathing sequence, rib cage positioning and abdominal function exercise progressions were initiated.
2. Isotonic (concentric/eccentric) and reaction-based exercises to promote improved shoulder girdle positioning, strengthening and stabilisation were introduced.

3. Exercises to specifically target the subscapularis and associated tissue stabilising the anterior shoulder capsule were selected and implemented. These particular exercises focused on solidifying proper abdominal function and rib cage control while maintaining upper R apical breathing expansion capability with simultaneous scapular positioning and open-chained concentric/eccentric resisted shoulder rotational movement.

4. Various pitching simulation drills were introduced later in the healing process utilising implements and external constraints to bridge the gap between rehabilitation and performance to optimise pitching mechanic efficiency.

The aforementioned treatment and rehabilitation programme was progressed in volume and intensity over the course of several weeks. A follow-up MRI completed at the 4{1/2} week mark post-injury revealed full resolution of the previous injury. At 5-week post-injury, an interval throwing programme was initiated. Return to competition was based on adequate healing time, elimination of symptoms and tolerance of functional and baseball activity progression.

SUMMARY

Athletic injuries present the practitioner with many different scenarios. As each athlete responds in a unique way, it is necessary to adapt the skills employed through knowledge and experience to meet the individual needs of the athlete, specific injury and surrounding variables.

MET, if utilised appropriately, can play a very important role in the overall healthcare of athletes. Further understanding of MET and other related therapies is an ever-evolving process for the sports practitioner.

REFERENCES

Andrews, J.R., Kupferman, S.P., Dillman, C.J., 1991. Labral tears in throwing and racquet sports. Clin. Sports Med. 10 (4), 901–911.

Borsa, P.A., Dover, G.C., Wilk, K.E., Reinold, M.M., 2006. Glenohumeral range of motion and stiffness in professional baseball pitchers. Med. Sci. Sports Exerc. 38 (1), 21–26.

Borsa, P.A., Scibek, J., Wilk, K.E., Jacobson, J.A., Reinold, M., Andrews, J., 2004. Instrumented measurement of gleno-humeral translation in professional baseball pitchers. Med. Sci. Sports Exerc. 36, S200.

Borsa, P.A., Wilk, K.E., Jacobson, J.A., Scibek, J.S., Dover, G.C., Reinold, M.M., et al., 2005. Correlation of range of motion and glenohumeral translation in professional baseball players. Am. J. Sports Med. 33 (9), 1392–1399.

Burkhart, S.S., Morgan, C.D., Kibler, W.B., 2000. Shoulder injuries in overhead athletes. The 'dead arm' revisited. Clin. Sports Med. 19 (1), 125–158.

Burkhart, S.S., Morgan, C.D., Kibler, W.B., 2003. The disabled throwing shoulder: spectrum of pathology. Part I, II, III. Arthroscopy, 19 (4), 19 (5), 19 (6).

Boyle, M., 2004. Functional training for sports. Human Kinetics Publishers.

Calder, A., 1990. Recovery: restoration and regeneration as essential components within training programmes. Excel 6 (3), 15–19.

Chaitow, L., 1994. Integrated neuromuscular inhibition technique. Br. J. Osteopathy 13, 17–20.

Chaitow, L., 2001. Muscle Energy Techniques, second ed. Churchill Livingstone, Edinburgh.

Chaitow, L., DeLany, J.W., 2002. Clinical Application of Neuromuscular Techniques. The Lower Body 2.

Chek, P., 2003. Certified high-performance exercise kinesiology practitioner certification level 1. Peak Performance, Manhattan, 10–19 November 2003.

Cools, A.M., Witvrouw, E.E., Declercq, G.A., Vanderstraeten, G.G., Cambier, D.C., 2004. Evaluation of isokinetic force production and associated muscle activity in the scapular rotators during a protraction-retraction movement in overhead athletes with impingement symptoms. Br. J. Sports Med. 38, 64–68.

Cools, A.M., Witvrouw, E.E., Mahieu, N.N., Danneels, L.A., 2005. Isokinetic scapular muscle performance in overhead athletes with and without impingement symptoms. J. Athl. Train. 40 (2), 104–110.

Crockett, H.C., Gross, L.B., Wilk, K.E., Schwartz, M.L., Reed, J., O'Mara, J., et al., 2002. Osseous adaptation and range of motion at the glenohumeral joint in professional baseball pitchers. Am. J. Sports Med. 30 (1), 20–26.

Dale, R.B., Kovaleski, J.E., Ogletree, T., Heitman, R.J., Norrell, P.M., 2007. The effects of repetitive overhead throwing on shoulder rotator isokinetic work-fatigue. N. Am. J. Sports Phys. Ther. 2 (2), 74–80.

Farfan, H.F., 1996. Biomechanics of the spine in sports. In: Watkins, R.G. (Ed.). The Spine in Sports, Mosby, St Louis, pp. 13–20.

Frederick, A., Frederick, C., 2006. Stretch to Win: Flexibility for Improved Speed, Power, and Agility. Human Kinetics, Champaign.

Fritz, S., Grosenbach, J.M., 2004. Mosby's Essential Sciences for Therapeutic Massage, second ed. Mosby, St Louis.

Gibson, M.H., Goebel, G.V., Jordan, T.M., Kegerreis, S., Worrell, T.W., 1995. A reliability study of measurement techniques to determine static scapular position. J. Orthop. Sports Phys. Ther. 21 (2), 100–106.

Gleim, G.W., McHugh, M.P., 1997. Flexibility and its effects on sports injury and performance. Sports Med., New Zealand 24 (5), 289–299.

Greenfield, B., Catlin, P.A., Coats, P.W., Green, E., McDonald, J.J., North, C., 1995. Posture in patients with shoulder overuse injuries and healthy individuals. J. Orthop. Sports Phys. Ther. 21 (5), 287–295.

Hodges, P., 2001. Postural activity of the diaphragm is reduced in humans when respiratory demand increases. J. Physiol. 537 (3), 999–1008.

Janda, V., 1987. Muscles and motor control in low back pain: assessment and management. In: Twomey, L.T. (Ed.), Physical Therapy of the low back. Churchill Livingstone, New York, pp. 253–278.

Janda, V., 1988. Muscles and cervicogenic pain syndromes. In: Grand, R. (Ed.), Physical Therapy of the Cervical and Thoracic Spine. Churchill Livingstone, New York, pp. 153–166.

Johnson, M.P., McClure, P.W., Karduna, A.R., 2001. New method to assess scapular upward rotation in subjects with shoulder pathology. J. Orthop. Sports Phys. Ther. 31 (2), 81–89.

Kapandji, I.A., 1982. The Physiology of the Joints Volume 1: Upper Limb, fifth ed. Churchill Livingstone, London.

Kebaetse, M., McClure, P., Pratt, N., 1999. Thoracic position effect on shoulder range of motion, strength, and three-dimensional scapular kinetics. Arch. Phys. Med. Rehabil. 80 (8), 945–950.

Kolar, P., 2007. Facilitation of agonist-antagonist co-activation by reflex stimulation methods. In: Liebenson, C. (Ed.), Rehabilitation of the Spine: A Practitioner's Manual, second ed. Lippincott Williams & Wilkins, Philadelphia, pp. 531–565.

Kolar, P., 2010. Dynamic neuromuscular stabilisation according to Kolar (DNS): a developmental kinesiology approach. Presentation, DNS Basic Course "A", 10 November 2010.

Kraemer, W.J., Gomez, A.L., 2001. Establishing a solid fitness base. In: Foran, B. (Ed.), High Performance Sports conditioning, 3–17.

Kurz, T., 1994. Stretching Scientifically: A Guide to Flexibility Training. Stadion, Island Pond.

Liebenson, C., 2007. A modern approach to abdominal training. J. Bodyw. Mov. Ther. 11, 194–198.

Lewit, K., 1999. Manipulative Therapy in Rehabilitation of the Motor System, third ed. Butterworths, London.

Ludewig, P.M., Cook, T.M., 2000. Alterations in shoulder kinematics and associated muscle activity in people with symptoms of shoulder impingement. Phys. Ther. 80 (3), 276–291.

Lukasiewicz, A.C., McClure, P., Michener, L., Pratt, N., Sennett, B., 1999. Comparison of 3-dimensional scapular position and orientation between subjects with and without shoulder impingement. J. Orthop. Sports Phys. Ther. 29 (10), 574–586.

Magee, D.J., 2008. Orthopaedic Physical Assessment, second ed. Saunders Elsevier, St. Louis.

McAtee, R.E., 1993. Facilitated Stretching. Human Kinetics, Champaign.

Meister, K., 2005. Throwing adaptations in youth and adolescents in baseball. Presentation, American Sports Medicine Institute Injuries in Baseball Course, 15 January 2005.

Moore, S.D., Laudner, K.G., McLoda, T.A., Shaffer, M.A., 2011. The immediate effects of muscle energy technique on posterior shoulder tightness: a randomised controlled trial. J. Orthop. Sports Phys. Ther. 41 (6), 400–407.

Mullaney, M.J., McHugh, M.P., Donofrio, T.M., Nicholas, S.J., 2005. Upper and lower extremity muscle fatigue after a baseball pitching performance. Am. J. Sports Med. 33 (1), 108–113.

Myers, J.B., Laudner, K.G., Pasquale, M.R., Bradley, J.P., Lephart, S.M., 2005. Scapular position and orientation in throwing athletes. Am. J. Sports Med. 33 (2), 263–271.

Myrland, S., 2004. No ice? No problem! Train. Cond. 24 (7), 43–47.

Nagrale, A., Glynn, P., Joshi, A., Ramteke, G., 2010. The efficacy of an integrated neuromuscular inhibition technique on upper trapezius trigger points in subjects with non-specific neck pain: a randomised controlled trial. J. Man. Manip. Ther. 18 (1), 38–44.

Norris, C.M., 2004. Sports Injuries, Diagnosis and Management, third ed. Butterworth-Heinemann, London.

Osbahr, D.C., Cannon, D.L., Speer, K.P., 2002. Retroversion of the humerus in the throwing shoulder of college baseball pitchers. Am. J. Sports Med. 30, 347–353.

Parmar, S., Shyam, A., Sabnis, S., Sancheti, P., 2011. The effect of isolytic contraction and passive manual stretching on pain and knee range of motion after hip surgery: a prospective, double-blinded, randomised study. Hong Kong Physiother. J. 29 (1), 25–30.

Pieper, H.G., 1998. Humeral torsion in the throwing arm of handball players. Am. J. Sports Med. 26, 247–253.

Reagan, K.M., Meister, K., Horodyski, M.B., Werner, D.W., Carruthers, C., Wilk, K., 2002. Humeral retroversion and its relationship to gleno-humeral rotation in the shoulder of college baseball players. Am. J. Sports Med. 30 (3), 354–360.

Riley, J., Bommarito, P., 2004. Position specific training for football: an application to the high school, college, and professional levels. Presentation. National Strength and Conditioning Association Sports Specific Conference, Orlando 10 January 2004.

Rothbart, B.A., 2002. Medial column foot systems: an innovative tool for improving posture. J. Bodyw. Mov. Ther. 6 (1), 37–46.

Selye, H., 1956. The Stress of Life. McGraw Hill, New York.

Spina, A., 2013a. Functional Range Conditioning BioFlow Redefining the Human Canvas. Functional Anatomy Seminars, 2013 pp. 1–18 Course Pack.

Spina, A., 2013b. Functional Range Conditioning Physiology of Stretching. Functional Anatomy Seminars, 1–13. Course Pack.

Spina, A., 2013c. Functional Range Conditioning PAILs/RAILs. Functional Anatomy Seminars, pp. 1–16 Course Pack.

Spina, A. 2013d. PAIL's and RAIL's for Rehab. Functional Anatomy Seminars. https://functionalanatomyseminars. com/frc-members-area/frc-members-lecture-videos/.

Spina, A. 2013e. FRC PAIL's/RAIL's. Functional Anatomy Seminars. https://functionalanatomyseminars.com/ frc-members-area/frc-members-lecture-videos/.

Stecco, L., Stecco, C., 2009. Fascial manipulation: Practical part. Piccin, Italy.

Thacker, S.B., Gilchrist, J., Stroup, D.F., Dexter Kimsey Jr., C., 2004. The impact of stretching on sports injury risk: a systematic review of the literature. Med. Sci. Sports Exerc. 36 (3), 371–378.

Thompson, B., 2005. Ankle pain (chronic) with associated low back pain. In: Chaitow, L., DeLany, J. (Eds.), Clinical Application of Neuromuscular Techniques – Practical Case Study Exercises. Churchill Livingstone, Edinburgh.

Warner, J.J., Micheli, L.J., Arsianian, L.E., Kennedy, J., Kennedy, R., 1992. Scapulothoracic motion in normal shoulders and shoulders with glenohumeral instability and impingement syndrome. Clin. Orthop. Relat. Res. 285, 191–199.

Wilk, K.E., 2004. Rehabilitation guidelines for the thrower with internal impingement. Presentation, American Sports Medicine Institute Injuries in Baseball Course, 23 January 2004.

Wilk, K.E., Meister, K., Andrews, J.R., 2002. Current concepts in the rehabilitation of the overhead athlete. Am. J. Sports Med. 30 (1), 136–151.

Wilk, K.E., Reinold, M.M., Dugas, J.R., Arrigo, C.A., Moser, M.W., Andrews, J.R., 2005. Current concepts in the recognition and treatment of superior labral (SLAP) lesions. J. Orthop. Sports Phys. Ther. 35 (5), 273–291.

Young, W.B., Behm, D.G., 2002. Should static stretching be used during a warm up for strength and power activities? Strength Cond. J. 24 (6), 33–37.

FURTHER READING

Anderson, J.E., 1983. Grant's Atlas of Anatomy, eighth ed. Williams and Wilkins, Baltimore.

Anderson, M.K., Hall, S.J., 1995. Sports Injury Management. Williams and Wilkins, Baltimore.

Andrews, J.R., Harrelson, G.L., Wilk, K.E., 2004. Physical Rehabilitation of the Injured Athlete, third ed. Saunders, Philadelphia.

Apostolopoulos, N., 2001. Performance flexibility. In: Foran, B. (Ed.), Performance flexibility. High Performance Sports Conditioning, 49–61.

Bandy, W.D., Irion, J.M., Briggler, M., 1998. The effect of static stretch and dynamic range of motion training on the flexibility of hamstring muscles. J. Orthop. Sports Phys. Ther. 27 (4), 295–300.

Basmajian, J.V., DeLuca, C.J., 1985. Muscles Alive, fifth ed. Williams and Wilkins, Baltimore.

Bompa, T.O., 1999. Periodization Training for Sports. Human Kinetics, Champaign.

Brotzman, S.B., Wilk, K.E., 2003. Clinical Orthopaedic Rehabilitation. Mosby, Philadelphia.

Chaitow, L., 2002. Positional Release Techniques, second ed. Churchill Livingstone, Edinburgh.

Chaitow, L., 2003. Palpation and Assessment Skills, second ed. Churchill Livingstone, Edinburgh.

Chaitow, L., DeLany, J.W., 2001. Clinical Application of Neuromuscular Techniques, Vol. 1: The Upper Body, second ed. Churchill Livingstone, Edinburgh.

Church, J.B., Wiggins, M.S., Moode, F.M., Crist, R., 2001. Effect of warm-up and flexibility treatments on vertical jump performance. J. Strength Cond. Res. 15 (3), 332–336.

Cook, G., 2001. Baseline sports-fitness testing. In: Foran, B. (Ed.), High Performance Sports Conditioning. Human Kinetics, Champaign, pp. 19–48.

Cramer, J.T., Housh, T.J., Johnson, G.O., Miller, J.M., Coburn, J.W., Beck, T.W., 2004. Acute effects of static stretching on peak torque in women. J. Strength Cond. Res. 18 (2), 236–241.

Derosa, C., Porterfield, J.A., 1998. Mechanical Low Back Pain: Perspectives in Functional Anatomy, second ed. Saunders, Philadelphia.

Ellenbecker, T.S., 2001. Restoring performance after injury. In: Foran, B. (Ed.), High Performance Sports Conditioning. Human Kinetics, Champaign, pp. 327–344.

Frederick, G.A., Syzmanski, D.J., 2001. Baseball (part I): dynamic flexibility. Strength Cond. J. 23 (1), 21–30.

Fritz, S., 2000. Mosby's Fundamentals of Therapeutic Massage, second ed. Mosby, St Louis.

Jones, L.H., Kusunose, R., Goering, E., 1995. Jones strain-counterstrain. Boise: Jones Strain Counterstrain Incorporated.

Janda, V., 1978. Muscles central nervous regulation and back problems. In: Korr, I. (Ed.), Neurobiological Mechanisms in Manipulative Therapy. Plenum Press, New York.

Kain, K., Berns, J., 1997. Ortho-bionomy: A Practical Manual. North Atlantic Books, Berkeley.

Kendall, F.P., McCreary, E.K., 1983. Muscle Testing and Function, third ed. Williams and Wilkins, Baltimore.

Knudson, D.V., Noffal, G.J., Bahamonde, R.E., Bauer, J.A., Blackwell, J.R., 2004. Stretching has no effect on tennis serve performance. J. Strength Cond. Res. 18 (3), 654–656.

Korr, I., 1980. Neurobiological Mechanisms in Manipulation. Plenum Press, New York.

Leahy, P.M., Mock, L.E., 1991. Altered biomechanics of the shoulder and subscapularis. Chiropr. Sports Med. 5 (3), 62–66.

Liebenson, C., 1990a. Muscular relaxation techniques. J. Manipulative Physiol. Ther. 12 (6), 446–454.

Liebenson, C., 1990b. Active muscular relaxation techniques (Part 2). J. Manipulative Physiol. Ther. 13 (1), 2–6.

Liebenson, C., 1996. Rehabilitation of the Spine. Williams and Wilkins, Baltimore.

Liebenson, C., 2001. Sensory motor training. J. Bodyw. Mov. Ther. 5 (1), 21–27.

Lukasiewiscz, A.C., McClure, P., Michener, L., Pratt, N., Sennett, B., 1999. Comparison of 3-dimensional scapular position and orientation between subjects with and without shoulder impingement. J. Orthop. Sports Phys. Ther. 29 (10), 574–586.

Lum, L.C., 1987. Hyperventilation syndromes in medicine and psychiatry: a review. J. R. Soc. Med. 80 (4), 229–231.

Magee, D., 1997. Orthopaedic Physical Assessment, third ed. Saunders, Philadelphia.

McGill, S., 2004. Ultimate Back Fitness and Performance. Wabuno, Waterloo.

Myers, T., 2002. Anatomy Trains Myofascial Meridians for Manual and Movement Therapists. Churchill Livingstone, Edinburgh.

Norris, C., 2000. Back Stability. Human Kinetics, Champaign.

Peri, M.A., Halford, E., 2004. Pain and faulty breathing: a pilot study. J. Bodyw. Mov. Ther. 8 (4), 297–306.

Sahrmann, S.A., 2002. Diagnosis and Treatment of Movement Impairment Syndromes. Williams and Wilkins, Baltimore.

Shrier, I., 1999. Stretching before exercises does not reduce the risk of local muscle injury; a critical review of the clinical and basic science literature. Clin. J. Sports Med. 9 (4), 221–227.

Simons, D., Travell, J., Simons, L., 1999. Myofascial Pain and Dysfunction: The Trigger Point Manual, second edUpper Half of Body1. Williams and Wilkins, Baltimore.

Solem-Bertott, E., Thuomas, K.A., Westerberg, C.E., 1993. The influence of scapular retraction and protraction on the width of the subacromial space: an MRI study. Clin. Orthop. 296 (Nov), 99–103.

Travell, J., Simons, D., 1993. The Lower Extremities. Myofascial Pain and Dysfunction; The Trigger Point Manual, vol. 2. Williams and Wilkins, Baltimore.

Warner, J.P., Micheli, L.J., Arslanian, L.E., Kennedy, J., Kennedy, R., 1992. Scapulothoracic motion in normal shoulders and shoulders with glenohumeral instability and impingement: a study using Moire topographic analysis. Clin. Orthop. 285 (Dec), 191–199.

Wenos, D.L., Konin, J.G., 2004. Controlled warm up intensity enhances hip range of motion. J. Strength Cond. Res. 18 (3), 529–533.

Integrated Neuromuscular Inhibition Technique (INIT) and Myofascial Pain

Leon Chaitow, Sandy Fritz

CHAPTER CONTENTS

EVIDENCE-INFORMED PRACTICE FOR MYOFASCIAL PAIN

Myofascial pain and myofascial trigger points (MTrPs) phenomena have been the focus of research for years. It is important to acknowledge that the mechanisms for the development of myofascial pain and for the benefits of various treatments remain elusive. There continues to be ongoing research on this topic (Abd El-Azeim et al., 2019; El-Hafez et al., 2020; Galasso et al., 2020; Yoosefinejad et al., 2021).

Multiple studies indicate that combined multi-modal treatment approaches tend to be the most successful (El-Hafez, et al., 2020; Lu et al., 2020; Arun & Kumar, 2020; Ortega-Santiago et al., 2020). Integrated neuromuscular inhibition technique (INIT) provides a structure for such an integrated and multimodal approach (Chaitow, 1994b; Saadat et al., 2018; Metgud et al., 2020).

LOCAL FACILITATION

According to research by Korr, a trigger point is a local-ised, commonly peripheral, area of somatic dysfunction which behaves in a facilitated (i.e. sensitised) manner, that will amplify and be affected by any form of stress imposed on the individual, whether this is physical, chemical or emotional (Korr, 1976). Korr's early work is confirmed by that of Mense (2008), Ge et al. (2009) and Affaitati et al. (2011). In Affaitati et al. (2020) state: 'The pathophysiology of these pain associations is complex and probably multifactorial; among the possible processes underlying the mutual influence of symptoms recorded in the associations is modulation of central sensitisation phenomena by nociceptive inputs from one or the other condition' (Srbely et al., 2010). Similar conclusions are reached in Donald Murphy's discussion of nociplasticity in Chapter 8.

While the exact pathophysiology of myofascial pain is not clear, the energy crisis theory is widely accepted.

Based on this theory, MTrPs are caused by a recurring trauma to the muscle tissue leading to an excessive release of calcium and shortening of the sarcomeres resulting in decreased blood supply, causing inadequate adenosine triphosphate (ATP) synthesis. As a result, the sarcomeres affected do not return to a normal resting length. This sustained contraction causes metabolic waste products to accumulate, which results in pain. In addition, the motor endplate theory describes that MTrPs are formed due to the abnormal and excessive release of acetylcholine from the motor endplate – even during relaxation (Huguenin, 2004; Wendt & Waszak, 2020). For years a correlation has been identified between motor points, innervation zones and the location of trigger points (Akamatsu et al., 2015; Pinheiro et al., 2020; Wada et al., 2020). Motor points are the surface projection onto the skin of the muscle zone of innervation. The location correlation occurs at a site where a branch of a muscle's motor nerve enters the muscle and terminates in a number of motor endplates. At this site there is also a neurovascular bundle, containing large and small sensory nerves, the latter having terminal nociceptors and blood vessels with closely associated autonomic nerve fibres (Mense et al., 2021). Minerbi and Vulfsons (2018) suggest that postural muscles, in which motor units are recruited in rotation, may be part of a causal relationship between muscle load, muscle strength and the evolution of an energy crisis, as well as providing a logical mechanism for the threshold properties of the energy crisis phenomenon and, consequently, of the myofascial pain syndrome.

In addition, tenderness at the MTrP site is also attributed to the release of neuropeptides, cytokines, inflammatory substances (substance P), calcitonin gene-related peptide, interleukin-1a, bradykinin and protons that create local acidity. Oxidative stress, inflammation and glial cell in the central nervous system are factors related to the persistence of pain sensation that later on lead to the myofascial trigger point (Shah and Gilliams, 2008; Widyadharma, 2020).

Another factor in myofascial syndromes appears to be the amount and viscosity of hyaluronic acid in an area. Hyaluronic acid (HA) acts as a lubricant for muscle sliding. HA is produced in higher amounts during overuse of muscles, increasing viscosity, thus impairing muscle and connective tissue sliding function which then stimulates mechanoreceptors and nociceptors causing pain and limited movements (Qureshi et al., 2019).

The long-standing description of a trigger point as an indurated, localised, painful entity, with a reference (target) area to which pain or other symptoms are referred (Chaitow, 1991a) remains a valid working definition. Trigger points in muscles are located either close to the centre of the muscle, near the motor endpoint or close to attachments. Simons et al. (1999) have suggested that care is needed in treating attachment points as these tissues are prone to inflammatory responses (enthesitis), and that deactivation of centrally located points (by means of treatment, see below, or by elimination or modification of aggravating factors) tends to halt the activity of attachment points.

Management of trigger points by manual means (neuromuscular approaches) has been fully described elsewhere (Chaitow & DeLany, 2000, 2002, 2008, 2011; Chaitow, 2003, 2011).

Muscles housing trigger points can frequently be identified as being unable to achieve their normal resting length using standard muscle evaluation procedures (Janda, 1983), as described in Chapter 6. The trigger point itself always lies in hypertonic tissue, and not uncommonly in fibrotic or scar tissue, which has evolved as the result of exposure of the tissues to diverse forms of stress, as outlined above.

Musnick (2008) has summarised the need to remove the stressors, adaptive demands that feed into the aetiology and the maintenance of myofascial pain. Many of these are amenable to the employment of Muscle Energy Techniques in one form or another:

- Reduce the synergistic inputs to the pain process (i.e. modify adaptive demands)
- Deactivate trigger points (see below in this chapter)
- Remove noxious input from scars (see below in this chapter)
- Enhance spinal and general joint functionality (as described in Chapters 6, 7, 8 and 9)
- Improve muscle recruitment, strength and flexibility (as described in Chapters 5 and 6)
- Pay attention to exacerbating factors in diet, lifestyle and habits (sleep, exercise, posture, balance, breathing)
- Consider emotional/psychological factors.

LOCATING TRIGGER POINTS

STAR Palpation

In osteopathic medicine, the acronym 'STAR' is used as a reminder of the characteristics of somatic dysfunction, such as myofascial trigger points. STAR stands for:

- **S**ensitivity (or 'Tenderness')[1] – this is the one feature that is almost always present when there is soft tissue dysfunction.
- **T**issue texture change – the tissues usually 'feel' different, for example, they may be tense, fibrous, swollen, hot, cold or have other 'differences' from normal; and/or the skin overlying dysfunctional tissues usually palpates as different from surrounding tissues (Lewit, 1999).
- **A**symmetry – there will commonly be an imbalance on one side, compared with the other, but this is not always the case.
- **R**ange of motion reduced – muscles will probably not be able to reach their normal resting length, or joints may have a restricted range.

If two or three of these features are present this is sufficient to confirm that there is a problem, a dysfunction.

Research by Fryer et al. (2004) has confirmed that this traditional osteopathic palpation method is valid. When tissues in the thoracic paraspinal muscles were found to be 'abnormal' (tense, dense, indurated) the same tissues (using an algometer) were also found to have a lowered pain threshold. See discussion on assessment accuracy in Chapter 4.

While the 'tenderness', altered texture and range of motion characteristics, as listed in the STAR (or TART) acronym, are *always* true for trigger points, additional trigger point changes have been listed by Simons et al. (1999):

- The soft tissues housing the trigger point will demonstrate a painful limit to stretch range of motion – whether the stretching is active or passive.
- In such muscles, there is usually pain or discomfort when it is contracted against resistance, with no movement taking place (i.e. an isometric contraction).
- The amount of force the muscle can generate is reduced when it contains active trigger points (or latent ones, i.e. trigger points that do not produce symptoms with which the patient is familiar) – and will usually test as being weaker than a normal muscle.
- There is a taut band, housing an exquisitely tender nodule, commonly located by palpation unless the trigger lies in very deep muscle and is therefore inaccessible to palpation.

---

[1]The acronym STAR is modified in some texts to 'TART' (**T**enderness – **A**symmetry – **R**ange of movement modified – **T**issue texture change).

- Pressure on an active trigger point produces pain familiar to the patient, and often a painful response ('jump sign').

Drag Palpation

It is possible to assess the skin for variations in skin friction, by lightly running a fingertip across the skin surface (no lubricant should be used). This palpation method can be used to compare areas that are palpated as 'different' from surrounding tissues or to rapidly investigate any local area for trigger point activity.

- The degree of pressure required is minimal – skin touching skin is all that is necessary – a 'feather-light touch'.
- Movement of a single palpating digit (pad of the index or middle finger is best) should be purposeful, not too slow and certainly not very rapid. Around 3 to 5 cm (1 to 2 inches) per second is a satisfactory speed. (If movement is too slow it will not easily pick up differences, and if too fast information may be missed.)
- What is being sought is any sense of 'drag', suggesting a resistance to the easy, smooth passage of the finger across the skin surface.
- A sense of 'dryness', 'sandpaper', a slightly harsh or rough texture, may all indicate an increased presence of hydrosis (sweat) on, or increased fluid in, the tissues.

The method of drag palpation is extremely accurate and speedy. It is thought to indicate a localised area of increased sympathetic activity, manifested by sweat. Lewit (1999) describes such regions as 'hyperalgesic skin zones'. A trigger point will commonly be found in such zones.

TRIGGER POINT TREATMENT METHODS

A wide variety of treatment methods have been advocated in the past and continue to be used for treating trigger points, including:

- Inhibitory (ischaemic compression) pressure methods (Nimmo, 1966; Lief, 1982/1989; Fernandez-de-las-Peñas et al., 2006)
- Acupuncture and/or ultrasound (Kleyhans, 1974; Gam et al., 1998)
- Chilling and stretching of the muscle in which the trigger lies (Hou et al., 2002)
- Dry needling (Gerwin & Dommerholt, 2002; Ong & Claydon, 2014; Liu et al., 2015)
- Procaine or xylocaine injections (Slocumb, 1984; Scott, 2009)
- Active or passive stretching (Lewit, 1999; Sherman et al., 2006)

- Massage and proprioceptive neuromuscular facilitation (PNF) style stretching (Trampas et al., 2010)

Clinical experience has shown that while all or any of these methods can successfully inhibit trigger point activity short-term, in order to completely eliminate the noxious activity of the structure, more is often needed (Galasso et al., 2020; Urits et al., 2020).

Travell and Simons (1983, 1992) have shown that whatever initial treatment is offered to inhibit the neurological overactivity of the trigger point, the muscle in which it lies has to be made capable of reaching its normal resting length following such treatment or else the trigger point will rapidly reactivate.

In treating trigger points, the method of chilling the offending muscle (which contains the trigger), while holding it at stretch in order to achieve this end, was advocated by Simons et al. (1999), while Lewit (1999) recommends Muscle Energy Techniques in which a physiologically induced postisometric relaxation (or reciprocal inhibition) response is created, prior to passive stretching. Both methods are commonly successful, although a sufficient degree of failure occurs (trigger rapidly reactivating or failing to completely 'switch off') to require investigation of more successful approaches. One reason for failure may be the possibility that the tissues being stretched were not the precise structures housing the trigger point.

THE STRETCHING EFFECT OF ISOMETRIC CONTRACTIONS

As described in Chapter 2, isometric contractions, as used in muscle energy technique (MET), have a direct lengthening effect on sarcomeres shortened as a result of the trigger point contracture. An isometric contraction introduces a lengthening of the series elastic component (fascial, tendinous structures), while the parallel elastic component of the sarcomere shortens, as actin and myosin slide across each other – so that the muscle overall does not change length.

Repeated isometric contractions effectively lengthen the *series elastic* structures – particularly if active or passive stretching is subsequently added (Lederman, 1997, 2005).

In this way, both the active and passive phases of MET can be seen to contribute to muscle elongation (Milliken, 2003).

HYPOTHESIS

The principal author Leon Chaitow hypothesised that partial contraction (using no more than 20% to 30% of patient strength, as is the norm in MET procedures) may sometimes fail to achieve activation of the fibres housing the trigger point being treated since the light contractions used in MET of this sort fail to recruit more than a percentage of the muscle's potential. Subsequent stretching of the muscle may therefore only marginally involve the critical tissues surrounding and enveloping, the myofascial trigger point.

It is also suggested that when a muscle, such as hamstrings or upper trapezius, is stretched as a whole, the tissues in which the trigger point is embedded may not lengthen specifically, and that localised stretches would seem to offer a more certain way of achieving lengthening of the taut, short, myofascial tissues surrounding the trigger point.

Failure to actively stretch the muscle fibres in which the trigger is housed – for whatever reason – may account for the not infrequent recurrence of trigger point activity in the same site following treatment. Repetition of the same stress factors that produced it in the first place could undoubtedly also be a factor in such recurrence – emphasising the need for re-education in rehabilitation. Indeed, it has been suggested that removal of the irritating stress factors (such as excessive use of particular muscle groups), that result in and maintain, the painful and other influences of active trigger points, is often all that is required. Nevertheless, because trigger points can create so much distress it is frequently important to deactivate them manually, or by other means (injection, dry needling, etc.). A method that achieves precise focus on the target tissues (in terms of tonus release and subsequent stretching) is clearly desirable (see INIT method described later in this chapter).

SELYE CONCEPTS

Selye has described the progression of changes in tissue which is being locally stressed (see Chapter 5 for more detail). There is an initial alarm (acute inflammatory) stage, followed by a stage of adaptation or resistance when stress factors are continuous or repetitive, at which time muscular tissue becomes progressively fibrotic as we have seen in earlier chapters. If this change is taking place in a muscle which has a predominantly postural rather than a phasic function, the entire muscle structure will shorten (Selye, 1984; Janda, 1985).

Such hypertonic, and possibly fibrotic tissue, lying in altered (shortened) muscle, may not be easily able to 'release' itself in order to allow the muscle to achieve its normal resting length which, as has been noted, is a prerequisite of normalisation of trigger point activity.

Along with various forms of stretch (passive, active, MET, PNF, etc.), it has been noted above that inhibitory pressure is commonly employed in the treatment of trigger points. Such pressure technique methods (analogous to acupressure or shiatsu methodology) are often successful in achieving at least a short-term reduction in trigger point activity and have variously been dubbed 'neuromuscular techniques' (Chaitow, 1991b).

ISCHAEMIC COMPRESSION VALIDATION

Researchers at the Department of Physical Medicine and Rehabilitation, University of California, Irvine, evaluated the immediate benefits of treating an active trigger point in the upper trapezius muscle by comparing four commonly used approaches, as well as a placebo treatment (Hong et al., 1993). The methods used included:

1. Ice spray and stretch (Simons et al. (1999) approach)
2. Superficial heat applied by a hydrocollator pack (20 to 30 minutes)
3. Deep heat applied by ultrasound (1.2 to 1.5 watt/cm² for 5 minutes)
4. Dummy ultrasound (0.0 watt/cm²)
5. Deep inhibitory pressure soft tissue massage (10 to 15 minutes of modified connective tissue massage and shiatsu/ischaemic compression).[2]

For the study, 24 patients were selected who had active triggers in the upper trapezius which had been present for not less than 3 months and who had had no previous treatment for these for at least 1 month prior to the study (as well as no cervical radiculopathy or

myelopathy, disc or degenerative disease). The following measurements were carried out:

- The pain threshold of the trigger point area was measured using a pressure algometer three times pre-treatment and within 2 minutes of treatment.
- The average was recorded on each occasion.
- A control group were similarly measured twice (30 minutes apart); this group received no treatment until after the second measurement.

The results showed that:

- All methods (but not the placebo ultrasound) produced a significant increase in pain threshold following treatment, with the greatest change being demonstrated by those receiving deep pressure treatment.
- The spray and stretch method was the next most efficient in achieving a reduction in pain threshold.

Why is the deep pressure technique more effective than other methods? The researchers suggest that:

Perhaps deep pressure massage, if done appropriately, can offer better stretching of the taut bands of muscle fibres than manual stretching because it applies stronger pressure to a relatively small area compared to the gross stretching of the whole muscle. Deep pressure may also offer ischemic compression which [has been shown to be] effective for myofascial pain therapy.

Simons (1989)

More current studies continue to validate findings from the studies conducted in the 1980s to 1990s, though higher quality research continues to be necessary (Saadat et al., 2018; Kaprail et al., 2019; Rezaei et al., 2020).

ISCHAEMIC COMPRESSION IN TRIGGER POINT DEACTIVATION

There is an apparent contradiction in applying deep pressure to already ischaemic tissues, as originally suggested by Travell and Simons (1983), since the effect of this would seem to be to reduce blood flow even more (McPartland, 2004). Indeed, in the second edition of that 1983 text, Simons et al. (1999) modified their suggested digital pressure approach (which they now describe as 'trigger point pressure release'), recommending a lighter compression, meeting tissue tension, engaging the restriction barrier and allowing gentle stretching of the affected tissues.

---

[2]Application of inhibitory pressure may involve elbow, thumb, finger or mechanical pressure (a wooden rubber-tipped T-bar is commonly employed in the USA), or cross-fibre friction. Such methods are described in detail in a further text in this series (Chaitow, 2003).

Australian research has validated Simons et al.'s (1999) suggested methodology (Fryer & Hodgson, 2005). The pressure pain threshold (PPT) of latent trigger points in the upper trapezius of 37 individuals was recorded pre- and post-intervention, using a digital algometer (Box 14.1). It was found that there was a significant increase in the mean PPT of trigger points following the use of ischaemic compression ($P > .001$). The researchers report that pressure was monitored and maintained during the application of treatment and a reduction in perceived pain and a significant increase in tolerance to treatment pressure ($P > .001$) appeared to be caused by a change in tissue sensitivity, rather than any unintentional reduction of pressure by the examiner.

Spanish research (de las Peñas et al., 2006) has also confirmed that PPTs reduced significantly (measured by an algometer and also using a visual analogue scale – see Box 14.1 on algometrics) when active and latent trigger points in the upper trapezius were treated using either ischaemic compression or cross-fibre friction massage methods.

The results showed a significant improvement in the PPT ($P = .03$), and a significant decrease in the visual analogue scale ($P = .04$) within each group. No differences were found between the improvements noted in both groups.

Effects of Sustained or Intermittent Compression?

- Ischaemia: reduces local circulation until pressure is released, after which a flushing of fresh oxygenated blood occurs (Simons et al., 1999)
- 'Neurological inhibition' as a result of a sustained volley of messages to the central nervous system (efferent barrage) (Ward, 1997)
- Mechanical stretching starts as 'creep' of connective tissue (Cantu & Grodin, 1992)
- Piezoelectric effects modify the 'gel' (hardened) state of tissues to a more solute ('sol' or softer) state (Barnes, 1996). While the evidence base for physiologically significant piezoelectric responses in tissue is lacking, difficulties in quantifying the physiological response and imperfect measurement techniques may have underestimated the property (Poillot et al., 2021.)
- Rapid nerve (mechanoreceptor) impulses interfere with slower pain messages reducing the amount of pain messages reaching the brain ('gate theory') (McMahon et al., 2013)

- Pain-relieving hormones (endorphins, enkephalins, endocannabinoids) released (Baldry, 1993; McPartland, 2008)
- Taut bands associated with trigger points release spontaneously when compressed (Simons et al., 1999)
- Traditional Chinese medicine (TCM) suggests modification of energy flow through tissues following pressure application. Guan et al. (2020) studied simulated Chinese medical manipulation (also known as Tuina). Tuina manipulations can activate internal biological pathways through coordinated and rhythmic pressure stimulation on the body (Zhang et al., 2016). The mechanical effects of the manipulations on human tissue involve periodic force changes, and then the mechanical effects are converted into the biological effects to relieve clinical symptoms (Guan et al., 2020).

BOX 14.1 The Use of Algometrics in Treating Trigger Points

An area of concern in trigger point evaluation lies in the non-standard degree of pressure being applied to tissues when they are being tested manually. In order to establish the 'type' and behaviour of trigger points, various researchers have evaluated the usefulness of an algometer in the process (Fryer & Hodgson, 2005; Bordeniuc et al., 2020; Jerez-Mayorga et al., 2020).

A basic algometer is a hand-held, spring-loaded, rubber-tipped, pressure-measuring device, which offers a means of achieving standardised pressure application. Using an algometer, sufficient pressure to produce pain is applied to preselected points. The measurement is taken when pain is reported. When the point is retested at a subsequent visit, if the same amount of pressure activates the patient's pain then the trigger point was not successfully deactivated previously. Ideally, there should be a measurable increase in the pain threshold, requiring greater pressure to produce the characteristic pain.

Baldry (1993) suggests that algometers should be used to measure the degree of pressure required to produce symptoms, 'before and after deactivation of a trigger point' because when treatment is successful, the pressure threshold over the trigger point increases.

A variety of algometer designs exist, including sophisticated versions that are attached to the thumb or finger, with a lead running to an electronic sensor that is itself connected to a computer. This gives very precise readouts of the amount of pressure being applied by the finger or thumb during treatment.

AN ALTERNATIVE METHODOLOGY

In the application of INIT (described below) an alternative method of ischaemic compression is suggested, in which firm pressure is applied to the trigger point, but not sustained. Rather an on-and-off pressure application is suggested, 5 seconds of pressure, 2 to 3 seconds release, followed by a further 5 seconds of pressure, and so on, repeated until a perceptible change is palpated, or the patient reports a change in the perceived pain sensation.

The alternating pressure allows a pumping effect, a flushing, as the ischaemic compression is released. This allows a circulatory influence on the previously ischaemic tissues, alongside the other obvious effects of pressure, including the release of pain-relieving opioid peptides (endorphin, enkephalin, endocannabinoids) (Thompson, 1984; Baldry, 1993, 2001; McPartland, 2008), mechanoreceptor stimulation, and hence an influence on pain perception (McMahon et al., 2013), as well as myofascial stretching of the tissues (Barnes, 1997).

ASSOCIATED METHODS

It is worth recalling that the stretching methods advocated by Travell and Simons, subsequent to applied pressure on trigger points, were derived from muscle energy procedures, something they acknowledged in Volume 2 of their text (1992), having earlier (1983) ascribed the methods to Lewit, who had in fact studied with the original developers of MET, including Fred L. Mitchell (McPartland, 2004). MET can therefore be seen to offer benefits in trigger point treatment. It forms a major element of the INIT approach described below, as does intermittent compression.

By combining the methods of direct inhibition (pressure mildly applied, continuously or in a make-and-break pattern), along with the concept of strain/counterstrain (see below) and MET, a specific targeting of dysfunctional soft tissues can be achieved (Chaitow, 1994a).

Strain/Counterstrain (SCS) Briefly Explained

Jones (1981) has shown that particular painful 'points' relating to joint or muscular strain, chronic or acute, can be used as 'monitors' – pressure being applied to them as the body or body part is carefully positioned in such a way as to remove or reduce the pain felt in the palpated point.[3]

When the position of ease is attained (using what is known in SCS terminology as 'fine tuning') in which pain vanishes from the palpated monitoring tender point, the stressed tissues are felt to be at their most relaxed – and clinical experience indicates that this is so since they palpate as 'easy' rather than having a sense of being 'bound' or tense (see Chapter 5 for a more detailed discussion of this phenomenon).

SCS is thought to achieve its benefits by means of an automatic resetting of muscle spindles, which help to dictate the length and tone in the tissues. This resetting apparently occurs only when the muscle housing the spindle is at ease, and usually results in a reduction in excessive tone and release of spasm. When positioning the body (part) in strain/counterstrain methodology, a sense of 'ease' is noted as the tissues reach the position in which pain vanishes from the palpated point. (See further discussion of the use of SCS in the INIT sequence in Chapter 13.)

INIT Method

1. Locate the trigger point, by means of palpation, using methods as described in relation to 'STAR' or 'drag'.
2. Apply ischaemic compression (sustained or intermittent) until the pain changes or until a significant 'release' is noted in the palpated tissues.
3. Positionally release trigger point tissues. Pressure is applied and the patient is asked to ascribe this a value of '10', and then tissues are repositioned (fine-tuned) until the patient reports a score of '2' or less.
4. With the tissues held in this 'folded' ease position a local-focused isometric contraction of these tissues is created.
5. This is followed by a local stretch of the tissues housing the trigger point, in the direction of the muscle fibres.
6. The whole muscle is then contracted isometrically as in all MET procedures (see Chapter 5).
7. This is followed by a stretch of the whole muscle, as in all MET procedures for muscles.

---

[3]These tender points, as described by Jones, are found in tissues which are short rather than being stretched at the time of injury (acute or chronic) and are usually areas in which the patient is unaware of pain previous to their being palpated. They seem to equate in most individuals with spontaneously tender 'Ah shi' points in traditional Chinese medicine.

8. Facilitation of the antagonists may then be considered, as a means of having the patient perform home exercises to encourage inhibition of the muscle housing the trigger point (see below).

Discussion

It is reasonable to assume, and palpation confirms, that when a trigger point is being palpated by direct finger or thumb pressure, and when the very tissues in which the trigger point lies are positioned in such a way as to take away the pain (entirely or at least to a great extent), that the most (dis)stressed fibres in which the trigger point is housed will be in a position of relative ease.

The trigger point would by then have received direct inhibitory pressure (mild or perhaps intermittent (Fig. 14.1A – see discussion earlier in this chapter) and (using positional release/SCS methods) would have been positioned so that the tissues housing it are relaxed (relatively or completely) (see Fig. 14.1B).

Following a period of 10 to 15 seconds (or longer, depending on the level of discomfort) in this 'position of ease' – accompanied by palpatory pressure – the patient would be asked to introduce an isometric contraction into the tissues housing the trigger (currently resting 'at ease') and to hold this for 7 seconds or so, so contracting the very fibres that had been repositioned to obtain

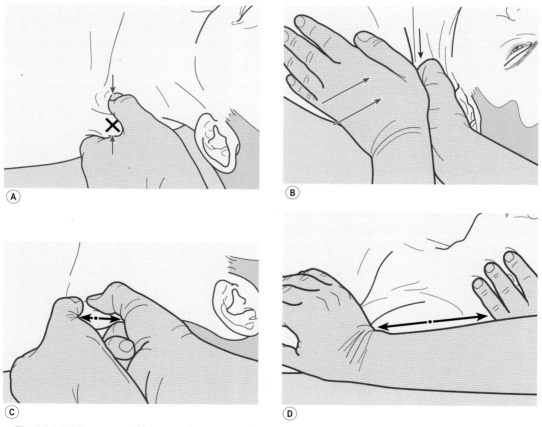

Fig. 14.1 (A) First stage of integrated neuromuscular inhibition technique (INIT) in which a tender/pain/trigger point in the upper trapezius is located and ischaemically compressed, either intermittently or persistently. (B) The pain is removed from the tender/pain/trigger point by finding a position of ease, which is held for at least 15 to 20 seconds, following which an isometric contraction is induced involving the tissues which house the tender/pain/trigger point. (C) Following the holding of the isometric contraction for 5 to 7 seconds, the muscle housing the trigger point is stretched. (D) Finally, a whole muscle (upper trapezius) contraction is requested, followed by stretching the muscle.

the strain/counterstrain release. The palpating finger(s) would determine that the contraction was focused precisely in the tissues around the trigger point.

Following the isometric contraction, there would be a reduction in tone in these tissues and they could then be gently stretched locally (see Fig. 14.1C).

Subsequently, after a more general, whole muscle, isometric contraction – as in any MET procedure (as described in previous chapters) – the entire muscle would be stretched (see Fig. 14.1D).

Ruddy's pulsed MET can be used to facilitate weak antagonists to complete the INIT sequence. The methods of pulsed MET as developed by Ruddy (1962) are discussed in earlier chapters (see Chapters 6 and 7 for examples). To complete the INIT sequence, pulsating contractions of the weak antagonists to muscles housing trigger points would further inhibit these muscles, as well as help to tone and proprioceptively re-educate the antagonists.

Validation of INIT

The integrated use of inhibitory pressure, strain/counterstrain and MET (INIT), has the advantage of allowing precise targeting of trigger points or other areas of soft tissue dysfunction involving pain or restriction of range of motion of soft tissue origin (Ginszt et al., 2020).

Intermittent ischaemic compression affects pain reduction through stimulating A-beta fibres which influence pain gate during pressure, as well as increasing circulation when the pressure is released. Strain counterstrain allows pain reduction, functional and range of motion (ROM) enhancement, and muscle amplitude improvement. By placing the muscle at the passive shortened position, circulation to the muscle may be increased and muscle spindle normalisation supported.

This integrated technique supports pain relief, as well as functional and ROM improvement (Nagrale et al., 2010) through working on autogenic muscle inhibition and supporting increased tolerance to stretching. Additionally, the MET component can be used to normalise joint function and ROM through changing muscle extensibility, reflex relaxation, and connective tissue viscoelasticity (Al-Najjar et al., 2020; Dayanır et al., 2020).

SUMMARY

The integrated use of inhibitory pressure and strain/counterstrain together with muscle energy technique, applied to a trigger point or other area of soft tissue

dysfunction involving pain or restriction of range of motion (of soft tissue origin), is a logical approach since it has the advantage of allowing precise targeting of the culprit tissues. There exists a legacy from a variety of clinicians and a research lineage that supports INIT as an important aspect of manual therapy into the future.

REFERENCES

Abd El-Azeim, A.S., Elhafez, H.M., Ahmed, S.E.B., Draz, A.H., Kattabei, O.M., 2019. Efficacy of Kinesio tape on pressure pain threshold and normalized resting myoelectric activity on upper trapezius myofascial trigger points (a randomized clinical trial). J. Adv. Pharm. Educ. Res. 9 (3), 28–33.

Affaitati, G., Costantini, R., Fabrizio, A., Lapenna, D., Tafuri, E., Giamberardino, M.A., 2011. Effects of treatment of peripheral pain generators in fibromyalgia patients. Eur. J. Pain 15 (1), 61–69.

Affaitati, G., Costantini, R., Tana, C., Cipollone, F., Giamberardino, M.A., 2020. Co-occurrence of pain syndromes. J. Neural. Transm. 127 (4), 625–646.

Akamatsu, F.E., Ayres, B.R., Saleh, S.O., Hojaij, F., Andrade, M., Hsing, W.T., et al., 2015. Trigger points: an anatomical substratum. Biomed. Res. Int 2015, 623287. doi:10.1155/2015/623287.

Al-Najjar, H.M.M., Mohammed, A.H., Mosaad, D.M., 2020. Effect of ice massage with integrated neuromuscular inhibition technique on pain and function in subjects with mechanical neck pain: randomized controlled trial. Bullet. Fac. Phys. Ther. 25 (1), 1–7.

Arun, B., Kumar, R.K.P., 2020. Effect of Ischemic Compression and Infrared Radiations on Myofascial Trigger Point of Trapezius. Int. J. Sport Exerc. Health Res. 4 (2), 69–72. doi:10.31254/sportmed.4208.

Baldry, P., 1993. Acupuncture, Trigger Points and Musculo-Skeletal Pain. Churchill Livingstone, Edinburgh.

Baldry, P., 2001. Myofascial Pain and Fibromyalgia Syndromes. Churchill Livingstone, Edinburgh.

Barnes, J., 1996. MFR in treatment of thoracic outlet syndrome. J. Bodyw. Mov. Ther. 1 (1), 53–57.

Barnes, M., 1997. The basic science of myofascial release. J. Bodyw. Mov. Ther. 1 (4), 231–238.

Bordeniuc, G., Lacusta, V., Fala, V., 2020. Evaluation of different instruments for quantifying pain in patients with masticatory muscle pain. In Congresul consacrat aniversării a 75-a de la fondarea Universității de Stat de Medicină și Farmacie „Nicolae Testemițanu" (pp. 694–694).

Cantu, R., Grodin, A., 1992. Myofascial Manipulation. Aspen Publications, Gaithersburg, MD.

Chaitow, L., 1991. Palpatory Literacy. Harper Collins, London.

Chaitow, L., 1991. Soft Tissue Manipulation. Healing Arts Press, Rochester, Vermont.

Chaitow, L., 1994a. INIT in treatment of pain and trigger points. Br. J. Osteopath. 13, 17–21.

Chaitow, L., 1994b. Integrated neuromuscular inhibition technique. Massage Ther. J. 33, 60–68.

Chaitow, L., 2003. Modern Neuromuscular Techniques, second ed. Churchill Livingstone, Edinburgh.

Chaitow, L., 2011. Modern Neuromuscular Techniques, third ed. Churchill Livingstone, Edinburgh.

Chaitow, L., DeLany, J., 2000. Clinical Applications of Neuromuscular Techniques, vol. 1. Upper Body. Churchill Livingstone, Edinburgh.

Chaitow, L., DeLany, J., 2002. Clinical Applications of Neuromuscular Techniques, vol. 2. Lower Body. Churchill Livingstone, Edinburgh.

Chaitow, L., DeLany, J., 2008. Clinical Applications of Neuromuscular Techniques, vol. 1. Upper Body, second ed. Churchill Livingstone, Edinburgh.

Chaitow, L., DeLany, J., 2011. Clinical Applications of Neuromuscular Techniques, vol. 2. Lower Body, second ed. Churchill Livingstone, Edinburgh.

Dayanır, I.O., Birinci, T., Kaya Mutlu, E., Akcetin, M.A., Akdemir, A.O., 2020. Comparison of three manual therapy techniques as trigger point therapy for chronic nonspecific low back pain: a randomized controlled pilot trial. J. Altern. Complement. Med. 26 (4), 291–299.

de las Penas, C.F., Alonso-Blanco, C., Fernández-Carnero, J., Miangolarra-Page, J.C., 2006. Immediate effects of ischemic compression technique and transverse friction massage on tenderness of active and latent myofascial trigger points: a pilot study. J. Bodyw. Mov. Ther. 10 (1), 3–9.

El-Hafez, H.M., Hamdy, H.A., Takla, M.K., Ahmed, S.E.B., Genedy, A.F., Shaymaa, Al, 2020. Instrument-assisted soft tissue mobilisation versus stripping massage for upper trapezius myofascial trigger points. J. Taibah. Univ. Med. Sci. 15 (2), 87–93.

Fernández-de-las-Peñas, C., Alonso-Blanco, C., Cuadrado, M.L., Gerwin, R. D., Pareja, J. A., 2006. Trigger points in the suboccipital muscles and forward head posture in tension-type headache. J Headache Pain 46 (3), 454–460.

Fryer, G., Hodgson, L., 2005. The effect of manual pressure release on myofascial trigger points in the upper trapezius muscle. J. Bodyw. Mov. Ther. 9, 248–255.

Fryer, G., Morris, T., Gibbons, P., 2004. Relation between thoracic paraspinal tissues and pressure sensitivity measured by digital algometer. J. Osteopath. Med. 7 (2), 64–69.

Galasso, A., Urits, I., An, D., Nguyen, D., Borchart, M., Yazdi, C., et al., 2020. A comprehensive review of the treatment and management of myofascial pain syndrome. Curr. Pain Headache Rep. 24 (8), 43. doi:10.1007/s11916-020-00877-5.

Gam, A.N., Warming, S., Larsen, L.H., Jensen, B., Høydalsmo, O., Allon, I., et al., 1998. Treatment of myofascial trigger-points with ultrasound combined with massage and exercise – a randomised controlled trial. Pain 77, 73–79.

Ge, H.Y., Nie, H., Madeleine, P., Danneskiold-Samsøe, B., Graven-Nielsen, T., Arendt-Nielsen, L., 2009. Contribution of the local and referred pain from active myofascial trigger points in fibromyalgia syndrome. Pain 147, 233–240.

Gerwin, R., Dommerholt, J., 2002. Treatment of myofascial pain syndromes. In: Weiner, R. (Ed.), Pain Management: A Practical Guide for Clinicians. CRC Press, Boca Raton, pp. 235–249.

Ginszt, M., Zieliński, G., Berger, M., Szkutnik, J., Bakalczuk, M., Majcher, P., 2020. Acute effect of the compression technique on the electromyographic activity of the masticatory muscles and mouth opening in subjects with active myofascial trigger points. Appl. Sci. 10 (21), 7750.

Hong, C.Z., Chen, Y.C., Pon, C.H., Yu, J., 1993. Immediate effects of various physical medicine modalities on pain threshold of an active myofascial trigger point. J. Musculoskelet. Pain 1 (2), 37–53.

Guan, H., Zhao, L., Liu, H., Xie, D., Liu, Y., Zhang, G., et al., 2020. Effects of intermittent pressure imitating rolling manipulation in traditional Chinese medicine on ultrastructure and metabolism in injured human skeletal muscle cells. Am. J. Transl. Res. 12 (1), 248–260.

Hou, C.R., Tsai, L.C., Cheng, K.F., Chung, K.C., Hong, C.Z., 2002. Immediate effects of various physical therapeutic modalities on cervical myofascial pain and trigger-point sensitivity. Arch. Phys. Med. Rehabil. 83, 1406–1414.

Huguenin, L.K., 2004. Myofascial trigger points: the current evidence. Phys. Ther. Sport 5 (1), 2–12.

Janda, V., 1983. Muscle Function Testing. Butterworths, London.

Janda, V., 1985. Pain in the locomotor system. In: Glasgow, E. (Ed.), Aspects of Manipulative Therapy. Churchill Livingstone, London.

Jerez-Mayorga, D., Dos Anjos, C.F., Macedo, M.C., Fernandes, I.G., Aedo-Muñoz, E., Intelangelo, L., et al., 2020. Instrumental validity and intra/inter-rater reliability of a novel low-cost digital pressure algometer. Peer J 8. e10162. https://doi.org/10.7717/peerj.10162.

Jones, L., 1981. Strain/Counterstrain. Academy of Applied Osteopathy. Colorado Springs.

Kaprail, M., Jetly, S., Sarin, A., Kaur, P., 2019. To study the effect of myofascial trigger point release in upper trapezius muscle causing neck disability in patients with chronic periarthritis shoulder. Sport Exerc. Med. Open J. 5 (1), 1–4.

Kleyhans, A., 1974. Digest of Chiropractic Economics (September).

Korr, I., 1976. Spinal Cord as Organiser of the Disease Process. Yearbook of the Academy of Applied Osteopathy, Newark, Ohio.

Lederman, E., 1997. Fundamentals of Manual Therapy. Churchill Livingstone, London, pp. 34.

Lederman, E., 2005. The Science and Practice of Manual Therapy. Elsevier, Edinburgh.

Lewit, K., 1999. Manipulation in Rehabilitation of the Locomotor System, third ed. Butterworths, London.

Lief, S., 1982. Described in: Chaitow L Neuromuscular Technique, 1982, revised as Soft Tissue Manipulation, 1989 (further revised in 1991). Thorsons, Wellingborough.

Liu, L., Huang, Q.M., Liu, Q.G., Ye, G., Bo, C.Z., Chen, M.J., et al., 2015. Effectiveness of dry needling for myofascial trigger points associated with neck and shoulder pain: a systematic review and meta-analysis. Arch. Phys. Med. Rehabil. 96 (5), 944–955. doi:10.1016/j.apmr.2014.12.015.

Lu, Z., Briley, A., Zhou, P., Li, S., 2020. Are there trigger points in the spastic muscles? Electromyographical evidence of dry needling effects on spastic finger flexors in chronic stroke. Front. Neurol., 11.

McMahon, S., Koltzenburg, M., Tracey, I., Turk, D.C., 2013. Wall and Melzack's Textbook of Pain, sixth ed. Elsevier, Philadelphia, PA.

McPartland, J., 2004. Travell trigger points – molecular and osteopathic perspectives. J. Am. Osteopath. Assoc. 104 (6), 244–249.

McPartland, J., 2008. Expression of the endocannabinoid system in fibroblasts and myofascial tissues. J. Bodyw. Mov. Ther. 12 (2), 169–182.

Mense, S., 2008. Muscle pain: mechanisms and clinical significance. Dtsch. Arztebl. Int. 105 (12), 214–219. doi:10.3238/artzebl.2008.0214.

Mense, S., Simons, D.G., Russell, I.J., 2001. Muscle Pain: Understanding its Nature, Diagnosis, and Treatment. Lippincott Williams & Wilkins.

Metgud, S.C., Monteiro, S.S., Heggannavar, A., D'Silva, P.V., 2020. Effect of integrated neuromuscular inhibition technique on trigger points in patients with nonspecific low back pain: randomized controlled trial. Indian J. Physiother. Occup. Ther. 2 (2), 99.

Milliken, K., 2003. The Effects of Muscle Energy Technique on Psoas Major Length. Unpublished Most Thesis, Unitec New Zealand, Auckland, New Zealand.

Minerbi, A., Vulfsons, S., 2018. Challenging the Cinderella hypothesis: a new model for the role of the motor unit recruitment pattern in the pathogenesis of myofascial pain syndrome in postural muscles. Rambam Maimonides Med. J. 9 (3).

Musnick, D., 2008. Pain Sensitization and Chronic Musculoskeletal Pain. 15th International Functional Medicine Symposium, Carlsbad CA May 22–25.

Nagrale, A.V., Glynn, P., Joshi, A., 2010. The efficacy of an integrated neuromuscular, inhibition technique on upper trapezius trigger, points in subjects with non-specific neck pain: a randomized controlled trial. J. Man. Manipul. Ther. 18 (1), 38–44.

Nimmo, R., 1966. Receptor tonus technique. Lecture notes Ruddy T. 1961. Osteopathic rhythmic resistive duction therapy. Yearbook of Academy of Applied Osteopathy. Indianapolis.

Ong, J., Claydon, L.S., 2014. The effect of dry needling for myofascial trigger points in the neck and shoulders: a systematic review and meta-analysis. J. Bodyw. Mov. Ther. 18 (3), 390–398. doi:10.1016/j.jbmt.2013.11.009.

Ortega-Santiago, R., González-Aguado, Á.J., Fernández-de-Las-Peñas, C., Cleland, J.A., de-la-Llave-Rincón, A.I., Kobylarz, M.D., et al., 2020. Pressure pain hypersensitivity and referred pain from muscle trigger points in elite male wheelchair basketball players. Braz. J. Phys. Ther. 24 (4), 333–341.

Pinheiro, R.P., Gaubeur, M.A., Itezerote, A.M., Saleh, S.O., Hojaij, F., Andrade, M., et al., 2020. Anatomical study of the innervation of the masseter muscle and its correlation with myofascial trigger points. J. Pain Res. 13, 3217.

Poillot, P., Le Maitre, C.L., Huyghe, J.M., 2021. The strain-generated electrical potential in cartilaginous tissues: a role for piezoelectricity. Biophys. Rev. 13 (1), 91–100.

Qureshi, N.A., Alsubaie, H.A., Ali, G.I., 2019. Myofascial pain syndrome: a concise update on clinical, diagnostic and integrative and alternative therapeutic perspectives. Neuropsychiatr. Dis. Treat. 13 (1), 1–14.

Rezaei, S., Shadmehr, A., Tajali, S.B., Moghadam, B.A., Jalaei, S., 2020. Application of combined laser and compression therapy on the pain and level of disability on trigger points in upper trapezius muscle. J. Modern Rehabil. 14 (2), 97–104.

Ruddy, T.J., 1962. Osteopathic Rhythmic Resistive Technic. Yearb. Acad. Appl. Osteopathy, 23–31.

Saadat, Z., Hemmati, L., Pirouzi, S., Ataollahi, M., Ali-Mohammadi, F., 2018. Effects of Integrated Neuromuscular Inhibition Technique on pain threshold and pain intensity in patients with upper trapezius trigger points. J. Bodyw. Mov. Ther. 22 (4), 937–940.

Scott, N.A., 2009. Trigger point injections for chronic non-malignant musculoskeletal pain: a systematic review. Pain Med 10 (1), 54–69.

Selye, H., 1984. The Stress of Life. McGraw Hill, New York.

Shah, J., Gilliams, E., 2008. Uncovering the biochemical milieu of myofascial trigger points using in vivo microdialysis: an application of muscle pain concepts to myofascial pain syndrome. J. Bodyw. Mov. Ther. 12, 371–384.

Sherman, K.J., Dixon, M.W., Thompson, D., Cherkin, D.C., 2006. Development of a taxonomy to describe massage treatments for musculoskeletal pain. BMC Complement Altern. Med. 6, 24. doi:10.1186/1472-6882-6-24.

Simons, D., 1989. Myofascial Pain Syndromes. Current Therapy of Pain. B C Decker, pp. 251–266.

Simons, D., Travell, J., Simons, L., 1999. Myofascial Pain and Dysfunction: The Trigger Point Manual, vol. 1. Upper Half of the Body, second ed. Williams and Wilkins, Baltimore.

Slocumb, J., 1984. Neurological factors in chronic pelvic pain. Am. J. Obstet. Gynaecol. 49, 536.

Srbely, J.Z., Dickey, J.P., Bent, L.R., 2010. Capsaicin-induced central sensitization evokes segmental, increases in trigger point sensitivity in humans. J. Pain 11 (7), 636–643.

Thompson, J., 1984. Opioid peptides. Br. Med. J. 288 (6413), 259–260.

Trampas, A., Kitsios, A., Sykaras, E., Symeonidis, S., Lazarou, L., 2010. Clinical massage and modified proprioceptive neuromuscular facilitation stretching in males with latent myofascial trigger points. Phys. Ther. Sport 11 (3), 91–98.

Travell, J., Simons, D., 1983. Myofascial Pain and Dysfunction: The Trigger Point Manual, Upper Half of the Body 1, first ed. Williams & Wilkins, Baltimore.

Travell, J., Simons, D., 1992. Myofascial Pain and Dysfunction: The Trigger Point Manual 2. Lower Extremities. Williams & Wilkins, Baltimore.

Urits, I., Charipova, K., Gress, K., Schaaf, A.L., Gupta, S., Kiernan, H.C., et al., 2020. Treatment and management of myofascial pain syndrome. Best Pract. Res.

Clin. Anaesthesiol. 34 (3), 427–448. doi:10.1016/j.bpa.2020.08.003.

Wada, J.T., Akamatsu, F., Hojaij, F., Itezerote, A., Scarpa, J.C., Andrade, M., et al., 2020. An anatomical basis for the myofascial trigger points of the abductor hallucis muscle. Biomed. Res. Int. 2020, 9240581.

Ward, R., 1997. Foundations of Osteopathic Medicine. Williams and Wilkins, Baltimore.

Wendt, M., Waszak, M., 2020. Evaluation of the combination of muscle energy technique and trigger point therapy in asymptomatic individuals with a latent trigger point. Int. J. Environ. Res. Public Health 17 (22), 8430.

Widyadharma, I.P.E., 2020. The role of oxidative stress, inflammation and glial cell in pathophysiology of myofascial pain. Adv. Psychiatry Neurol. 29 (3), 180–186. https://doi.org/10.5114/ppn.2020.100036.

Yoosefinejad, A.K., Samani, M., Jabarifard, F., Setooni, M., Mirsalari, R., Kaviani, F., et al., 2021. Comparison of the prevalence of myofascial trigger points of muscles acting on knee between patients with moderate degree of knee osteoarthritis and healthy matched people. J. Bodyw. Mov. Ther. 25, 113–118.

Zhang, H., Liu, H., Lin, Q., Zhang, G., Mason, D.C., 2016. Effects of intermittent pressure imitating rolling manipulation on calcium ion homeostasis in human skeletal muscle cells. BMC Complem. Altern. Med. 16, 314.

INDEX

Page numbers followed by '*f*' indicate figures, '*t*' indicate tables, and '*b*' indicate boxes.